Surgery of the Skull Base

Alexander König
Uwe Spetzger
Editors

Surgery of the Skull Base

Practical Diagnosis and Therapy

Springer

Editors
Alexander König
Neurochirurgische Klinik
Städtisches Klinikum Karlsruhe
Karlsruhe, Baden-Württemberg
Germany

Uwe Spetzger
Neurochirurgische Klinik
Klinikum Karlsruhe
Karlsruhe, Baden-Württemberg
Germany

ISBN 978-3-319-64017-4 ISBN 978-3-319-64018-1 (eBook)
https://doi.org/10.1007/978-3-319-64018-1

Library of Congress Control Number: 2017954377

Printed on acid-free paper

This Springer imprint is published by Springer Nature
The registered company is Springer International Publishing AG
The registered company address is: Gewerbestrasse 11, 6330 Cham, Switzerland

Contents

Contributors

Sinan Barazi
Department of Neurosurgery
King's College Hospital, Denmark Hill
London, SE5 9RS, UK
sbarazi@nhs.net

Konstantinos Barkas
Department of Neurosurgery
King's College Hospital, Denmark Hill
London, SE5 9RS, UK
konstantinos.barkas@nhs.net

Gerd Becker
RadioChirurgicum, CyberKnife®-Südwest
Eichertstr. 3, D-73035
Göppingen, Germany
becker@radiochirurgicum.de

Marcel Biegler
Neurochirurgische Klinik, Klinikum Karlsruhe,
Moltkestr. 90, D-76133
Karlsruhe, Germany
marcel.biegler@klinikum-karlsruhe.de

Martin Bleif
RadioChirurgicum, CyberKnife®-Südwest
Eichertstr. 3, D-73035
Göppingen, Germany
bleif@radiochirurgicum.de

Hamid Borghei-Razavi
Surgical Neuroanatomy Lab
Department of Neurological Surgery
UPMC Presbyterian, Suite B-400
200 Lothrop Street
Pittsburgh, PA 15213, USA
shbr61@yahoo.com

Juan Fernandez-Miranda
Surgical Neuroanatomy Lab
Department of Neurological Surgery
UPMC Presbyterian, Suite B-400
200 Lothrop Street
Pittsburgh, PA 15213, USA
fernandezmirandajc@upmc.edu

Kåre Fugleholm
Neurokirurgisk klinik, Rigshospitalet
Blegdamsvej 9, DK-2100
København Ø, Denmark
kaare.fugleholm.buch@regionh.dk

Takanori Fukushima
Division of Neurosurgery, Duke University
Medical Center, Carolina Neuroscience Institute
4030 Wake Forest Rd suite 115
Raleigh, NC 27612, USA
fukushima@carolinaneuroscience.com

Nikolai Hopf
NeuroChirurgicum, Maybachstraße 50
D-70469, Stuttgart, Germany
hopf@neurochirurgicum.com

Goh Inoue
Department of Neurosurgery
Duke University, INERF
4030 Wake Forest Road Suite 115
Raleigh, NC 27609, USA
inoue5@tsc.u-tokai.ac.jp

Alexander König
Neurochirurgische Klinik, Klinikum Karlsruhe
Moltkestr. 90, D-76133
Karlsruhe, Germany
alexander.koenig@klinikum-karlsruhe.de

Peter Kurucz
Neurochirurgische Klinik, Klinikum Stuttgart
Katharinenhospital
Kriegsbergstraße 60
D-70174, Stuttgart, Germany
p.kurucz@klinikum-stuttgart.de

Torstein Meling
Nevrokirurgisk avdeling, Rikshospitalet
Sognsvannsveien 20, N-0372
Oslo, Norway
tmeling@ous-hf.no

Anthony Mélot
Service de Neurochirurgie
Hôpital Nord
F-13015, Marseille, France
anthony.melot@ap-hm.fr

Yoichi Nonaka
Department of Neurosurgery
Fukushima Takanori Skull Base Center
Shin-yurigaoka General Hospital
255 Furusawa Asao-ku, Kawasaki
Kanagawa, 215-0026, Japan
ynonaka1971@yahoo.co.jp

Sebastian Ranguis
Department of Otolaryngology
Head and Neck Surgery
St. Vincent's Hospital Sydney
390 Victoria St
Darlinghurst, NSW 2010, Australia
scranguis@gmail.com

Robert Reisch
ENDOMIN - Zentrum für endoskopische
und minimalinvasive Neurochirurgie
Witellikerstrasse 40
CH -8032, Zürich, Switzerland
robert.reisch@hirslanden.ch

Pierre-Hugues Roche
Service de Neurochirurgie, Hôpital Nord
F-13015, Marseille, France
proche@ap-hm.fr

Uta Schick
Neurochirurgie, Clemenshospital
Düesbergweg 124
D-48153, Münster, Germany
neurochirurgie@clemenshospital.de

Outouma Soumare
Service de Neurochirurgie, Hôpital Nord
F-13015, Marseille, France
outouma.soumare@ap-hm.fr

Uwe Spetzger
Neurochirurgische Klinik
Klinikum Karlsruhe
Moltkestr. 90
D-76133, Karlsruhe, Germany
uwe.spetzger@klinikum-karlsruhe.de

Nick Thomas
Department of Neurosurgery
King's College Hospital, Denmark Hill
London, SE5 9RS, UK
nick.thomas1@nhs.net

Lucas Troude
Service de Neurochirurgie, Hôpital Nord
F-13015, Marseille, France
lucas.troude@hotmail.fr

Ali Zomorodi
Department of Neurosurgery
Duke University, INERF
4030 Wake Forest Road Suite 115
Raleigh, NC, 27609, USA
lori@carolinaneuroscience.com

Introduction into Skull Base Surgery

Uwe Spetzger

Electronic Supplementary Material The online version of this chapter (https://doi.org/10.1007/978-3-319-64018-1_1) contains supplementary material, which is available to authorized users.

A. König, U. Spetzger (eds.), *Surgery of the Skull Base*,
https://doi.org/10.1007/978-3-319-64018-1_1

1.1 Concepts and Strategies in Skull Base Surgery

Modern skull base surgery has developed to a multidisciplinary specialty with a specific collaboration between several diagnostic and therapeutic medical disciplines. Due to the complex anatomy and important functional structures, there are specific conditions for surgical procedures at the skull base. They require a maximum of precision, persistency and well-grounded anatomical knowledge. Furthermore, a skilled tactile surgical realisation of the treatment strategy is required for the maintenance of neurological functions.

In this book therapeutical concepts and treatment strategies are depicted from the perspective of a neurosurgeon but with appropriate cross references to interdisciplinary «interfaces» and further medical specialties. Therefore, in every chapter selected and experienced, skull base surgeons describe therapeutical concepts in cases of tumourous, traumatic, vascular or congenital triggered diseases of the skull base including brilliant photographic images of surgical procedures. By means of clinical cases, the diagnostics, planning of treatment and steps of surgical procedures are depicted consecutively and with relation to clinical practice. For all relevant skull base pathologies, surgical strategies and alternative modern treatment concepts are described, and, finally, a future perspective about the further development of skull base surgery is given.

1.2 From Function-Preserving to Function-Improving Skull Base Surgery

In principle, skull base surgery has experienced a basic strategical change in the last 25 years. The dogma of maximum radicalness with the goal of complete and radical tumour removal has given way to the principle of function-preserving skull base surgery. Today the treatment philosophy in modern skull base surgery can be formulated so that by an optimisation of surgical approaches with all technical possibilities the surgeon tries to remove the tumour or lesion at best and keeping in mind that the main goal is preserving neurological function but not maximum radicalness. That means that vascular structures, cranial nerves and functional areas of the brain have to be treated with care and if necessary a multimodal and repeated treatment strategy with different therapeutical methods such as endovascular embolisation or radiosurgery has to be applied.

With a historical view on the development of skull base surgery, a big milestone was the introduction of the operating microscope that enabled better visualisation and thereby a more precise microsurgical dissection and preservation of relevant structures while resecting skull base pathologies. The introduction of microsurgery and the refinement of microsurgical techniques brought an important improvement of surgical results and a significant reduction of surgical morbidity and mortality. On the other hand, due to the improved visualisation skull base surgery became a more and more aggressive surgery in the 1980s and 1990s because the microscopical view enabled more invasive and more aggressive approaches. Especially the surgery in the region of the cavernous sinus reached a technical overkill that resulted in increased morbidity in the publications from that period without resulting in a significant improvement of the patients' long-term prognosis.

The introduction of navigation technology can be considered as the next milestone. It offered a better planning, simulation and an image-guided demonstration of the several surgical steps. At the same time the multimodal intraoperative electrophysiological monitoring was significantly improved which resulted in further risk minimisation and improvement of surgical results.

Due to the interdisciplinary collaboration of the different medical specialties, the surgical expertise for the treatment of skull base lesion has been continuously improved. A good example for this is the increasing use of endoscopic techniques in skull base surgery whereupon from a neurosurgical point of view the transnasal approach to the pituitary gland and to the anterior skull base as well as the combination of endoscopy and microsurgical techniques play the most important role.

A further improvement resulted from the optimisation of the delineation of cranial nerves in high-resolution MR imaging. Hereby, it will result in a more detailed visualisation and delineation and, thus, a more precise navigation. But also the increasing therapeutical expertise of interventional radiologists in vascular skull base surgery will be of relevance. The highly precise and selective embolisation techniques or the vessel wall reconstruction by individualised crafted stents and flow diverters for the treatment of vascular lesions and aggressive skull base tumours infiltrating main blood vessels will bring a significant improvement.

An increasing and important contribution comes from highly precise irradiation techniques in which an exact three-dimensional dose planning is possible with modern stereotactic radiosurgery (Gammaknife and CyberKnife). Thus, the combination of radiosurgery and image-guided microsurgery will open a wide field and bring further benefit for our patients. In the course of further spreading of modern skull base surgery, the specific surgical education and training has to undergo further structuring and improvement.

Skull base surgery is an interdisciplinary domain since it requires surgical expertise from different specialties: neurosurgery, ENT surgery, maxillofacial surgery and ophthalmology. Due to the fact that an increasing number of endovascular procedures are used for the treatment of skull base pathologies, interventional neuroradiologists become more and more involved. Furthermore, oncologists with an expertise in the treatment of head and neck neoplasms as well as radiotherapists performing stereotactic radiosurgery are part of the skull base team.

With a balanced corporate action and interdependent trustful collaboration, the optimum treatment for the patient is achieved. Therefore personal communication and a good understanding of the different surgical methods of the several disciplines are crucial. It is well proven to determine the course of surgery in terms of chronology and organisation. That means that the members of the surgical team and the leading specialty are appointed and the sequence of who is doing what is determined.

From this follows that a complex skull base operation depends on qualified single surgical steps, like in a well-rehearsed orchestra where the individual contributions of soloists result in a magnum opus. In this respect, the basic principle is that the specialist with the highest expertise for a certain anatomical area will do the part of the surgical procedure there. This kind of interdisciplinary skull base surgery requires a cooperative and respectful behaviour as well as a mutual trust. Especially in the case of surgically induced morbidity, the complication management can be a big challenge.

The use of computer-assisted surgery also had an important impact on the interdisciplinary cooperation in skull base surgery. The platform of navigation allows the different disciplines an optimal image-guided planning with precise delineation of the pathology and possible approaches by computer-assisted simulation. Thus, by means of navigation, the exact surgical strategy can be determined by the surgeons at the computer screen. During computer-assisted simulation, specific problems and different surgical approaches can be discussed. Finally, interdisciplinary planning with the navigation system allows the determination of a perfect individual course of surgery.

This book about skull base surgery focuses on the neurosurgical therapeutic options but again and again shows the relevant interfaces to other specialties at the same time. Exemplarily three selected clinical cases are presented that are characteristic for interdisciplinary collaboration and show the neurosurgical point of view as well as the therapeutical strategy.

1.3 Illustrative Cases

1.3.1 Neuroma of the Maxillary Nerve

Interdisciplinary treatment planning by neuroradiology, maxillofacial surgery, ENT surgery, neurosurgery and radiotherapy

Due to massive facial pain in the region of the maxilla, our 45-year-old patient underwent dental examination and, finally, a cranial MRI. The latter showed a space-occupying lesion in the pterygopalatine fossa (◻ Fig. 1.1).

After an interdisciplinary conference with colleagues from ENT surgery, a surgical procedure with direct approach to the tumour through the maxillary sinus was planned (◻ Fig. 1.2). The planning included an intraoral incision by maxillofacial surgeons and was conducted with the help of a BrainLab navigation system (BrainLab, München, Germany) which was also used for intraoperative orientation (◻ Fig. 1.3).

As planned, the intraoral incision and the skull base approach through the maxillary sinus were performed by maxillofacial surgeons. After

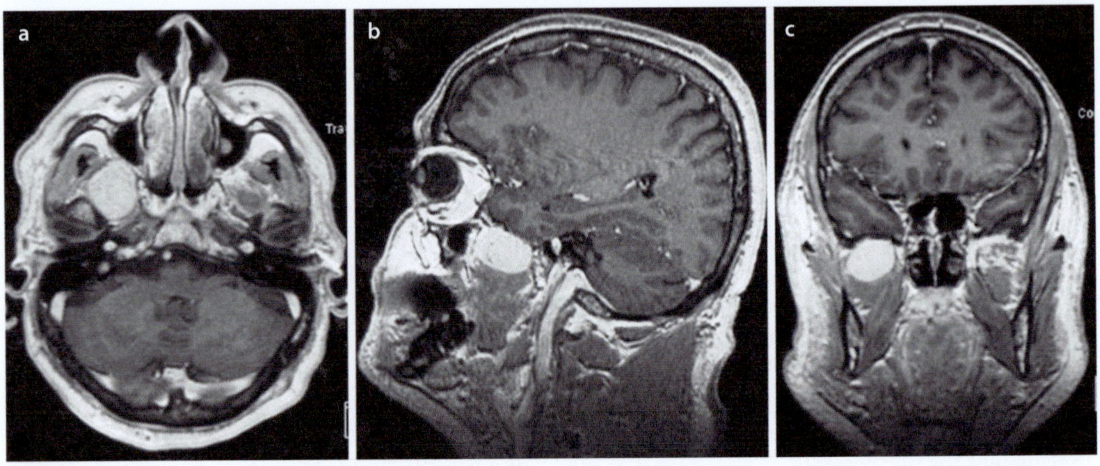

Fig. 1.1 MRI with contrast in the axial **a**, sagittal **b**, and coronal plane **c** shows a tumour mass with contrast enhancement in the right pterygopalatine fossa that was suspected to be a neuroma of the second branch of the trigeminal nerve

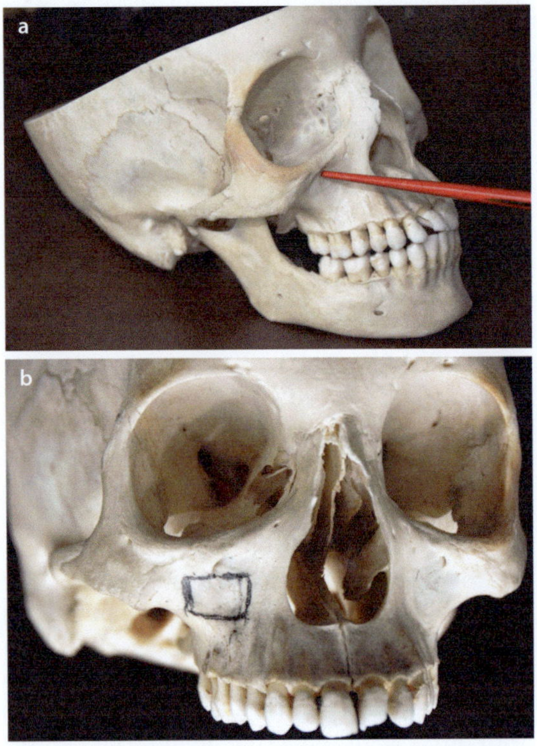

Fig. 1.2 Demonstration of the planned surgical approach with a trajectory through the maxillary sinus **a**. Designated opening of the anterior wall of the maxillary sinus directly below the foramen of the right infraorbital nerve **b**

dissection of the oral mucosa, the anterior wall of the maxillary sinus was cut out with a piezo-driven ultrasonic saw just below the foramen of the infraorbital nerve and, thus, the nerve could be preserved. Under microscopic view after the removal of the mucosa inside the maxillary sinus, the posterior wall of the maxillary sinus was resected with a 3-mm diamond drill which enabled a direct view onto the tumour. The lesion was then reduced in size by using an ultrasonic surgical aspirator (CUSA), a bipolar forceps and tumour forceps as it can be seen in the accompanying surgical video. Afterwards the tumour was microsurgically dissected from the maxillary nerve and removed from the pterygopalatine fossa. Intraoperative histological analysis confirmed the diagnosis of a benign neuroma (schwannoma).

Maxillary nerve and infraorbital nerve, respectively, could be preserved in their course at the roof of the maxillary sinus. Postoperatively the patient's facial pain disappeared within 2 days with preserved sensory function in the V_2 dermatome. The only postoperative deficits were a mild hypaesthesia and dysaesthesia at the right upper lip.

1.3.2 Partially Thrombosed Giant Aneurysm of the Left Vertebral Artery

Interdisciplinary treatment planning by oncology, neuroradiology and neurosurgery

A 57-year-old female patient had previous surgery for a tonsillar carcinoma (staging: T2N2M0-G3). Due to a slight gait ataxia and per-

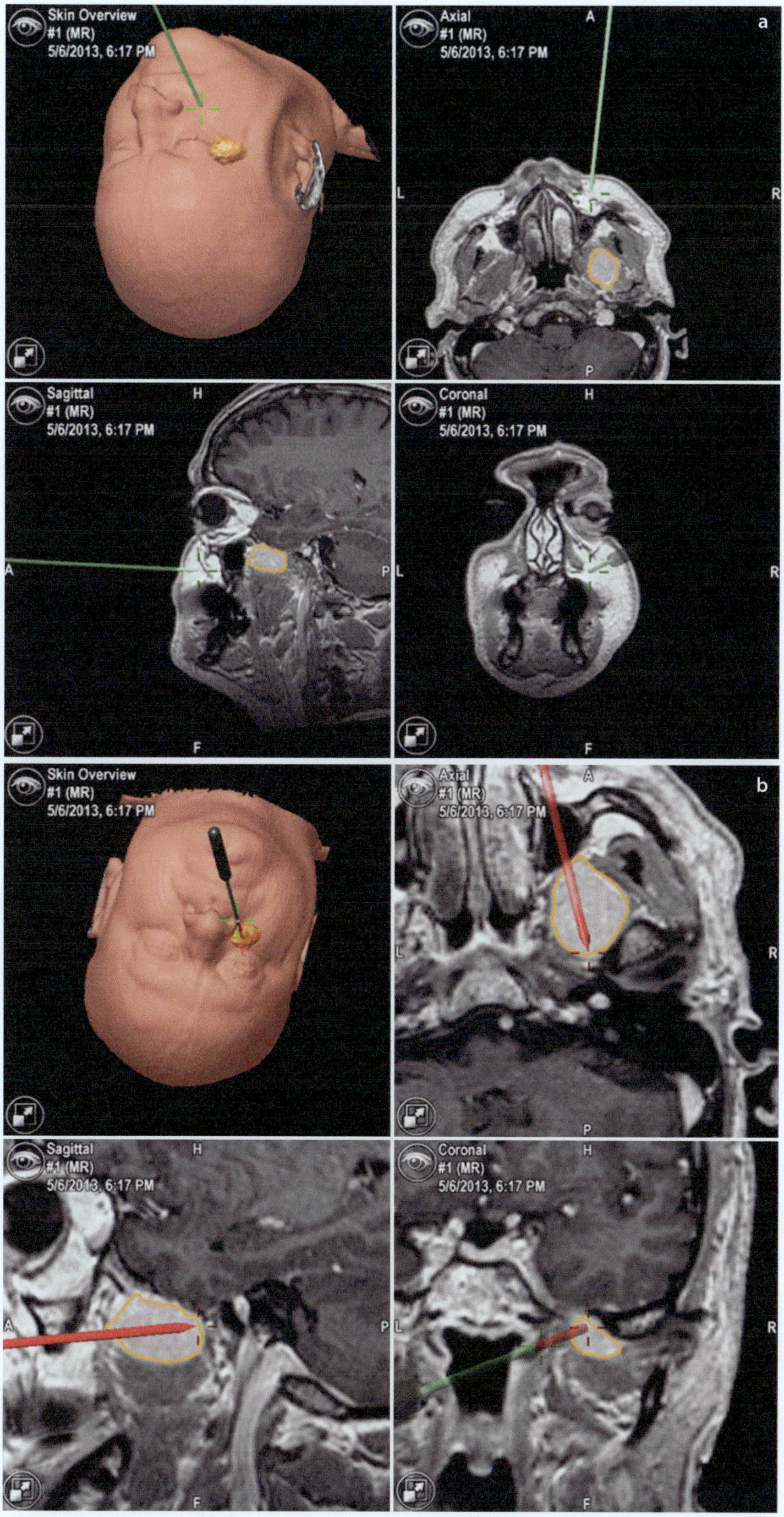

Fig. 1.3 Intraoperative planning of the approach by using neuronavigation. The pointer is positioned at the lower edge of the maxillary sinus after lifting the upper lip **a**. Intraoperative planning of the trajectory and simulation of the surgical approach through the maxillary sinus with virtual elongation of the pointer (*red*) until the posterior edge of the tumour into the direction of the foramen rotundum **b**. Surgical field of the transoral transmaxillary approach during tumour resection while the tip of the pointer is located at the temporal skull base close to the upper posterior edge of the right maxillary sinus **c**. View into the resection cavity through the maxillary sinus after total resection of the neuroma. The posterior wall of the maxillary sinus was reconstructed with TachoSil **d**

Fig. 1.3 (continued)

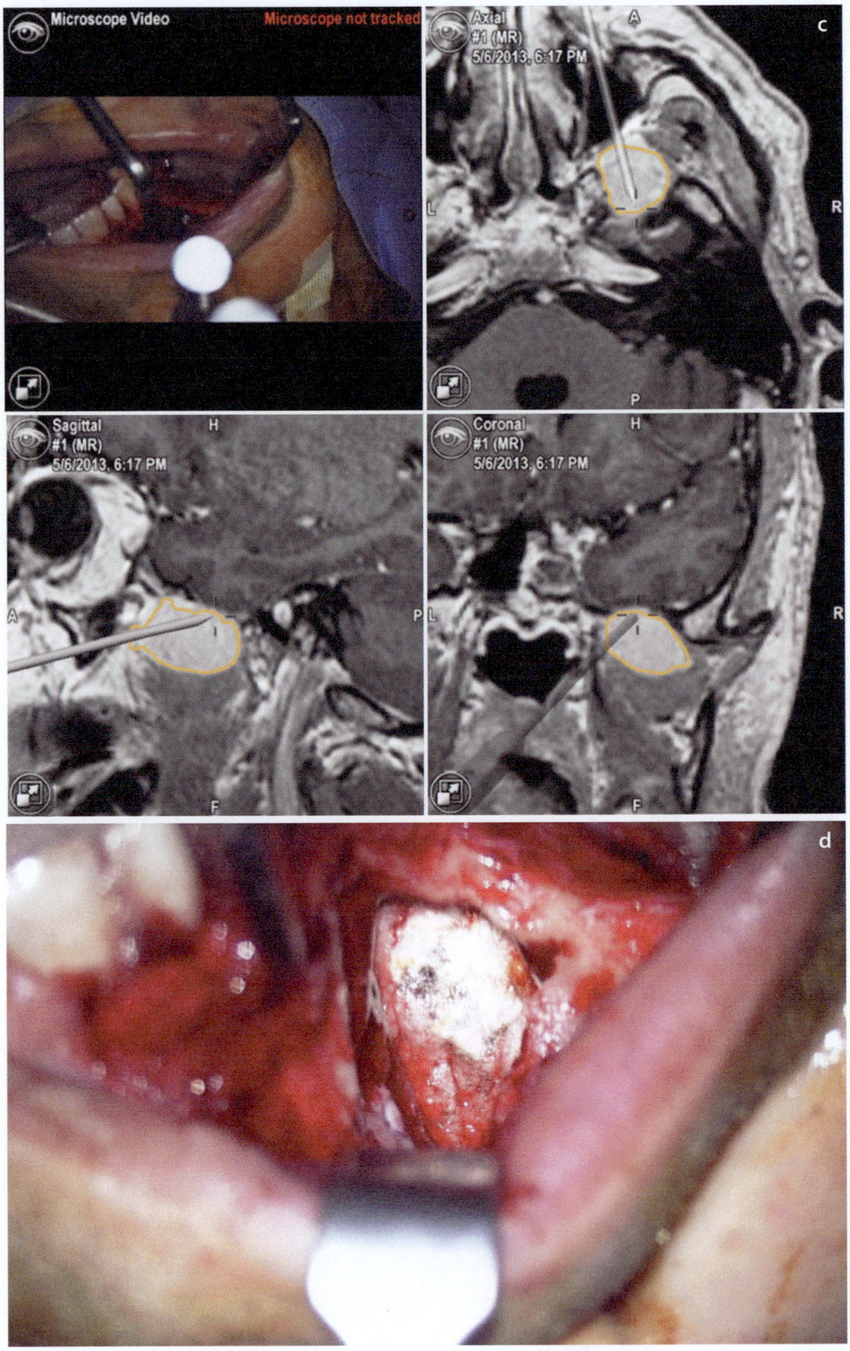

sisting dysphagia, our oncologic colleagues initiated a cranial MRI to rule out cerebral metastases. MRI showed a partially thrombosed giant aneurysm of the left vertebral artery with compression of the lower cranial nerves and the brainstem (■ Figs. 1.4, 1.5, 1.6, and 1.7). Cerebral digital subtraction angiography confirmed the relatively small part of the aneurysm neck with blood flow and showed the origin of the posterior inferior cerebellar artery (PICA) right beside the aneurysm neck as well as irregularities of the tunica intima of the left vertebral artery. This case with

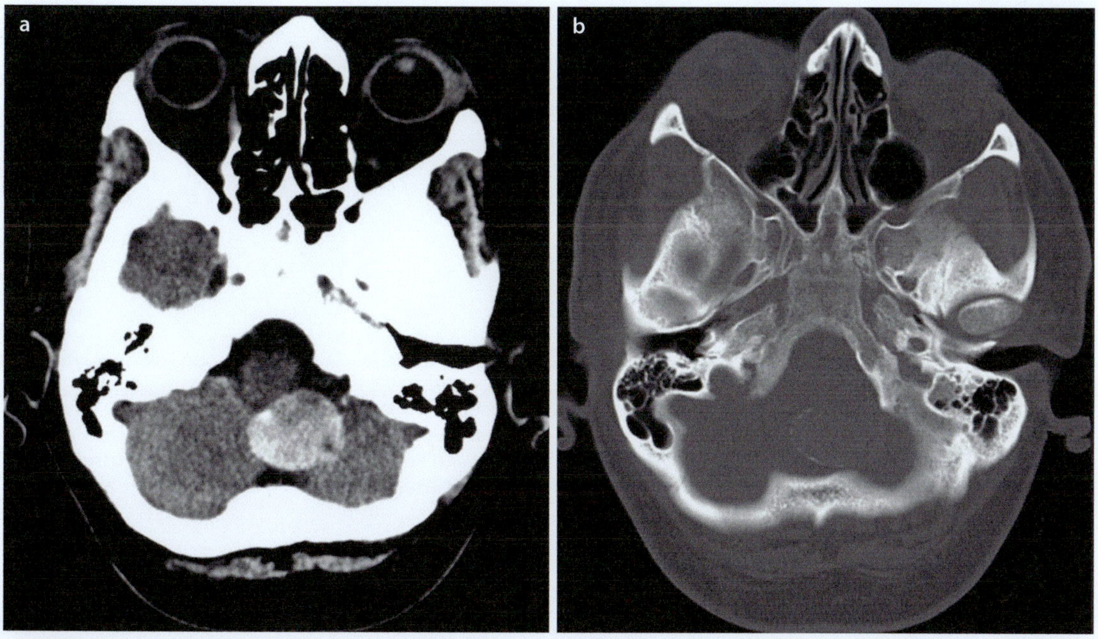

Fig. 1.4 Preoperative cranial CT scan. The axial slices show the thrombotic giant aneurysm in the posterior fossa with contact to the medulla oblongata **a**. In the bone window CT scan, the calcifications of the aneurysm wall can be visualised **b**

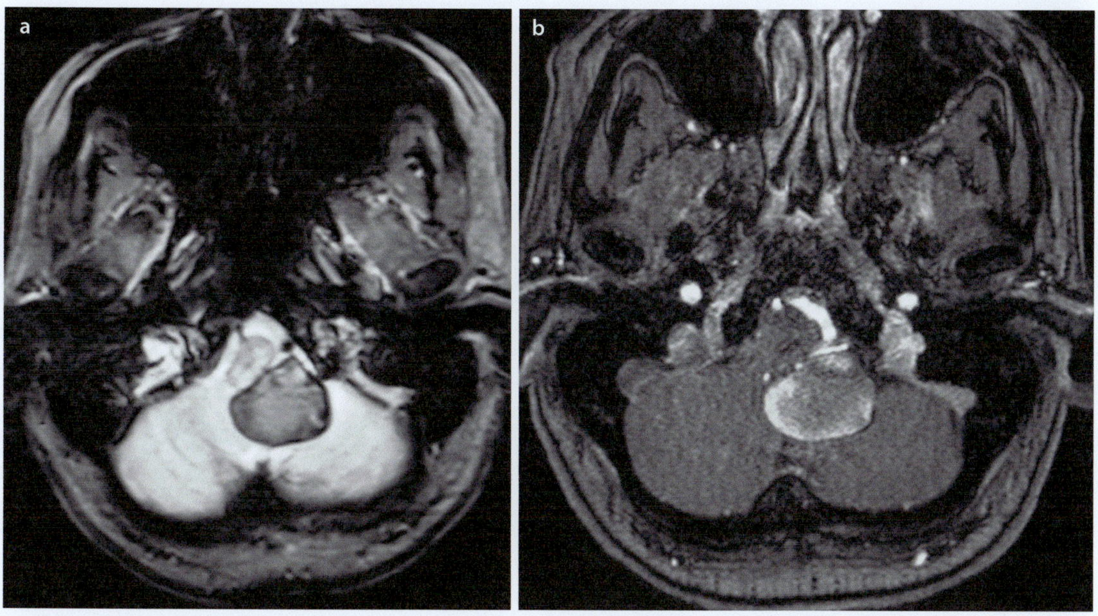

Fig. 1.5 Axial MRI. The T2-fl2d image shows the thrombotic part of the aneurysm as well as the space-occupying effect inside the cerebellum with consecutive compression of the brainstem **a**. The TOF-3D MRI shows the thick left vertebral artery with the crossing PICA course **b**

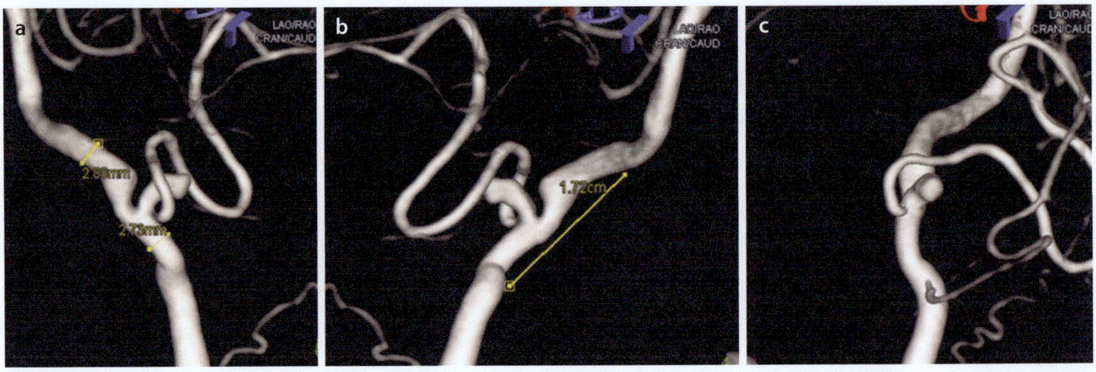

Fig. 1.6 Reconstructed images of the digital 3D rotational angiography. The relatively small perfused aneurysm neck, the irregularities in the diameter of the vertebral artery and the origin of the PICA are shown in different projections **a-c**. Length and diameters were measured to plan a potential endovascular treatment with stent-supported coil embolisation **a**, **b**. The PICA runs below and behind the aneurysm neck and crosses the vertebral artery **c**

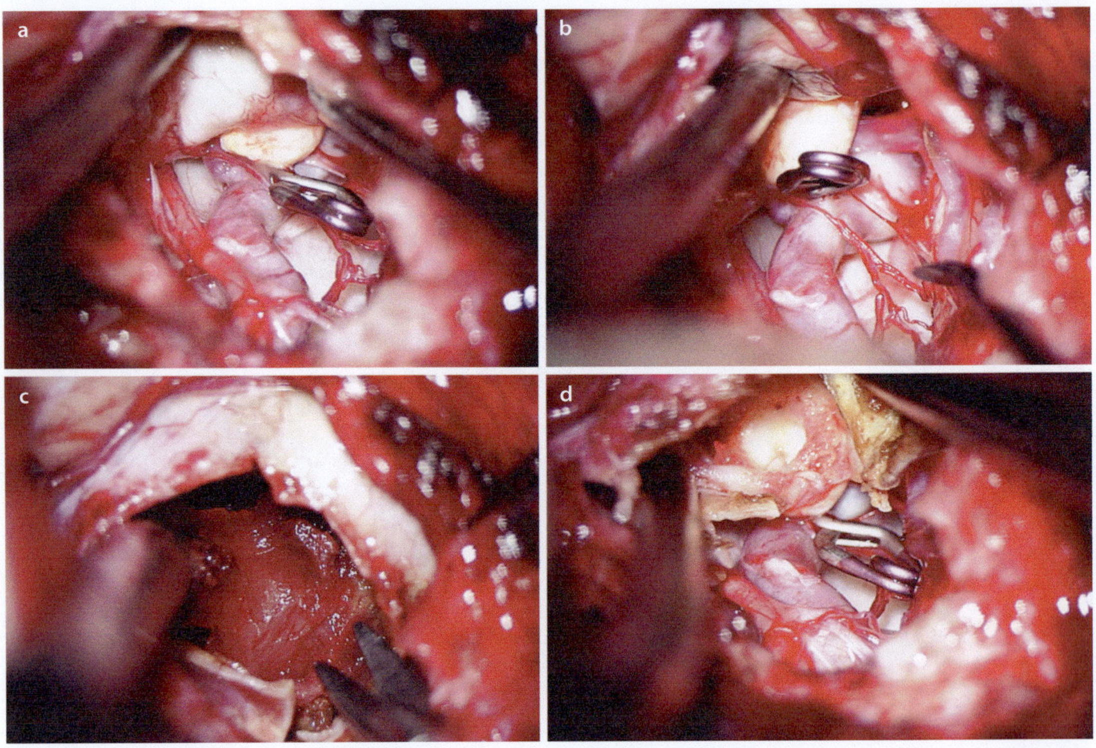

Fig. 1.7 Intraoperative images showing the microsurgical clipping of the partial thrombosed giant VA aneurysm. Application of a straight 7-mm Yasargil mini clip that completely occludes the point of rupture and the aneurysm neck **a**. The PICA which crosses behind the aneurysm and the small perforating arteries are intact **b**. Opening of the aneurysm and reduction of the solid thrombotic material with micro scissors to decompress the brainstem **c**. View in the formerly perfused part of the aneurysm after clipping of the aneurysm base and after partial resection of the aneurysm wall at the end of surgery **d**

slight clinical symptoms of brainstem compression and slowly developing dysfunction of lower cranial nerves is a classical example for an indication for microsurgical management of a giant aneurysm in the posterior fossa.

After discussion with neuroradiologist the therapeutical concept was determined as suboccipital craniotomy, clipping of the aneurysm and decompression of the brainstem under electrophysiological monitoring as the best strategy. Main arguments against an interventional endovascular procedure with stent-supported coil embolisation were the huge thrombotic part and the compressive and space-occupying effect of the aneurysm and the configuration of the aneurysm neck.

The surgical plan was primary opening of the aneurysm wall with resection of the big thrombotic part of the aneurysm and clipping of the neck after decompression. But intraoperatively an early rupture of the aneurysm during inspection and dissection of the neck and the origin of the PICA occurred (see ▫ Video 1.2). Therefore primary clipping of the aneurysm neck was necessary, and then aneurysm resection was possible by using ultrasound surgical aspirator, curettes, forceps and sucker.

1.3.3 Palsy of the Trochlear Nerve

Interdisciplinary treatment planning by ophthalmology, neurology, neuroradiology, ENT surgery, neurosurgery and radiotherapy

The 53-year-old male patient had been suffering from a slowly increasing retrobulbar globus sensation on the left side and, therefore, was initially treated under the suspected diagnosis of glaucoma by ophthalmologists. In the further course of disease, the patient suffered from massive attacks of headaches that he localised behind the left eye. Furthermore, redness of the eye and lacrimation occurred. A cranial CT scan did not show any pathological findings. Under the suspected diagnosis of cluster headaches (Bing-Horton neuralgia), the patient saw a neurologist. Medical treatment with analgesics and inhalation of oxygen did not show any improvement of the symptoms. In the further course of disease, diplopia when looking downwards appeared. Then cerebral MRI showed a space-occupying lesion in the left cavernous sinus (▫ Fig. 1.8). Clinical examination showed a palsy of the left trochlear nerve and minimal dysaesthesia in the left V_2 dermatome.

By MRI and MR angiography, a cavernous ICA aneurysm could be ruled out. We discussed the further diagnostic and possible therapeutic options with the patient. Finally, a navigation-guided endonasal microsurgical biopsy and partial resection was indicated and performed (▫ Figs. 1.9, 1.10, 1.11, and 1.12).

The postoperative course was without any complication; the pre-existing palsy of the trochlear nerve and the sensory disorder in the V_2 dermatome did not show any changes. After confirmation of the histological result of a schwannoma type Antoni A 6 weeks after biopsy, a stereotactic radiosurgical therapy with the CyberKnife (18 Gy single shot) was performed (▫ Fig. 1.13).

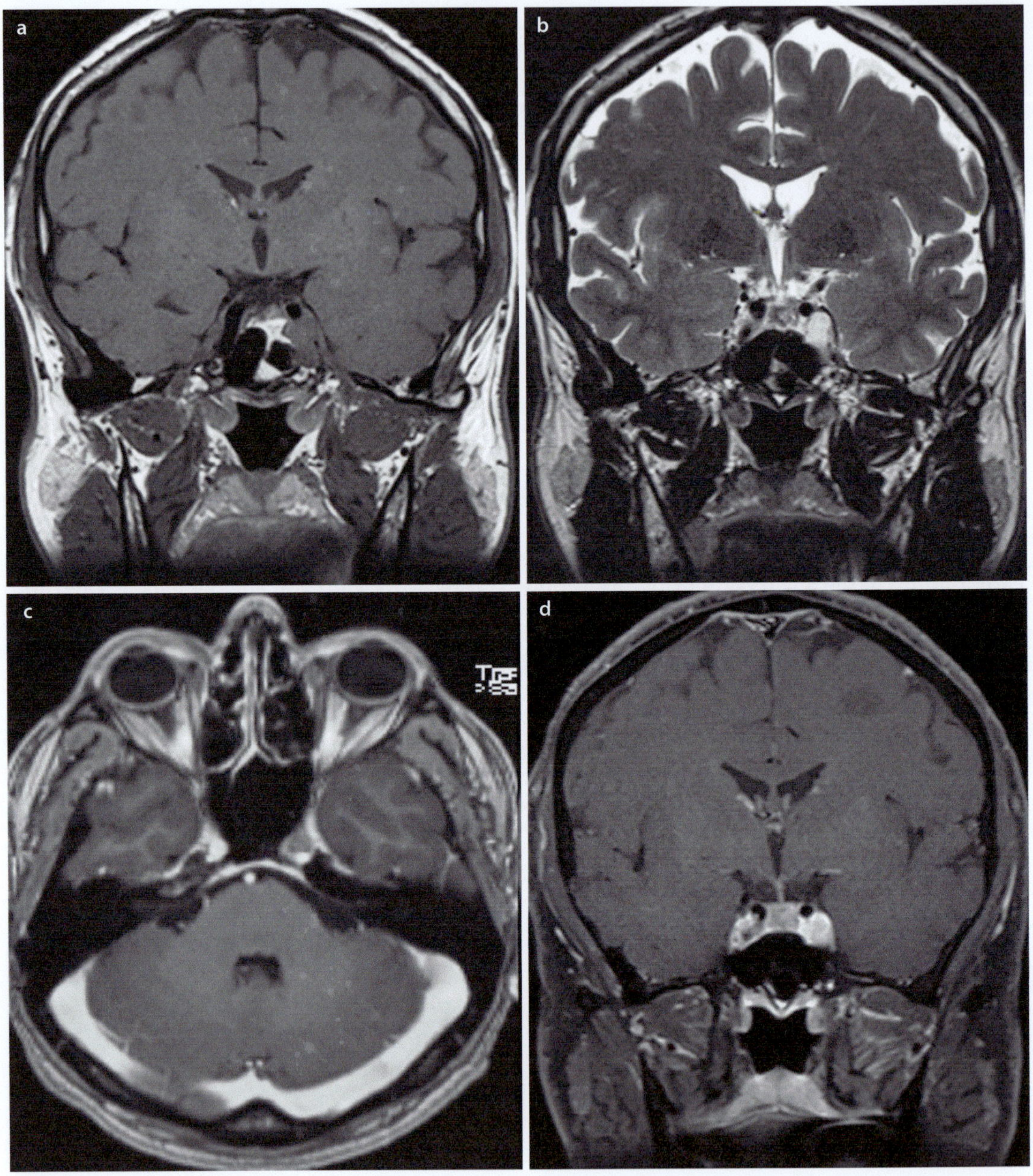

Fig. 1.8 MRI native and with contrast agent in different sequences and planes. The coronal T1-weighted native sequence **a** and the coronal T2-weighted native sequence **b** show the isointense and in T2 hypointense space-occupying lesion with enlargement of the left cavernous sinus. In the axial T1-weighted sequence with contrast agent, an inhomogeneous contrast enhancement with posterior displacement of the left ACI can be seen **c**. The coronal T1-weighted sequence with contrast agent shows a homogeneous contrast enhancing intracavernous space-occupying lesion with displacement of the left ACI and enlargement of the lateral wall of the cavernous sinus **d**

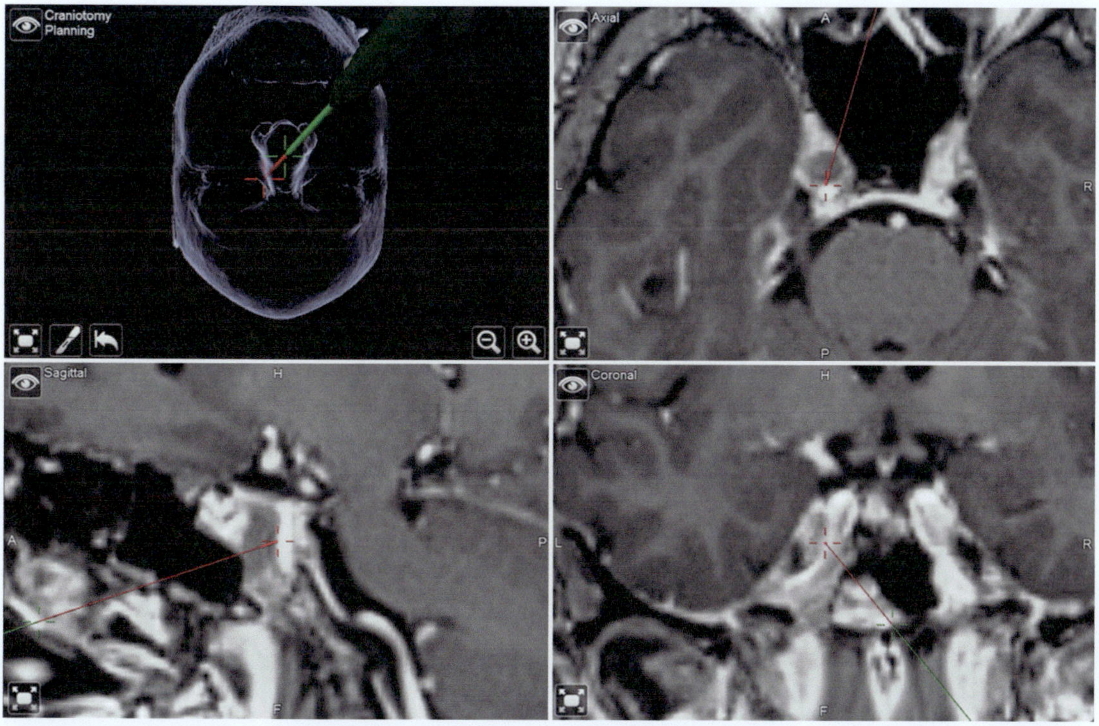

Fig. 1.9 Intraoperative images show the planning of the approach with an endonasal placed pointer of the navigation system. The surgical approach was placed through the right nasal cavity, and the tip of the pointer is virtually elongated through the tumour onto the wall of the left ACI

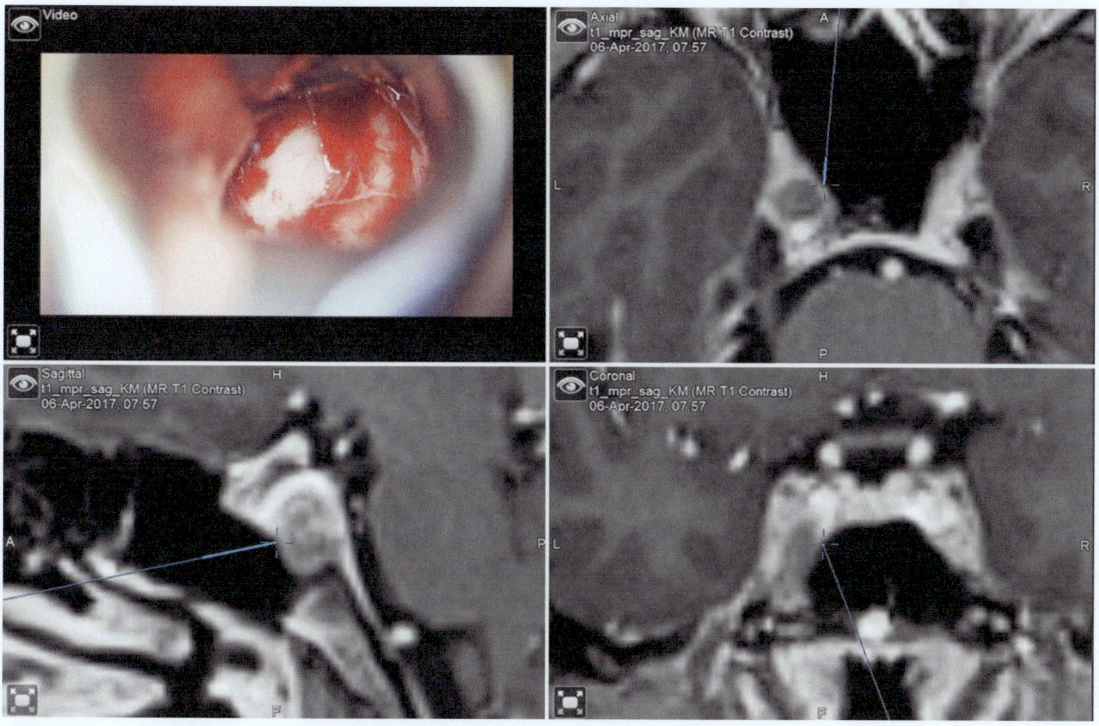

Fig. 1.10 Intraoperative view through the nasal speculum. The operating microscope is connected and referenced with the navigation system. Target point and focus is the posterior wall of the left sphenoid sinus which is the bony border of the tumour

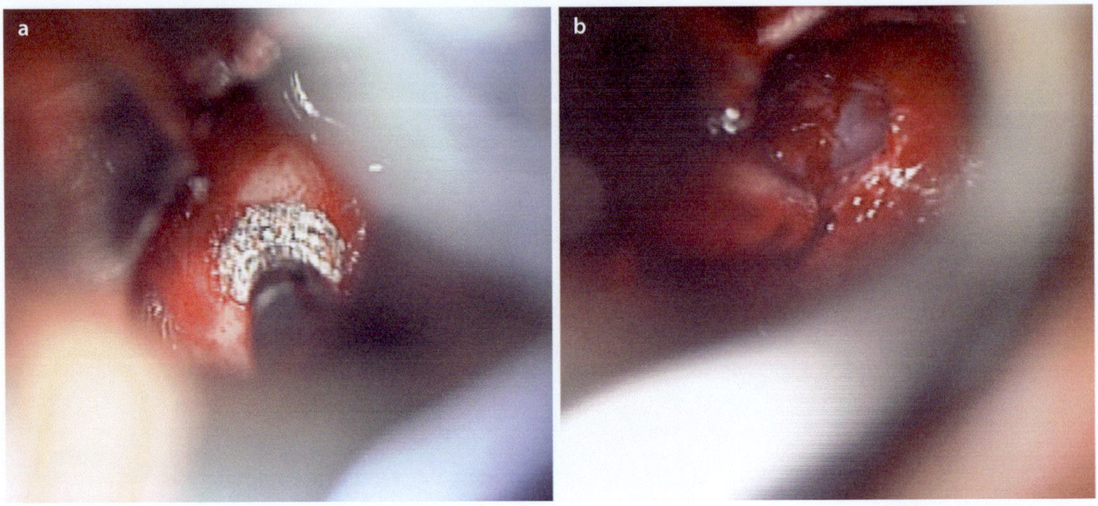

Fig. 1.11 Opening of the posterior wall of the sphenoid sinus with a diamond drill **a** and exposition of the tumour capsule **b**

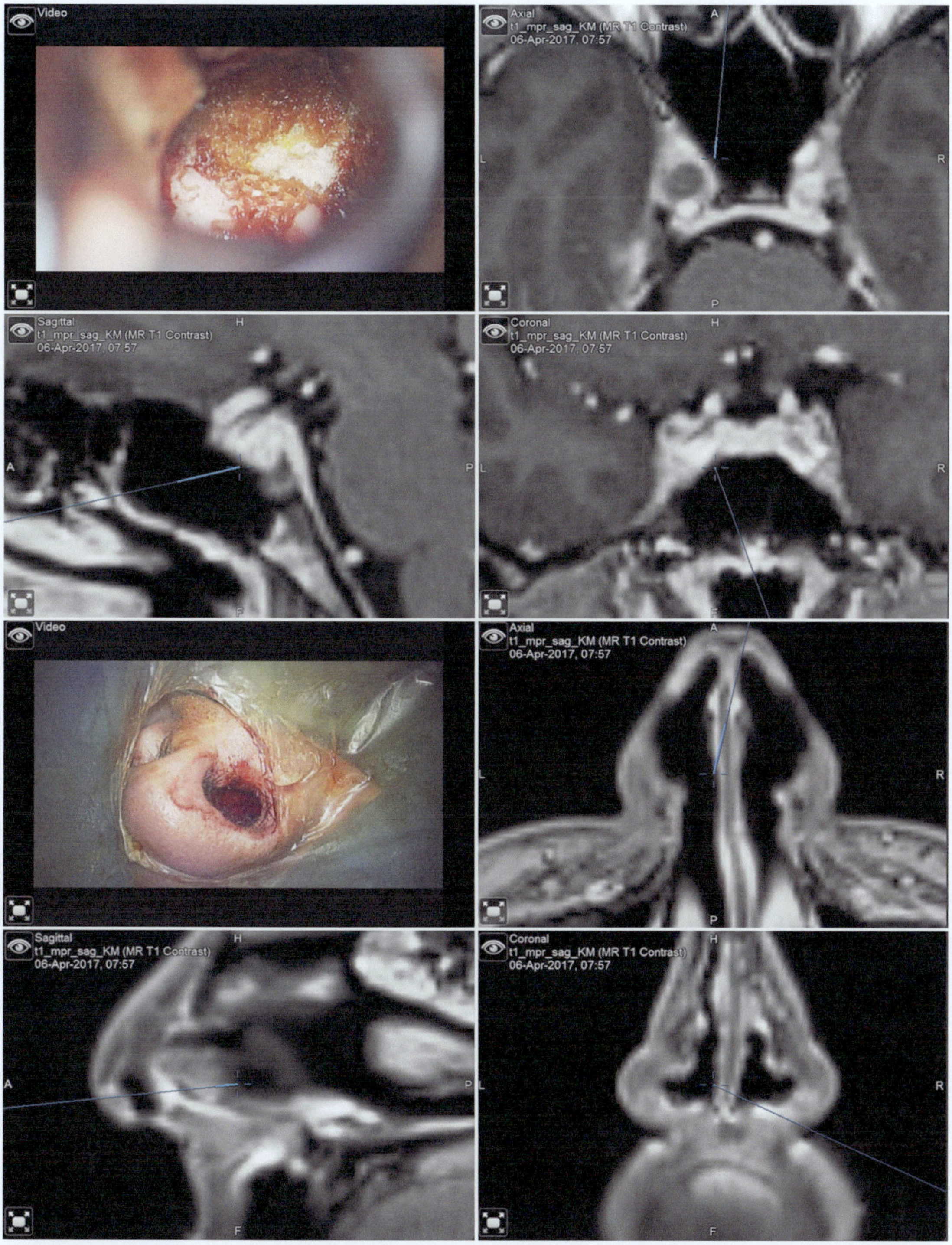

Fig. 1.12 Osseous reconstruction of the posterior wall of the sphenoid sinus with application of glueing material and removal of the speculum

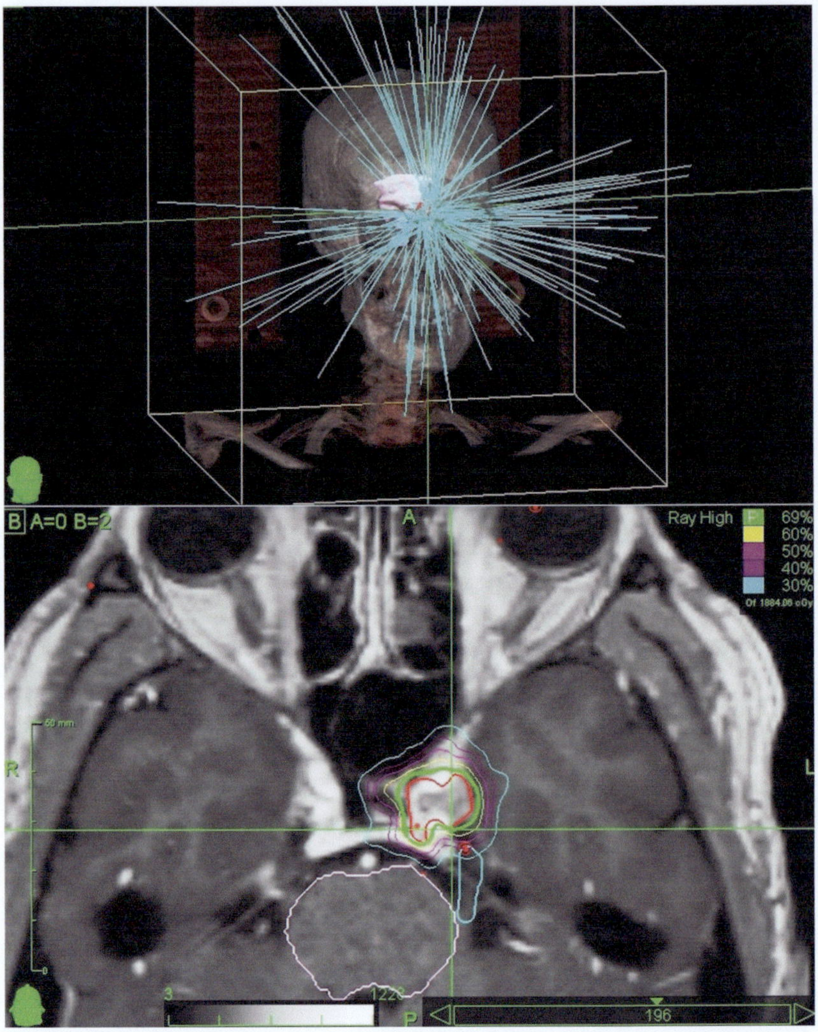

Fig. 1.13 Planning of isodoses and simulation of radiation trajectories for robot-assisted single shot radiosurgery

Clinical Anatomy

Hamid Borghei-Razavi, Marcel Biegler, Alexander König, and Juan Fernandez-Miranda

The original version of this chapter was revised. An erratum to this chapter can be found at https://doi.org/10.1007/978-3-319-64018-1_9

Electronic Supplementary Material The online version of this chapter (https://doi.org/10.1007/978-3-319-64018-1_2) contains supplementary material, which is available to authorized users.

A. König, U. Spetzger (eds.), *Surgery of the Skull Base*,
https://doi.org/10.1007/978-3-319-64018-1_2

This chapter describes the anatomy of the osseous skull base and the neurovascular structures in the anterior, middle, and posterior cranial fossa with special emphasis on the clinical and surgical meaning of their morphology.

Editor's Comment

Detailed anatomical knowledge is a basic precondition for planning and performing surgical procedures. Due to the complex anatomy and important functional areas, this is notably the case for skull base procedures.

The learning and consolidation of knowledge about the fascinating skull base anatomy is less complex when combining reading of anatomical descriptions and searching them on a bony human skull. Like in the famous scene of Shakespeare's Hamlet with the skull in one hand and the book in the other hand one can much easier learn human anatomy. Looking at the skull through the operating microscope as well as inspecting the skull base through an endoscope both give an insight and illustrate the microsurgical anatomy in three dimensions in the classical sense. Furthermore, to extend his or her knowledge, the skull base surgeon should study the microsurgical anatomical books of Wolfgang Seeger (*Anatomical Dissection for the Use in Neurosurgery*) that are rich in detail, the well-illustrated work of Gazi Yasargil (*Microsurgery* Volume 4), or the microsurgically oriented publication by Takanori Fukushima (*Manual of Skull Base Dissection*). In all of the books, one will recognize the direct clinical relevance of microsurgical skull base anatomy. For vascular lesions at the skull base the book *Neurovascular Surgery* by Robert Spetzler and for the anatomy of the cerebellopontine angle the book *Surgery of Cerebellopontine Lesions* by Madjid Samii are recommended.

The chapter about clinical anatomy of the skull base can, of course, only give an overview and should be stimulus for self-studying and reading the accompanying literature.

2.1 Anterior Cranial Fossa and Frontal Skull Base

2.1.1 Osseous Components

The os frontale (frontal bone) makes up the largest portion of the anterior cranial fossa and the osseous frontal base. It forms the predominant portion of the orbital roofs (Fig. 2.1). Only at the transition from the anterior to the middle cranial fossa (lateral) and in the orbital apex area (medial) portions of the orbital roofs consist of the os sphenoidale (sphenoid bone). The latter also forms the planum sphenoidale as the dorsal section of the median frontal base. The limbus sphenoidale separates the planum sphenoidale (anterior fossa) from the pre-chiasmatic sulcus (middle fossa) and continues laterally with the anterior roof of the optic canal (Fig. 2.2). The lamina cribrosa below the olfactory cortex area is formed by the os ethmoidale (ethmoid bone) [12].

2.1.2 Foramina and Their Contents

The lamina cribrosa (cribriform plate of the ethmoid bone) possesses multiple openings for the filia olfactoria of the olfactory nerve (CN I). The anterior meningeal artery, a branch of the anterior ethmoidal artery, runs intracranially through the lamina cribrosa. The anterior ethmoidal nerve, a branch of the nasociliary nerve (from the ophthalmic nerve [V1]), initially goes through the cribriform plate intracranially, and from there peters out extracranially to the nasal mucosa. The optic nerve (CN II) and the ophthalmic artery reach the inferior part of the orbital cavity through the optic canal (Figs. 2.1, 2.2, 2.3, and 2.4).

The oculomotor nerve originates from the anterior aspect of the midbrain. It runs anteriorly, passing below the posterior cerebral artery and above the superior cerebellar artery. The nerve pierces the dura mater and enters the lateral aspect of the cavernous sinus at the oculomotor triangle. This triangle consists of three ligaments as shown in Fig. 2.5: anterior petroclinoid ligament, posterior petroclinoid ligament, and interclinoid ligament. Opening and cutting these ligaments is necessary in different approaches to the cavernous sinus.

The ophthalmic artery is a branch of the supraclinoid portion of the internal carotid artery in most cases. This vessel follows the optic nerve into the optic canal and orbit and is responsible for the supply of the orbital structures. The origin of the ophthalmic artery is usually medial to the anterior clinoid process and below the optic nerve. At the level of the optic canal, this artery has passed to a position lateral

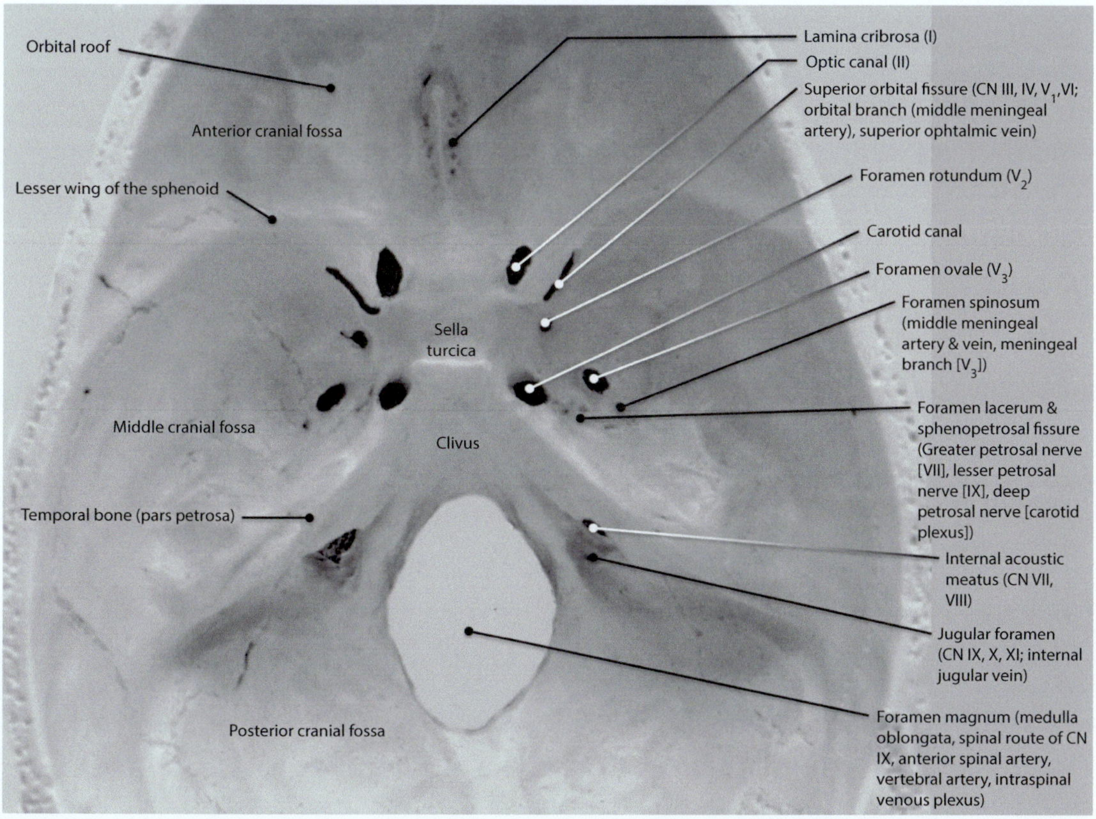

Fig. 2.1 Foramina of the osseous skull base specifying the pervading neurovascular structures

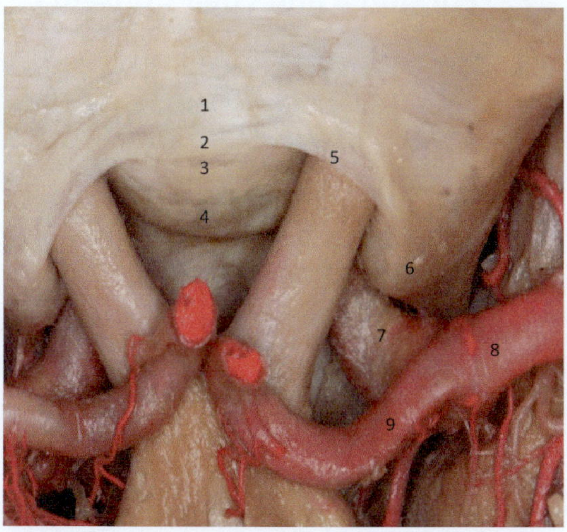

Fig. 2.2 Overview of the anterior-middle fossa junction and components: *1* planum sphenoidale, *2* limbus sphenoidale, *3* prechiasmatic sulcus, *4* tuberculum sellae, *5* falciform ligament, *6* anterior clinoid process, *7* internal carotid artery (supraclinoid segment), *8* middle cerebral artery (M1 segment), *9* anterior cerebral artery (A1 segment)

to the nerve. This anatomical fact must be kept in mind during the opening of the falciform ligament to avoid an iatrogenic lesion of this artery (Fig. 2.5b).

2.2 Middle Cranial Fossa, Sellar Region, and Temporal Base

2.2.1 Osseous Components

The middle cranial fossa is formed in its anterior portion by the greater and lesser wings of the sphenoid bone, whereby the lesser wing represents the border between middle and anterior cranial fossa. The temporal bone (os temporale) forms the major portion of the middle cranial fossa. The tip of the petrous part of the temporal bone represents the boundary to the posterior cranial fossa (Fig. 2.1).

The sella turcica is completely formed by the medial portions of the sphenoid bone. Important

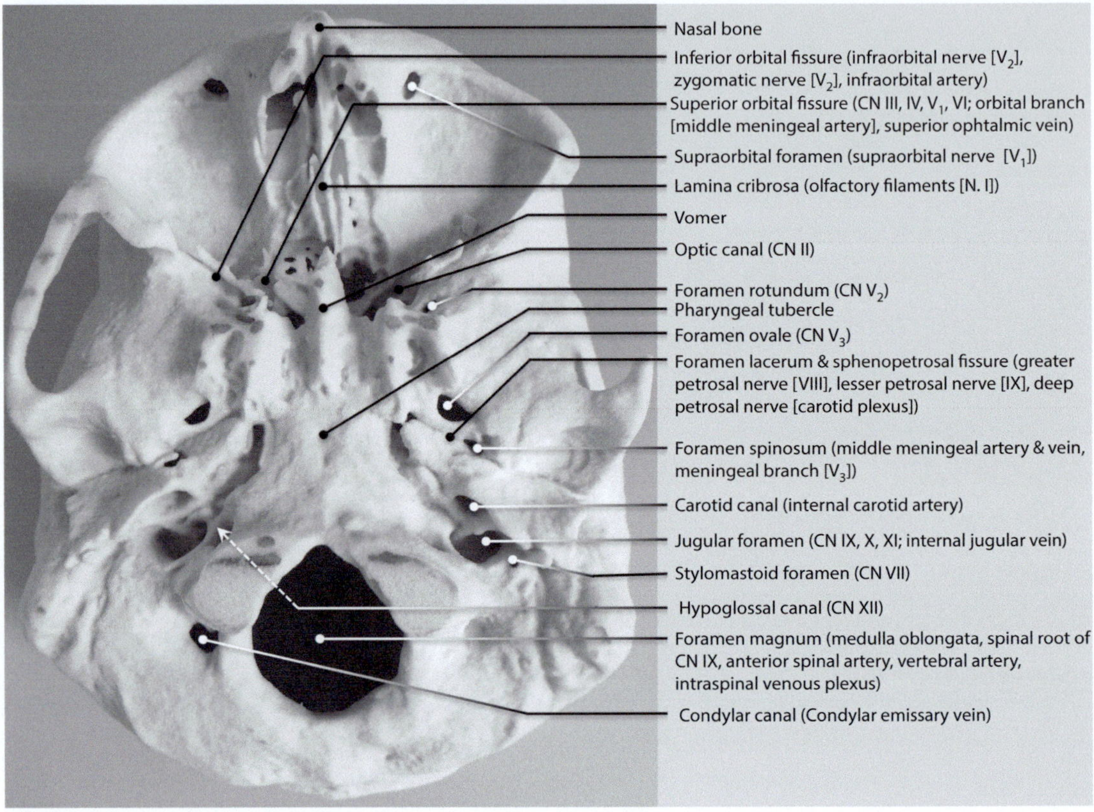

Fig. 2.3 Osseous skull base, inferior view, with foramina

landmarks here are the anterior, middle, and posterior clinoid processes (Figs. 2.2, 2.5, and 2.6) [4, 9, 17].

The middle clinoid process is an osseous prominence that arises from the body of the sphenoid bone at the anterolateral margin of the sella turcica. It is identifiable in 60% of the normal population (bilateral in 35%). Recognition of this structure, especially when there is a caroticoclinoid ring, is very important in the surgical planning of endoscopic endonasal surgeries in the perisellar region (Fig. 2.6) [7].

The prechiasmatic sulcus is a groove on the upper surface of the sphenoid bone running transversely between the optic canals bounded anteriorly by the sphenoidal limbus and posteriorly by the tuberculum sellae; the optic chiasm is located just above the prechiasmatic sulcus (Figs. 2.2 and 2.6) [2].

2.2.2 Foramina and Their Contents

Numerous structures permeate the superior orbital fissure (Figs. 2.1 and 2.4):

- Oculomotor nerve (CN III)
- Trochlear nerve (CN IV)
- Abducens nerve (CN VI)
- Nasociliary nerve (branch from CN V_1)
- Lacrimal nerve (branch from CN V_1)
- Frontal nerve (branch from CN V_1)
- Superior ophthalmic vein

The cranial nerves III, IV, and VI control the oculomotor system, while cranial nerve III also controls the pupillomotor system. The branches from the ophthalmic nerve (V_1) have sensory fibers from the cornea and upper facial area. The lacrimal nerve additionally has attached sympathetic and parasympathetic fibers for the lacrimal gland.

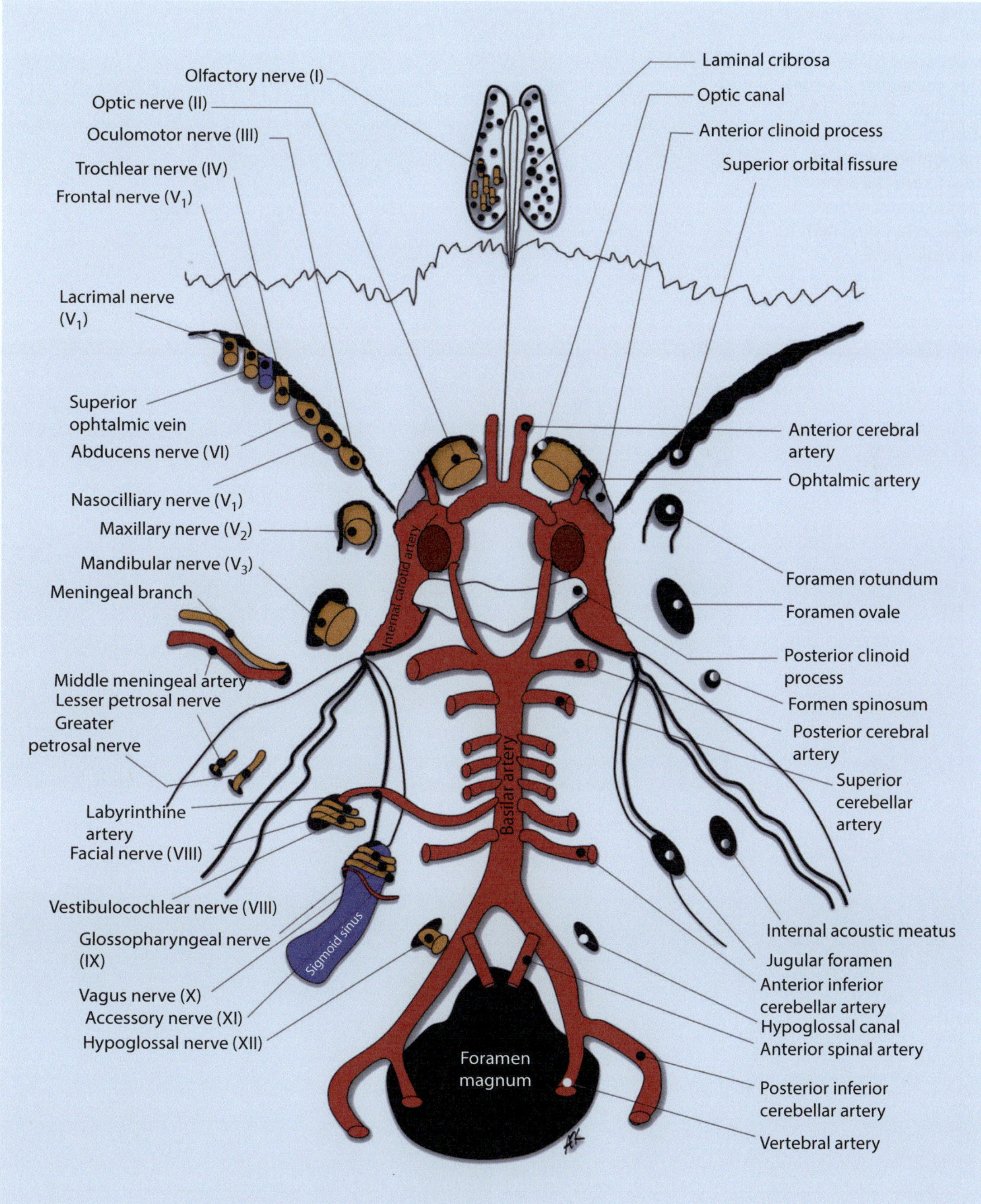

Fig. 2.4 Schematic drawing of the most important neurovascular structures of the skull base

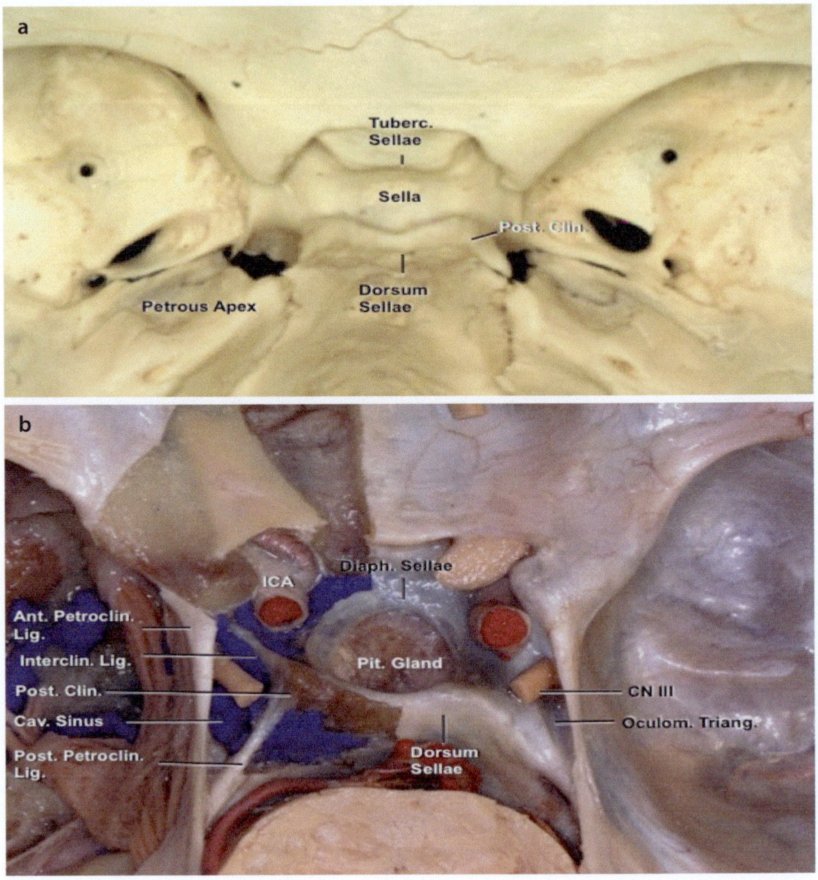

Fig. 2.5 Overview of the cavernous sinus, oculomotor triangle, and their correlations. **a** Bony structures, **b** anatomical structures: pay attention to the ophthalmic artery origin from the internal carotid artery at the left side and its correlation to the optic nerve

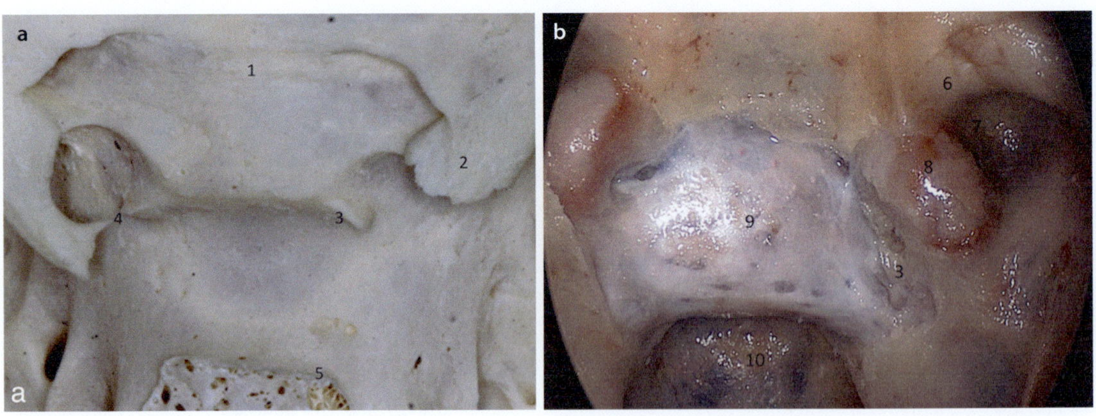

Fig. 2.6 Intracranial **a** and transnasal endoscopic **b** view of the middle clinoid process. *1* prechiasmatic sulcus, *2* anterior clinoid process, *3* middle clinoid process, *4* carotidoclinoid ring, *5* posterior clinoid process, *6* optic nerve, *7* lateral opticocarotid recess, *8* internal carotid artery (supraclinoid segment), *9* sella turcica, *10* clivus recess

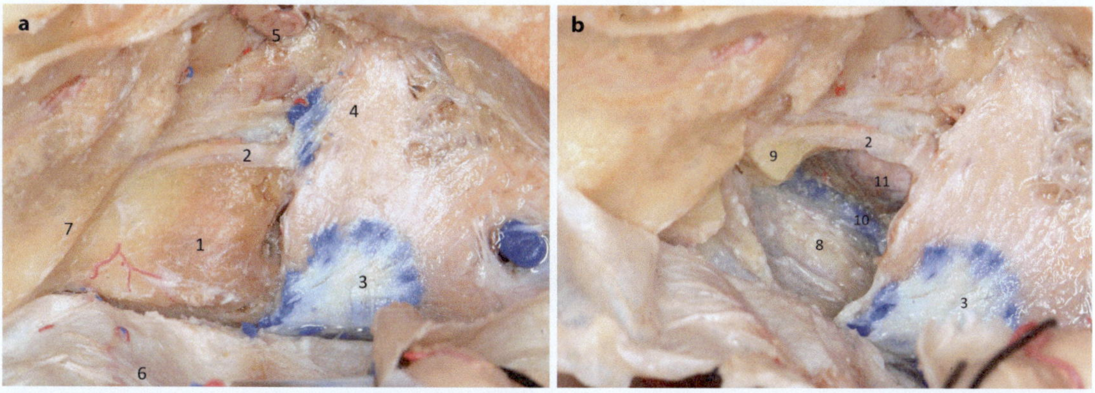

Fig. 2.7 Extradural exposure of the middle fossa floor and Kawase triangle **a**. Exposure of the posterior fossa dura after drilling the Kawase triangle **b**. *1* Kawase triangle (KT), *2* greater petrosal nerve (lateral border of KT), *3* Gasserian ganglion, *4* V_1 nerve (anterior border of KT), *5* middle meningial artery, *6* middle fossa dura, *7* arcuate eminence (posterior border of KT), *8* posterior fossa dura, *9* cochlea, *10* inferior petrosal sinus, *11* internal carotid artery (intrapetrosal part)

The inferior orbital fissure contains:

- Infraorbital nerve (branch from V_2)
- Zygomatic nerve (branch from V_2)
- Infraorbital artery
- Parasympathetic fibers from the pterygopalatine ganglion

Both nerve branches from V_2 are the sensory provision for the middle facial region. The zygomatic nerve receives parasympathetic fibers at the pterygopalatine ganglion for the lacrimal gland, which it passes on to the lacrimal nerve.

The maxillary nerve (V_2) and mandibular nerve (V_3) each possess their own foramina in the middle cranial fossa — foramen rotundum and foramen ovale (Figs. 2.1, 2.3, and 2.4).

The maxillary nerve is the sensory provision for the middle third of the face, as well as the gums and teeth of the upper jaw.

The mandibular nerve is the sensory provision for the lower facial region and tongue, as well the motor provision for the masticatory muscles, portions of the muscles in the base of the mouth, the tensor tympani muscle, and the tensor veli palatini muscle [5, 10, 13].

The greater petrosal nerve leaves the petrous portion of the temporal bone at its anterior side (Figs. 2.4 and 2.7) and draws on the floor of the middle cranial fossa toward the foramen lacerum, through which it reaches the outer cranial base. Beyond the synapses of its parasympathetic fibers in the pterygopalatine ganglion, it reaches the lacrimal gland and the glands of the nasal mucosa, gums, and epipharynx via branches of the maxillary nerve [8, 15]. This nerve is especially of importance during the anterior transpetrosal approach as a reliable lateral landmark of the Kawase triangle (Fig. 2.7) [3].

The lesser petrosal nerve (Jacobson anastomosis) leads parasympathetic fibers from the glossopharyngeal nerve and leaves the petrous portion of the temporal bone at its anterior surface (Fig. 2.4). It leaves the middle cranial fossa via the foramen lacerum and the sphenopetrosal fissure and draws through the infratemporal fossa to the otic ganglion (switching of the parasympathetic fibers). It reaches the parotid gland via anastomoses with the auriculotemporal nerve (from V_3) and with the facial nerve (CN VII) [18].

The greater superficial and deep petrosal nerves join to form the vidian nerve at the level of the foramen lacerum around the ICA. The vidian nerve enters the sphenoid bone, passes through the pterygoid canal, and ends in the pterygopalatine ganglion, where the parasympathetic fibers synapse. Sympathetic and parasympathetic fibers exit the ganglion and join the nerves that supply the orbit, nasal cavity, and palate. The vidian nerve has an important role in maintaining normal lacrimation and nasopharyngeal physiology.

The vidian nerve is a landmark for safe identification of the petrous internal carotid artery during endoscopic endonasal approaches (EEAs) to the skull base (Fig. 2.8) [1, 14].

The pterygosphenoidal fissure (curved line in Fig. 2.8) is the best landmark to find the foramen lacerum segment of the internal carotid artery.

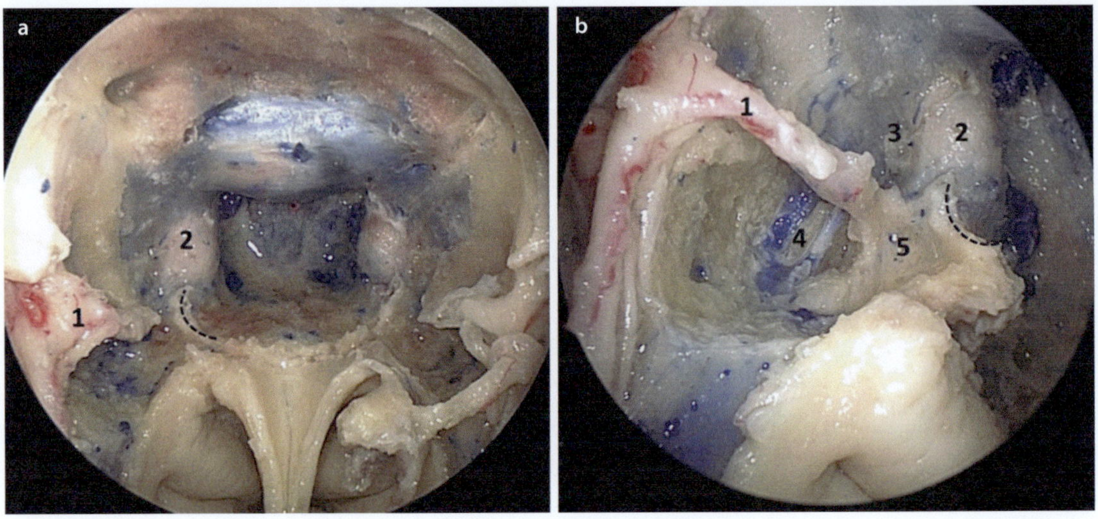

Fig. 2.8 Transsphenoidal transpterygoid exposure of the vidian nerve along with other anatomical landmarks **a**, **b**. *1* vidian nerve; *2* paraclival internal carotid artery, curved line, pterygosphenoidal fissure; *3* lingual process of the sphenoid bone; *4* mandibular strut; *5* foramen lacerum fibrocartilaginous

2.3 Cranial Base of the Posterior Cranial Fossa

2.3.1 Osseous Components

The posterior cranial fossa, including the foramen magnum and the caudal clivus, is primarily formed by the occipital bone. The posterior surface of the petrous bone is part of the temporal bone and anterolateral border of posterior fossa.

2.3.2 Foramina and Their Contents

The foramen magnum represents the connection of the intracranial space with the spinal canal (Figs. 2.4, 2.9, 2.10, and 2.11). It contains the medulla oblongata, the spinal roots of CN XI, the anterior spinal artery, the vertebral arteries, and the marginal sinus.

The hypoglossal canal enables the hypoglossal nerve (XII) to pass through the cranial base. Its function is the motor innervation of the tongue.

Fig. 2.9 Osseous skull base in a CT scan with important foramina for the passage of neurovascular structures

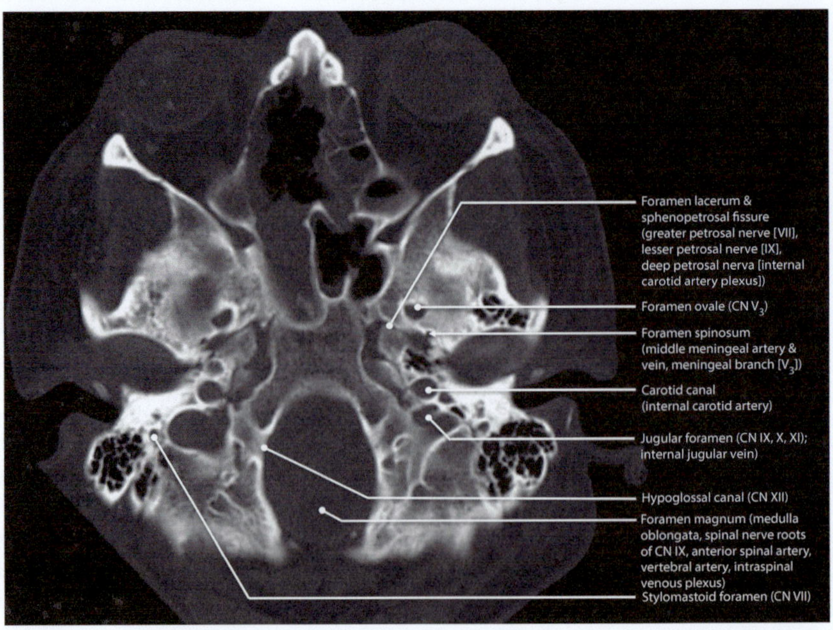

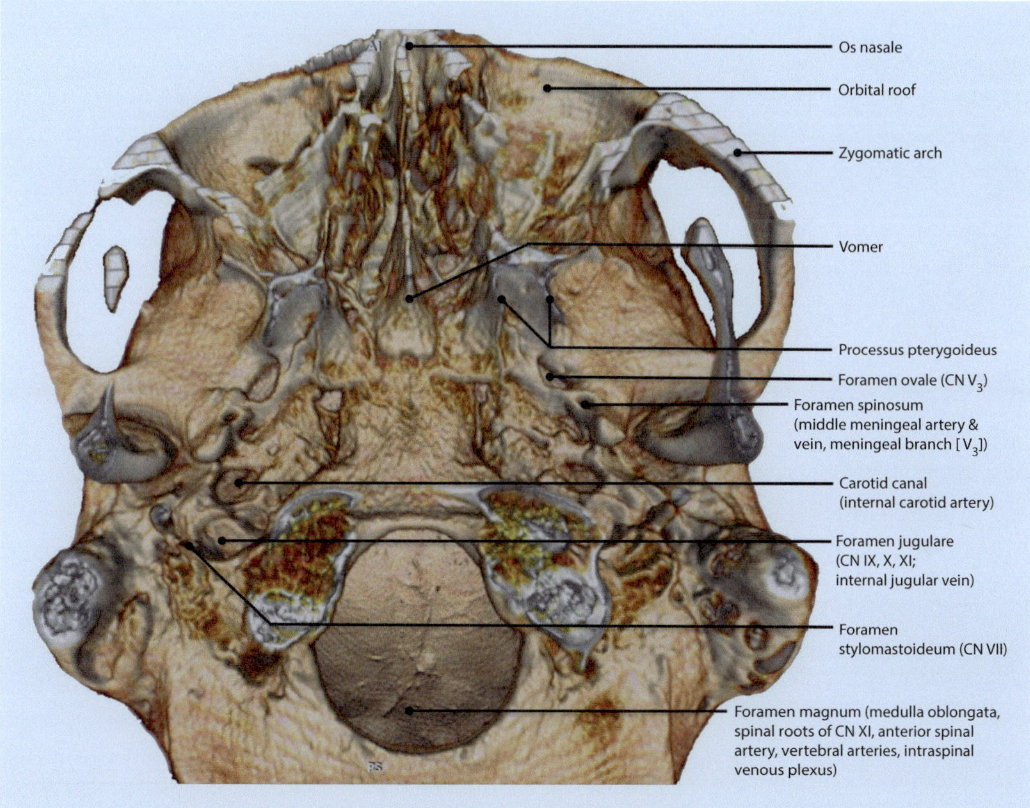

Fig. 2.10 Inferior view of the osseous skull base with anatomical landmarks and the most important openings for the passage of neurovascular structures (3D reconstruction of a skull base CT scan)

The internal jugular vein, the glossopharyngeal nerve (IX), the vagus nerve (X), and the accessory nerve (XI) leave the intracranial space via the jugular foramen, while the posterior meningeal artery (arises from the ascending pharyngeal artery) enters the skull base here [10, 11, 13].

The glossopharyngeal nerve leads sensory, motor, and parasympathetic fibers for the tongue, pharynx, and parotid gland. Impulses from pressoreceptors run from the carotid sinus to the medulla oblongata via this nerve.

The vagus nerve (CN X) is the most important nerve of the parasympathetic nervous system, ensuring extensive vegetative control of internal organs. It operates on a motor, sensory, viscerosensory, and visceromotor basis. It is involved in the innervation and control of the following organs: larynx, pharynx, upper esophagus, heart, trachea, bronchia, stomach, proximal intestine, liver, spleen, and kidneys.

The accessory nerve (CN XI) provides innervation for the voluntary motor control of the sternocleidomastoid and trapezius muscles.

2.3.3 Anatomy in the Cerebellopontine Angle

The cerebellopontine angle possesses great clinical importance, because it is the origin for a series of pathologies and their clinical manifestations. Various types of tumors can be found here, e.g., vestibular schwannomas (acoustic neuromas), epidermoids, and meningiomas arising from the posterior surface of the petrous bone or tentorium or even neurovascular conflicts such as trigeminal neuralgia, hemifacial spasms, or glossopharyngeal neuralgia [6, 12].

The drainage patterns of the superior petrosal venous complex are defined on the basis of the relationship between their site of entry into the superior petrosal sinus, Meckel's cave, and the internal acoustic meatus.

The drainage pattern of the superior petrosal vein appears to vary among the different CP angle pathologies. In general, preservation of the superior petrosal vein is not always achiev-

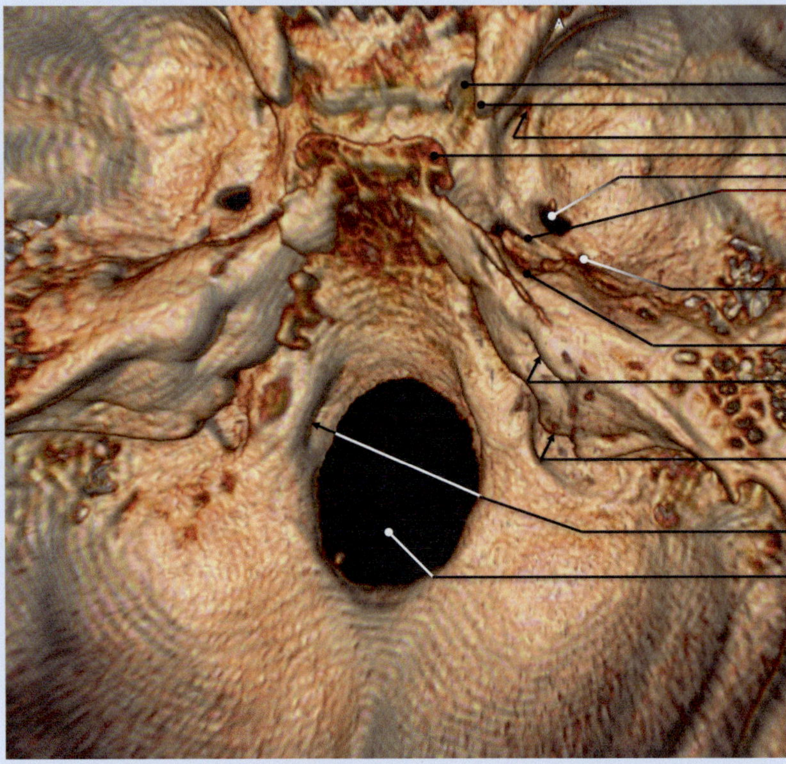

Fig. 2.11 Interior view of the skull base with the most important openings for the passage of neurovascular structures (3D reconstruction of a skull base CT scan)

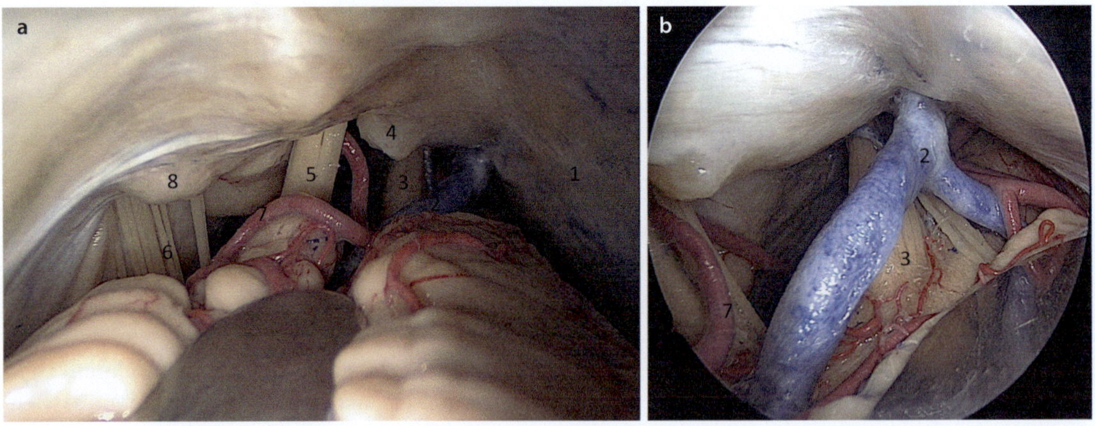

Fig. 2.12 Anatomy of the cerebellopontine angle, overview **a** and close up view on the superior petrosal vein (Dandy's vein) **b**. *1* tentorium; *2* superior petrosal vein; *3* trigeminal nerve (CN V); *4* suprameatal tubercle; *5* CN VII/VIII complex; *6* CN IX, X, XI complex entering the jugular foramen; *7* anterior-inferior cerebellar artery (AICA); *8* jugular tubercle

able in neurosurgical procedures, especially when the standard suboccipital approach is modified with suprameatal and/or supratentorial extension [16].

The retrosigmoidal access is considered as the standard surgical approach to the CPA. Here, the cranial nerves and vessels represented in Fig. 2.12 can be identified [6, 11, 12].

References

1. Alfieri A, Jho HD, Schettino R, Tschabitscher M. Endoscopic endonasal approach to the pterygopalatine fossa: anatomic study. Neurosurgery. 2003;52(2):374–8.
2. Abhinav K, Acosta Y, Wang WH, Bonilla LR, Koutourousiou M, Wang E, Synderman C, Gardner P, Fernandez-Miranda JC. Endoscopic endonasal approach to the optic canal: anatomic considerations and surgical relevance. Neurosurgery. 2015;11(Suppl 3):431–45.
3. Borghei-Razavi H, Tomio R, Fereshtehnejad SM, Shibao S, Schick U, Toda M, Kawase T, Yoshida K. Anterior petrosal approach: the safety of Kawase triangle as an anatomical landmark for anterior petrosectomy in petroclival meningiomas. Clin Neurol Neurosurg. 2015;139:282–7.
4. Cheng Y, Chen Y, Zhou Z, Zhu J, Feng Y, Zhao G. Anatomical study of posterior clinoid process (PCP) and its clinical meanings. J Craniofac Surg. 2015;26(2):537–40.
5. Chotai S, Kshettry VR, Petrak A, Ammirati M. Lateral transzygomatic middle fossa approach and its extensions: surgical technique and 3D anatomy. Clin Neurol Neurosurg. 2015;130:33–41.
6. Colasanti R, Tailor AR, Gorjian M, Zhang J, Ammirati M. Microsurgical and endoscopic anatomy of the extended retrosigmoid inframeatal infratemporal approach. Neurosurgery. 2015;11(Suppl 2):181–9.
7. Fernandez-Miranda JC, Tormenti M, Latorre F, Gardner P, Snyderman C. Endoscopic endonasal middle clinoidectomy: anatomic, radiological, and technical note. Neurosurgery. 2012;71(2 Suppl Operative):233–9.
8. Jiang Y, Chen Y, Yao J, Tian Y, Su L, Li Y. Anatomic assessment of petrous internal carotid artery, facial nerve, and cochlea through the anterior transpetrosal approach. J Craniofac Surg. 2015;26(7):2180–3.
9. Kimball D, Kimball H, Matusz P, Tubbs RS, Loukas M, Cohen-Gadol A. Ossification of the posterior petroclinoid dural fold: a cadaveric study with neurosurgical significance. J Neurol Surg B Skull Base. 2015;76(4):272–7.
10. Kirsch CF. Advances in magnetic resonance imaging of the skull base. Int Arch Otorhinolaryngol. 2014;18(Suppl 2):S127–35.
11. Komune N, Matsushima K, Matsushima T, Komune S, Rhoton AL Jr. Surgical approaches to jugular foramen schwannomas: an anatomic study. Head Neck. 2015;38(Suppl 1):E1041–53.
12. Patel CR, Fernandez-Miranda JC, Wang WH, Wang EW. Skull base anatomy. Otolaryngol Clin N Am. 2016;49(1):9–20.
13. Prevedello LM. Advances in computed tomography evaluation of skull base diseases. Int Arch Otorhinolaryngol. 2014;18(Suppl 2):S123–6.
14. Prevedello DM, Pinheiro-Neto CD, Fernandez-Miranda JC, Carrau RL, Snyderman CH, Gardner PA, Kassam AB. Vidian nerve transposition for endoscopic endonasal middle fossa approaches. Neurosurgery. 2010;67(2 Suppl Operative):478–84.
15. Rigante L, Herlan S, Tatagiba MS, Stanojevic M, Hirt B, Ebner FH. Petrosectomy and topographical anatomy in traditional Kawase and Posterior Intradural Petrous Apecectomy (PIPA) approach: an anatomical study. World Neurosurg. 2015;86:93–102.
16. Watanabe T, Igarashi T, Fukushima T, Yoshino A, Katayama Y. Anatomical variation of superior petrosal vein and its management during surgery for cerebellopontine angle meningiomas. Acta Neurochir. 2013;155:1871–8.
17. Wright E, Spetzler RF. The expanded endoscopic endonasal approach to petroclival lesions: a useful adjunct to traditional skull base approaches. World Neurosurg. 2015;84(2):224–5.
18. Young C. Temporal bone CT: anatomy, technique, and associated pathophysiology. Radiol Technol. 2015;86(5):535CT–55CT.

Therapeutical Principles in the Treatment of Skull Base Pathologies

Uwe Spetzger, Martin Bleif, and Gerd Becker

A. König, U. Spetzger (eds.), *Surgery of the Skull Base*,
https://doi.org/10.1007/978-3-319-64018-1_3

3

3.1 Surgical Principles

In cases of complex skull base tumours, the primary interdisciplinary discussion among different medical specialties is a basic principle. Preserving and improving neurological function have become the highest dictum when planning treatment. Generally, the individualisation of the therapeutical concept according to all clinical and radiological data represents another principle of modern skull base surgery that can be gently put into practice by the continuous improvement of preoperative diagnostics, therapy simulation and intraoperative visualisation with modern endoscopy which is associated with a miniaturisation of surgical approaches.

Editor's Comment
Uwe Spetzger

As mentioned above this book mainly represents a neurosurgeon's point of view onto modern skull base surgery. But nowadays of course, modern skull base surgery can only be performed in close cooperation with all disciplines that diagnostically and therapeutically deal with disease of head and neck. Here strategical principle is similar to the treatment of skull base lesions by other disciplines whereupon the main goal is avoiding any harm to the patient due to the treatment.

Therapeutical procedures are affected by the ongoing innovation and technical progress in neuroradiology which has significant improvement of diagnostic and interventional procedures. The paradigm shift of minimising surgical approaches to reduce invasiveness of skull base surgery is closely connected with technical innovations. Basically, the trend to smaller approaches will continue and even move away from surgical incision like it was already achieved with stereotactic radiosurgery using the CyberKnife. Application of energy into the tumour for local destruction like the use of focussed ultrasound will be a continuously growing and important therapeutical principle in skull base surgery, too.

A relevant and strategically important principle is training and further education in the specialty of skull base surgery. It summarises the education of interdisciplinary thinking and acting as well as the specific neurosurgical training. In the future the specific and well-grounded surgical training of the young generation of neurosurgeons will become more difficult due to a decreasing number of cases, shortened working time and increasing number of therapeutic alternatives especially in skull base surgery.

The strategical principles in skull base surgery do not differ significantly from the general principles in modern neurosurgery. In cases of complex skull base tumours an interdisciplinary discussion with experts from other specialties is a basic principle. Thus, after adequate clinical, neurological and radiological diagnostics as well as after additional assessment by ophthalmologists, ENT surgeons, maxillofacial surgeons, oncologists and radiation therapists, a comprehensive multidisciplinary therapeutical plan is established. In general, this book is focused on the neurosurgical aspect of skull base surgery.

3.1.1 Risks of Treatment Versus Surgical Radicalness

Basically, skull base tumours should be resected as radically as possible, and vascular lesions should be eliminated completely. There are several methods in recent skull base surgery that are often combined or used consecutively to achieve this aim.

The basic therapeutical strategy is to reach maximum radicalness with minimum effort and risk, thus, with the least amount of morbidity.

According to this nowadays, the supreme principle is maintaining or even improving neurological function. There has been a paradigm shift compared to the last decades so that surgical radicalness is not the main goal anymore but a low surgical morbidity if ever possible and a high level of the patient's quality of life [2–4, 20, 32].

In general, the individualisation of treatment concepts according to all available clinical and radiological data is a basic principle of modern skull base surgery.

This individualised therapeutical concept is the basis for the determination of the aim of surgery whereupon the basic principle «maintenance of function» is of higher importance than «radicalness». In this process histology is often decisive, and it can be determined by a biopsy if this can be done with low morbidity. Otherwise modern MR spectroscopy can be used preoperatively to narrow the number of differential diagnoses [24].

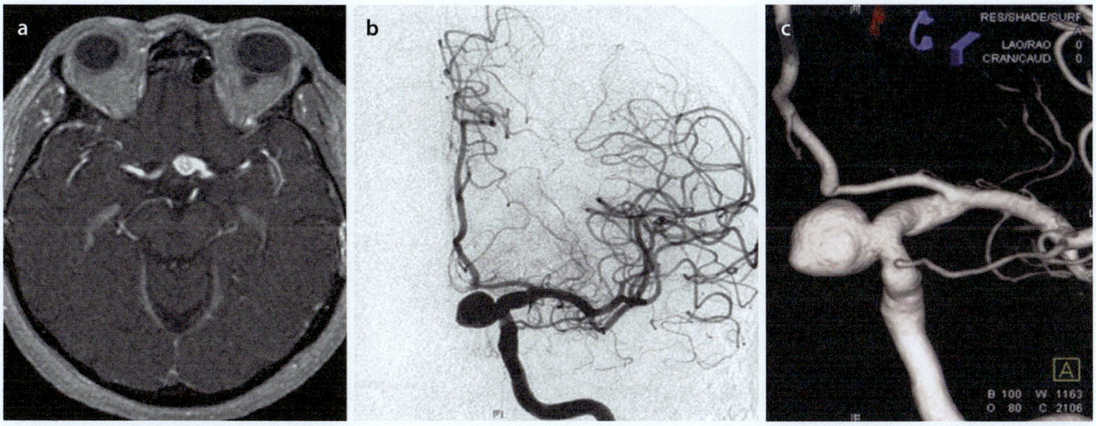

Fig. 3.1 Multimodal neuroradiological diagnostics in the case of a 56-year-old patient with left-sided progressive visual disorder due to compression of the left optic nerve by a complex ICA aneurysm. Axial contrast-enhanced MRI due to the initial suspicion of a tumourous lesion **a**. DSA confirming the left-sided ICA aneurysm **b**. 3D reconstruction of the rotational angiographical data **c**

3.1.2 Comprehensive Neuroradiological Diagnostics

Comprehensive neuroradiological diagnostics is the basic prerequisite for adequate planning and operative performance in cases of skull base tumours. In most cases a combination of CT and MRI scan is used for the optimum visualisation of bony and neural structures [5]. Depending on the individual pathology, different examination protocols and MR sequences are required [5, 24]. Recently, an MPR data set for optimum 3D visualisation and as a basis of image-guided preoperative planning as well as intraoperative surgical navigation have become an important principle and a universal neuroradiological strategy in cases of skull base lesions [6].

Nowadays only in select cases a thin-sliced CT scan of the orbits is performed to reduce the exposition of eyes and lenses to radiation all the more so since modern image converting algorithms can fuse MRI and CT data with high precision.

Especially in cases of vascular lesions of the skull base like large aneurysms, angiomas or highly vascularised tumours, the vascular anatomy and the individual vascular structure as well as their selective and detailed visualisation play an important role in the preoperative work-up. In those cases, CT angiography and MR angiography cannot completely replace the conventional digital subtraction angiography (DSA) which is nowadays usually conducted as 3D rotational angiography [19].

The DSA delivers essential information about haemodynamics and the flow properties inside of a lesion which is not possible with CT or MR angiography (Figs. 3.1 and 3.2). With this information, possibly concepts for revascularisation, e.g. as a bypass for an obstructed artery, can make up a therapeutical concept. Beside the well-established balloon occlusion under clinical and/or electrophysiological monitoring, also up-to-date blood flow simulations on the basis of MR data play an increasing role.

Modern flow analysis programmes that work with time-of-flight MR data and 2D phase contrast MR date enable a blood flow quantification by using complex calculating algorithms. These quantifications play an increasing role in the planning of intracranial bypasses in revascularising surgery [16, 40, 47].

3.1.3 Computer-Assisted and Navigation-Guided Skull Base Surgery

After the multidisciplinary treatment planning, the actual operative simulation of the therapeutical concept can be done by using a 3D simulation based on CT and MRI imaging as well as on data from angiograms and nuclear medicine. The DICOM compatible data are fused on a workstation enabling a multimodal data set for the

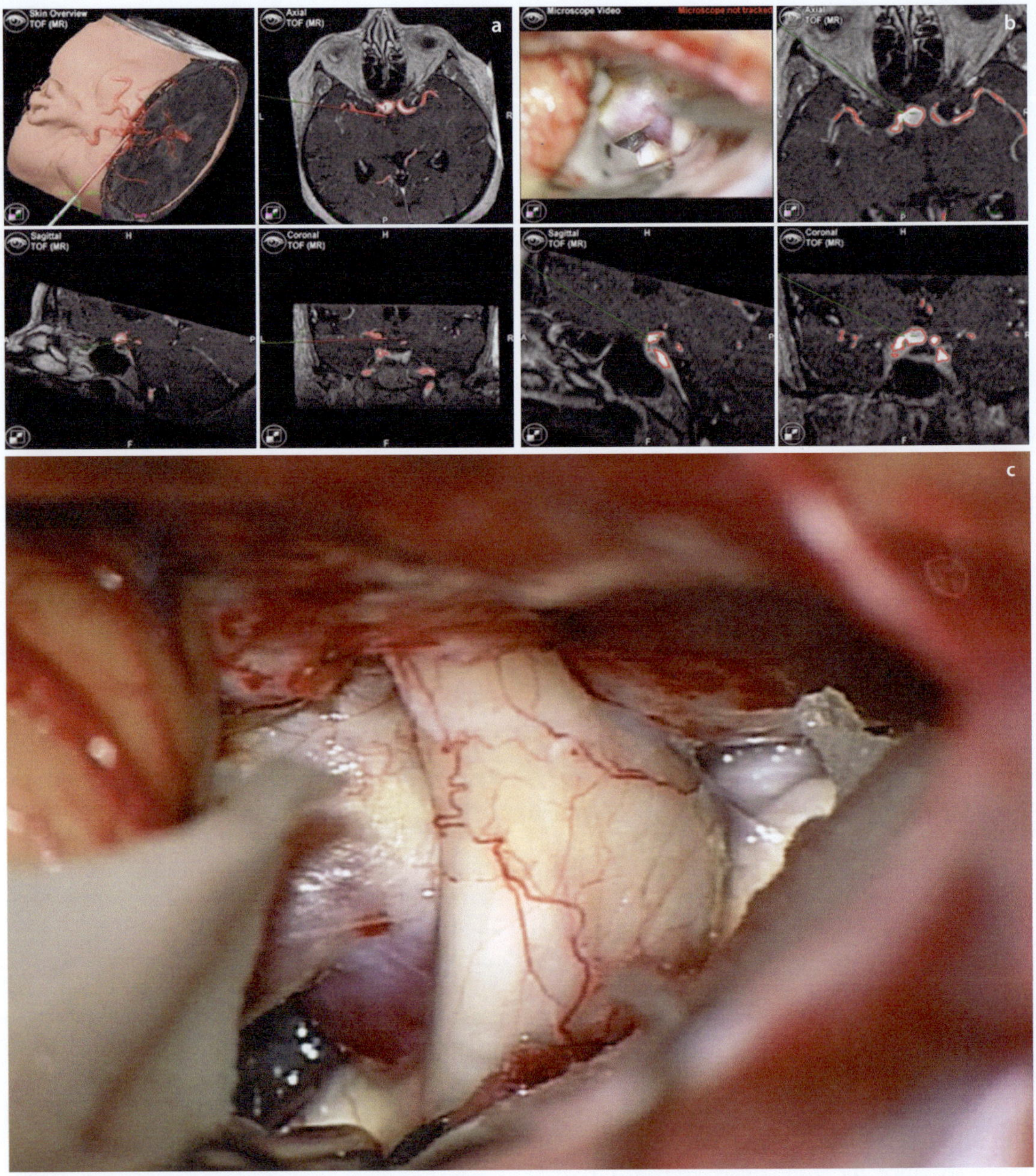

Fig. 3.2 MRI 3D MPR data set with contrast enhancement **a**. Segmentation of blood vessels and simulation of the surgical approach **b**. Intraoperative navigation guidance with exposure of the aneurysm neck **c**. The intraoperative image shows the massive compression of the left optic nerve by the medially oriented ACI aneurysm

simulation including 3D visualisation, image editing, segmentation of crucial structures and designation of anatomical landmarks. This individually edited data set is the basis for intraoperative navigation. Thus, computer-assisted multimodal simulation and surgical planning using navigation data have been established as a basic principle in modern skull base surgery (Fig. 3.3). The use of navigation systems has been accepted as an important strategy in modern skull base surgery [28, 33, 44].

3.1.4 Radiation Therapy and Stereotactic Radiosurgery

Postoperative adjuvant radiation therapy and specific chemotherapies are becoming more and

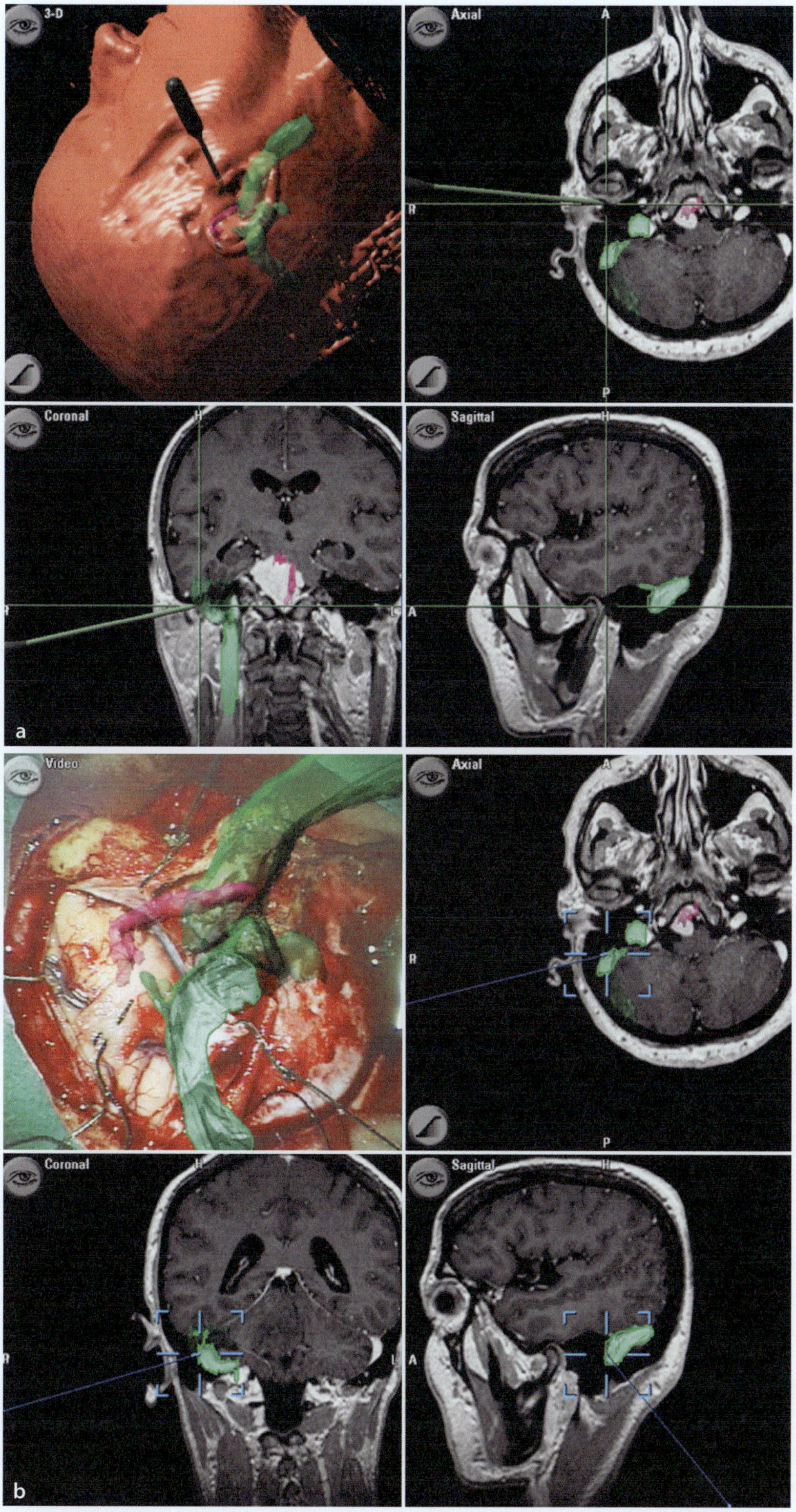

Fig. 3.3 Navigation-guided combined temporobasal anterosigmoidal approach for the resection of petroclival meningioma. Planning of the approach with segmentation of the sigmoid sinus, transverse sinus and basilar artery in relation to the tumour **a**. Finished approach with dural opening **b**. With the use of virtual reality, the segmented vascular anatomy can be mirrored into the microscopic view

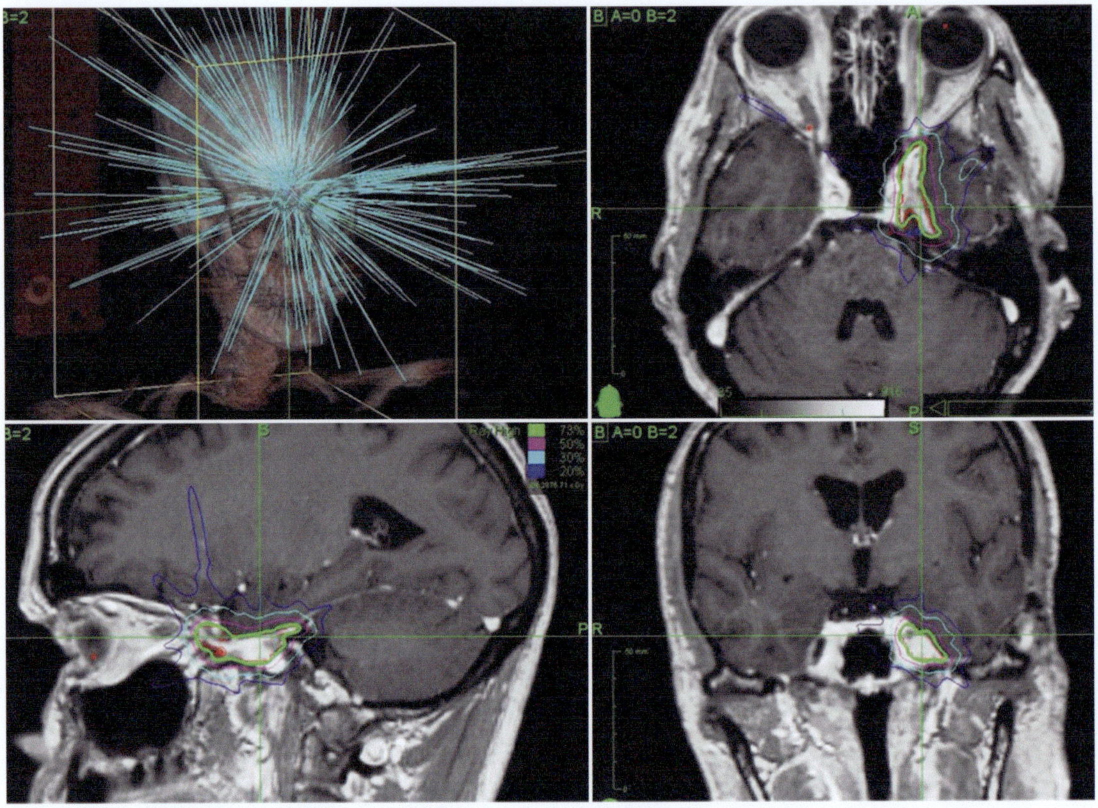

Fig. 3.4 Treatment plan for robot-assisted radiosurgery using the CyberKnife for the therapy of an extensive recurrent meningioma of the sphenoid wing with infiltration of the left sigmoid sinus and Meckel's cave showing the distribution of isodoses and simulation of multiple radiation angles

more important, not only for the treatment of malign skull base tumours. Also the concept of radiosurgical treatment especially in cases of complex skull base meningiomas is of increasing importance. The stereotactical radiation as a primary treatment option or the combination of surgery and radiosurgery with the Gamma Knife or the robot-assisted CyberKnife is an optimisation of the treatment concept (Fig. 3.4). This therapeutical option which has become an established concept is appreciated in this book with a standalone chapter [9, 10, 27, 42, 65].

3.1.5 Special Techniques and Modern Technologies

Another strategy in skull base surgery is the improvement of surgical techniques as well as the use of specially designed instruments and tools.

A milestone in skull base surgery is the use of navigation as a basic principle for preoperative planning and intraoperative orientation. Furthermore, the refinement of intraoperative electrophysiological monitoring and anaesthesiological procedures contributed to an improvement of postoperative outcome and clinical results. The use of technical innovations, modifications and improvements of anaesthesia, cranial nerve monitoring and blood flow measurement as well as the establishment of ICG angiography as a monitoring procedure in aneurysm surgery and blood flow simulation in bypass surgery are just a few examples that have become strategical basic principles in skull base surgery [18, 23].

Furthermore, the gentle removal of bone tissue adjacent to blood vessels and cranial nerves by using Piezo ultrasound will become a technical standard and surgical strategy in skull base surgery [15].

And also innovations in haemostasis and new dura closure compounds are of importance. The avoidance of CSF fistulas by harvesting autologous tissues like fascia lata will disappear in the medium term since modern

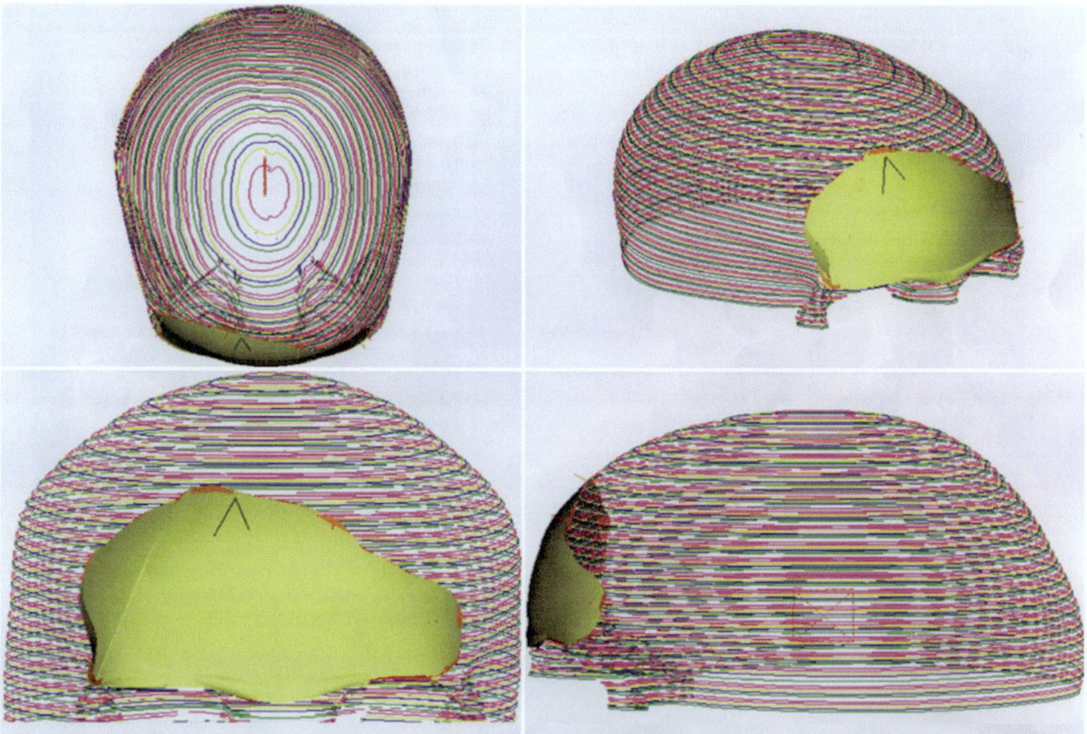

Fig. 3.5 Simulation and planning of an individualised cranial CAD/CAM titanium implant. The simulation was based on a 1 mm thin-sliced CT data set

and biocompatible dura replacements are available, and, thus, the invasiveness of surgeries will decrease [17].

An important contribution to accurate and patient-individual reconstruction of the scull has been given by modern implant technology [36]. Nowadays very precise computer-aided manufactured implants enable an improvement of cosmetic results as well as an exact reconstruction of the skull base [21, 30, 45]. In the future 3D printing technologies will lead to a faster manufacturing and the use of different materials for the reconstruction of the skull base ([38]; Figs. 3.5, 3.6, and 3.7).

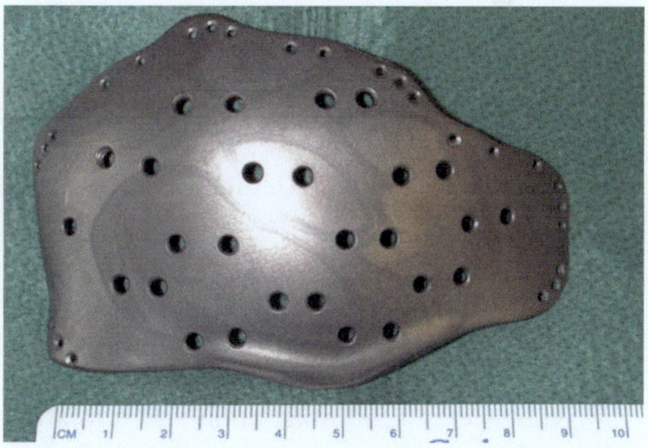

Fig. 3.6 Finalised CAD/CAM titanium implant for the reconstruction of the frontal skull and skull base

3.1.6 Era of Miniaturisation

With time a basic change of surgical strategy in terms of surgical radicalness has occurred. Some decades ago the radical resection of the lesion was the main goal of surgery, and, thus, complex and extensive surgical approaches had been developed and brought to perfection. Especially extensive midfacial approaches and surgeries inside of the cavernous sinus resulting from that time are nowadays only used in a few selected cases and have been widely replaced by less invasive techniques. Especially radiosurgery plays an important role in the treatment of complex skull base lesions [14, 26].

During the last few years, there has been a basic strategy in skull base surgery of diminishing radical approaches [46]. Nevertheless, the basic princi-

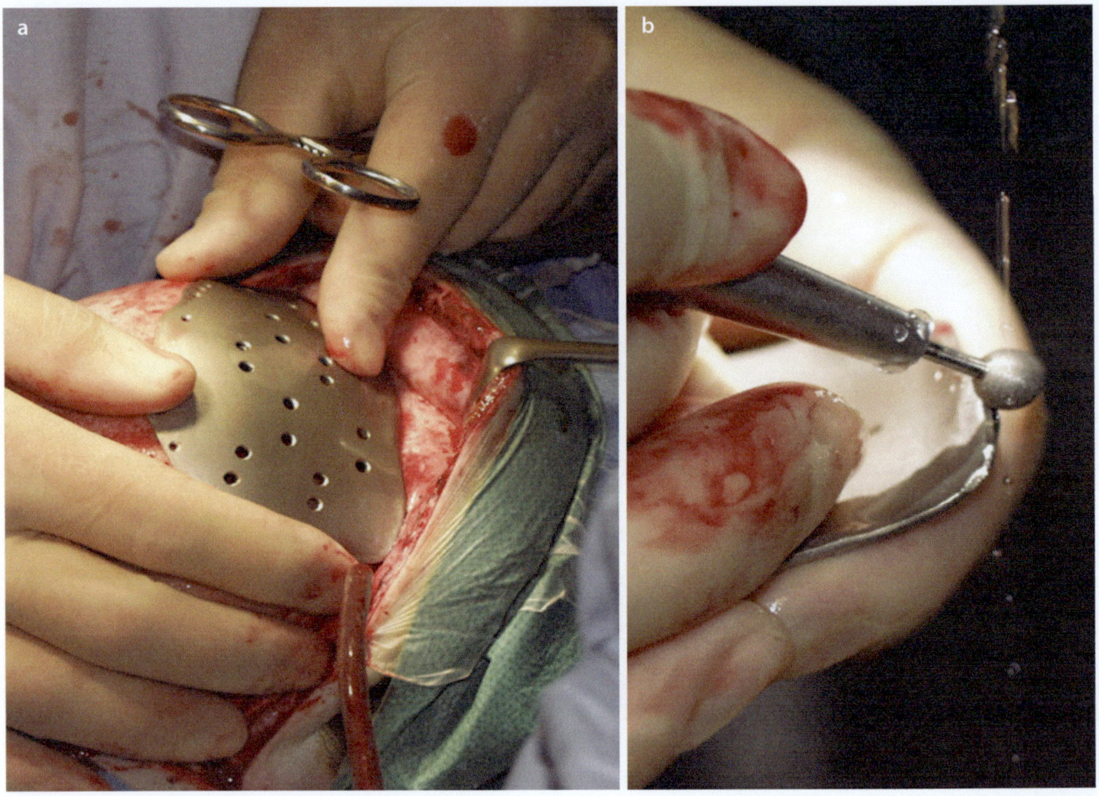

Fig. 3.7 Intraoperative image after implantation and reconstruction of osteoclastic skull base defect **a**. Minimal adaption by drilling the edge of the implant with a diamant burr for better fitting accuracy **b** which is much more difficult than in cases of more recently used materials like PMMA

ple of «aggressive to the bone, smooth to the brain» is still valid. The actual common orbitozygomatic approaches or the combined temporal retrosigmoid or anterosigmoid resulted from these principles, and they have several modifications that are further individualised to the patient's anatomy and the configuration of the skull base lesion by using navigation systems [29, 31, 35].

The new era of minimalisation and miniaturisation of skull base surgery has already begun. Personal clinical experience as well as the literature show that the minimalisation of surgical approaches reduces the trauma to muscles, especially to the temporal muscle and the neck muscles, resulting in faster convalescence and a better subjective well-being after surgery. Furthermore, smaller dural openings and smaller craniotomies are recognised as less surgery-related stress by the patient [25, 41].

Thus, in the future there will be a further individualisation and downsizing of skull base approaches. Modern endoscopy with its significantly improved visualisation will make a substantial contribution to this development [39].

Already today surgical approaches to pituitary adenomas and anterior skull base tumours can be significantly reduced by using endoscopically assisted microsurgery or even pure endoscopic surgery. Beside anterior skull base tumours, this strategy is also increasingly used for lesions of the petrous bone and retrosigmoid approaches. Improved visualisation as well as the training and education of younger colleagues and the expected innovation boost by 3D endoscopy will enhance this trend even further. Neuroendoscopy and the accompanying miniaturisation of surgical approaches will obviously be one of the relevant future strategies in skull base surgery [1, 8].

3.1.7 Training and Further Education

The rapid development of endovascular techniques with an increasing number of coils and stents for the treatment of vascular malformations and stenoses will reduce but not completely replace the number of microsurgical vascular procedures [12, 13, 34, 43]. Thus, an important strategy in skull base surgery is the education and surgical training of younger skull base surgeons who have to be able to treat complex vascular and neoplastic lesions.

In general, highly qualified operative training and continuing education will continue to be a basic principle in this subspecialty. Computer-aided training models on the basis of virtual reality, intense microsurgical training using plastic and animal models especially in vascular microsurgery as well as hands-on workshops with practical microsurgical exercises using cadaveric specimen are methods for training and further education ([7, 11, 22, 37]; ◘ Fig. 3.8).

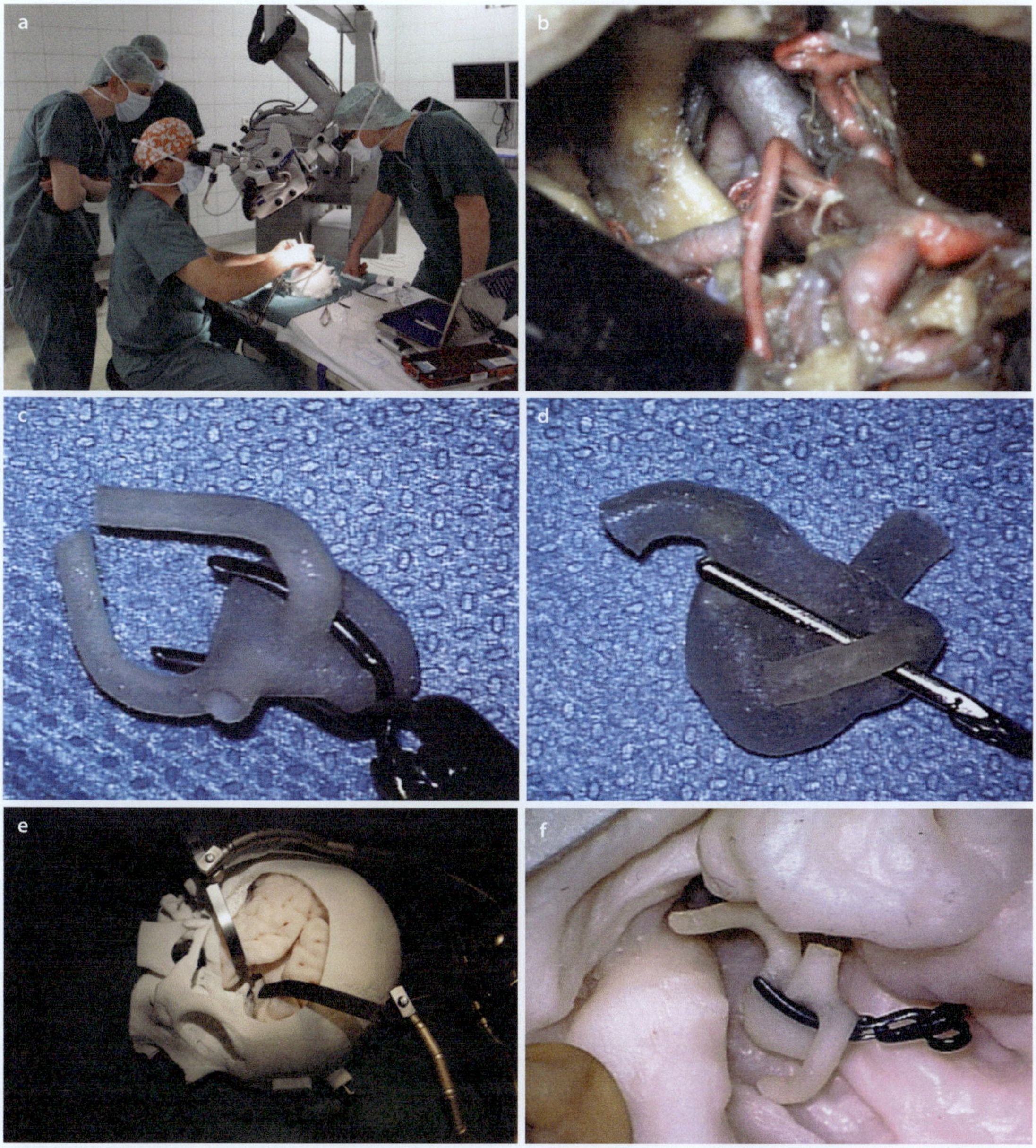

◘ **Fig. 3.8** Practical microsurgical education and «non-bloody» training using models **a**. Dissection of blood vessels in a cadaveric specimen **b**. Clipping on a 3D aneurysm model made of plastic **c**. Checking of the correct clip position and the vascular reconstruction **d**. Extensive osteoclastic craniotomy and spatula retraction of the Sylvian fissure on a realistic plastic model (Kezlex, Tokyo, Japan) **e**. Clipping of an artificial 3D aneurysm in the depth of the Sylvian fissure **f**

3

3.1.8 Function-Preserving and Function-Improving Skull Base Surgery

The fast ongoing development of the methods and techniques mentioned above will lead to a reduction of surgical morbidity by miniaturisation of surgical approaches which results in the resent development from function-preserving to function-improving skull base surgery.

3.2 Radiosurgical Principles

Radiosurgery is a very effective option for the definitive treatment of primary tumours of the skull base. Radiosurgery can be used as a sole treatment modality for tumours of the skull base in patients who are poor candidates for surgery, for recurrent tumours after primary surgery and as an adjunct to surgery in a combined bimodal treatment concept which is increasingly used to avoid mutilating surgery and provides a high chance for long-term tumour control.

Main indications for radiosurgery are schwannomas of the vestibular nerve and – less frequent – other cranial nerves, meningiomas of the skull base, pituitary gland adenomas and paragangliomas.

Radiosurgery is classically applied as a single-session treatment using dedicated devices like the Gamma Knife, the CyberKnife or the modified linear accelerators (LINACs). There are almost no randomised study data available yet directly comparing the efficacy of the different radiosurgical devices and techniques with each other or with conventionally fractionated treatment.

In current practice small tumours up to 30 mm are often treated with single-fraction stereotactic radiosurgery, whereas the treatment of very large tumours >50 mm is a domain for conventionally fractionated regimen. The Gamma Knife was the first dedicated tool designed for single-fraction radiosurgery. However, since more than a decade, other specialised tools for radiosurgery like the CyberKnife system and specifically adapted LINACs are available. The development of frameless radiosurgery without rigid fixation provides the possibility to apply hypo-fractionated schedules with three or five fractions, which widens the indication for radiosurgery of skull base tumours. These tools opened the possibility also to treat larger tumours of the skull base (>30 mm) and tumours in close proximity to the optic pathway by radiosurgery with ablative doses using hypo-fractionated regimen with three to five fractions.

Editor's Comment
Uwe Spetzger

Stereotactic radiosurgery using the Gamma Knife or CyberKnife made the big step from adjunct radiation therapy to a primary treatment option for tumours of the skull base. Especially in the treatment of acoustic neuromas as well as of tumours invading the cavernous sinus, stereotactic radiosurgery plays an increasing role as primary treatment option. This phenomenon is the result of the good treatment results as well as of the acceptance by patients who more and more prefer radiosurgery since they consider an incision and craniotomy as much more invasive than radiosurgery.

Stereotactic radiosurgery in skull base tumours is underrepresented in neurosurgical training and will gain an importance with networking and integration of neurosurgeons in such highly specialised treatment centres. The interdisciplinary and corporate treatment planning as well as the specific consideration and decision algorithm for microsurgery or primary radiosurgery requires adequate expertise and should be made with consensus since this optimises the quality of treatment for the patient. This structure was proven of value during my training and work at the Department of Neurosurgery of RWTH Aachen University with the local Gamma Knife Centre, and I experience this nowadays with the CyberKnife Centre Southwest in Göppingen as an optimum constellation for innovative treatment of complex skull base lesions.

3.2.1 Principles and Methods of Radiosurgery

The Biological Basis of Radiosurgery

In conventional radiotherapy the treated volume is manifold larger than the gross volume of the tumour. Set-up errors, patient movements and tumour movements relative to the patient add spatial uncertainties which demand safety margins of at least 5–10 mm, sometimes more, around the tumour to ensure reliable coverage of the target.

Even in cranial radiotherapy using mask fixation and conformational planning techniques, safety margins of 3–5 mm are not uncommon. Moreover, due to the physics of photon dose distribution and the limited number of beamlets, the lack of conformity to the tumour will additionally increase the volume of healthy tissue within the isodoses that are prescribed to the target.

The need for safety margins and the gradient for dose fall-off beyond the target normally results in a considerable spatial overlap between tumour and dose-limiting normal tissue within the treated volume.

Therefore, to overcome this problem and to widen the therapeutic window, the concept of «conventional fractionation» has introduced into radiation oncology almost 90 years ago.

The term «conventional or normo-fractionation» is related to treatment schedules which distribute the overall dose upon a series of small fractions of 1.8–2 Gy, which are applied five times weekly with a 24-h gap.

The rationale for fractionation relies on biological differences between tumour and dose-limiting normal tissue. In case of cranial irradiation, the dose-limiting normal tissues (DLNT) include vascular structures, grey and white matter, cranial nerves, inner ear and visual pathway including the eyes. These are slow-growing, so-called «late-reacting,» normal tissue cells with intact DNA repair cope and low DNA turnover rates, which cope much better with sublethal ray damage compared to fast-growing tumour cells with a high DNA turnover rate which harbour often a variety of different DNA repair deficits.

Radiobiology has provided various mathematical models to estimate the fractionation sensitivity of different tissue types. The most commonly used in clinical practice is the so-called α-/β-model. The α-/β-value of a certain tissue type reflects the degree of sensitivity to fractionation. In most cases of cancer treatment, the therapeutic target is characterised by fast-growing tumours with high α-/β-values of 6–10 Gy, whereas the dose prescription to this target is mainly limited by late reaction tissues like nerves with low α-/β-values of 2–3 Gy. In such a setting, the therapeutic index, defined as the ratio between local control (LC) and normal tissue complication probability (NTCP), is increased by normo-fractionation. In these situations, fractionation can be considered as a biological strategy to widen the therapeutic window.

However, the situation may be different for the mostly benign tumour entities of the skull base. For instance, for acoustic neuromas (AN) alpha/beta values between 1.77 and 2.4 Gy and for meningiomas alpha/beta values between 3.3 and 3.6 Gy have been estimated. In such a setting, the benefit of fractionation is questionable since there is hardly no difference between the fractionation sensitivity of the tumour and the limiting normal tissues [121].

Target Volume Concepts in Cranial Radiosurgery

The concept of radiosurgery tries to solve the problem by a «physical» strategy. Radiosurgery aims to separate the target volume spatially from the DLNT. To this end set-up errors must be reduced to submillimetre ranges, so that safety margins can be more or less omitted. This requires a highly reliable and reproducible positioning of the patient, often including rigid fixation and/or the possibility of real-time online correction. Moreover, to avoid an overlap of high-dose regions and DLNT, the treatment plans used for radiosurgery must provide a very steep dose fall-off and a high degree of conformity, even when irregular targets are treated.

These are the prerequisites for the application of high single ablative doses. Keeping these challenges in mind, it is not surprising that radiosurgery was initially restricted to the treatment of intracranial targets with limited volumes (e.g. <30 mm diameter). The reasons are easily understandable: Cranial radiosurgery deals with static targets with a rigid spatial relation to the surrounding bony skull. Therefore, the localisation of the skull, which can be identified very precisely by imaging techniques (X-ray and/or computed tomography (CT), can serve as surrogate for the target. The identification of the target during the planning process relies on additional imaging modalities (MRI, angiography, etc.) which are fused to the planning CT scan.

In the pre-image-guidance era when correction of set-up errors by real-time image guidance was not available submillimetre accuracy could only be achieved by rigid fixation by using an invasive stereotactic frame. Rigid fixation is invasive, time consuming and grossly limited to cranial radiotherapy. These constraints were best resolved by using a single dose, thus defining the term radiosurgery as single-fraction stereotactic radiotherapy. In adequately selected patients, radiosurgery provides a variety of advantages compared to conventionally fractionated regimen: Single-fraction radiosurgery is convenient and cost-effective. In addition, single-fraction radiosurgery (or hypo-fractionated) radiosurgery is highly efficient in terms of local control. At least for tumours with low alpha/beta values, the use of SRS may sometimes enable higher biologically equivalent doses (BED) compared to normofractionated regimen. Moreover, high single doses may provide additional biological effects like induction of apoptosis, damage of tumour vasculature, lack of repair and repopulation [121].

The concept of single-fraction radiosurgery was established in the mid-1970s when the Gamma Knife came into clinical practice. More than 10 years later, first attempts have been made to establish this concept also on modified linear accelerators by using rigid frames with invasive fixation. When orthovolt image guidance became available at the end of the 1990s, non-invasive masks were introduced into cranial radiosurgery, but only the combination of real-time image guidance and the possibility of online correction of set-up errors by robotic couches or by robotic radiosurgery systems like the CyberKnife provided a comparable accuracy like invasive fixation. The benefit of these newer system compared to the first to third generation of the Gamma Knife or modified LINACs using invasive frames relies on the flexibility in terms of fractionation. Thus, extremely hypo-fractionated stereotactic radiotherapy/radiosurgery concepts came into practice. With these concepts tumours larger than 30 mm and/or in close proximity to the visual pathway (<3 mm) came into the range of radiosurgery.

Tools for Radiosurgery

Gamma Knife

The Gamma Knife was the first system dedicated to radiosurgery, developed and introduced in the mid-1970s by Lars Leksell. It is the only cobalt-based system still in use for radiosurgery. The initial system underwent various modifications and optimisations. The most up-to-date model is the Leksell Gamma Knife (LGK) Perfexion, which was introduced in 2006; however, the previous model, the LGK 4C, is still widely in use.

The therapeutic gamma ray photons are generated by numerous cobalt sources to produce gamma rays which are collimated and directed to converge precisely at a single point or «isocentre». Accuracy is achieved by eliminating almost any patient movement during treatment by means of a rigid stereotactic head frame. This frame has to be fixed under local anaesthesia. Immediately after fixation computed tomography and/or magnetic resonance imaging is taken for treatment dose planning.

The LGK 4C model includes 201 cobalt sources and collimators arranged in a hemispherical «helmet». Four individual «helmets» with 201 collimators are available to provide beam diameters of 4, 8, 14 or 18 mm each. The LGK 4C has a fixed 40 cm source-to-focal point distance.

The more recent Perfexion model relies on 192 cobalt sources. These cobalt sources are arranged in a cylindrical configuration of five rings. The source-to-focus distance for each ring varies from 37.4 to 43.3 cm. Instead of four different collimator helmets, in the Perfexion model, a single collimator unit is installed which enables the automatic changing of beam sizes between 4, 8 and 16 mm diameters. The advantage of this arrangement lies on the greater flexibility in composite dose distribution shaping, because the beams of different beam diameters can be combined in one treatment session.

In the most recent version, an additional relоca, non-invasive frame is available. In principle, however still time consuming, this device allows also hypo-fractionated therapy on the Gamma Knife. In addition, with this frame also, targeting of more caudal cervical spine locations is feasible. This new frame has a vacuum bite-block, which ensures as demonstrated by a study of the pre-commercial version hypo-fractionation with sub-millimetre displacement.

CyberKnife

The CyberKnife system (Accuray, Sunnyvale, CA, USA) is a non-invasive system designed for both intracranial and extracranial radiosurgery [48] (◘ Figs. 3.9, 3.10, 3.11, and 3.12). It combines a 6 mV, flattening filter-free LINAC mounted on an industrial robot (Kuka, Augsburg, Germany) with an orthogonal X-ray system (amorphous silicon detectors) which enables real-time image guidance with high frequency and tumour tracking during the whole treatment.

The kV X-ray imaging system consists of two cameras in the ceiling directed obliquely towards amorphous silicon detectors integrated into the

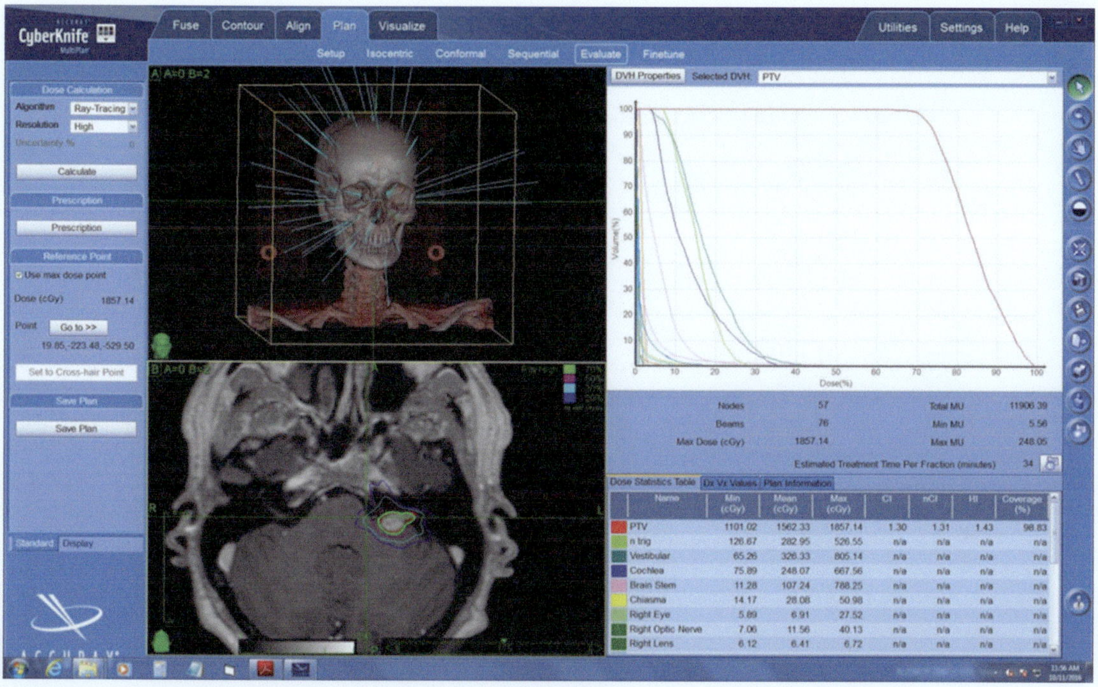

Fig. 3.9 Radiosurgical planning for the treatment of a vestibular schwannoma (©RadioChirurgicum/CyberKnife Südwest)

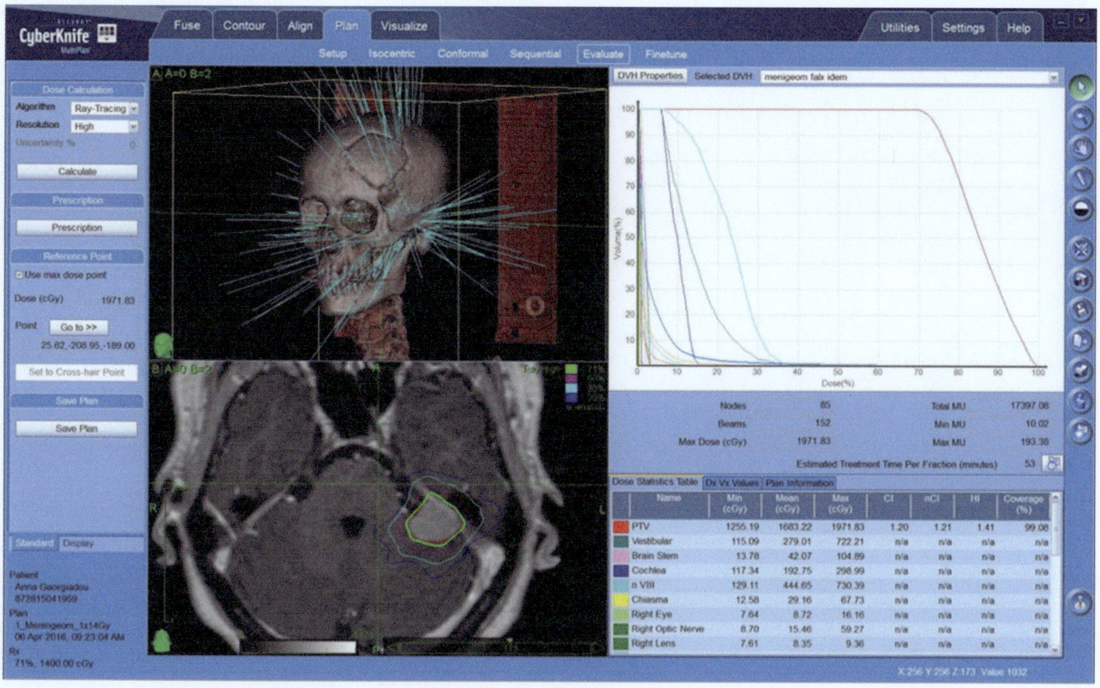

Fig. 3.10 Radiosurgical planning for the treatment of a meningioma (©RadioChirurgicum/CyberKnife Südwest)

3

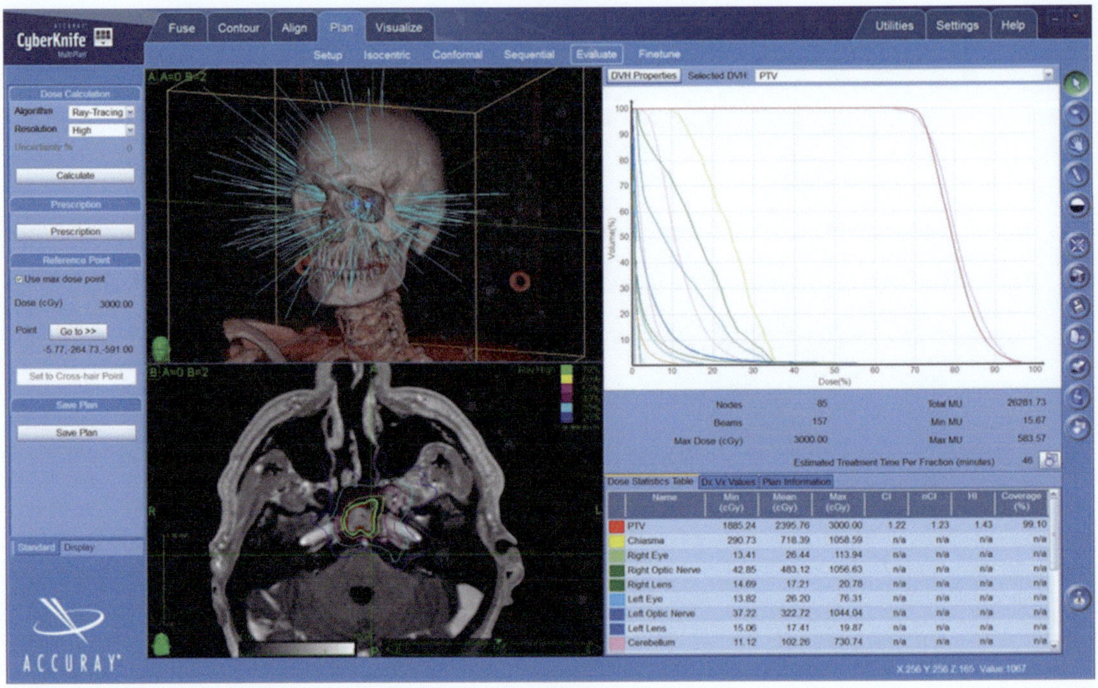

Fig. 3.11 Radiosurgical planning for the treatment of a pituitary adenoma (©RadioChirurgicum/CyberKnife Südwest)

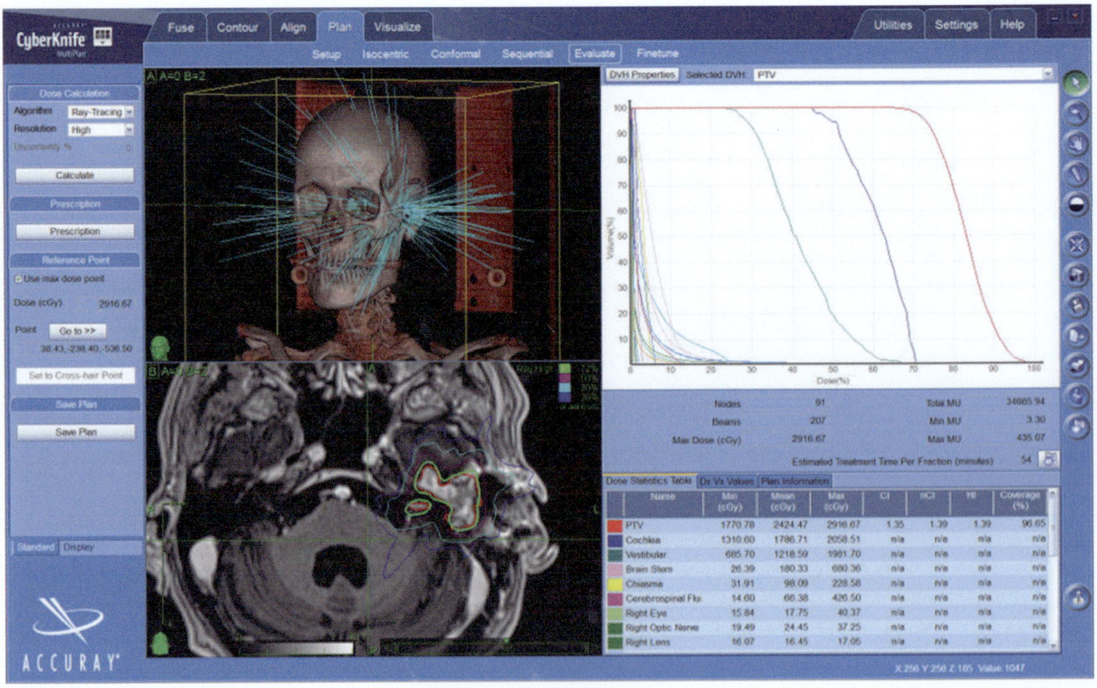

Fig. 3.12 Radiosurgical planning for the treatment of a glomus tumour (©RadioChirurgicum/CyberKnife Südwest)

floor. This imaging system is used for 2D-3D image registration of the live images to a digitally reconstructed radiograph which determines the patient position in near real-time and is used to correct patient motions during treatment.

In cranial radiosurgery a so-called 6D skull algorithm is used which is based on bone correlation between the CT planning DRR and the real-time kV images and automatic real-time set-up correcting throughout the whole treatment by the robot.

The treatment table has 5° of freedom for automatic repositioning, and the robot's arm has 6° of freedom, providing up to 2000 treatment positions with 5–60 mm collimators, a flexible IRUC collimator and – in the most recent version (M6) – a multi-leaf collimator.

A principle design advantage of the CyberKnife system lies in its method of active image guidance during treatment delivery. The system is capable of imaging before every single-treatment beam, although in clinical practice, imaging often can be reduced to intervals of every third to fifth beam or every 15–60 s without losing accuracy. These short imaging intervals in combination with the robot-based online correction of set-up errors achieve a spatial accuracy which is comparable to rigid fixation of the skull. The targeting error of the system lies within a submillimetre range [55].

According to our own experience and the literature, the observed accuracy for intracranial target ranges from 0.2 to 0.3 and even for extracranial target from 0.4.to 0.7 mm [96].

The accuracy of the system is defined by the end-to-end test. This test takes a phantom through the complete treatment planning and delivery process comparing the location of the delivered isodose with the planned dose.

It is often thought that the CyberKnife is a stereotactic system and can only treat small tumours; however, the system is able to treat quite large tumours (up to 2500 cm^3) if they are appropriately planned. Since there is no need for rigid fixation in theory, every kind of fractionation regimen is feasible which is an advantage when larger tumours have to be treated. In theory, every fractionation schedule is applicable, even conventionally fractionated concepts. In the clinical practice, however, the system is used mostly for single-fraction radiosurgery and hypo-fractionated concepts with 3–5 fractions. This is recommendable not only due to economic reasons. Also the normal tissue dose constraints for radiosurgery and hypo-fractionated stereotactic radiotherapy are mainly related to these fractionation schedules [178].

Typical treatment times for cranial radiosurgery are about 20–50 min for each fraction. In contrast to conventional radiotherapy, the treatment planning is usually non-isocentric, and the dose prescription does not follow the ICRU guidelines (dose prescription to the 95% isodose). The treatment doses are prescribed usually to an isodose line between 65% and 80% of the maximum dose. This strategy is used because the dose fall-off in the range between the 60% and 75% isodose is often steeper than the range between the 90% and 100% isodose.

But in principle, like the fractionation schedule, also the dose prescription is flexible and should be adapted to the clinical situation. In some cases the CyberKnife is used to emulate brachytherapy dose distribution so the prescription isodose is around 50% like in the Gamma Knife, whereas in other clinical situations, when normal tissue is located within the target as in arteriovenous malformations, prescription isodoses of 80% and higher are used to achieve a higher degree of homogeneity.

Linear Accelerators (LINACs) Modified for SRS

At the time when the Gamma Knife was introduced in the mid-1970s, linear accelerators (LINACs) were used for conventional radiotherapy. In the early 1980s, the first reports had been published about LINACs adapted for SRS purposes. Pioneers in this field were the groups of Oswaldo Betti and Federico Colombo [105, 161]. In 1991 the first commercially developed LINAC dedicated to SRS, the Varian 600 SR system, became available. The initial LINAC-based radiosurgery systems were «retrofitted» conventional LINACs with modifications including circular collimator cones with various diameters, monitoring devices for couch motion and an attachment to connect the couch in a rigid manner with a stereotactic head frame. Planning systems were developed to support treatment planning, which is based on the combination of various noncoplanar arcs.

Due to the rigid fixation of the bony skull throughout the treatment, these systems did not depend on image guidance and the possibility of online corrections of patient movements during treatment. Spherical targets within the brain could be treated with such devices with high precision and satisfactory coverage and conformity, but the systems were limited when irregular targets should be covered adequately. They were inconvenient and time consuming and not suitable for multisession or extracranial radiosurgery.

With the development of image guidance based on kV or mV cone-beam CT or additionally installed X-ray systems in combination with high-definition micro-MLCs and forward or inverse treatment planning systems allowing the planning of intensity-modulated radiotherapy (IMRT), the practice of LINAC-based SRS changed.

Whereas the first-generation LINACs for SRS often used a set of fixed collimators, later generations are more flexible due to the addition of multi-leaf collimators which allow targeting of larger and more complexly shaped lesions. Intensity-modulated radiotherapy was developed in 1992. Since then the intensity of the radiation beam was also able to be dynamically changed with the multi-leaf collimators. Therefore, not only the shape but the dose distribution could be better tailored to irregular targets.

The development of image-guided radiation therapy (IGRT) added the possibility of correction of set-up errors immediately before or even during treatment. Imaging can be obtained by many methods, including radiography, fluoroscopy or cone-beam tomography. These images are then correlated with the treatment planning images to correct changes in target location due to patient motion or natural movement of the target.

With the introduction of image guidance, invasive frame-based fixation was mostly substituted by thermoplastic relocatable masks. The planning as well as the treatment process became much faster and much more convenient for both, staff and patient.

However, since thermoplastic masks allow some motion relative to the system and many devices for image guidance are not able to provide a high-frequency real-time online control throughout the whole treatment, the price for this gain could be a loss of a little bit of accuracy. Thus, many LINAC-based systems add 1 up to 2 mm safety margins to the clinical target volume to compensate inaccuracy.

To ensure precise positioning comparable to invasive systems, more sophisticated masks with bite-block systems have been developed to overcome this problem, but they are not widely used for LINAC-based SRS.

Currently various commercial systems, both dedicated devices for SRS use, and devices that can deliver both conventional radiotherapy and SRS, are available (▫ Tables 3.1 and 3.2). Whereas the Gamma Knife depends on rays generated by

▫ **Table 3.1** A comparison of conceptual differences between radiosurgery and conventionally fractionated radiotherapy

Radiosurgery (single session)	Conventional fractionated RT
1-day outpatient procedure	25–28 fractions, 5 times weekly
Requirement of rigid frame or dedicated online imaging and correction	Non-invasive relocatable frame
No additional margins to correct for set-up errors	1–3 mm margins to correct for set-up errors
Limited to smaller tumours (e.g. <30 mm)	Ability to treat larger tumours with signs of compression
No improvement of therapeutic ratio with fractionation in slow-growing tumours with low alpha/beta values	Improvement of therapeutic ratio with fractionation in fast-growing tumours with high alpha/beta values
Growth rate/repopulation does not matter	Growth rate/repopulation matters
Lack of reoxygenation in apparently hypoxic (malignant) tumours	Reoxygenation
Lethal DNA damage; additional death pathways (e.g. apoptosis) triggered by high single doses	Additive sublethal DNA damage
Damage of vasculature	Apparently no effects on tumour vasculature

Table 3.2 Characteristics of various SRS systems

System	Source or radiation	Patient immobilisation	Extracranial radiosurgery	Fractionation	Collimators	Image guidance
Gamma Knife 4C	1.25 mV Co60 (*N* = 201)	Invasive frame	No	No	4,8,14,18 mm	No
Gamma Knife Perfexion	1.25 mV Co60 (*N* = 192)	Invasive frame or relocatable non-invasive frame	Caudal cervical spine only	Possible	4,8,16 mm	No
CyberKnife	6 mV LINAC	Frameless	Yes	Yes	5–60 mm	Orthogonal kV X-ray
Novalis	6 mV LINAC	Frameless	Yes	Yes	3 mm MLC	Orthogonal kV X-ray + infrared cameras
Novalis TX	6/15 mV LINAC	Frameless	Yes	Yes	2.5 mm MLC	Orthogonal kV X-ray kV CBCT
Synergy S	6 mV LINAC	Frameless	Yes	Yes	4 mm MLC	kV X-ray + kV CBCT
Trilogy	6 mV LINAC	Frameless	Yes	Yes	5 mm MLC	kV X-ray + kV CBCT
Artiste	6/18 mV LINAC	Frameless	Yes	Yes	5 mm MLC	kV + mV CBCT
Tomo-Therapy	6 mV LINAC	Frameless	Yes	Yes	6.25 mm MLC	mV CT

cobalt decay (1.17 and 1.33 mV), the X-rays produced by LINACs are over a range of energies which are usually higher (4–6 mV).

In general, the LINAC gantry rotates around the patient on a fixed arch. When noncoplanar beam ankles shall be added, the patient couch has to be rotated in the horizontal plane. The intersecting noncoplanar arches deliver a high dose to an isocentric target similar in concept to the intersecting beams produced by the Gamma Knife, but the number of beams is usually lower when static beams are used.

One of the first commercial LINAC-SRS systems was the Novalis (BrainLab, Heimstetten, Germany). BrainLab added an automated tertiary micro-multi-leaf collimator with leaf widths of 3, 4.5 and 5.5 mm for the Varian 600SR and renamed it the Novalis shaped beam radiosurgery unit. The Novalis system is based on a 6 mV LINAC. Image guidance is performed with two infrared cameras and kilovoltage X-rays.

Newer LINAC-based SRS systems include CT-IGRT like Varian Novalis TX (Varian, BrainLab, Palo Alto, CA, USA), Trilogy (Varian), Siemens Artiste (Siemens OCS, Concord, CA, USA) and TomoTherapy Hi-ART (TomoTherapy, Inc., Madison, WI, USA).

The Elekta Synergy (Elekta, Stockholm, Sweden) system was the first one to incorporate cone-beam CT for image guidance for SRS. It uses a kilovoltage cone-beam CT (CBCT) imaging system perpendicular to the treatment beam and a flat-panel detector. The Synergy also has a 4 mm micro-multi-collimator. Its imaging is capable of radiography and fluoroscopy in addition to CBCT. The advantage of CBCT is that a 3D volumetric imaging can be acquired with a single rotation of the gantry.

The Novalis TX differs from other devices due to its high-definition multi-leaf collimator with the smallest leafs with 2.5 mm width. Moreover, it also can deliver radiation in three energy modes: 6 mV photon energy, 15 mV photon energy and 6 mV photon energy with a 1000 MU/min dose rate.

The Novalis TX and the Varian Trilogy have hybrid systems with both kV orthogonal X-ray imaging and CBCT. The TomoTherapy Hi-ART has high-energy mV single-slice CT image guidance. The Siemens Artiste has both kV and mV imaging capabilities. mV imaging has some advantages when high-density surgical hardware has been implanted, but usually this is relevant in some cases of body SRS but not for cranial SRS.

Technical Issues of Radiosurgery for Skull Base Tumours: Treatment Planning, Imaging and Definition of the Target Volume

In the pre-MRI era, target volume definition relied solely on contrast-enhanced high-resolution CT scans of the skull base. Since MRT has been available, the delineation of the target and the organs at risk (OAR) should be based on high-resolution 3D MRI scans that are fused to a planning CT.

All patients are initially fitted with a fixation system, either a rigid frame or a relocatable mask to ensure consistent correct positioning throughout the whole radiological imaging, planning and treatment process. Patients then undergo contrast-enhanced axial computerised tomography.

Prior to delineation of the target and the organs at risk additional imaging is fused with the planning CT. The target volume definition should be based on a high-resolution MRI 3D data set with 0.75–1.5 mm slice thickness including post-contrast T1, T2 and T2-CISS sequences. Brainstem, ipsilateral trigeminal and facial nerve, cochlea and vestibular organ, brain, optic pathway, eyes including the eye lens and pituitary gland should be delineated as organs of risk.

Target planning is usually accomplished by combining pretreatment MR and CT imaging. In tumours with involvement of osseous structures as it is the case in some meningioma, it may be helpful to adjust the treatment planning CT to visualise the bone. In vestibular schwannomas the internal auditory canal can be used as landmark for an exact definition of the intracanalicular part of the tumour. Therefore, also in this case, planning CT should be adjusted to visualise the bone. In addition, the cochlea is better defined when the CT is set for bone visualisation and to be used as a landmark for the quality of image fusion.

Neuromas and meningiomas are best seen on MRI with contrast. But for selected basal tumours, fat suppression imaging may be helpful. For radiosurgery of meningiomas, the limitation of the treated volume is crucial. Therefore, in contrast to fractionated radiotherapy usually only small parts of the dural tail in close proximity of the tumour are included into the GTV. Interestingly, recurrences in the penumbra of the «dural tail» are uncommon [58]. This may be explained by the fact that biopsies of dural tail tissue at resection often show only hyperemic dura and not tumour.

A gross tumour volume (GTV) is defined by integration of all imaging modalities. Due to the set-up error of the different devices for SRS, an additional margin of 0–2 mm has to be added to create the planning target volume (PTV).

Brainstem, ipsilateral trigeminal and facial nerve, cochlea and vestibular organ, brain, optic pathway, eyes including the eye lens and pituitary gland should be delineated as organs of risk.

A maximum tolerable dose is assigned to the principal critical structures based on the volume of the tumour and history of previous radiation treatment. The primary goal of planning for acoustic neuroma radiosurgery is to deliver a sufficient radiosurgical dose to the target volume that conforms closely to the surface of the tumour and spares thereby the adjacent neural structures.

During the individual planning process trade-offs have to be considered between the various organs at risk, e.g. the cochlea, the brainstem and the facial and trigeminal nerve. The evaluation of the plan is based on an analysis of the volumetric dose, including dose-volume histogram analyses of the target volume and critical normal structures.

3.2.2 Vestibular Schwannoma and Schwannomas of Other Cranial Nerves

Introduction

Vestibular schwannomas, also termed acoustic neuromas, are benign tumours of Schwann cell origin. They count for 5–10% of all intracranial tumours; however, they represent 80–90% of tumours of the cerebellopontine angle. Mostly they occur unilateral. Bilateral tumours are hallmarks of neurofibromatosis type 2 (NF-2). The estimated incidence of vestibular schwannomas is 2 per 100,000 person-years, and the prevalence is currently approximately 2 in 10,000 people [145].

Some authors report about an increasing incidence of diagnosed vestibular schwannomas over recent years, but it is unclear whether this simply reflects the increasingly used modern sensitive MRI imaging techniques for patients with respective symptoms and due to other reasons.

The overall prognosis of the disease is good in terms of survival. With the availability of modern techniques for early diagnosis, monitoring and treatment, vestibular schwannomas are usually not live limiting; however, they may have a significant impact on quality of life (QoL) due to hearing loss, tinnitus and dizziness.

The primary goal of treatment is local tumour control; however, secondary goals like the preservation of hearing, release of disease-related symptoms, QoL after treatment and treatment-related adverse effect are additional parameters which must be taken into account for treatment decision making.

Currently there is no international consensus and no high-level evidence in the literature about the appropriate treatment strategy. Management options include observation, microsurgical resection and stereotactic radiosurgery. Moreover, further reports in the literature describe the use of hypo-fractionated radiosurgery or conventionally fractionated conformal radiotherapy. The data about fractionated radiotherapy are sparse, and the published trials altogether encompass a very limited number of patients compared to the number of patients treated with microsurgical resection or single-fraction radiosurgery worldwide [108, 128]. Any randomised data comparing the different strategies to each other are still lacking [145].

Since many of these tumours grow slowly over years or may not grow at all for a period of time, not only the choice of the treatment strategy but also the optimal time point for treatment is a matter of debate. In elderly patients with asymptomatic or minimal symptoms and in selected patients with bilateral NF-2 tumours, observation may be an appropriate strategy, but in most cases, early therapeutic intervention appears to be the best strategy to preserve functional hearing [51].

Surgery appears to be the treatment of choice for very large tumours (>30 mm) with brainstem compression and/or obstructive hydrocephalus. For small to intermediate tumours, stereotactic radiosurgery provides similar tumour control rates of more than 90% compared to microsurgical resection [144]. There may be a trend for better preservation of hearing in patients treated with radiosurgery, but this statement should be made with caution since the hearing preservation rates differ between different surgical approaches, and currently we have no data available which addressed this issue in a randomised trial.

Results of Radiosurgery of Vestibular Schwannoma: Local Control, Functional Outcome and Adverse Effects

The use of stereotactic single-session radiosurgery for vestibular schwannomas was first described by Lars Leksell [125]. Since then this technique with some modifications has been increasingly used as an alternative to microsurgical resection in patients with small and moderate size tumours [94, 114, 144]. Currently there is a common consensus that tumours up to 3 cm in diameter when including the internal auditory canal in the measurement can be successfully controlled in the majority of patients with single-fraction RS. The largest body of evidence for single-session RS comes from Gamma Knife radiosurgery. Currently more than 80,000 patients have been treated worldwide since the introduction of the technique in the 1970s. When the technique was established at the Karolinska Institute, few initial patients were treated with very high doses of 25–35 Gy. Since short-term local control was good but post-treatment hearing loss was reported in the majority of these patients, the prescribed doses were

3

Table 3.3 Early SRS trial for VS using higher single doses[a]

Author	Median FU (months)	Patients (N)	Marginal dose (Gy)	Prescription isodose (%)	Local control (%)	CN V preservation (%)	CN VI preservation (%)	Useful hearing preservation (%)
Leksell 1971 [125]	44.4	160	18–25	NA	81	82	86	20
Flickinger 1993 [79]	24	134	17 (median)	50	89.2	67.1	71	35
Foote 1995 [80]	16	36	16–20	50	100	41.4	33.5	41
Mendenhall 1994 [134]	>12	56	10–22.5	80	95	>78	>78	NA
Kondziolka 1998 [118]	>60	162	16.6 (median)	50	98	73	73	51
Suh 2000 [177]	49	29	8–24; 16 (median)	80	94	85	68	26

[a]All trials Gamma Knife, except Mendenhall and Suh (modified LINAC)
Modified according to Murphy et al. [143]

stepwise reduced. Early Gamma Knife and LINAC trials including patients treated in the 1980s used doses of about 14–18 Gy which are still higher than those used in current concepts (see Table 3.3). This must be taken into account when clinical results are analysed and compared to each other. For instance, Kondziolka and associates treated 162 consecutive patients in the years between 1987 and 1992 with a mean transverse tumour diameter of 2.2 cm and an average dose to the tumour margins of 16 Gy.

The follow-up included patients between 5 and 10 years after radiosurgery. Tumour control defined as failure of progression requiring surgery was excellent at 98%. However, the functional outcome was still not satisfying. They reported about comparably high rates of post radiosurgery cranial neuropathies involving the facial of the trigeminal nerve of more than 20% and a drop of 67% in their Gardner-Robertson hearing level [118].

In the 1990s radiosurgery came down to single doses of 12–13 Gy, usually prescribed to the 50% isodose levels in case of Gamma Knife treatment or to the 80 up to 90% isodose in cases of LINAC-based radiosurgery. Imaging and planning quality was also improved, and the planning for schwannomas became more and more conformal. The results published by the University of Pittsburgh may serve as an example for what can be achieved by «up-to-date» radiosurgery of vestibular schwannomas: About 313 patients were treated in Pittsburgh with radiosurgery single doses of 12–13 Gy in the years between 1991 and 2001. The actuarial clinical tumour control rate of these patients was 98.6% after 7 years with unchanged rates of facial strength, facial sensation, stable hearing levels and useful hearing preservation rates after 7 years of 100%, 95,6%, 70.3% and 78,6%, respectively. These excellent results were reproduced by other groups like [99, 100, 142]. In the year 2011, Murphy et al. [143] reviewed present studies of SRS for VS; both concepts form the «high-dose» and the «low-dose» era [144]. They included 13 trials ($N = 10$ trials with 1324 patients based on the Gamma Knife; $N = 3$ trails with 340 patients based on dedicated LINAC systems) with modern dose concepts. They found progression-free survival rates of 91% up to 100% when doses of 12–13 Gy are prescribed to the PTV (50–80% ID) (see Table 3.4).

Table 3.4 Long-term results of SRS trials for VS using lower single doses[a]

Author	Median FU (years)	Patients (N)	Marginal dose (Gy) (median)	Local control (%)	CN V preservation (%)	CN VI preservation (%)	Useful hearing preservation (%)
Prasad 2000 [160]	4.27	153	13	92	98.3	98.4	58
Unger 2002 [180]	6.3	100	13	96	100	98	55
Chopra 2007 [67]	5.7	216	13	98.3	94.9	100	44
Hasagawa 2005 [93]	>5	317	13.2	93	96/98 (>/<13Gy)	94/99 (>/<13Gy)	13/68 (>/<13Gy)
Myrseth 2005 [146]	>3–4	103	12.2	93	NA	94.8	32
Kim 2007 [115]	6	59	12	97	100	98.3	33.3
Iwai 2008 [99]	7.4	25	12	100	100	100	64
Niranjan 2008 [149]	3.5	96	13	99	100	100	64.5
Fukuoka 2009 [83]	>5	152	12	94	97.4	100	71
Murphy 2010 [143]	3.6	103	13	91.1	99	95	NA
Coombs 2006 [69]	9	26	13	91.1	92	95	55
Friedman 2006 [81]	3.3	296	12.5	99	99.3	99.3	NA
Kalogeridi 2009 [111]	4.6	19	11–12	100	100	100	NA

[a]Modified according to Murphy and Suh [144]

The preservation of functional hearing was in the range of 44–71% when doses ≤13 Gy are used. Not only functional hearing was much better than in the older trials but also the neuropathy rates came down to below 5%. Facial nerve preservation was in a range of 95% up to 100%, and also much lower rates of trigeminal neuropathy of between 0% and 8% were observed in these trials [92, 114, 144]. These favourable functional results were confirmed by two large meta-analyses: A review of 23 articles representing 2204 patients revealed an overall facial nerve preservation rate of 96.2% after Gamma Knife radiosurgery [189], and a review of 45 articles representing 4234 patients showed an overall hearing preservation rate of 51% [190].

After the introduction of the CyberKnife® by John Adler in 1997, a further device dedicated for radiosurgery was available which provides comparable accuracy and quality of treatment plan for brain tumours compared to the Gamma Knife [187].

Since then the CyberKnife is increasingly used for single-session radiosurgery of vestibular schwannoma [74], the dose concepts were comparable to Gamma Knife treatment; however, CyberKnife normally uses prescription isodoses between 65% and 75%. The group of Wowra which collected experience with both techniques analysed in detail a cohort of 386 patients treated between 1995 and 2008, 257 of them with the Gamma Knife and 159 with the CyberKnife. The patient characteristics as well as the treatment parameters showed no significant difference between both groups with the exception of the prescription isodoses that were 53.5 (52.7–54.3) Gy for the GK patients and 68.2 (67.5–68.9) CyberKnife. They achieved comparable good results in terms of local control and functional outcome which were in the line of the Pittsburgh data described above.

Tsai et al. [179] also reported excellent tumour control rates of 99.1% with a mean imaging follow-up of 61.1 months using the CyberKnife technique. In their cohort 81.5% of the patients' initial hearing according to the Gardener-Robertson scale I–II maintained GR I or II hearing after CK, with a mean audiometric follow-up of 64.5 months.

In contrast to the first-generation Gamma Knifes, CyberKnife radiosurgery is frameless and does not need rigid fixation. Therefore, hypofractionated regimens are also feasible. This has been evaluated by various groups either to treat larger tumours greater than 25 or 30 mm of maximum diameter or to improve the rates of serviceable hearing.

Three to five fraction schedules with doses of 3 × 6–7 Gy or 5 × 4–5 Gy have been evaluated. The Stanford group introduced a three-fraction schedule and reported comparable high rates of local control (98%) as in single-session RS with a very good functional outcome. No trigeminal dysfunction was observed, and only two patients showed a transient facial palsy. Of the 63 patients under evaluation, 74% presented with serviceable hearing (GR class I–II) after a mean follow-up of 48 months [62]. Other groups have also reported about the efficacy and feasibility of hypofractionated regimen. With regard to hearing, the results are inconsistent. The rate of hearing preservation was in the range of other published data, but currently there is no clear indication that hypo-fractionation will improve the functional outcome compared to modern single-session concepts [112, 140, 183].

A small series of patients treated with the Gamma Knife either with one session (mean dose 12.6 Gy) or with three sessions (overall dose of 18 Gy) showed no significant differences between both schedules [114]. However especially the Vincenza group demonstrated that hypofractionation may be a way to treat patients safely with large VS which are poor candidates for surgery [59].

The aetiology of hearing loss after radiotherapy is a matter of debate. The posttreatment hearing function is a multiparametric issue which is influenced by both treatment- and patient-related factors. Patients with a Gardener-Robertson (GR) hearing class of I or II definitively have a better prognosis than patients with pretreatment GR scales of III or IV. Maybe even more relevant, it has been demonstrated that patients with a pretreatment speech discrimination score (SDS) of >70% were 11.1 times more likely to maintain serviceable hearing following SRS compared to patients with an SDS <70%.

With regard to treatment-related factors, the mean cochlea dose is considered to be the most meaningful parameter. Recently, a meta-analysis of hearing preservation after radiosurgery for vestibular schwannomas has been published in two articles including nearly 6000 patients. A 57% preservation rate of serviceable hearing was reported. Amazingly, patient age and tumour size had no significant effect on hearing preservation, but radiation dose did matter.

In this regard, the question arises in which way mean cochlea dose and the dose prescribed to the target are correlating. It is important to keep in mind that the mean cochlea dose is of course correlated to the dose prescribed to the target, but this relation is strongly influenced by other cofounding factors like the size of the target, its extension with the internal auditory canal and the quantity of the plan, its gradient index in direction to the cochlea and the conformity of the plan. It is not clear yet whether size and location of the tumour or the prescribed overall dose are independent factors which are relevant for hearing preservation or if they are just co-factors which have an impact on the mean cochlear dose. It cannot be ruled out that also the maximum on the cochlear nerve of its DVH will have an addition impact on hearing, an issue, which has been poorly evaluated yet.

Nevertheless, there are various reports which demonstrate that a mean cochlear dose higher than 3.0 up to 4.2 Gy (depending on the threshold for discrimination chosen by the respective study) and a maximum cochlear dose higher than 6.9 Gy were significantly associated with post-SRS hearing worsening. An analysis by Baschnagel et al. [54] reported about a very favourable rate of 2-year serviceable hearing preservation rate of 90% in the subgroup of patients who received a mean cochlea dose of 3 Gy. Therefore, it is our policy is to keep the maximum dose to the cochlea under 7.0 Gy and the mean dose under 3.0 of 4.0 Gy whenever possible.

A matter of concern has been the possible induction of malignancy in vestibular schwannomas after radiosurgery [167]. However, the causal role of radiation is still not quite clear. In fact, few case reports have been published about malignant transformation of VS after radiosurgery. Seferis et al. [167] recently described a new case of verified induction of malignant peripheral nerve sheath tumour (MPNST) in a vestibular schwannoma. This patient is currently the 26th reported case of verified malignant transformation after radiation.

However, most of the cases were patients with NF-2, which has an inherent enhanced risk for malignant transformation to MPNSTs. More important, additional 20 cases of malignant transformation of VS have been reported yet in patients who had not been irradiated before. Seferis et al. [167] concluded that despite recent reports of malignant transformation in vestibular schwannomas after radiation, only in NF-2 cases the incidence of malignancies appears to be notable in relation to the number of patients treated. Even in this group malignant transformation is rare event.

The overall risk appears to be small in the region of 0.01–0.02%. At least in patients which are no candidates for watch and wait strategies, this risk has to be counterbalanced with a reported mortality rate after craniotomies of about 1% [167].

Posttreatment Follow-Up

Clinical Evaluation

During the first 2 years after radiosurgery, ENT and neurological examination and audiograms are performed every 6 months. After the first 2 years, audiograms are obtained annually, after 4 years and depending on the clinic, every 2 years. Speech discrimination, speech reception threshold and pure tone averages should be evaluated from each audiogram. Whenever possible, patients should obtain audiograms at the same facility to minimise errors in technique. Physical examination along these intervals includes neurological examination and testing of the fifth, seventh and eighth cranial nerves.

Radiological Evaluation

The radiological follow-up should follow the same schedule. For the first 2 years after radiosurgery, gadolinium-enhanced MRI scans be should performed every 6 months, in the third and fourth years after initial treatment every 12 months and thereafter in patients without new symptoms every 2 years. Tumour size is measured in three orthogonal dimensions on each follow-up. MRI scans are compared with the previous measurements and the MRI scan used for planning.

Currently there is no consensus about the appropriate length of follow- up. Most of the data regarding local control report about 5- or 10-year local control rates. Some groups advocate a 10-year period of follow-up; some performed after an 8-year follow-up period another MRI 16 years after initial treatment.

Very few reports focus on long follow-up intervals. One series analysed changes in MRI and clinical status in a period of more than 10 years after the initial treatment in 80 patients with unilateral vestibular schwannomas. Tumour progression after 10 years was an infrequent; however, surgical removal was necessary in 3.8% (3/80) at 143, 151 and 167 months. Of notice, no new cranial nerve symptom without tumour growth and no malignant transformation of the tumour were observed more than 10 years after SRS [147].

Conclusions and Implications for Practice

Stereotactic radiotherapy is increasingly used in the management of patients with small to intermediate size vestibular schwannomas. With modern dose concepts and treatment techniques, it is an effective technique providing high rates of local control, comparable to the control rates which can be achieved by microsurgical resection. In addition, the functional outcome is satisfactory with preservation rates of functional hearing of between 50% and 70%, whereas facial nerve palsy and trigeminal dysfunction occur in only 1% up to 5% of the patients.

Since hearing preservation is better with early intervention, watchful waiting strategies should be restricted to elderly patients without or with minimal symptoms.

Until now, there are no randomised studies available which compare various treatment strategies to each other. Therefore, the choice of the treatment modality should be made on an individual basis taking into consideration the patient's preferences, medical history and individual disease-related parameters.

Surgical resection should be preferred in large tumours >30 m and/or in tumours with acute signs of compression as well as in patients who present with severe dizziness as the leading symptom. Hypo-fractionated radiosurgery of conventionally fractionated radiotherapy may be options for patients with large tumours and contraindication for surgery, but the optimal fractionation regimen still needs to be evaluated.

3.2.3 Skull Base Meningiomas

Introduction

Microsurgery is still the mainstay for the treatment of meningiomas. However, in the recent years, there has been a shift away from aggressive surgical approaches aimed to remove the tumour completely if ever possible to treatment strategies with lower invasiveness providing better functional outcomes. Nowadays there is a major emphasis on the patient's quality of life and the avoidance of postoperative neurological deficits. Particularly in critical anatomical regions like the skull base, the cavernous sinus and the petroclival region, complete surgical removal of meningiomas is not feasible or can be associated with severe postoperative neurological deficits. Since incompletely resected skull base meningioma carries a significant risk for symptomatic recurrences, primary radiosurgery or combined approaches including tumour debulking and postoperative radiosurgery are increasingly used. Long-term follow-up studies have demonstrated that radiosurgery has an important role in completing microsurgery in these cases by providing postoperative long-term tumour control.

Pretreatment Patient Evaluation

The indication for treatment should be based on up-to date magnetic resonance imaging and a throughout clinical evaluation. CT is helpful in cases of infiltration of osseous structures. The extension of the tumour and its spatial relation to critical skull base structures, namely, the optic pathway, have to be determined in three dimensions. Prior to treatment, clinical evaluation of the cranial nerves and a comprehensive physical and neurological examination have to be done. In meningiomas adjacent to the optic pathway and the pituitary gland, additional pretreatment ophthalmological and endocrinological evaluation of the pituitary axes is mandatory. Trigeminal nerve function is graded on a semi-quantitative scale as normal sensation, decreased sensation or no sensation. Facial nerve function can be graded on the House-Brackmann scale.

Results of Radiosurgery: Local Control, Functional Outcome and Adverse Effects

To date, however, no formal randomised study comparing surgical resection with radiotherapy or radiosurgery with other forms of radiotherapy techniques has been published. Nevertheless, single-session radiosurgery has become a generally accepted technique for managing a small inaccessible benign skull base meningioma (WHO grade I and II) [50, 63, 64, 70, 71, 82, 119, 120].

For radiosurgery local control rates of 92–100% have been reported when single doses between 12 and 16 Gy for grade I meningiomas and between 14 and 20 Gy for grade II prescribed to the 50 or 70% isodose are applied. The overall toxicity and especially the toxicity to the cranial nerves are commonly kept below 5% when modern techniques and dose concepts are used which respect the dose constraints for cranial nerves and brain tissue. Even for meningiomas at the cerebellopontine angle, facial nerve morbidity is an infrequent event. Especially for parasellar meningiomas, the tolerance of the optic pathway is one of the most critical issues. Maximum point doses should be kept below 10 Gy (single fraction) to optic pathway structures in patients without pretreatment. Other cranial nerves obviously tolerate slightly to moderately higher single doses [141].

These satisfactory results reported from various single institutions are in accordance with the largest corpus of date regarding radiosurgery of meningiomas published in 2012. A retrospective multicentre observational analysis included 4565 consecutive patients harbouring 5300 benign meningiomas. All patients were treated with single-fraction radiosurgery with a median prescription dose of 14 Gy. The median tumour volume was 4.8 cm^3, and the median imaging follow-up 63 months. After exclusion of the patients with an imaging follow-up of less than 24 months, 3768 remaining meningiomas (71%) were available for evaluation [165].

The overall tumour control rate was 92.5% defined by no change or shrinkage of the tumour. In 58% of all cases, the volume of treated tumour tissue decreased and remained unchanged in 34.5%. The reported 5- and 10-year progression-free survival rates were 95.2% and 88.6%, respectively.

Favourable prognostic factors for local control were grade I histology, female sex, sporadic meningioma and skull base location. The permanent morbidity rate was 6.6% at the last follow-up. This study also identified prognostic factors for adverse effects. Patients with peritumoural oedema being present prior to treatment had a 4.58 higher risk for an aggravation of the oedema. In the group of meningiomas without initial peritumoural swelling, an oedema occurred only in 13.1%.

Low-grade meningiomas have a very slow growth rate. Therefore, long-term follow-up data are crucial for a realistic estimation of local efficacy of radiosurgery. Since the Gamma Knife was historically the first tool used for routine cranial radiosurgery, most long-term data rely on this technique. A trial published by a British group has reported about the clinical outcome of 86 patients with a median follow-up period of 10 years. This study documented a persistent high local tumour control even after more than 10 years after treatment [165]. The local control rate was 87.8% for those patients and thereby only slightly lower than in other published observations with shorter follow-up. Those patients who received a dose below the median prescription dose of 13.4 Gy exhibited significantly higher rates of local recurrences than the group treated with less than 13.4 Gy (7.1% vs. 24%, $p = 0.0096$). The median time between initial treatment and recurrence was 5.8 years in this trial which is in accordance to the observations from other groups. Of note, out of field recurrences were documented in this cohort at a median of 7.5 years in 15.1% of patients.

The low rate of late progression after radiosurgery is confirmed by the data of Pollock et al. [158]. They monitored the outcome after radiosurgery in some patients for even more than 20 years. The median treatment volume was 6.1 cm^3 (range 0.3–35.4 cm^3); the mean tumour margin dose was 16.0 Gy (range 12–20 Gy). In a cohort of 255 patients treated between 1990 and 2008, the tumour size decreased in 181 patients (72.1%) and was unchanged in 67 patients (26.7%). Only three patients (1.2%) had in-field tumour progression at 28, 145 and 150 months, respectively. The 1- and 5-year complication rates in these cases were 8.3% and 11.5%, respectively. The radiation-related adverse effects were associated with convexity/falx tumours, but not in the skull base region, and increased with tumour volume on multivariate analysis.

Not only tumours of higher volume (e.g. >10–12 cm or larger than 30 mm in diameter) but also tumours in close proximity to the optic pathway are a particular challenge for radiosurgery. It is widely acknowledged that the radiation sensitivity of the normal optic apparatus precludes single-session radiosurgery when the lesion is within 2 mm of the anterior visual pathways. In such cases, tumour debulking prior to radiosurgery may be a feasible strategy. Non-radical surgery reduces tumour volume and may create larger distances between the target volume and the visual pathway thereby providing favourable conditions for consolidating radiosurgery [88].

Since frameless and especially robotic-guided systems have been introduced, not only single-session radiosurgery but also hypo-fractionated radiosurgery concepts have become feasible. Regimen with three up to five sessions may be an alternative for intermediate size meningiomas or tumours in the vicinity of the optic pathway.

One of these first reported experiences regarding hypo-fractionated radiosurgery for skull base tumours came from John Adler and colleges from Stanford [49]. Forty-nine consecutive patients had skull base tumours closer than 2 mm to the optic pathway, whereas 27 of these patients had meningiomas. All were treated with multisession robotic-guided radiosurgery of two to five sessions to a cumulative average marginal dose of 20.3 Gy. The average tumour volume was 7.7 cm^3. Although a significant part of the patients was pretreated (39 had previous subtotal surgical resection and 6 had even previously been treated with conventional fractionated radiotherapy), the outcome regarding preservation of vision was very satisfactory: After a mean visual field follow-up of 49 months (range 6–96 months), vision was unchanged after radiosurgery in 38 patients, improved in 8 (16%) and worsened only in three (6%). The concept was not only feasible; after a mean imaging follow-up period of 46 months, the tumour volume was stable or smaller in all other cases.

Since the latest-generation Gamma Knife also allows multisession stereotactic treatment, however less convenient, there are some experiences with hypo-fractionation in Gamma Knife radiosurgery. Han et al. [91] reported about 42 patients with larger meningiomas (median tumour volume 15.2 ml, range 2.1–53.2 ml) who received median single doses of 6 Gy delivered over a median of 2.7 median sessions and had a median follow-up of 32.8 months. The intermediate time local efficacy was similar compared to single-fraction radiosurgery and to the results of Adler et al. [49] with a local tumour control rate of 97.2%. The tumour volume decreased (>25%) in 22.2%, remained stable in 75% and increased (>25%) in 2.8%.

Losa et al. [131] published a series of 97 patients with meningiomas adjacent to the anterior visual pathway (mean tumour volume 8.28 [0.33–34.2] cm^3, mean follow-up 26.4 months). Gamma Knife radiosurgery was delivered in three sessions with a mean prescription dose of 6.8 Gy per session (range 6–7 Gy) and a mean overall prescription dose of 20.4 Gy (range 18–21 Gy). The maximum dose to the optic apparatus was kept always below 7 Gy for each session. At last follow-up, tumour volume was unchanged in 50.5%, decreased in 47.4% and increased in 3.1%. 35.1% of the patients had an improvement of previous palsies, but 5.4% developed new cranial nerves palsies following treatment. Among the patients with visual deficits prior to treatment, 23.8% had an improvement of vision, while it worsened in 2.4% of these patients.

In summary, single-fraction radiosurgery provides a safe and efficient option for small- to medium-sized irresectable meningiomas of the skull base. Currently single-fraction doses of 13–14 Gy for grade I and 18 Gy for grade II tumours are widely accepted concepts. The introduction of hypo-fractionated concepts with three to five sessions provides further options for larger meningiomas (>8–10 cm^3 or >30 mm in diameter) and/or for tumours in close proximity to the visual pathway. We currently treat such tumours with 3 × 7 or 5 × 5 Gy for grade I and 3 × 8 or 5 × 6 Gy for grade II meningiomas.

Posttreatment Follow-Up

Clinical Evaluation

During the first 2 years after treatment, follow-up intervals of 6 months are recommended. The follow-up should include a throughout clinical neurological examination with special emphasis on cranial nerve function. In tumours adjacent to the optic pathway and/or the pituitary gland, additional visual testing and an endocrinological evaluation of the pituitary axes should be performed.

After the first 2 years depending on the clinical situation, the follow-up intervals can be extended to 1 year. After 4 years two-year intervals may be sufficient in asymptomatic patients.

Radiological Evaluation

The radiological follow-up should follow the same schedule. For the first 2 years after radiosurgery, gadolinium-enhanced MRI scans should be performed every 6 months, in the third and fourth year after initial treatment every 12 months and thereafter in patients without new symptoms every 2 years. Tumour size is measured in three orthogonal dimensions on each follow-up. MRI scans have to be compared with the previous measurements and the MRI scan used for planning.

Currently there is no consensus about the appropriate length of follow- up. Most of the data regarding local control report about 5- or 10-year local control rates. Some groups advocate a 10-year period of follow-up; some others performed after an 8-year follow-up period another MRI 16 years after initial treatment.

As mentioned above, very few reports focus on follow-up intervals longer than 120 months. According to the above cited data by Pollock et al. [158] which showed that long-term recurrences can occur, however infrequently, and due to the fact that meningioma patients exhibit an increased risk of de novo growth of additional out of filed lesions, we recommend longer follow-up intervals but with reduced imaging frequency [164].

Conclusions and Implications for Practice

Radiosurgery proved to be a safe and effective method for treating benign meningiomas in patients who are no good candidates for complete surgical resection. Even in a long-term perspective, the local efficacy is high with control rates of more than 90% in appropriately selected patients.

The rate of severe late adverse effects is acceptable. Cranial nerve palsies as well as symptomatic oedema usually occur in less than 5% of the patients when the appropriate normal tissue constraints are considered. The risk for symptomatic oedema increases when larger tumours (>7–10 cm) are treated, in patients with pre-existing oedema and/or in tumours with hemispheric of midline location.

The introduction of hypo-fractionated regimen with three to five sessions opened an additional window for radiosurgical treatment of tumours which are no ideal candidates for single-fraction radiosurgery due to the tumour volume or the location in close proximity to the visual pathway. Furthermore, radiosurgery is a useful tool in combined concepts as a consolidation treatment after function-preserving non-radical microsurgery.

3.2.4 Pituitary Gland Adenomas

Introduction

Pituitary adenomas can either be classified according to their size into microadenomas (<1 cm) and macroadenomas (>1 cm) and/or functionally according to their clinical presentation, hormone levels and immunohistochemical staining characteristics. The latter classification constitutes two major groups, the so-called nonsecretory (nonfunctioning) and the group of secretory (functioning) adenomas.

The first group does not produce excessive pituitary hormones. While nonsecretory microadenomas are asymptomatic and usually remain undetected, the clinical problems caused by nonsecretory macroadenomas are consequences of tumour mass effects, mainly to the optic pathway and the pituitary gland itself leading to visual disturbances and endocrine deficiencies.

Fifty to sixty percent of all patients with macroadenomas (secretory and nonsecretory) present with visual field abnormalities due to compression of optic nerve structures. Invasion of the cavernous sinus may cause other visual symptoms (ophthalmoplegia, diplopia, ptosis) or facial numbness or pain.

In line with these problems, first-line therapy is the microsurgical resection of the tumours with the goal of surgical decompression of the affected adjacent structures while preserving or restoring normal neurologic and endocrine function.

The group of secretory or functioning adenomas includes the different types of hormonal hypersecretion, including the prolactin-producing tumours (prolactinoma), the growth hormone (GH)-producing adenoma and the adenoma with excessive production of the adrenocorticotrophic hormone (ACTH). These tumours, of course, can also cause problems by mass effects, but in most cases, they are detected earlier because of the clinical consequences of the related endocrinopathies.

Prolactinomas are the most common pituitary adenomas. They account for 45% of pituitary tumours. The clinical consequences of long-lasting hyperprolactinaemia are hypogonadism together with decreased libido and impotence in males as well as amenorrhea, galactorrhoea, infertility and osteoporosis in women.

The first-line treatment for these tumours is based on dopamine agonists such as bromocriptine or cabergoline which normalise the PRL levels in 80–90% with higher success rates in the treatment of microadenomas. The remaining group of 10–20% of patients in whom PRL levels fail to normalise following maximal medical therapy is treated with resection and/or radiosurgery. In addition, local treatment is indicated in those patients who cannot tolerate dopamine agonists due to their side effects.

The excessive production of growth hormone (GH) from pituitary adenomas results in acromegaly in adults, an endocrine disorder characterised by progressive somatic disfigurement or gigantism in children and adolescents. The patients suffer from pituitary gigantism, changes of voice, diabetes mellitus, hypertension, sleep apnoea and cardiomyopathy which lead to increased mortality rates secondary to the systemic effects of chronically elevated GH and its primary mediator insulin-like growth factor-1 (IGF-1).

Surgery was the first treatment available for GH-producing adenomas. The effect of surgery is favourable in GH-producing microadenomas with cure rates of approximately 75–95%, as defined by local tumour control and the normalisation of the hormone hypersecretion. However, due to the insidious nature of the disease, the majority of the patients present with macroadenomas. In those patients the cure rates by surgery alone is in the range of only 40–68%. Surgical debulking can lead to improved medical management, but the majority of these patients are still dependent on somatostatin analogues and GH antagonists for life, which are very costly and may lead to problems due to drug-associated adverse effects and/or suboptimal suppression of growth hormone.

ACTH-secreting pituitary adenomas account for approximately 80% of newly diagnosed cases of Cushing's syndrome (excessive systemic cortisol from any source). Patients with ACTH oversecretion from a pituitary adenoma may present with Cushing's disease or, less frequent, with Nelson's syndrome, depending on the functionality of the adrenal glands. Functional ACTH-staining adenomas represent approximately 14% of all surgically resected pituitary adenomas. The majority of ACTH adenomas are microadenomas that do not cause a substantial degree of mass effect on surrounding structures. In these cases, the primary goal of treatment is the induction of endocrinological remission as defined by normalisation (or preferably subnormal levels) of serum and urine cortisol.

Surgery is still the primary option for most patients with a new diagnosis of Cushing's disease. Especially in patients with microadenomas, transsphenoidal resection is a procedure with excellent outcomes and low surgical risks which provides postoperative hormonal remission rates between 70% and 90% of all patients, depending on tumour size and degree of invasion into surrounding regions.

Nevertheless, the remaining group of patients which do not achieve satisfactory hormonal remission needs further adjunct therapy. Adjunctive treatments following surgical management may include medical therapy, radiosurgery or other radiation-based treatments and/or bilateral adrenalectomy.

Radiosurgery for Cushing's disease is often an adjuvant to surgical resection of ACTH-secreting adenomas which do not achieve remission or in case of tumour recurrences that are observed in up to 30% of cases following initial successful transsphenoidal resection.

Pretreatment Patient Evaluation

Treatment decision should rely on up-to-date magnetic resonance imaging and a throughout neurological and the endocrinological evaluation of the functions of the different pituitary hormonal axes. The indication for radiosurgery is made in an interdisciplinary setting including endocrinologists, neurosurgeons, radiologists and radiotherapists.

The extension of the tumour and its spatial relation to critical skull base structures, namely, the optic pathway, have to be determined in three dimensions. Prior to treatment, clinical evaluation of the cranial nerves and a comprehensive physical neurological examination should be performed. In tumours adjacent to the optic pathway, additional pretreatment ophthalmological examination is mandatory.

Results of Radiosurgery: Local Control, Functional Outcome and Adverse Effects

Nonsecretory Pituitary Adenomas

In patients with nonsecretory macroadenomas, radiosurgery can be performed as a primary treatment, as an alternative to surgery in poor surgical candidates, as an immediate adjunct treatment after incomplete resection or in case of recurrence or progression of residual tumours.

After subtotal resection the optimal moment for treatment is a matter of debate. The direct comparison of retrospective series investigating progression rates after surgery is difficult as each study includes patients with variable extents of resection. Therefore, a wide range of 10-year recurrence risk following surgery alone of between 2% and 80% has been reported. Retrospective analyses indicate that in patients with radiographic evidence of residual tumour, the progression rate is typically about 50% at 5–10 years. The factors mostly associated with the risk of growth are invasion into parasellar structures such as the cavernous sinus.

The early use of radiotherapy appears to lead to better tumour control supporting the notion of early radiation treatment for tumour control rather than a «wait-and-see» policy [150, 157, 171, 181].

The efficacy of radiosurgery of nonsecretory macroadenomas is well documented. Numerous reports to date have assessed the long-term tumour control of SRS in such patients. Although the majority of the studies have used Gamma Knife radiosurgery (GKRS), other modalities of radiosurgery including CyberKnife and, less frequently, linear accelerator-based (LINAC) radiosurgery, both as single-dose treatments and hypo-fractionated schemes, have been published [94, 157, 173, 181].

The retrospective Gamma Knife series have the longest follow-up with the majority of studies reporting about more than 60 months of follow-up. The reported tumour control rates are in a range between 83% and 100% with a trend towards lower control rates in the studies with the longest follow-up. The dose concepts for single-session RS are variable. The mean/median margin dose used in the GKRS-based publications ranged from 13 to 24 Gy, with the majority of groups reporting a mean/median margin dose of approximately 14–20 Gy. In newer studies there is a trend towards lower doses in the range of 14–16 Gy.

The primary goal of treatment is usually tumour control (or prevention of tumour growth). However, many studies have also reported about rates of reduction in tumour size. The shrinkage of the tumour is far more variable compared to local control with rates ranging from 42% to 89%. In this regard, the definition of tumour shrinkage may in part account for the reported heterogeneity since some groups define shrinkage as a reduction in tumour size of at least 20–25%, whereas others count any reduction in total tumour size on magnetic resonance imaging as remission.

Although the CyberKnife patients usually have shorter follow-up periods, the published data are more or less comparable with the Gamma Knife results. The results are fairly satisfactory with promising intermediate time local control rates of over 92–100% [65, 109, 113, 152, 162].

Prolactinomas

Radiosurgery is an option for patients which fail to normalise prolactin following medical treatment or which do not tolerate the adverse effects of drug treatment and are not suitable for surgery. It can be applied as adjunct after non-radical resection, in case of relapse or as or as primary local treatment when medical therapy fails. In contrast to non-functioning pituitary adenomas, the primary goal or local treatment is twofold: Local therapy should stop tumour growth and should reverse the excessive hormonal production.

The latter goal needs usually higher doses than local control of nonsecreting adenomas. Therefore, median peripheral radiation doses used for prolactinoma are in the range of 25 Gy, but the variation of doses is high (13 up to 34 Gy) not only between different studies but also between individual patients within one study. The median time to remission is in the range of 30–36 months, but there is a trend to higher remission rates in the studies with longer follow-up.

Beside the follow-up period, the applied dose may be a main cause for the large variability of hormonal remission rates.

The success rate of hormone ablation is a function of dose, but often the prescription of single doses over 22–24 Gy is hindered by the proximity of critical structures, mainly the optic pathway. Therefore, dose prescription is often a result of «inverse planning,» so that doses are prescribed which keep the maximum point dose on the optic pathway under 10 Gy.

In accordance with the wide range of applied doses, the reported rates of complete endocrine normalisation are quite variable.

The remission criteria are generally defined as prolactin levels within normal limits (often <20 ng/ml), but the interpretation of the different results is hindered by the fact

that not all groups published their remission criteria, and minimally elevated prolactin levels may be due to stalk injury without residual tumour.

The endocrine normalisation rates are far from ideal; however, the picture turns more optimistic when also the rates of significant reduction of prolactin levels without complete endocrine normalisation are taken into account. This is observed in up to 80% of all treated patients. Microadenomas appear to be more responsive than macroadenomas with remission rates of 70% versus 30%, respectively. Patients with tumours smaller than 3 cm^3 and who are not receiving dopamine agonists at the time of SRS will likely benefit the most from SRS. It has been hypothesised that suspending dopamine agonist therapy prior to SRS may increase tumour cell susceptibility to radiosurgery, and various groups have published findings to support this. Therefore, it is recommended to interrupt treatment with dopamine agonists in a period between 6 weeks before until 6 weeks after radiosurgery.

The success rate regarding the local control is much more favourable. Control rates as defined by no further growth of the tumour approach almost 100%; however, tumour shrinkage occurs in only 20–50% of patients.

Growth Hormone-Producing Adenomas (Acromegaly)

Radiosurgery is currently proposed for patients with persistent active disease after surgery and/or during medical therapy or patients not suitable for surgery. A variety of studies have been published about radiosurgery of GH-producing pituitary adenomas. The majority of these trials used single doses of 20–25 Gy which is slightly lower compared to the doses used for prolactinomas; however, in a subset of patients, margin doses up to 35 Gy had been applied.

The reported tumour growth control following SRS in patients with acromegaly is between 95% and 100% [52, 61] with regard to median follow-up period of 31 up to 60 months (see ◘ Tables 3.5). As in other pituitary adenomas, the reduction of tumour size after treatment is much more variable with observed rates in 30–60% of the patients after treatment.

Biochemical remission of the disease has been reported in 35–100% of patients with GH-secreting adenomas after radiosurgery. The variable rates of biochemical control may again reflect the different lengths of follow-up but also the different dose concepts and the different criteria used to define the biochemical control of disease.

◘ **Table 3.5** Radiosurgery of growth hormone-secreting adenomas

Author	Patients (N)	Dose (Gy)	FU (months)	Tumour control (%)	Biochemical remission (%)	Late toxicity (visual) (%)	Late toxicity (hypopituitarism) (%)
Attanasio 2003 [52]	30	20	48	100	30 (5y)	0	6.7
Jane 2003 [104]	64	15	>18	NA	36	0	28
Castinetti 2005 [60]	82	26	49.5	NA	17	1.2	17
Gutt 2005 [90]	44	23	22	100	48	NA	NA
Kobayashi 2005 [117]	67	18.9	63	100	17	11	
Jezkova 2006 [106]	96	32	53.7	100	44 (5y)	0	27.1
Voges 2006 [184]	64	16.5	54.3	97	14 (3y) 33 (5y)	0	13 (3y) 18 (5y)
Pollock 2007 [155]	46	20	63	100	11 (2y) 60 (5y)	3.8	33 (5y)
Vik-Mo 2007 [182]	53	26.5	67	100	58 (5y) 86 (10y)	4	10 (5y)
Roberts 2007 [162]	9	22	25.4	100	44.4	0	33
Jagannathan 2008 [103]	95	22	57	98	53	0	34
Losa 2008 [131]	83	21.5	69	97	52 (5y) 82 (10y)	0	10 (10y)
Ronchi 2009 [163]	35	20	114	100	46 (10y)	0	50
Wan 2009 [185]	103	21.4	67	95	37	0	6
Hayashi 2010 [94]	25	25.2	36	100	40	0	0
Iwai 2010 [100]	26	20	84	96	17 (5y) 47 (10y)	0	8

Modified according to Minniti et al. [136]

Moreover, the baseline levels of GH prior to radiosurgery have emerged as predictors of endocrine response to SRS in acromegaly. Various groups have reported that lower baseline levels of GH and/or IGF-1 at the time of radiosurgery were a positive predictor of endocrine response to SRS.

When stringent criteria of biochemical remission as defined by suppressed GH levels during OGTT and normal age-corrected IGF-1 levels are considered, a 5-year actuarial biochemical remission has been reported in 30–60% of patients following SRS including patients who achieved normal GH/IGF-1 levels during medical treatment with somatostatin analogues. In patients with remission, the normalisation of GH/IGF-1 levels continues throughout the follow-up period [110].

The stepwise increase of biochemical remission rate with time after treatment was shown by Losa et al. [131] and Jagannathan et al. [103]. The Milan group [131] analysed 83 patients with acromegaly treated with Gamma Knife radiosurgery and reported actuarial biochemical remission rates of 30%, 52% and 85% at 3, 5 and 10 years, respectively. Jagannathan et al. [103] observed normalisation of the serum IGF-1 in 53% of 95 patients treated with radiosurgery. The mean time to remission was 30 months; 12 patients achieved endocrine remission within the first year of treatment, 28 within 2 years and 34 within 3 years, respectively.

Like in radiosurgery for prolactinoma, cessation of antihormonal treatment seems to increase the efficacy of radiosurgery. Some authors reported that the cessation of somatostatin analogues or GH antagonists prior to radiosurgery resulted in a beneficial response [123, 155].

The mechanism behind the medication status is a matter of debate. Maybe adenoma cells not being suppressed by medication are actively proliferating, and thus, they are more susceptible to the effects of radiation. However, the effect could also be based on a simple selection bias since the observation is made by retrospective studies. Possibly, patients who could actually tolerate being off medications may have a less aggressive form of the disease. Although somatostatin analogue withdrawal before SRS is increasingly used in clinical practice, future prospective studies are needed to clarify that issue.

Adrenocorticotrophic Hormone-Producing Adenomas (Cushing's Disease)

Radiosurgery for Cushing's disease is often an adjuvant to microsurgical resection of ACTH-secreting adenomas, less frequently as primary alternative to surgery. Failure to achieve remission or tumour recurrence occurs in up to 30% following initial successful transsphenoidal resection of ACTH-secreting tumours in Cushing's disease patients. A less common clinical issue is the so-called Nelson's syndrome: Bilateral adrenalectomy for the treatment of Cushing's syndrome may lead to uncontrolled growth of any pre-existing pituitary adenoma due to the lack of negative feedback from endogenous cortisol. The resulting tumours of Nelson's syndrome are often aggressive and difficult to control. SRS has been reported to be less effective in Nelson's syndrome than Cushing's disease with cure rates in less than 36% of patients despite lower ACTH levels in approximately 70% of patients and tumour growth control in up to 90% of patients. Fortunately, because of improvements in the management of ACTH-secreting tumours and more stringent indications for performing bilateral adrenalectomies, Nelson's syndrome has become a relatively uncommon entity [53].

▣ Table 3.6 summarises the results of 29 trials including 445 patients regarding radiosurgery of ACTH-producing adenomas that were treated surgically with postoperative radiosurgery or with primary radiosurgery. The prescribed margin doses used for radiosurgery of ACTH-producing adenomas are variable and range from 9 to 32 Gy, but the vast majority used doses of 20–25 Gy which reflects probably the adequate dose range when the relevant constraints are met with this prescription doses.

Fifteen studies used the 24-h urine cortisol concentration as part of the criteria for endocrine evaluation, eight studies did not report the methodology employed to establish endocrine remission or failure and the remainder used a combination of endocrine tests [192].

In most trials the tumour control rate is more than 90% with a variable rate of decreased adenoma volume. Again, tumour control is defined as a reduction in tumour volume or

3

Table 3.6 Radiosurgery of ACTH-secreting adenomas

Author	Patients (N)	Dose (Gy)	FU (Months)	Tumour control (%)	Biochemical remission (%)
Ganz 1993 [84]	4	25	18	100	50
Martinez 1998 [133]	3	24	36	100	100
Lim 1998 [127]	4	25	26	66	25
Mitsumori 1998 [137]	5	15	47	91	40
Morange-Ramos 1998 [139]	6	28	20	NA	67
Witt 1998 [186]	25	19	32	94	28
Yoon 1998 [191]	1	17	49	NA	NA
Hayashi 1999 [95]	10	24	16	92	10
Inoue 1999 [98]	3	20	>24	100	100
Lim 1998 [127]	8	29	27	NA	62
Laws 1999 [124]	50	NA	NA	NA	58
Mokry 1999 [138]	5	17	56	98	33
Izawa 2000 [101]	12	22	28	83	17
Sheehan 2000 [170]	43	20	44	100	63
Shin 200 [174]	7	32	88	100	50
Hoybye 2001 [97]	18	NA	204	NA	83
Feigl 2002 [77]	4	15	55	94	NA
Kobayashi 2002 [116]	20	29	64	100	35
Pollock 2002 [153]	9	20	42	100	78
Wong 2003 [188]	5	14.8–19.9	38	NA	80
Petrovic 2003 [151]	4	15	41	50	50
Choi 2003 [66]	5	28.5	42.5	97	56
Devin 2004 [73]	35	14.7	42	91	49
Colin 2005 [72]	12	NA	80	98	100
Kajiwara 2005 [109]	2	17.5	35.3	95	50
Kong 2007 [122]	7	9–30	36.7	100	100
Colin 2005 [72]	40	29.5	54.7	NA	43
Jagganathan 2007 [102]	90	23	45	95	54
Pollock 2008	8	22	56	100	87

Modified according to Zada

stability of tumour volume on postradiosurgical neuroimaging.

Radiosurgery achieves normalisation of ACTH levels in a median time of approximately 7.5–58 months. Success rates of hormone normalisation by radiosurgery are variable and difficult to interpret given the lack of standardised criteria for postoperative hormone control (e.g. 24-h urinary free cortisol vs. serum ACTH vs. basal serum cortisol). Moreover, many studies did not mention whether medical therapy is ongoing during the postoperative period. Complete endocrine remission has been reported in 17–100% of patients, however, most reports showing remission rates of approximately 40–65%. Radiosurgical parameters that affect the rate of endocrine remission remain a matter of debate. Some reports have found no relationship between radiosurgical treatment parameters and remission (possibly just due to the small size of the treated cohort), whereas others have found a correlation between remission and treatment dose, maximal dose, margin dose, tumour invasiveness and absence of hormone-suppressive medications at the time of radiosurgery. None of the trials observed a correlation between decrease in tumour volume and endocrine remission.

Similar to other functioning adenomas, microadenomas are associated with a better response rate than macroadenomas, and remission rates may be improved by continuing medical therapy in the postoperative period.

Tumour recurrence can present late with recurrent hypercortisolism being reported as late as 8 years postoperatively. These findings suggest that despite evidence of endocrine remission following SRS, Cushing's patients may require lifelong follow-up.

In the largest study to date, Jagannathan et al. [102] and colleagues treated 90 evaluable Cushing patients with a mean dose of 23 Gy (median 25 Gy) and a mean endocrine follow-up of 45 months. They reported normalisation of 24-h urinary free cortisol in 54% of patients with an average time to remission of 13 months (range 2–67 months).

Treatment-Related Adverse Effects

Since the used doses do not differ significantly between the different hormone-secreting adenomas, the complication rates should be expected to be similar between these entities, whereas in theory somehow lower rates should be expected for non-functioning adenomas.

This might be true for the most common complication, the onset of new anterior pituitary deficits, which has been reported in 0–66% of patients, because the prescription of doses is usually not limited by constraints of the pituitary. The reported incidence of new anterior pituitary deficits is quite variable which may reflect the fact that it probably relies on patient-related factors, treatment doses, treated volumes and especially length of the follow-up.

The rate of pituitary insufficiency seems to be a function of time since the group that reported the highest incidence of new pituitary deficits had the longest follow-up period; however, treatment technique, conformity, size of the tumour and prescribed doses surely may play a role as well. Pollock et al. [157] reported that one third of 39 patients with acromegaly had a new pituitary deficit following radiosurgery with an actuarial incidence of new anterior pituitary deficits of 10% at 2 years and 33% at 5 years, respectively. Similar incidences of hypopituitarism at 5 years in the region of 20–40% have been observed in other series, suggesting that it will likely increase significantly over time.

In this regard a long-term study from the Karolinska Institute with a mean follow-up of 17 years is of special interest because it demonstrated a comparably high incidence of pituitary hormone deficiency of 72%. However, the observed difference to the other trials should not be explained only by the time factor since the patients in the Karolinska trial received higher doses than current radiosurgery and were at least in part targeted using outdated imaging modalities.

The reported incidence of cranial nerve deficits, especially treatment-related visual dysfunction, relies mainly on the dose-volume histogram of the respective organs at risk and does not systematically differ between the various types of adenomas. The most challenging adverse effect may be visual dysfunction, which has also been reported following stereotactic radiosurgery for all types of pituitary adenomas. In summary, the rate of visual dysfunction is low in patients with no visual dysfunction prior to treatment.

In the literature, there are about 30 reported cases of new onset of visual dysfunction after radiosurgery of pituitary adenomas. The postradiosurgical deficits varied from quadrantanopsia to complete visual loss. The mentioned radiosurgical doses associated with visual field loss varied from 0.7 to 12 Gy so that at least for the lower dose a causal relationship between treatment and adverse effect is questionable [176].

A recent Mayo Clinic study evaluated the risk of radiation-induced optic neuropathy in 222 patients, 78 of them with pituitary adenoma, treated with single-session radiosurgery. The mean clinical and imaging follow-up periods were 83 and 123 months, respectively. Only one patient (0.5%) who received a maximum radiation dose of 12.8 Gy to the anterior visual pathway (AVP) developed unilateral blindness 18 months after SRS. The chance of radiation-induced optical neuropathy (RION) according to the maximum radiation dose received by the anterior visual pathway was 0% for patients receiving less than 8 Gy, (95% confidence interval [CI] 0–3.6%), 0% for patients receiving between 8.1 and 10.0 Gy (95% CI 0–10.7%), 0% for patients receiving between 10.1 and 12.0 Gy (95% CI 0–9.0%) and 10% for patients receiving more than 12 Gy, respectively. The cumulative overall risk of RION in patients receiving >8 Gy to the AVP was 1.0% (95% CI 0–6.2%); however, this risk relied on patients who received more than 12 Gy.

These data are more or less in accordance with the study of Skeie et al. [175] and Cifarelli et al. [68]. Skeie et al. [175] reported about 100 patients with cavernous sinus meningiomas treated with Gamma Knife SRS. Two patients (2%) developed optic neuropathy. One patient received 8.6 Gy to the AVP; the other patient underwent radiosurgery three times in addition to prior stereotactic fractionated radiotherapy. Cifarelli et al. [68] evaluated 217 patients undergoing radiosurgery for recurrent pituitary adenomas (secretory $n = 131$, nonsecretory $n = 86$). Two patients (0.9%) developed a permanent optic neuropathy. Again, prior radiation exposure increased the risk of AVP in this series.

On the other hand, also improvement in visual acuity and fields has been noted following radiosurgery in 10–20% patients with pituitary adenomas with tumour compression of the optic pathway and pretreatment visual deficits which may be a result of tumour shrinkage and optic nerve decompression.

Taken together, most authors advocate that single maximum doses of less than 8–10 Gy are fairly safe for the optic pathway in non-pretreated patients.

Especially the cavernous sinus is frequently irradiated at high doses in patients with residual pituitary adenoma so that other cranial neuropathies may occur. Indeed, neuropathies including oculomotor, trochlear, trigeminal or abducens nerves have been reported; however, many of those were transient. In the trial of Cifarelli et al. [68], nine patients (4%) developed new or worsened dysfunction of the cranial nerves II, III, IV or VI.

Cavernous carotid artery injury is rare following radiosurgery. Four cases have been reported with two resulting in symptomatic stenosis [170]. Pollock et al. [156, 157] have recommended limiting the radiation coverage to the internal carotid artery to not more than 50% of the vessel diameter whenever possible, whereas Shin et al. [174] recommended restricting the dose to the internal carotid artery to less than 30 Gy. None of these complications occurred in patients treated for a pituitary adenoma.

Posttreatment Follow-Up

Clinical and Endocrinological Evaluation

During the first 2 years after treatment, follow-up intervals of 6 months are recommended. The follow-up should include a throughout clinical neurological and ophthalmological examination with special emphasis on the patient's visus and other cranial nerve functions. In addition, a detailed endocrinological evaluation of the pituitary gland should be performed.

After the first 2 years depending on the clinical situation, the follow-up intervals can be extended to once a year. After 2 years two-year intervals may be sufficient in asymptomatic patients. The endocrinological function should be monitored lifelong.

Radiological Evaluation

The radiological follow-up should follow the same schedule. Gadolinium-enhanced MRI scans should be performed every 6 months, in the third and fourth after treatment every 12 months and thereafter in patients without new symptoms every 2 years. Currently there is no consensus about the appropriate length of follow-up. Most of the data regarding local control report about 5- or 10-year local control rates. Some groups advocate a 10-year period of follow-up; some performed after an 8-year follow-up period another MRI 16 years after initial treatment.

Conclusions and Implications for Practice

Despite advances in endoscopic techniques, intraoperative imaging and microsurgical methods, there is still a significant cohort of patients with subtotal resection of pituitary adenomas or recurrent tumour on account of invasion into parasailer structures. Patients who have undergone surgical resection with residual, recurrent or progressive endocrinological disease or radiographical progression should be considered for radiotherapy.

Radiosurgery is a safe and effective adjuvant or salvage treatment for patients with small to intermediate size pituitary adenomas presenting with residual or recurrent tumour after surgery, with persistent or recurrent hormone hypersecretion.

Furthermore, it is suitable as a primary treatment for patients with small to intermediate size pituitary adenomas, which are unsuitable surgical candidates. Single-fraction radiosurgery is preferred for small pituitary adenomas that are not closer than 2 mm to the optic pathway. Compared to fractionated radiotherapies, radiosurgery is much less time consuming and has been shown to have lower rates of endocrinopathies and faster times to remission of hypersecretion than conventional radiotherapy. Hypo-fractionated radiosurgery with three to five sessions may be an option for lager tumours and/or tumours in the close vicinity to the optic pathway when further debulking is not feasible. However, further trials regarding hypo-fractionated radiosurgery for a better definition of the appropriate patient cohort and the optimal treatment schedule are needed.

3.2.5 Paraganglioma (Glomus Jugulare and Glomus Tympanicum Tumours)

Introduction

Paragangliomas (glomus jugulare and glomus tympanicum tumours) are highly vascularised tumours that arise from the paraganglionic tissue of the ninth or tenth cranial nerves. When populated by chromaffin cells, they can secrete catecholamines leading to instable blood pressure and tachycardia. They are considered as benign tumours; however, infrequently they may involve regional lymph nodes. The symptoms associated with the condition are predominantly a consequence of the tumour's mass effect on adjacent structures such as the lower cranial nerves.

Surgery is the mainstay of treatment; however, due to their location in the skull base, complete microsurgical resection of these tumours often carries considerable risks of morbidity and mortality including cerebrospinal fluid leaks and lower cranial nerve deficits. Therefore, often only an incomplete resection can be achieved and even after macroscopical complete removal of the tumour the recurrence rate is about 20% [168].

Adjuvant external beam radiotherapy and also primary conventionally fractionated external beam radiotherapy were successfully applied and provide high rates of local control. Although this approach achieves satisfactory tumour control rates, large treatment planning margins were required resulting in high radiation doses to the adjacent structures.

Therefore, radiosurgery is an attractive option for the primary treatment of small to intermediate size paragangliomas of the skull base, either for primary treatment or for treatment of recurrent or residuals tumours after surgery [107]. Radiosurgery provides a high degree of accuracy and rapid dose fall-off at the periphery allowing the clinician to deliver a high radiation dose to neoplastic tissue and spare healthy brain tissue. Moreover, the high single doses may provide additional beneficial effects on the tumour vessels.

Despite these theoretical benefits of radiosurgery, only a limited number of studies regarding SRS have been published yet, and no randomised controlled trials (RCTs) comparing the use of radiosurgery and other treatment modalities are available. Since surgery is still considered as the reference standard initial treatment, the results are possible biases, since patients treated with radiosurgery in such studies were possibly either poor surgical candidates or patients with recurrent disease after microsurgical resection which makes the direct comparison of the results between surgery and radiosurgery difficult.

Pretreatment Patient Evaluation

Tumour size and location should be evaluated by magnetic resonance imaging which should be not older than 3 months. In lesions adjacent to the inner ear and/or the inner auditory canal, pretreatment audiograms should be performed prior to treatment to document baseline hearing. The hearing can be document by means of the Gardner-Robertson scale. Careful clinical neurological examination is needed as a baseline examination with special regard to the function of the cranial nerves. Depending on the location of the tumours, trigeminal nerve function can be graded on a semi-quantitative scale as normal sensation, decreased sensation or no sensation, and facial nerve function can be graded by the House-Brackman scale.

Results of Radiosurgery: Local Control, Functional Outcome and Adverse Effects

Stereotactic radiosurgery is being increasingly used for both: as the upfront management modality and as a complementary or salvage treatment option for glomus jugulare or glomus tympanicum tumours (◘ Table 3.7) [56, 76, 78]. A meta-analysis published in 2011 summarised the results of radiosurgery of 335 patients in altogether 19 studies [89].

Treatment efficacy was determined by local tumour control and the clinical control of symptoms. The tumour control after radiosurgery for paragangliomas was defined as an unchanged or a reduced tumour volume of the glomus jugulare tumour as assessed by MR imaging. According to these criteria, the meta-analysis revealed a tumour control rate of 97% (95% confidence interval [CI], 95–99%). The clinical control rate defined as unchanged or improved clinical status after radiosurgery was 95% (95% CI, 92–97%). Eight of the included studies documented a mean or median follow-up time of more than 36 months. This subgroup achieved similar rates of clinical tumour control of 96% and 98%, respectively. This suggests a durable effect of radiosurgery.

In summary, the results of this meta-analysis suggest that radiosurgery is a highly efficacious modality in the management of glomus jugulare tumours. Treatment efficacy has always to be balanced against the treatment that revealed adverse effects. However, also in this read, radiosurgery for small to intermediate size paragangliomas seems to provide promising results, also when compared with the effects of surgery [57].

The overall rate of significant late effects was low. Six out of 19 studies reported no late effects, the other 13 studies about overall late effect rates of 7–25%, but many of these were of transient nature (see table). According to the size and location of the tumour transient facial palsy, permanent facial palsy, trigeminal neuralgia, transient tongue weakness, hearing loss, transient vocal cord paresis, transient low-grade nausea, vertigo and headache have been reported.

The rate of severe permanent damage of cranial nerves was in the range of 0–7%. Leakage of cerebrospinal fluid was not reported.

Since then some further single-centre studies have been published. Their results are mainly in accordance with the meta-analysis. El Majdoub et al. [75] presented long-term data of his cohort: Twenty-seven patients with a follow-up longer than 5 years (median 11 years, range 5.3–22.1 years) were selected for a retrospective analysis. The median therapeutical single dose applied to the tumour surface was 15 Gy (range 11 to 20 Gy), and the median tumour volume was 9.5 ml (range 2.8–51 ml). They reported that 10 of 27 patients showed a significant improvement of their previous neurological complaints, whereas 12 patients remained unchanged. MR imaging showed a partial remission in 12 and stable disease in 15 patients. No tumour progression was observed.

Licsak et al. [130] updated their results that confirm more or less their initial experience. Forty-six patients with glomus tumours treated with doses between 10 and 30 Gy (median 20 Gy) were analysed. They observed that neurological deficits improved in 19 (42%) of the 45 patients and deteriorated in 2 patients (4%), tumour size decreased in 34 (77%) of 44 patients with imaging follow-up, while an increase in volume was observed in 1 patient (2%) 182 months after radiosurgery. Seven patients died between 22 and 96 months after radiosurgery but all for unrelated reasons. They also concluded that radiosurgery has proved to be a safe treatment with a low morbidity rate and a reliable long-term anti-proliferative effect.

Posttreatment Follow-Up

Clinical and Endocrinological Evaluation

Follow-up intervals of 6 months are recommended within the first 2 years after initial treatment. Follow-up should include ENT and neurological examinations. In lesions close to the inner ear and/or the eighth cranial nerve, additional audiograms should be performed every 6 months. After the first 2 years, audiograms are obtained annually, after 4 years and according to clinical symptoms every 2 years. Whenever possible patients should obtain audiograms at the same facility to minimise errors in technique. Physical examination along these intervals

Table 3.7 Radiosurgery of paragangliomas

Author	Year	Fractions (N)	Average marginal dose (Gy)	Patients (N)	Follow-up (month)	Local control (%)	Symptom control (%)	Adverse effects
Navarro	2010	1	14	10	10	100	100	None
Genc	2010	1	15.6	18	53	94	94	None
Miller	2009	1	15	5	34	100	100	None
Ganz	2009	1	13.6	14	28	100	100	Transient facial palsy (1/14)
Sharma	2008	1	16.4	24	26	100	100	Trigeminal neuralgia (1/24)
Lim	2007	1	20.4	18	60	100	100	Transient tongue weakness/hearing loss (2/18) Transient vocal cord paresis (1/18)
Gerosa	2006	1	17	20	50	100	100	None
Varma	2006	1	15	17	48	76	76	None
Poznanovic	2006	1	15.1	8	16	100	100	Vertigo (1/8), transient neuropathy IX, X, XI ((1/8)
Bitaraf	2006	1	18	16	19	100	100	Vertigo (1/18)
Feigl	2006	1	17	12	33	100	100	Transient facial spasm (1/12), transient hoarseness (1/12), vertigo (1/12), nausea (1/12)
Sheehan	2005	1	15	8	28	100	100	None
Pollock	2004	1	14.9	42	44	97	97	Hearing loss (1/42) complete (5/42) partial, facial numbness (1/42),
Maarouf	2003	1	15	14	48	100	100	Facial palsy (1/14)
Feigenberg	2002	1	15	5	27	80	80	Transient facial palsy (1/5)
Saringer	2001	1	12	13	50	80	100	Transient facial palsy (1/13), transient dysphagia (1/13)
Jordan	2000	1	16.3	8	27	100	100	Vertigo (1/8)
Liscak	1999	1	16.5	66	24		100	Tinnitus (1/66), hearing loss (2/66) vertigo (2/66), facial palsy (2/66), inner ear inflammation (2)

Modified according to Guss et al. [89]

3

includes neurological examination and testing of the fifth, seventh and eighth cranial nerves [85].

Radiological Evaluation

The radiological follow-up should follow the same schedule. Gadolinium-enhanced MRI scans should be performed every 6 months, in the third and fourth after initial treatment every 12 months and thereafter in patients without new symptoms every 2 years. Currently there is no consensus about the appropriate length of follow-up. Most of the data regarding local control report about 5- or 10-year local control rates. Some groups advocate a 10-year period of follow-up; some performed after an 8-year follow-up period another MRI 16 years after initial treatment.

Conclusions and Implications for Practice

At present, radiosurgery is usually reserved for patients with contraindications for conventional surgery or with recurrent or residual disease after surgical resection. However, the published results suggest that single-session radiosurgery is a highly efficacious modality in the management of small- to intermediate-sized skull base paragangliomas [86, 87]. The high success rates in tumour and clinical control in both the GK and the LINAC/CK studies for >300 patients suggest that either modality is suitable for the management of glomus jugulare tumours [126, 129, 132, 135, 148, 154, 159, 166, 169, 172]. The published trials used doses between 1 × 12 Gy up to 1 × 20 Gy with a median of 15 Gy. Since the series are too small, neither for adverse effects nor for local control, a reliable dose effect relationship could not be extracted from these data. However, single doses of 14–16 Gy either prescribed to the 50% or 70% isodoses can be considered as safe and effective.

References

Surgical Principles

1. Altieri R, Tardivo V, Pacca P, Pennacchietti V, Penner F, Garbossa D, Ducati A, Garzaro M, Zenga F. 3D HD endoscopy in skull base surgery: from darkness to light. Surg Technol Int. 2016;XXIX:359–65.
2. Amit M, Abergel A, Fliss DM, Gil Z. The clinical importance of quality-of-life scores in patients with skull base tumors: a meta-analysis and review of the literature. Curr Oncol Rep. 2012;14(2):175–81.
3. Ausman JI. A revolution in skull base surgery: the quality of life matters! Surg Neurol. 2006;65(6):635–6.
4. Bambakidis NC, Kakarla UK, Kim LJ, Nakaji P, Porter RW, Daspit CP, Spetzler RF. Evolution of surgical approaches in the treatment of petroclival meningiomas: a retrospective review. Neurosurgery. 2007;61(5 Suppl 2):202–9.
5. Bi WL, Brown PA, Abolfotoh M, Al-Mefty O, Mukundan S Jr, Dunn IF. Utility of dynamic computed tomography angiography in the preoperative evaluation of skull base tumors. J Neurosurg. 2015;123(1):1–8.
6. Blitz AM, Aygun N, Herzka DA, Ishii M, Gallia GL. High resolution three-dimensional MR imaging of the skull base: compartments, boundaries, and critical structures. Radiol Clin N Am. 2017;55(1):17–30.
7. Cabrilo I, Sarrafzadeh A, Bijlenga P, Landis BN, Schaller K. Augmented reality-assisted skull base surgery. Neurochirurgie. 2014;60(6):304–6.
8. Cappabianca P, Doglietto F, Gentili F, Nicolai P. Endoscopic skull base surgery: where on the parabola? J Neurosurg Sci. 2016;60(4):438–40.
9. Cho YH, Lee JM, Lee D, Park JH, Yoon K, Kim SO, Kwon DH, Kim JH, Kim CJ, Roh SW. Experiences on two different stereotactic radiosurgery modalities of gamma knife and Cyberknife in treating brain metastases. Acta Neurochir. 2015;157(11):2003–9.
10. Colombo F, Casentini L, Cavedon C, Scalchi P, Cora S, Francescon P. Cyberknife radiosurgery for benign meningiomas: short-term results in 199 patients. Neurosurgery. 2009;64(2 Suppl):A7–13.
11. Da Cruz MJ, Francis HW. Face and content validation of a novel three-dimensional printed temporal bone for surgical skills development. J Laryngol Otol. 2015;129(Suppl 3):S23–9.
12. Dengler J, Heuschmann PU, Endres M, Meyer B, Rohde V, Rufenacht DA, Vajkoczy P, Giant Intracranial Aneurysm Study Group. The rationale and design of the giant intracranial aneurysm registry: a retrospective and prospective study. Int J Stroke. 2011;6(3):266–70.
13. Dengler J, Maldaner N, Gläsker S, Endres M, Wagner M, Malzahn U, Heuschmann PU, Vajkoczy P, Giant Intracranial Aneurysm Study Group. Outcome of surgical or endovascular treatment of Giant intracranial aneurysms, with emphasis on age, aneurysm location, and unruptured aneuryms–a systematic review and meta-analysis. Cerebrovasc Dis. 2016;41(3–4):187–98.
14. Dolenc V. Direct microsurgical repair of intracavernous vascular lesions. J Neurosurg. 1983;58(6):824–31.
15. Grauvogel J, Grauvogel TD, Kaminsky J. Piezosurgical lateral suboccipital craniectomy and opening of the internal auditory canal in the rat. J Neurosurg Sci. 2014;58(1):17–22.
16. Hage ZA, Alaraj A, Arnone GD, Charbel FT. Novel imaging approaches to cerebrovascular disease. Transl Res. 2016;175:54–75.
17. Hayashi N, Mitsuya K, Gorai K, Inoue K, Ito I, Nakagawa M, Nakasu Y. A novel graft material for preventing cerebrospinal fluid leakage in skull base reconstruction: technical note of perifascial areolar tissue. J Neurol Surg B Skull Base. 2015;76(1):7–11.

18. Hide T, Yano S, Shinojima N, Kuratsu J. Usefulness of the indocyanine green fluorescence endoscope in endonasal transsphenoidal surgery. J Neurosurg. 2015;122(5):1185–92.
19. Hochmuth A, Spetzger U, Schumacher M. Comparison of three-dimensional rotational angiography with digital subtraction angiography in the assessment of ruptured cerebral aneurysms. AJNR Am J Neuroradiol. 2002;23(7):1199–205.
20. Jones SH, Iannone AF, Patel KS, Anchouche K, Raza SM, Anand VK, Schwartz TH. The impact of age on long-term quality of life after endonasal endoscopic resection of skull base meningiomas. Neurosurgery. 2016;79(5):736–45.
21. König SA, Ranguis S, Gramlich V, Spetzger U. Reconstruction of the anterior skull base after major trauma or extensive tumour resection. Acta Neurochir. 2015;157(1):139–44.
22. Krombach G, Ganser A, Fricke C, Rohde V, Reinges M, Gilsbach J, Spetzger U. Virtual placement of frontal ventricular catheters using frameless neuronavigation: an "unbloody training" for young neurosurgeons. Minim Invasive Neurosurg. 2000;43(4):171–5.
23. Lefaucheur JP, Neves DO, Vial C. Electrophysiological monitoring of cranial motor nerves (V, VII, IX, X, XI, XII). Neurochirurgie. 2009;55(2):136–41.
24. Mathur A, Jain N, Kesavadas C, Thomas B, Kapilamoorthy TR. Imaging of skull base pathologies: role of advanced magnetic resonance imaging techniques. Neuroradiol J. 2015;28(4):426–37.
25. Reisch R, Stadie A, Kockro R, Gawish I, Schwandt E, Hopf N. The minimally invasive supraorbital subfrontal key-hole approach for surgical treatment of temporomesial lesions of the dominant hemisphere. Minim Invasive Neurosurg. 2009;52(4):163–9.
26. Sachs ME, Conley J, Rabuzzi DD, Blaugrund S, Price J. Degloving approach for total excision of inverted papilloma. Laryngoscope. 1984;94(12 Pt 1):1595–8.
27. Sanli E, Mabhouti H, Cebe M, Codel G, Pacaci P, Serin E, Kucuk N, Kucukmorkoc E, Doyuran M, Canoglu D, Altinok A, Acar H, Caglar Ozkok H. SU-F-SPS-10: the dosimetric comparison of GammaKnife and Cyberknife treatment plans for brain SRS treatment. Med Phys. 2016;43(6):3352.
28. Schipper J, Maier W, Arapakis I, Spetzger U, Laszig R. Navigation as a tool to visualize bone-covered hidden structures in transfrontal approaches. J Laryngol Otol. 2004a;118(11):849–56.
29. Schipper J, Ridder GJ, Maier W, Spetzger U. The anterosigmoidal approach. A function-preserving surgical method for petroclival tumors. HNO. 2004b;52(11):984–7.
30. Schipper J, Ridder GJ, Spetzger U, Teszler CB, Fradis M, Maier W. Individual prefabricated titanium implants and titanium mesh in skull base reconstructive surgery. A report of cases. Eur Arch Otorhinolaryngol. 2004c;261(5):282–90.
31. Schipper J, Spetzger U, Tatagiba M, Rosahl S, Neumann HP, Boedeker CC, Maier W. Juxtacondylar approach in temporal paraganglioma surgery: when and why? Skull Base. 2009;19(1):43–7.
32. Seifert V. Clinical management of petroclival meningiomas and the eternal quest for preservation of quality of life: personal experiences over a period of 20 years. Acta Neurochir. 2010;152(7):1099–116.
33. Spetzger U, Laborde G, Gilsbach JM. Frameless neuronavigation in modern neurosurgery. Minim Invasive Neurosurg. 1995;38(4):163–6.
34. Spetzger U, Reul J, Weis J, Bertalanffy H, Thron A, Gilsbach JM. Microsurgically produced bifurcation aneurysms in a rabbit model for endovascular coil embolization. J Neurosurg. 1996;85(3):488–95.
35. Spetzger U, Hubbe U, Struffert T, Reinges MH, Krings T, Krombach GA, Zentner J, Gilsbach JM, Stiehl HS. Error analysis in cranial neuronavigation. Minim Invasive Neurosurg. 2002;45(1):6–10.
36. Spetzger U, Vougioukas V, Schipper J. Materials and techniques for osseous skull reconstruction. Minim Invasive Ther Allied Technol. 2010;19(2):110–21.
37. Spetzger U, von Schilling A, Brombach T, Winkler G. Training models for vascular microneurosurgery. Acta Neurochir Suppl. 2011;112:115–9.
38. Spetzger U, Frasca M, König SA. Surgical planning, manufacturing and implantation of an individualized cervical fusion titanium cage using patient-specific data. Eur Spine J. 2016;25(7):2239–46.
39. Snyderman CH, Wang EW, Fernandez-Miranda JC, Gardner PA. The making of a skull base team and the value of multidisciplinary approach in the management of sinonasal and ventral skull base malignancies. Otolaryngol Clin North Am. 2017;50(2):457–65. https://doi.org/10.1016/j.otc.2016.12.017.
40. Tantongtip D, Fratianni A, Jenkner J, Arnold S, Spetzger U. Surgical treatment of inadvertent internal carotid artery lesion by extraintracranial high-flow bypass. A case report and review of the literature. J Neurol Surg Rep. 2015;76(1):e100–4.
41. Thaher F, Hopf N, Hickmann AK, Kurucz P, Bittl M, Henkes H, Feigl G. Supraorbital keyhole approach to the skull base: evaluation of complications related to CSF fistulas and opened frontal sinus. J Neurol Surg A Cent Eur Neurosurg. 2015;76(6):433–7.
42. Tuniz F, Soltys SG, Choi CY, Chang SD, Gibbs IC, Fischbein NJ, Adler JR Jr. Multisession cyberknife stereotactic radiosurgery of large, benign cranial base tumors: preliminary study. Neurosurgery. 2009;65(5):898–907.
43. von Schilling A, Spetzger U. Clipping of a partially thrombosed giant VA aneurysm. Neurosurg Focus. 2015;38(VideoSuppl1):Video18.
44. Vougioukas VI, Hubbe U, Schipper J, Spetzger U. Navigated transoral approach to the cranial base and the craniocervical junction: technical note. Neurosurgery. 2003;52(1):247–50.
45. Vougioukas VI, Hubbe U, van Velthoven V, Freiman TM, Schramm A, Spetzger U. Neuronavigation-assisted cranial reconstruction. Neurosurgery. 2004;55(1):162–7.
46. Yagmurlu K, Safavi-Abbasi S, Belykh E, Kalani MY, Nakaji P, Rhoton AL Jr, Spetzler RF, Preul MC. Quantitative anatomical analysis and clinical experience with mini-pterional and mini-orbitozygomatic approaches for intracranial aneurysm surgery. J Neurosurg. 2016;18:1–14.

47. Zhao M, Amin-Hanjani S, Ruland S, Curcio AP, Ostergren L, Charbel FT. Regional cerebral blood flow using quantitative MR angiography. AJNR Am J Neuroradiol. 2007;28(8):1470–3.

Radiosurgical Principles

48. Adler JR Jr, Chang SD, Murphy MJ, Doty J, Geis P, Hancock SL. The Cyberknife: a frameless robotic system for radiosurgery. Stereotact Funct Neurosurg. 1997;69:124–8.
49. Adler JR Jr, Gibbs IC, Puataweepong P, Chang SD. Visual field preservation after multisession cyberknife® radiosurgery for perioptic lesions. Neurosurgery. 2006;59:244–54.
50. Aichholzer M, Bertalanffy A, Dietrich W, Roessler K, Pfisterer W, Ungersboeck K, Heimberger K, Kitz K. Gamma knife radiosurgery of skull base meningiomas. Acta Neurochir. 2000;142:647–52.
51. Akpinar B, Mousavi SH, McDowell MM, Niranjan A, Faraji AH, Flickinger JC, Lunsford LD. Early radiosurgery improves hearing preservation in vestibular schwannoma patients with normal hearing at the time of diagnosis. Int J Radiat Oncol Biol Phys. 2016;95(2):729–34.
52. Attanasio R, Epaminonda P, Motti E, Giugni E, Ventrella L, Cozzi R, Farabola M, Loli P, Beck-Peccoz P, Arosio M. Gamma-knife radiosurgery in acromegaly: a 4-year follow-up study. J Clin Endocrinol Metab. 2003;88:3105–12.
53. Banasiak MJ, Malek AR. Nelson syndrome: comprehensive review of pathophysiology, diagnosis, and management. Neurosurg Focus. 2007;23(3):E13.
54. Baschnagel AM, Chen PY, Bojrab D, Pieper D, Kartush J, Didyuk O, Naumann IC, Maitz A, Grills IS. Hearing preservation in patients with vestibular schwannoma treated with gamma knife surgery. J Neurosurg. 2013;118(3):571–8.
55. Benedict SH, Yenice KM, Followill D, Galvin JM, Hinson W, Kavanagh B, Keall P, Lovelock M, Meeks S, Papiez L, Purdie T, Sadagopan R, Schell MC, Salter B, Schlesinger DJ, Shiu AS, Solberg T, Song DY, Stieber V, Timmerman R, Tomé WA, Verellen D, Wang L, Yin FF. Stereotactic body radiation therapy: the report of AAPM Task Group 101. Med Phys. 2010;37(8):4078–101.
56. Bitaraf MA, Alikhani M, Tahsili-Fahadan P, Motiei-Langroudi R, Zahiri A, Allahverdi M, Salmanian S. Radiosurgery for glomus jugulare tumors: experience treating 16 patients in Iran. J Neurosurg. 2006;105(Suppl):168–74.
57. Borba LA, Araújo JC, de Oliveira JG, Filho MG, Moro MS, Tirapelli LF, Colli BO. Surgical management of glomus jugulare tumors: a proposal for approach selection based on tumor relationships with the facial nerve. J Neurosurg. 2010;112:88–98.
58. Bulthuis VJ, Hanssens PE, Lie ST, van Overbeeke JJ. Gamma knife radiosurgery for intracranial meningiomas: do we need to treat the dural tail? A single-center retrospective analysis and an overview of the literature. Surg Neurol Int. 2014;5(Suppl 8):S391–5.
59. Casentini L, Fornezza U, Perini Z, Perissinotto E, Colombo F. Multisession stereotactic radiosurgery for large vestibular schwannomas. J Neurosurg. 2015; 122:818–24.
60. Castinetti F, Taieb D, Kuhn JM, Chanson P, Tamura M, Jaquet P, Conte-Devolx B, Régis J, Dufour H, Brue T. Outcome of gamma knife radiosurgery in 82 patients with acromegaly: correlation with initial hypersecretion. J Clin Endocrinol Metab. 2005;90:4483–8.
61. Castinetti F, Nagai M, Dufour H, Kuhn JM, Morange I, Jaquet P, Conte-Devolx B, Regis J, Brue T. Gamma knife radiosurgery is a successful adjunctive treatment in Cushing's disease. Eur J Endocrinol. 2007; 156:91–8.
62. Chang SD. Staged stereotactic irradiation for acoustic neuroma. Neurosurgery. 2005;56:1254–63.
63. Chen JC, Giannotta SL, Yu C, Petrovich Z, Levy Aichholzer M, Bertalanffy A, Dietrich W, Roessler K, Pfisterer W, Ungersboeck K, Heimberger K, Kitz K. Gamma knife radiosurgery of skull base meningiomas. Acta Neurochir. 2000;142:647–52.
64. Chen JC, Giannotta SL, Yu C, Petrovich Z, Levy ML, Apuzzo ML. Radiosurgical management of benign cavernous sinus tumors: dose profiles and acute complications. Neurosurgery. 2001;48:1022–30.
65. Cho CB, Park HK, Joo WI, Chough CK, Lee KJ, Rha HK. Stereotactic radiosurgery with the CyberKnife for pituitary adenomas. J Korean Neurosurg Soc. 2009;45:157–63.
66. Choi JY, Chang JH, Chang JW, Ha Y, Park YG, Chung SS. Radiological and hormonal responses of functioning pituitary adenomas after gamma knife radiosurgery. Yonsei Med J. 2003;44:602–7.
67. Chopra R, Kondziolka D, Niranjan A, Lunsford LD, Flickinger JC. Long-term followup of acoustic schwannoma radiosurgery with marginal tumor doses of 12 to 13 Gy. Int J Radiat Oncol Biol Phys. 2007;68:845–51.
68. Cifarelli CP, Schlesinger DJ, Sheehan JP. Cranial nerve dysfunction following gamma knife surgery for pituitary adenomas: long-term incidence and risk factors. J Neurosurg. 2012;116:1304–10.
69. Combs SE, Thilmann C, Debus J, Schulz-Ertner D. Long-term outcome of stereotactic radiosurgery (SRS) in patients with acoustic neuromas. Int J Radiat Oncol Biol Phys. 2006;64:1341–7.
70. Cohen-Inbar O, Tata A, Moosa S, Lee CC, Sheehan JP. Stereotactic radiosurgery in the treatment of parasellar meningiomas: long-term volumetric evaluation. J Neurosurg. 2017;24:1–11.
71. Combs SE, Ganswindt U, Foote RL, Kondziolka D, Tonn JC. State-of-the-art treatment alternatives for base of skull meningiomas: complementing and controversial indications for neurosurgery, stereotactic and robotic based radiosurgery or modern fractionated radiation techniques. Radiat Oncol. 2012;7:226.
72. Colin P, Jovenin N, Delemer B, Caron J, Grulet H, Hecart AC, Lukas C, Bazin A, Bernard MH, Scherpereel B, Peruzzi P, Nakib I, Redon C, Rousseaux P. Treatment of pituitary adenomas by fractionated stereotactic radiotherapy: a prospective study of 110 patients. Int J Radiat Oncol Biol Phys. 2005;62:333–41.
73. Devin JK, Allen GS, Cmelak AJ, Duggan DM, Blevins LS. The efficacy of linear accelerator radiosurgery in the management of patients with Cushing's disease. Stereotact Funct Neurosurg. 2004;82(5–6):254–62.

74. Dutta D, Balaji Subramanian S, Murli V, Sudahar H, Gopalakrishna Kurup PG, Potharaju M. Dosimetric comparison of Linac-based (BrainLAB®) and robotic radiosurgery (CyberKnife®) stereotactic system plans for acoustic schwannoma. J Neuro-Oncol. 2012;106(3):637–42.
75. El Majdoub F, Hunsche S, Igressa A, Kocher M, Sturm V, Maarouf M. Stereotactic LINAC-radiosurgery for glomus jugulare tumors: a long-term follow-up of 27 patients. PLoS One. 2015;10(6):e0129057.
76. Feigenberg SJ, Mendenhall WM, Hinerman RW, Amdur RJ, Friedman WA, Antonelli PJ. Radiation therapy for Paraganglioma of the temporal bone. Head Neck. 2002;24:384–9.
77. Feigl GC, Bonelli CM, Berghold A, Mokry M. Effects of gamma knife radiosurgery of pituitary adenomas on pituitary function. J Neurosurg. 2002;97(5 Suppl):415–21.
78. Feigl GC, Horstmann GA. Intracranial glomus jugulare tumors: volume reduction with gamma knife surgery. J Neurosurg. 2006;105(Suppl):161–7.
79. Flickinger JC, Lunsford LD, Linskey ME, Duma CM, Kondziolka D. Gamma knife radiosurgery for acoustic tumors: multivariate analysis of four year results. Radiother Oncol. 1993;27:91–8.
80. Foote RL, Coffey RJ, Swanson JW, Harner SG, Beatty CW, Kline RW, Stevens LN, Hu TC. Stereotactic radiosurgery using the gamma knife for acoustic neuromas. Int J Radiat Oncol Biol Phys. 1995;32:1153–60.
81. Friedman WA, Bradshaw P, Myers A, Bova FJ. Linear accelerator radiosurgery for vestibular schwannomas. J Neurosurg. 2006;105:657–61.
82. Friedman WA, Foote KD. Linear accelerator radiosurgery for skull base tumors. Neurosurg Clin North Am. 2000;11:667–80.
83. Fukuoka S, Takanashi M, Hojyo A, Konishi M, Tanaka C, Nakamura H. Gamma knife radiosurgery for vestibular schwannomas. Prog Neurol Surg. 2009;22:45–62.
84. Ganz JC, Backlund EO, Thorsen FA. The effects of gamma knife surgery of pituitary adenomas on tumor growth and endocrinopathies. Stereotact Funct Neurosurg. 1993;61(Suppl 1):30–7.
85. Ganz JC, Abdelkarim K. Glomus jugulare tumours: certain clinical and radiological aspects observed following gamma knife radiosurgery. Acta Neurochir. 2009;151:423–6.
86. Genç A, Bicer A, Abacioglu U, Peker S, Pamir MN, Kilic T. Gamma knife radiosurgery for the treatment of glomus jugulare tumors. J Neuro-Oncol. 2010;97:101–8.
87. Gerosa M, Visca A, Rizzo P, Foroni R, Nicolato A, Bricolo A. Glomus jugulare tumors: the option of gamma knife radiosurgery. Neurosurgery. 2006;59:561–9.
88. Goldsmith BJ, Wara WM, Wilson CB, Larson DA. Postoperative irradiation for subtotally resected meningiomas. A retrospective analysis of 140 patients treated from 1967 to 1990. J Neurosurg. 1994;80:195–201.
89. Guss ZD, Batra S, Limb CJ, Li G, Sughrue ME, Redmond K, Rigamonti D, Parsa AT, Chang S, Kleinberg L, Lim M. Radiosurgery of glomus jugulare tumors: a meta-analysis. Int J Radiat Oncol Biol Phys. 2011;81(4):e497–502.
90. Gutt B, Wowra B, Alexandrov R, Uhl E, Schaaf L, Stalla GK, Schopohl J. Gamma-knife surgery is effective in normalising plasma insulin-like growth factor I in patients with acromegaly. Exp Clin Endocrinol Diabetes. 2005;113:219–24.
91. Han MS, Jang WY, Moon KS, Lim SH, Kim IY, Jung TY, Jung SI. Fractionated gamma knife radiosurgery a safe and effective treatment approach for large-volume (>10 cm^3) intracranial meningiomas? World Neurosurg. 2017;99:477–83.
92. Hansasuta A, Choi CY, Gibbs IC, Soltys SG, Tse VC, Lieberson RE, Hayden MG, Sakamoto GT, Harsh GR 4th, Adler JR Jr, Chang SD. Multisession stereotactic radiosurgery for vestibular schwannomas: single-institution experience with 383 cases. Neurosurgery. 2011;69(6):1200–9.
93. Hasegawa T, Kida Y, Kobayashi T, Yoshimoto M, Mori Y, Yoshida J. Long-term outcomes in patients with vestibular schwannomas treated using gamma knife surgery: 10-year follow up. J Neurosurg. 2005;102:10–6.
94. Hayashi M, Chernov M, Tamura N, Nagai M, Yomo S, Ochiai T, Amano K, Izawa M, Hori T, Muragaki Y, Iseki H, Okada Y, Takakura K. Gamma Knife robotic microradiosurgery of pituitary adenomas invading the cavernous sinus: treatment concept and results in 89 cases. J Neuro-Oncol. 2010;98(2):185–94.
95. Hayashi M, Izawa M, Hiyama H, Nakamura S, Atsuchi S, Sato H, Nakaya K, Sasaki K, Ochiai T, Kubo O, Hori T, Takakura K. Gamma knife radiosurgery for pituitary adenomas. Stereotact Funct Neurosurg. 1999; 72(Suppl 1):111–8.
96. Ho AK, Fu D, Cotrutz C, Hancock SL, Chang SD, Gibbs IC, Maurer CR Jr, Adler JR Jr. A study of the accuracy of cyberknife spinal radiosurgery using skeletal structure tracking. Neurosurgery. 2007;60(2 Suppl 1):ONS147–56.
97. Höybye C, Grenbäck E, Rähn T, Degerblad M, Thorén M, Hulting AL. Adrenocorticotropic hormone-producing pituitary tumors: 12- to 22-year follow-up after treatment with stereotactic radiosurgery. Neurosurgery. 2001;49:284–91.
98. Inoue HK, Kohga H, Hirato M, Sasaki T, Ishihara J, Shibazaki T, Ohye C, Andou Y. Pituitary adenomas treated by microsurgery with or without gamma knife surgery: experience in 122 cases. Stereotact Funct Neurosurg. 1999;72(Suppl 1):125–31.
99. Iwai Y, Yamanaka K, Kubo T, Aiba T. Gamma knife radiosurgery for intracanalicular acoustic neuromas. J Clin Neurosci. 2008;15:993–7.
100. Iwai Y, Yamanaka K, Yoshimura M, Kawasaki I, Yamagami K, Yoshioka K. Gamma knife radiosurgery for growth hormone-producing adenomas. J Clin Neurosci. 2010;17(3):299–304.
101. Izawa M, Hayashi M, Nakaya K, Satoh H, Ochiai T, Hori T, Takakura K. Gamma knife radiosurgery for pituitary adenomas. J Neurosurg. 2000;93(Suppl 3):19–22.
102. Jagannathan J, Sheehan JP, Pouratian N, Laws ER, Steiner L, Vance ML. Gamma knife surgery for Cushing's disease. J Neurosurg. 2007;106:980–7.
103. Jagannathan J, Sheehan JP, Pouratian N, Laws ER Jr, Steiner L, Vance ML. Gamma knife radiosurgery for acromegaly: outcomes after failed transsphenoidal surgery. Neurosurgery. 2008;62:1262–9.
104. Jane JA Jr, Vance ML, Woodburn CJ, Laws ER Jr. Stereotactic radiosurgery for hypersecreting pituitary

3

tumors: part of a multimodality approach. Neurosurg Focus. 2003;14:e12.
105. Jayarao M, Chin LS. Robotics and its applications in stereotactic radiosurgery. Neurosurg Focus. 2007;23:E6.
106. Jezková J, Marek J, Hána V, Krsek M, Weiss V, Vladyka V, Lisák R, Vymazal J, Pecen L. Gamma knife radiosurgery for acromegaly–long-term experience. Clin Endocrinol. 2006;64:588–95.
107. Jordan JA, Roland PS, McManus C, Weiner RL, Giller CA. Stereotactic radiosurgery for glomus jugulare tumors. Laryngoscope. 2000;110:35–8.
108. Ju DT, Lin JW, Lin MS, Lee LM, Tseng HM, Wei CP, Yen CH, Hung CC, Hung KS, Lin CM, Lin TJ, Chiu WT, Tsai JT. Hypofractionated CyberKnife stereotactic radiosurgery for acoustic neuromas with and without association to neurofibromatosis Type 2. Acta Neurochir Suppl. 2008;101:169–73.
109. Kajiwara K, Saito K, Yoshikawa K, Kato S, Akimura T, Nomura S, Ishihara H, Suzuki M. Image-guided stereotactic radiosurgery with the CyberKnife for pituitary adenomas. Minim Invasive Neurosurg. 2005;48:91–6.
110. Kajiwara K, Saito K, Yoshikawa K, Ideguchi M, Nomura S, Fujii M, Suzuki M. Stereotactic radiosurgery/radiotherapy for pituitary adenomas: a review of recent literature. Neurol Med Chir (Tokyo). 2010;50:749–55.
111. Kalogeridi MA, Georgolopoulou P, Kouloulias V, Kouvaris J, Pissakas G. Long term results of LINAC-based stereotactic radiosurgery for acoustic neuroma: the Greek experience. J Cancer Res Ther. 2009;5:8–13.
112. Karam SD, Tai A, Strohl A, Steehler MK, Rashid A, Gagnon G, Harter KW, Jay AK, Collins SP, Kim JH, Jean W. Frameless fractionated stereotactic radiosurgery for vestibular schwannomas: a single-institution experience. Front Oncol. 2013;3:121.
113. Killory BD, Kresl JJ, Wait SD, Ponce FA, Porter R, White WL. Hypofractionated CyberKnife radiosurgery for perichiasmatic pituitary adenomas: early results. Neurosurgery. 2009;64(2 Suppl):A19–25.
114. Vermeulen S, Kim E. The stereotactic radiosurgical treatment of common benign brain tumors: pituitary adenomas, vestibular schwannoma and meningiomas. Translat Cancer Res. 2014;3(4):391–8.
115. Kim KM, Park CK, Chung HT, Paek SH, Jung HW, Kim DG. Long-term outcomes of gamma knife stereotactic radiosurgery of vestibular schwannomas. J Korean Neurosurg Soc. 2007;42:286–92.
116. Kobayashi T, Kida Y, Mori Y. Gamma knife radiosurgery in the treatment of Cushing disease: long-term results. J Neurosurg. 2002;97(5 Suppl):422–8.
117. Kobayashi T, Mori Y, Uchiyama Y, Kida Y, Fujitani S. Long-term results of gamma knife surgery for growth hormone-producing pituitary adenoma: is the disease difficult to cure? J Neurosurg. 2005;102(Suppl):119–23.
118. Kondziolka D, Lunsford LD, McLaughlin MR, Flickinger JC. Long-term outcomes after radiosurgery for acoustic neuromas. New Engl J Med. 1998;339:1426–33.
119. Kondziolka D, Levy EI, Niranjan A, Flickinger J, Lunsford LD. Long term outcomes after meningioma radiosurgery: physician and patient perspectives. J Neurosurg. 1999;91:44–50.
120. Kondziolka D, Nathoo N, Flickinger JC, Niranjan A, Maitz AH, Lunsford LD. Long-term results after radiosurgery for benign brain tumors. Neurosurgery. 2003;53:815–22.
121. Kondziolka D, Shin SM, Brunswick A, Kim I, Silverman JS. The biology of radiosurgery and its clinical applications for brain tumors. Neuro-Oncology. 2015;17(1):29–44.
122. Kong DS, Lee JI, Lim DH, Kim KW, Shin HJ, Nam DH, Park K, Kim JH. The efficacy of fractionated radiotherapy and stereotactic radiosurgery for pituitary adenomas: long-term results of 125 consecutive patients treated in a single institution. Cancer. 2007;110:854–60.
123. Landolt AM, Haller D, Lomax N, Scheib S, Schubiger O, Siegfried J, Wellis G. Stereotactic radiosurgery for recurrent surgically treated acromegaly: comparison with fractionated radiotherapy. J Neurosurg. 1998;88:1002–8.
124. Laws ER Jr, Vance ML. Radiosurgery for pituitary tumors and craniopharyngiomas. Neurosurg Clin N Am. 1999;10:327–36.
125. Leksell L. A note on the treatment of acoustic tumours. Acta Chir Scand. 1971;137:763–5.
126. Lim M, Gibbs IC, Adler JR Jr, Chang SD. Efficacy and safety of stereotactic radiosurgery for glomus jugulare tumors. Neurosurg Focus. 2004;17:E11.
127. Lim YL, Leem W, Kim TS, Rhee BA, Kim GK. Four years' experiences in the treatment of pituitary adenomas with gamma knife radiosurgery. Stereotact Funct Neurosurg. 1998;70(Suppl 1):95–109.
128. Lin VY, Stewart C, Grebenyuk J, Tsao M, Rowed D, Chen J, Nedzelski J. Unilateral acoustic neuromas: long-term hearing results in patient managed with fractionated stereotactic radiotherapy, hearing preservation surgery, and expectantly. Laryngoscope. 2005;115:292–6.
129. Liscák R, Vladyka V, Simonová G, Vymazal J, Janousková L. Leksell gamma knife radiosurgery of the tumor glomus jugulare and tympanicum. Stereotact Funct Neurosurg. 1998;70(Suppl. 1):152–60.
130. Liscak R, Urgosik D, Chytka T, Simonova G, Novotny J Jr, Vymazal J, Guseynova K, Vladyka V. Leksell gamma knife radiosurgery of the jugulotympanic glomus tumor: long-term results. J Neurosurg. 2014;121(Suppl): 198–202.
131. Losa M, Gioia L, Picozzi P, Franzin A, Valle M, Giovanelli M, Mortini P. The role of stereotactic radiotherapy in patients with growth hormone secreting pituitary adenoma. J Clin Endocrinol Metab. 2008;93: 2546–52.
132. Maarouf M, Voges J, Landwehr P, Bramer R, Treuer H, Kocher M, Müller RP, Sturm V. Stereotactic linear accelerator-based radiosurgery for the treatment of patients with glomus jugulare tumors. Cancer. 2003; 97:1093–8.
133. Martinez R, Bravo G, Burzaco J, Rey G. Pituitary tumors and gamma knife surgery. Clinical experience with more than two years of follow-up. Stereotact Funct Neurosurg. 1998;70(Suppl 1):110–8.
134. Mendenhall WM, Friedman WA, Bova FJ. Linear accelerator based stereotactic radiosurgery for acoustic schwannomas. Int J Radiat Oncol Biol Phys. 1994; 28:803–10.
135. Miller JP, Semaan MT, Maciunas RJ, Einstein DB, Megerian CA. Radiosurgery for glomus jugulare tumors. Otolaryngol Clin N Am. 2009;42:689–706.

136. Minniti G, Scaringi C, Enrici RM. Radiation techniques for acromegaly. Radiat Oncol. 2011;6:167.
137. Mitsumori M, Shrieve DC, Alexander E 3rd, Kaiser UB, Richardson GE, Black PM, Loeffler J. Initial clinical results of LINAC-based stereotactic radiosurgery and stereotactic radiotherapy for pituitary adenomas. Int J Radiat Oncol Biol Phys. 1998;42:573–80.
138. Mokry M, Ramschak-Schwarzer S, Simbrunner J, Ganz JC, Pendl G. A six year experience with the postoperative radiosurgical management of pituitary adenomas. Stereotact Funct Neurosurg. 1999;72(Suppl 1): 88–100.
139. Morange-Ramos I, Regis J, Dufour H, Andrieu JM, Grisoli F, Jaquet P, Peragut JC. Gamma-knife surgery for secreting pituitary adenomas. Acta Neurochir. 1998;140:437–43.
140. Morimoto M, Yoshioka Y, Kotsuma T, Adachi K, Shiomi H, Suzuki O, Seo Y, Koizumi M, Kagawa N, Kinoshita M, Hashimoto N, Ogawa K. Hypofractionated stereotactic radiation therapy in three to five fractions for vestibular schwannoma. Jpn J Clin Oncol. 2013; 43(8):805–12.
141. Morita A, Coffey RJ, Foote RL, Schiff D, Gorman D. Risk of injury to cranial nerves after gamma knife radiosurgery for skull base meningiomas: experience in 88 patients. J Neurosurg. 1999;90:42–9.
142. Muacevic A, Jess-Hempen A, Tonn JC, Wowra B. Results of outpatient gamma knife radiosurgery for primary therapy of acoustic neuromas. Acta Neurochir Suppl. 2004;91:75–8.
143. Murphy ES, Barnett GH, Vogelbaum MA, Neyman G, Stevens GH, Cohen BH, Elson P, Vassil AD, Suh JH. Long-term outcomes of gamma knife radiosurgery in patients with vestibular schwannomas. J Neurosurg. 2011;114(2):432–40.
144. Murphy ES, Suh JH. Radiotherapy for vestibular schwannomas: a critical review. Int J Radiat Oncol Biol Phys. 2011;79(4):985–97.
145. Muzevic D, Legcevic J, Splavski B, Cayé-Thomasen P. Stereotactic radiotherapy for vestibular schwannoma. Cochrane Database Syst Rev. 2014;(12).
146. Myrseth E, Møller P, Pedersen PH, Vassbotn FS, Wentzel-Larsen T, Lund-Johansen M. Vestibular schwannomas: clinical results and quality of life after microsurgery or gamma knife radiosurgery. Neurosurgery. 2005;56:927–35.
147. Nakamura H, Jokura H, Takahashi K, Boku N, Akabane A, Yoshimoto T. Serial follow-up MR imaging after gamma knife radiosurgery for vestibular schwannoma. Am J Neurorad. 2000;21:1540–6.
148. Navarro Martín A, Maitz A, Grills IS, Bojrab D, Kartush J, Chen PY, Hahn J, Pieper D. Successful treatment of glomus jugulare tumours with gamma knife radiosurgery: clinical and physical aspects of management and review of the literature. Clin Transl Oncol. 2010; 12:55–62.
149. Niranjan A, Mathieu D, Flickinger JC, Kondziolka D, Lunsford LD. Hearing preservation after intracanalicular vestibular schwannoma radiosurgery. Neurosurgery. 2008;63:1054–62.
150. Park P, Chandler WF, Barkan AL, Orrego JJ, Cowan JA, Griffith KA, Tsien C. The role of radiation therapy after surgical resection of nonfunctional pituitary macroadenomas. Neurosurgery. 2004;55:100–6.
151. Petrovich Z, Yu C, Giannotta SL, Zee CS, Apuzzo ML. Gamma knife radiosurgery for pituitary adenoma: early results. Neurosurgery. 2003;53:51–9.
152. Pham CJ, Chang SD, Gibbs IC, Jones P, Heilbrun MP, Adler JR Jr. Preliminary visual field preservation after staged CyberKnife radiosurgery for perioptic lesions. Neurosurgery. 2004;54:799–810.
153. Pollock BE, Young WF Jr. Stereotactic radiosurgery for patients with ACTH-producing pituitary adenomas after prior adrenalectomy. Int J Radiat Oncol Biol Phys. 2002;54:839–41.
154. Pollock BE. Stereotactic radiosurgery in patients with glomus jugulare tumors. Neurosurg Focus. 2004;17:E10.
155. Pollock BE, Jacob JT, Brown PD, Nippoldt TB. Radiosurgery of growth hormone-producing pituitary adenomas: factors associated with biochemical remission. J Neurosurg. 2007;106:833–8.
156. Pollock BE, Brown PD, Nippoldt TB, Young WF Jr. Pituitary tumor type affects the chance of biochemical remission after radiosurgery of hormone-secreting pituitary adenomas. Neurosurgery. 2008a;62:1271–6.
157. Pollock BE, Cochran J, Natt N, Brown PD, Erickson D, Link MJ, Garces YI, Foote RL, Stafford SL, Schomberg PJ. Gamma knife radiosurgery for patients with nonfunctioning pituitary adenomas: results from a 15-year experience. Int J Radiat Oncol Biol Phys. 2008b;70:1325–9.
158. Pollock BE, Stafford SL, Link MJ, Garces YI, Foote RL. Single-fraction radiosurgery for presumed intracranial meningiomas: efficacy and complications from a 22-year experience. Int J Radiat Oncol Biol Phys. 2012;83:1414–8.
159. Poznanovic SA, Cass SP, Kavanagh BD. Short-term tumor control and acute toxicity after stereotactic radiosurgery for glomus jugulare tumors. Otolaryngol Head Neck Surg. 2006;134:437–42.
160. Prasad D, Steiner M, Steiner L. Gamma surgery for vestibular schwannoma. J Neurosurg. 2000;92:745–59.
161. Rahman M, Murad GJ, Bova F, Friedman WA, Mocco J. Stereotactic radiosurgery and the linear accelerator: accelerating electrons in neurosurgery. Neurosurg Focus. 2009;27:E13.
162. Roberts BK, Ouyang DL, Lad SP, Chang SD, Harsh GR 4th, Adler JR Jr, Soltys SG, Gibbs IC, Remedios L, Katznelson L. Efficacy and safety of CyberKnife radiosurgery for acromegaly. Pituitary. 2007;10(1):19–25.
163. Ronchi CL, Attanasio R, Verrua E, Cozzi R, Ferrante E, Loli P, Montefusco L, Motti E, Ferrari DI, Giugni E, Beck-Peccoz P, Arosio M. Efficacy and tolerability of gamma knife radiosurgery in acromegaly: a 10-year follow-up study. Clin Endocrinol. 2009;71:846–52.
164. Sandström H, Nordström H, Johansson J, Kjäll P, Jokura H, Toma-Dasu I. Variability in target delineation for cavernous sinus meningioma and anaplastic astrocytoma in stereotactic radiosurgery with Leksell Gamma Knife Perfexion. Acta Neurochir. 2014;156(12):2303–12.
165. Santacroce A, Walier M, Régis J, Liščák R, Motti E, Lindquist C, Kemeny A, Kitz K, Lippitz B, Martínez Álvarez R, Pedersen PH, Yomo S, Lupidi F, Dominikus K,

3

Blackburn P, Mindermann T, Bundschuh O, van Eck AT, Fimmers R, Horstmann GA. Long-term tumor control of benign intracranial meningioma after radiosurgery in a series of 4565 patients. Neurosurgery. 2012;70:32–9.
166. Saringer W, Khayal H, Ertl A, Schoeggl A, Kitz K. Efficiency of gamma knife radiosurgery in the treatment of glomus jugulare tumors. Minim Invasive Neurosurg. 2001;44:141–6.
167. Seferis C, Torrens M, Paraskevopoulou C, Psichidis G. Malignant transformation in vestibular schwannoma: report of a single case, literature search, and debate. J Neurosurg. 2014;121(Suppl):160–6.
168. Semaan MT, Megerian CA. Current assessment and management of glomus tumors. Curr Opin Otolaryngol Head Neck Surg. 2008;16:420–6.
169. Sharma MS, Gupta A, Kale SS, Agrawal D, Mahapatra AK, Sharma BS. Gamma knife radiosurgery for glomus jugulare tumors: therapeutic advantages of minimalism in the skull base. Neurol India. 2008;56:57–61.
170. Sheehan JM, Vance ML, Sheehan JP, Ellegala DB, Laws ER Jr. Radiosurgery for Cushing's disease after failed transsphenoidal surgery. J Neurosurg. 2000;93:738–42.
171. Sheehan JP, Kondziolka D, Flickinger J, Lunsford LD. Radiosurgery for residual or recurrent nonfunctioning pituitary adenoma. J Neurosurg. 2002;97(5 suppl):408–14.
172. Sheehan J, Kondziolka D, Flickinger J, Lunsford LD. Gamma knife surgery for glomus jugulare tumors: an intermediate report on efficacy and safety. J Neurosurg. 2005;102(Suppl):241–6.
173. Sheehan JP, Pouratian N, Steiner L, Laws ER, Vance ML. Gamma knife surgery for pituitary adenomas: factors related to radiological and endocrine outcomes. J Neurosurg. 2011;114(2):303–9.
174. Shin M, Kurita H, Sasaki T, Tago M, Morita A, Ueki K, Kirino T. Stereotactic radiosurgery for pituitary adenoma invading the cavernous sinus. J Neurosurg. 2000;93(Suppl 3):2–5.
175. Skeie BS, Enger PO, Skeie GO, Thorsen F, Pedersen PH. Gamma knife surgery of meningiomas involving the cavernous sinus: long-term follow-up of 100 patients. Neurosurgery. 2010;66(4):661–8.
176. Stafford SL, Pollock BE, Leavitt JA, Foote RL, Brown PD, Link MJ, Gorman DA, Schomberg PJ. A study on the radiation tolerance of the optic nerves and chiasm after stereotactic radiosurgery. Int J Radiat Oncol Biol Phys. 2003;55:1177–81.
177. Suh JH, Barnett GH, Sohn JW, Kupelian PA, Cohen BH. Results of linear accelerator-based stereotactic radiosurgery for recurrent and newly diagnosed acoustic neuromas. Int J Cancer. 2000;90:145–51.
178. Tran TA, Stanley TR, Malhotra HK, De Boer SF, Prasad D, Podgorsak MB. Target and peripheral dose during patient repositioning with the Gamma Knife automatic positioning system (APS) device. J Appl Clin Med Phys. 2010;11(1):3150.
179. Tsai JT, Lin JW, Lin CM, Chen YH, Ma HI, Jen YM, Chen YH, Ju DT. Clinical evaluation of CyberKnife in the treatment of vestibular schwannomas. Biomed Res Int. 2013;2013:297093.
180. Unger F, Walch C, Schröttner O, Eustacchio S, Sutter B, Pendl G. Cranial nerve preservation after radiosurgery of vestibular schwannomas. Acta Neurochir Suppl. 2002;84:77–83.
181. van den Bergh AC, van den Berg G, Schoorl MA, Sluiter WJ, van der Vliet AM, Hoving EW, Szabó BG, Langendijk JA, Wolffenbuttel BH, Dullaart RP. Immediate postoperative radiotherapy in residual nonfunctioning pituitary adenoma: beneficial effect on local control without additional negative impact on pituitary function and life expectancy. Int J Radiat Oncol Biol Phys. 2007;67:863–9.
182. Vik-Mo EO, Oksnes M, Pedersen PH, Wentzel-Larsen T, Rødahl E, Thorsen F, Schreiner T, Aanderud S, Lund-Johansen M. Gamma knife stereotactic radiosurgery for acromegaly. Eur J Endocrinol. 2007;157:255–63.
183. Vivas EX, Wegner R, Conley G, Torok J, Heron DE, Kabolizadeh P, Burton S, Ozhasoglu C, Quinn A, Hirsch BE. Treatment outcomes in patients treated with CyberKnife radiosurgery for vestibular schwannoma. Otol Neurotol. 2014;35(1):162–70.
184. Voges J, Kocher M, Runge M, Poggenborg J, Lehrke R, Lenartz D, Maarouf M, Gouni-Berthold I, Krone W, Muller RP, Sturm V. Linear accelerator radiosurgery for pituitary macroadenomas: a 7-year follow up study. Cancer. 2006;107:1355–64.
185. Wan H, Chihiro O, Yuan S. MASEP gamma knife radiosurgery for secretory pituitary adenomas: experience in 347 consecutive cases. J Exp Clin Cancer Res. 2009;28:36.
186. Witt TC, Kondziolka D, Flickinger JC, et al. In: Lunsford LD, Kondziolka D, Flickinger J, editors. Gamma knife radiosurgery for pituitary tumors. gamma knife brain surgery progress in neurological surgery. Basel: Karger; 1998. p. 114–27.
187. Wowra B, Muacevic A, Tonn JC. Quality of radiosurgery for single brain metastases with respect to treatment technology: a matched-pair analysis. J Neuro-Oncol. 2009;94:69–77.
188. Wong GK, Leung CH, Chiu KW, Ma R, Cockram CS, Lam MJ, Poon WS. LINAC radiosurgery in recurrent Cushing's disease after transsphenoidal surgery: a series of 5 cases. Minim Invasive Neurosurg. 2003;46:32 7–30.
189. Yang I, Sughrue ME, Han SJ, Fang S, Aranda D, Cheung SW, Pitts LH, Parsa AT. Facial nerve preservation after vestibular schwannoma gamma knife radiosurgery. J Neuro-Oncol. 2009;93:41–8.
190. Yang I, Sughrue ME, Han SJ, Aranda D, Pitts LH, Cheung SW, Parsa AT. A comprehensive analysis of hearing preservation after radiosurgery for vestibular schwannoma. J Neurosurg. 2010;112:851–9.
191. Yoon SC, Suh TS, Jang HS, Chung SM, Kim YS, Ryu MR, Choi KH, Son HY, Kim MC, Shinn KS. Clinical results of 24 pituitary macroadenomas with linac-based stereotactic radiosurgery. Int J Radiat Oncol Biol Phys. 1998;41:849–53.
192. Zada G. Diagnosis and multimodality management of Cushing's disease: a practical review. Int J Endocrinol. 2013;2013:893781.

Trauma Traumatic Injuries of the Skull Base

Alexander König and Sebastian Ranguis

Electronic Supplementary Material The online version of this chapter (https://doi.org/10.1007/978-3-319-64018-1_4) contains supplementary material, which is available to authorized users.

A. König, U. Spetzger (eds.), *Surgery of the Skull Base*,
https://doi.org/10.1007/978-3-319-64018-1_4

The main indication for a surgical procedure after trauma in the area of the anterior cranial fossa (frontobasal injury) is a persisting rhinorrhoea of CSF with the potential of secondary meningitis. At the middle fossa and lateral skull base, indication for surgery is given in cases of epidural haematoma, rhinorrhoea or otorrhoea or injury of the facial nerve. In the posterior fossa, mainly epidural haematomas require surgery, whereupon the surgeon has to keep in mind that the haemorrhage can have its origin from an injury of a venous dural sinus. Significant instabilities of the craniocervical junction after trauma often require occipitocervical fusion.

Editor's Comment

The treatment of traumatic injuries of the skull base is only adequately possible with close cooperation with the different specialties being involved. Basically, the safeguarding of vital functions is the first essential step after severe head injury with injury of the skull base. After stabilisation of circulation and treatment of relevant bleedings, the next step in the emergency situation is a thin-sliced spiral CT scan with application of a contrast agent to visualise bony and vascular injuries as well. In this juncture it is crucial to detect injuries of the spine and craniocervical junction as well. The immediate emergency indication for the surgical treatment of space-occupying haematomas (epidural, subdural, intracerebral) can be all dominant for the whole further treatment. Depending on the CT findings in some cases, there is also an indication for the implantation of an ICP measuring probe or for CSF drainage.

The surgical treatment of skull base injuries is usually a secondary procedure. Depending on the pattern of injury, a multidisciplinary conference will define the treatment plan. The neurosurgeon usually has to collaborate with colleagues from neuroradiology, ophthalmology, maxillofacial surgery, ENT surgery and trauma surgery to establish an individual therapeutic algorithm and to define the urgency and the sequence of surgical procedures. The classification of the trauma is of importance here: Is it an open head injury with injury of the dura at the skull base with the risk of rhinorrhoea and meningitis or is it mainly a bony injury with significant negative functional or cosmetic effects for the patient? Basically, the discipline with the highest expertise for the injured anatomical region should be the trauma leader in the surgical treatment of skull base injuries keeping in mind that trauma mechanisms and fracture lines do not respect the borders of medical specialties.

Depending on the organisation of the local skull base centre and its constellation and expertise, there will be different treatment strategies and surgical procedures. However, the severity of intracranial injury defines the treatment algorithm and the indication for surgical procedures, and thus, it is a domain of neurosurgery in most cases.

4.1 Injuries of the Anterior Fossa

4.1.1 General Information

Severe injuries of the osseous structures of the midface are associated with a high incidence of frontobasal injuries because of the bony trajectories between skull base and midface [7]. The risk of a CSF leak with the potential risk of meningitis rises with associated fractures of the nasal sinuses [8].

The exact localisation of the fracture within the anterior skull base is crucial for the choice of operative treatment (open transcranial, endoscopic, unilateral or bilateral approach, etc.). Therefore, Oberascher [13] developed a classification to localise fractures of the anterior skull base with special emphasis on the different nasal sinuses (Table 4.1).

Table 4.1 Localisation of frontobasal fractures [13]

Region	Localisation
Region I	Anterior wall of the frontal sinus
Region II a	Lamina cribrosa
Region II b	Roof of the ethmoid bone
Region III a	Roof of the sphenoid sinus
Region III b	Lateral wall of the sphenoid sinus and adjacent petrous bone

Surgical revision is indicated for fractures of region I. The procedure for fractures of regions II a and II b depends on the size and number of defects. Smaller lesions can be treated endoscopically. In case of extended fractures, the authors recommend an open transcranial frontobasal revision. For regions III a and III b, an endoscopic procedure should be performed because of the difficulties when approaching these regions transcranially.

4.1.2 Clinical Signs and Symptoms

General clinical signs of a trauma of the anterior skull base are:

- Skin contusions of the forehead
- Haemorrhage from nose and/or throat
- Deformities of the nose and forehead
- «Racoon eyes» or unilateral orbital bruising
- Hyposphagma (subconjunctival haemorrhage)

Further symptoms of involvement of the nasal sinuses are:

- Rhinorrhoea
- Meningitis (if CSF leak has not been treated)
- Anosmia

In cases of involvement of the optic canal or the posterior orbit, additional symptoms occur due to lesions of the optic system:

- Visual disorders or loss of vision (lesion of optic nerve)
- Scotomas (lesion of optic nerve)
- Double vision (lesions of oculomotor, trochlear or abducens nerve)
- Mydriasis (lesions of oculomotor nerve)

In most cases frontobasal injuries do not cause any symptoms, especially during the first few hours or days after trauma. Therefore, the primary diagnosis is often made radiologically with a CT scan in the emergency room.

4.1.3 Investigations

Nowadays the initial trauma CT scan includes thin-sliced bone window image sequences in the axial and coronal planes. This enables the detection of thin fracture lines and intracranial air bubbles as signs of injury to the anterior skull base.

If there are clinical signs of a CSF leak from the nose, it is necessary to verify the beta trace protein in the fluid in question. This protein is a prostaglandin D synthase of which the concentration in CSF is 35 times higher than in serum [8].

In cases of a secondary CSF leak of unclear location of the origin, it might be helpful to perform an MRI scan in the prone position. During this examination, it is possible to detect fluid collections in the paranasal sinuses or the presence of CSF flow on T2 weighted image sequences.

If CT and MRI scans are not successful in detecting the location of the CSF leak, then the fluorescein technique is a very sensitive method for detecting a CSF fistula into the nasal sinuses [15]. This method uses a solution of 5% sodium fluorescein which is applied through a lumbar spinal tap. Following this, a nasendoscope with a blue filtered light source and a complementary blocking filter is used. Using this method even the smallest traces of fluorescein-stained CSF can be detected [15].

4.1.4 Therapeutic Options

Injuries of the anterior skull base bare the specific risk of a CSF leak into the frontal, ethmoid or sphenoid sinuses which may develop into secondary meningitis. Therefore, surgical intervention should be considered in most cases of persisting CSF leak. In cases of no CSF leak or CSF rhinorrhoea that resolves spontaneously within days, these injuries may be managed conservatively. Uncomplicated fractures of the orbital roof do not require surgical therapy. Orbital fracture reduction is required in significant dislocation of bony fragments into the orbit in the presence of symptomatic diplopia.

If there is evidence of dislocation of bony fragments into the optic canal with signs of impaired visual function, then an emergency surgical decompression of the optic nerve is indicated because of the risk to vision.

The surgical method depends on the extension and the location of the fracture. Small lesions with intact sense of smelling are treated minimally/invasively using endonasal endoscopy by an ENT surgeon [1, 4–6]. Lesions of the very

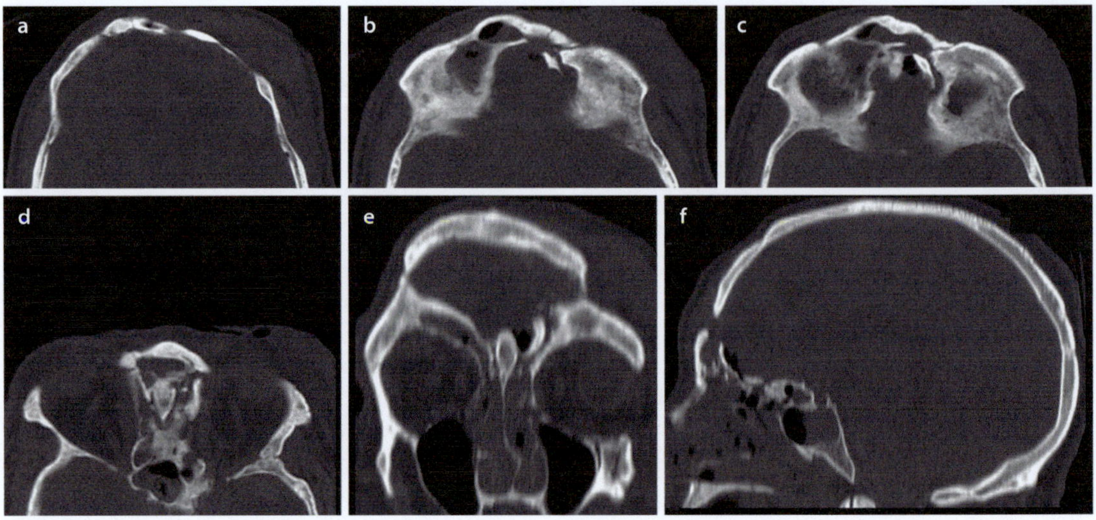

■ **Fig. 4.1** Left paramedian frontobasal fracture in the region of the Crista galli with clinical signs of rhinorrhoea following frontal **a**–**c** and frontobasal **d**–**f** traumatic injuries. CT scan (bone window) in axial **a**–**d**, coronal **e** and sagittal **f** planes

dorsally located sphenoid sinus should be treated endoscopically because a transcranial approach bears a relatively high risk of surgical morbidity. Fractures of the orbits especially with concomitant fractures of the midface are treated by maxillofacial surgeons.

In cases of extensive defects of the anterior skull base in region II a and II b (see above) with persisting CSF leak, the classical neurosurgical technique of transcranial frontobasal revision using a subfrontal approach is indicated (■ Figs. 4.1, 4.2, 4.3, and 4.4) [2, 12]. This technique enables a safe and watertight covering of the anterior skull base with a pericranial flap. When using this method, it is by its natures impossible to preserve sense of smell. Therefore, it should only be indicated in cases of previous traumatic anosmia. For a detailed description of the surgical technique, see ▶ Sect. 4.1.5.

For smaller open head injuries involving the frontal sinuses, it is possible to use a direct surgical approach (■ Figs. 4.5, 4.6, 4.7, 4.8, 4.9, 4.10, 4.11, and 4.12).

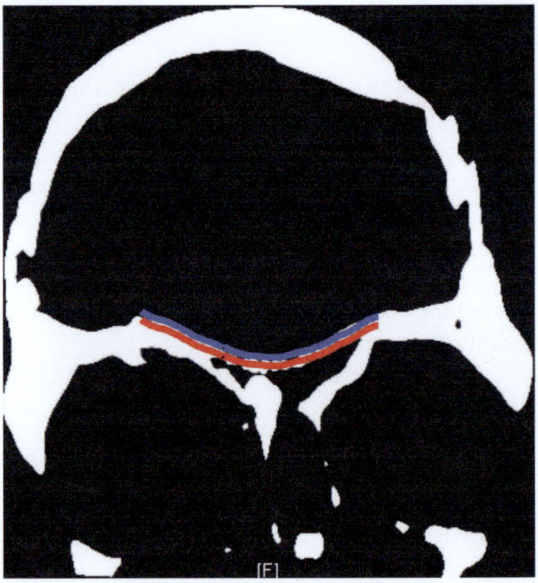

■ **Fig. 4.2** Scheme of the operative strategy with coverage of the anterior skull base with fascia lata (*red*) and titanium mesh (*blue*) that presses the duraplasty onto the orbital roofs. The frontobasal dura itself is covered with Tachosil™ (not shown in this image)

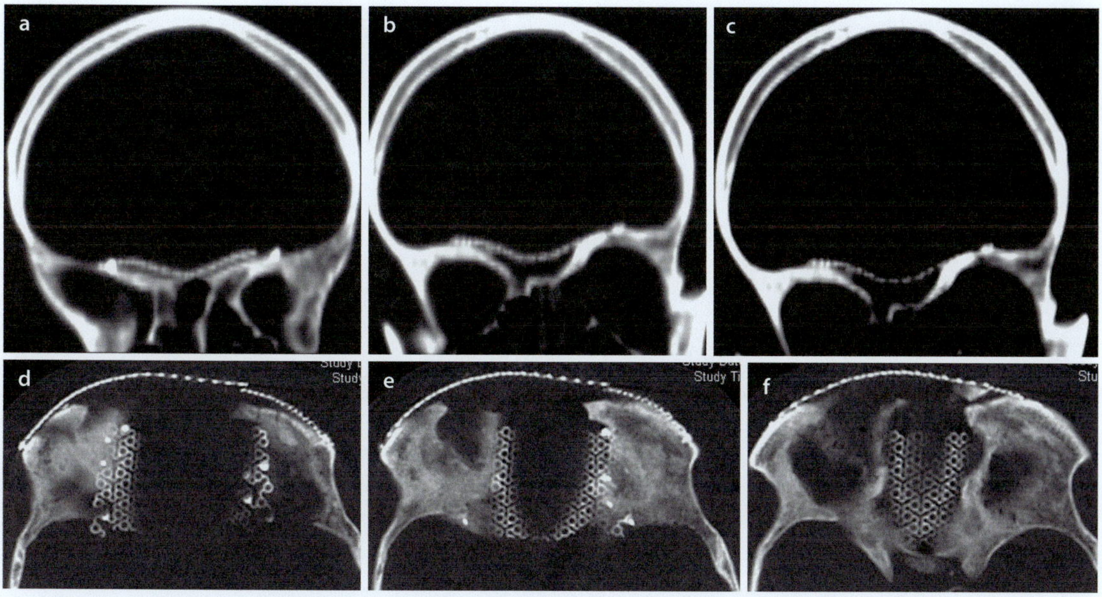

■ **Fig. 4.3** Postoperative result of the patient from ■ Figs. 4.1 and 4.2. Reconstruction of the anterior skull base and the frontal convexity with titanium mesh. Coronal **a–c** and axial **d–f** CT scans (bone window)

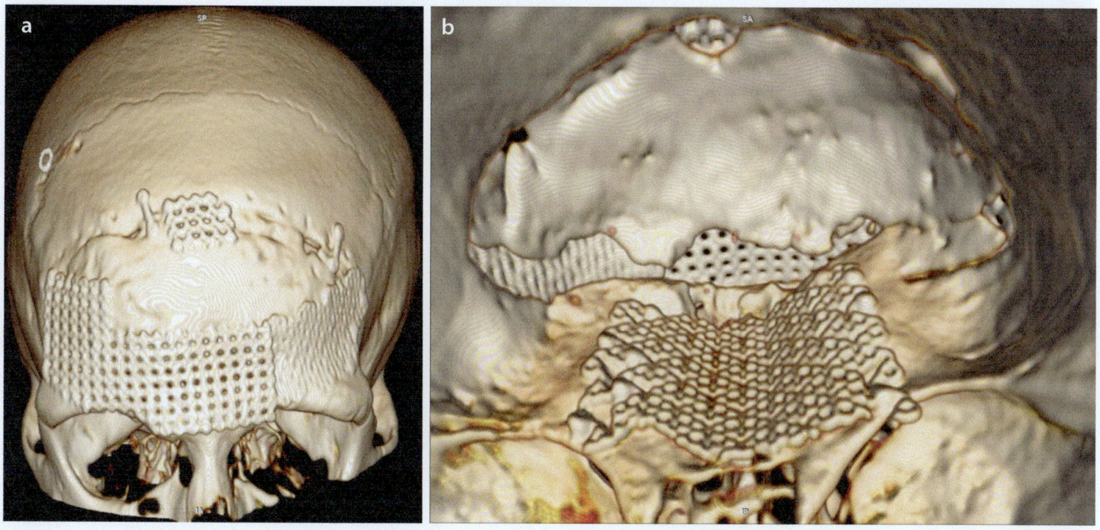

■ **Fig. 4.4** Postoperative result of the patient from ■ Figs. 4.1, 4.2, and 4.3. Reconstruction of the anterior skull base and the frontal convexity with titanium mesh. 3D volume rendering from CT data set

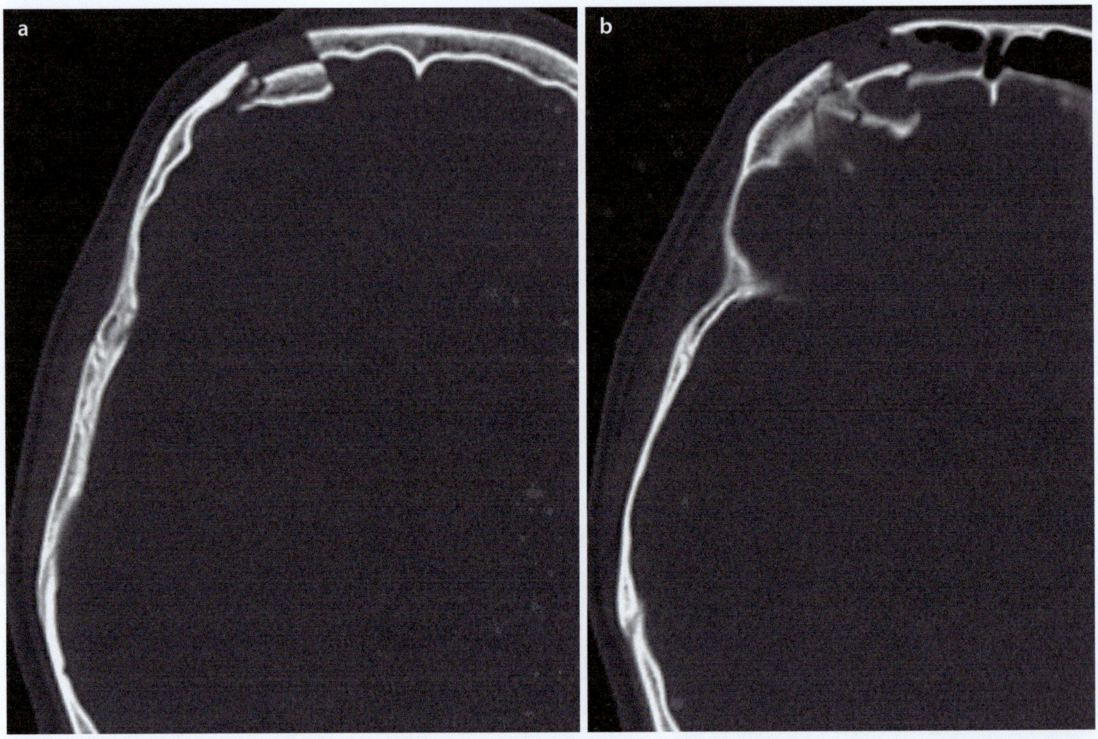

Fig. 4.5 Depressed frontal fracture **a** and frontobasal fracture with involvement of the anterior and posterior wall of the frontal sinus **b** following a motor vehicle accident. Bone window CT scan

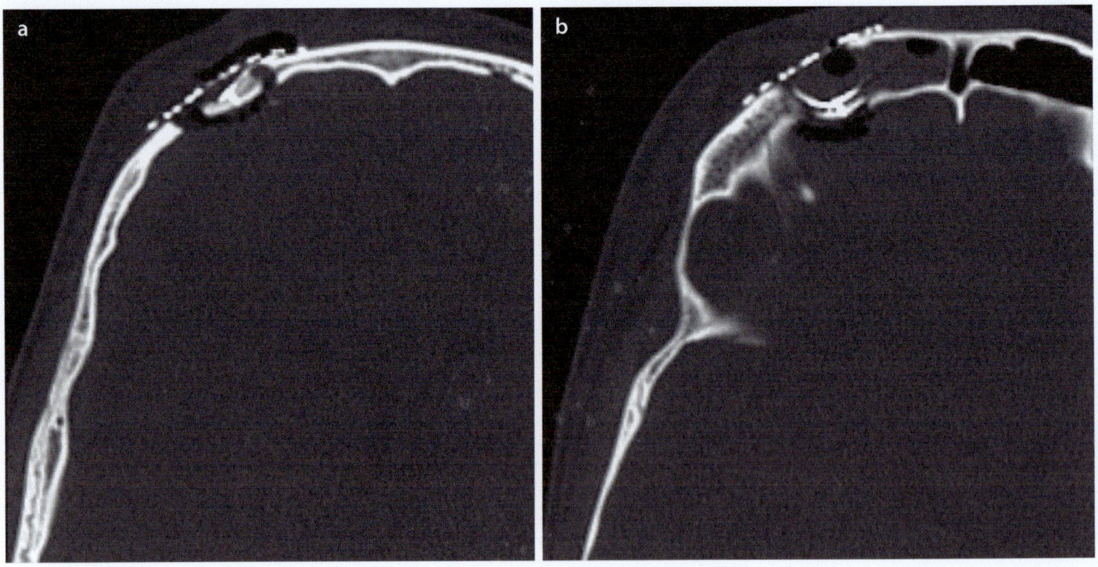

Fig. 4.6 Patient from Fig. 4.5. Postoperative CT scan showing the reconstruction of the convexity of the skull **a** and of the frontal sinus **b**. Bone window CT scan

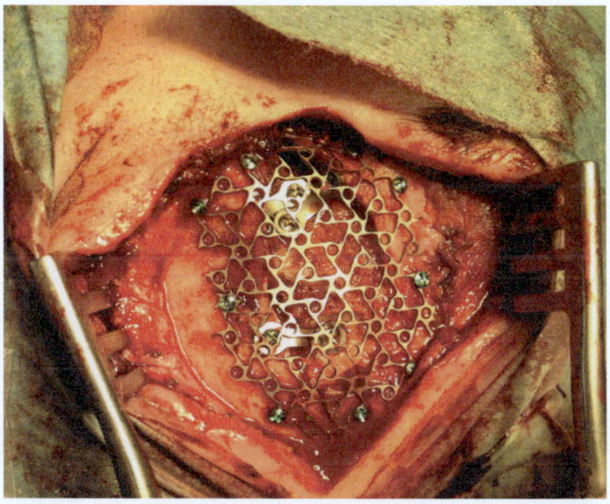

Fig. 4.7 Patient from **Figs.** 4.5 and 4.6. Intraoperative photograph demonstrating reconstruction of the convexity and the frontal sinus. The fragment of the frontal sinus' posterior wall could be refixed. The multiple fragments of the anterior wall had to be replaced by titanium mesh

4.1.5 Surgical Technique of Frontobasal Duraplasty and Cranioplasty

The surgical technique of frontobasal duraplasty is suited for reconstruction of the anterior skull base for traumatic injuries as well as following extensive tumour resections. After a bicoronal skin incision, the galea has to be dissected, reverted inferiorly and fixed with self-retracting hooks. The periosteum and the connective tissue of the aponeurosis of the skull are initially left in place and then dissected from the bone during the next step. This kind of dissection creates a so-called pericranial flap that has the capacity to cover the whole anterior skull base if necessary (Figs. 4.13, 4.14, 4.15, 4.16, and 4.17).

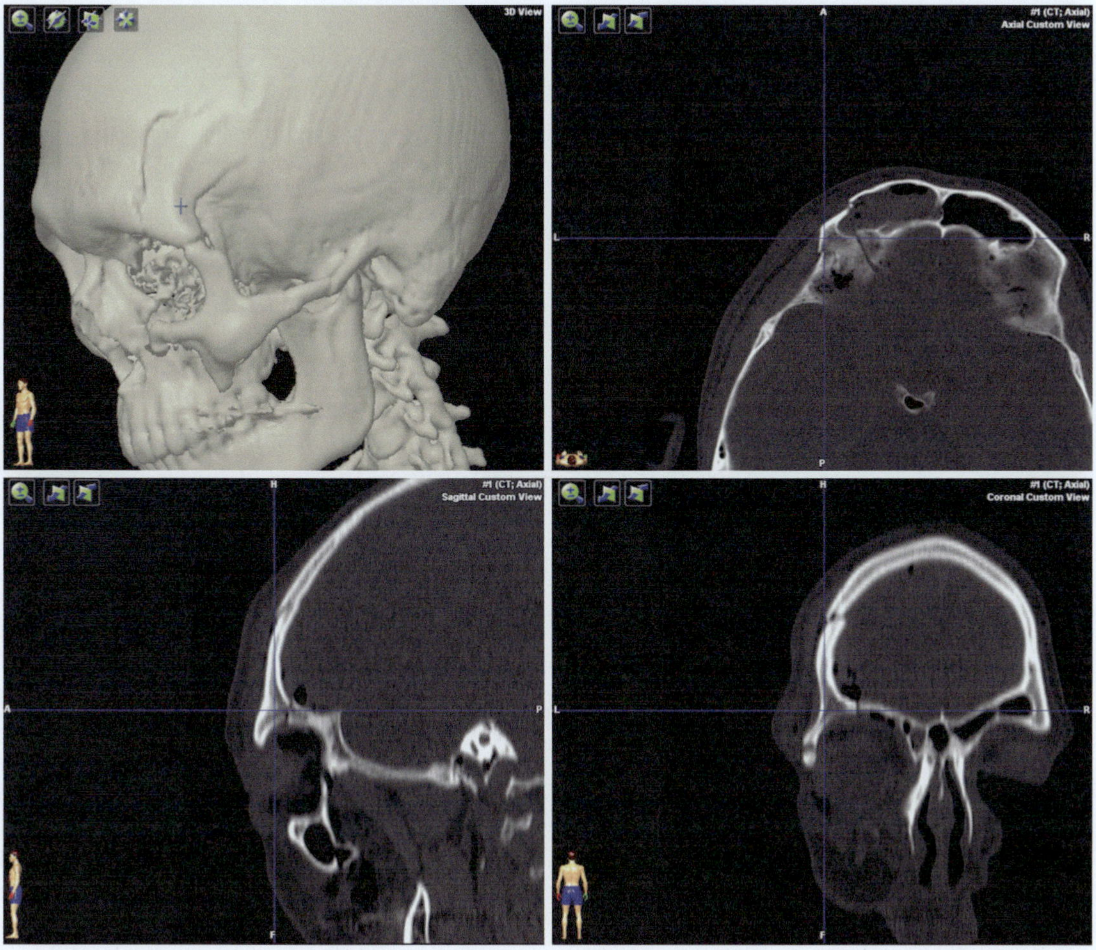

Fig. 4.8 Frontobasal injury including fractures of orbital roof, anterior and posterior wall of the frontal sinus as well as of the midface following a bicycle accident. There are intracranial air bubbles as a sign of skull base injury. 3D volume rendering and CT scan in three planes (bone window)

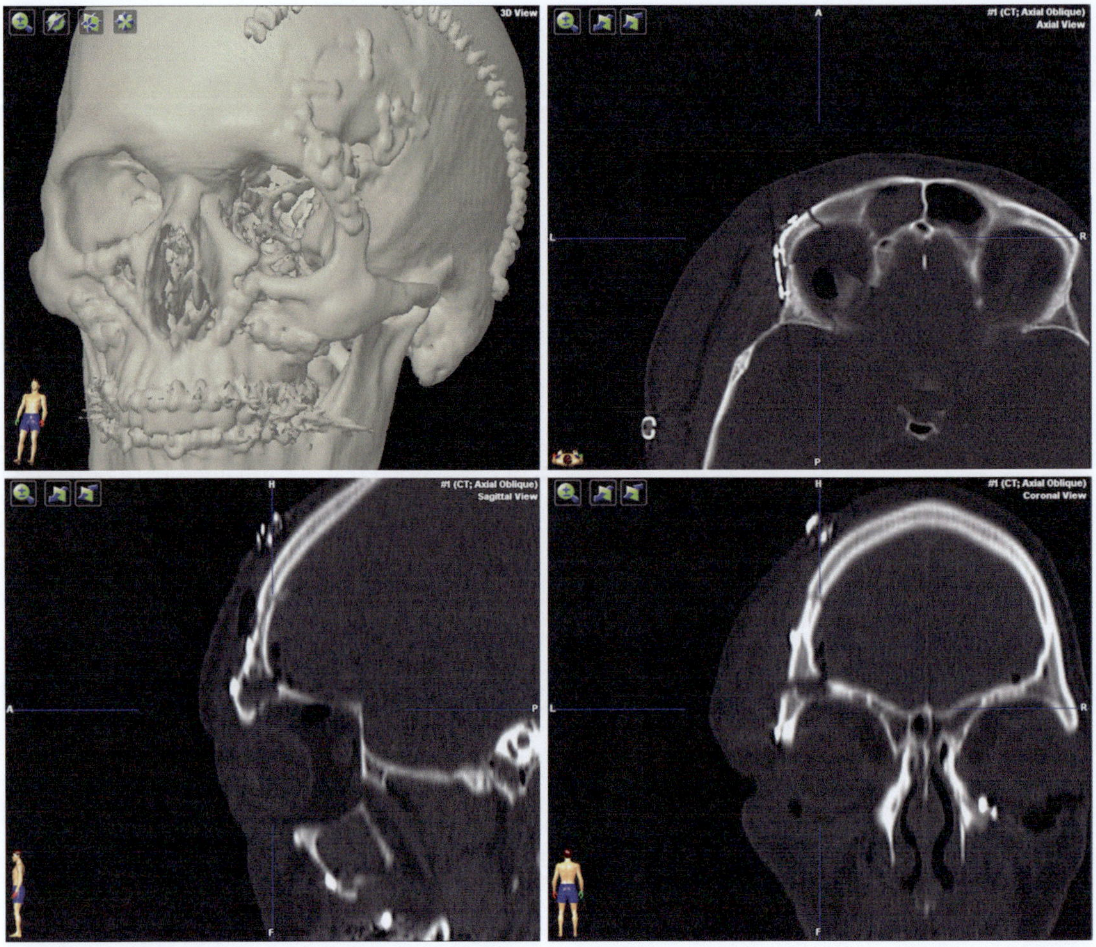

Fig. 4.9 Patient from the previous figure. Status after frontolateral craniotomy with duraplasty and osteosynthetic reconstruction of the frontobasal and midface fractures. 3D volume rendering and CT scan in three planes (bone window)

Usually a single frontal burr hole in the midline just over the superior sagittal sinus is sufficient to perform a bifrontal craniotomy. By using this burr hole, it is then necessary to carefully dissect the dura from the internal table to avoid dural injury or heavy epidural bleeding from an opened superior sagittal sinus during the craniotomy (Figs. 4.18, 4.19, 4.20, 4.21, 4.22, and 4.23).

In supine position gravity will pull the frontal lobes dorsally, and thus it is possible to inspect the anterior skull base using «dynamic» brain retraction with the surgeon's instruments (Figs. 4.24, 4.25, and 4.26). After inspection of the bony defects and dural injuries, the surgical technique to be used is decided upon. In cases of relatively small bony defects, the classical surgical technique is the method of choice even with relatively large dural injuries. In cases of bigger bony defects, especially with mobile fragments, the modified surgical technique as described below will be more successful. In cases of small medial injuries, the transnasal endoscopic technique as used by ENT surgeons is a minimally invasive method with very good results.

When using the classic technique, the dura is opened over the poles of both frontal lobes. The frontobasal dura including the defect(s) is then covered with the pericranial flap. In cases of larger bony injuries and defects (Figs. 4.12, 4.27, 4.28, and 4.29), a modified technique is recommended [11]. The frontopolar dura is not opened, but the frontobasal dura is dissected from the anterior skull base. Afterwards the pericranial flap is put on the anterior skull base and fixed with a

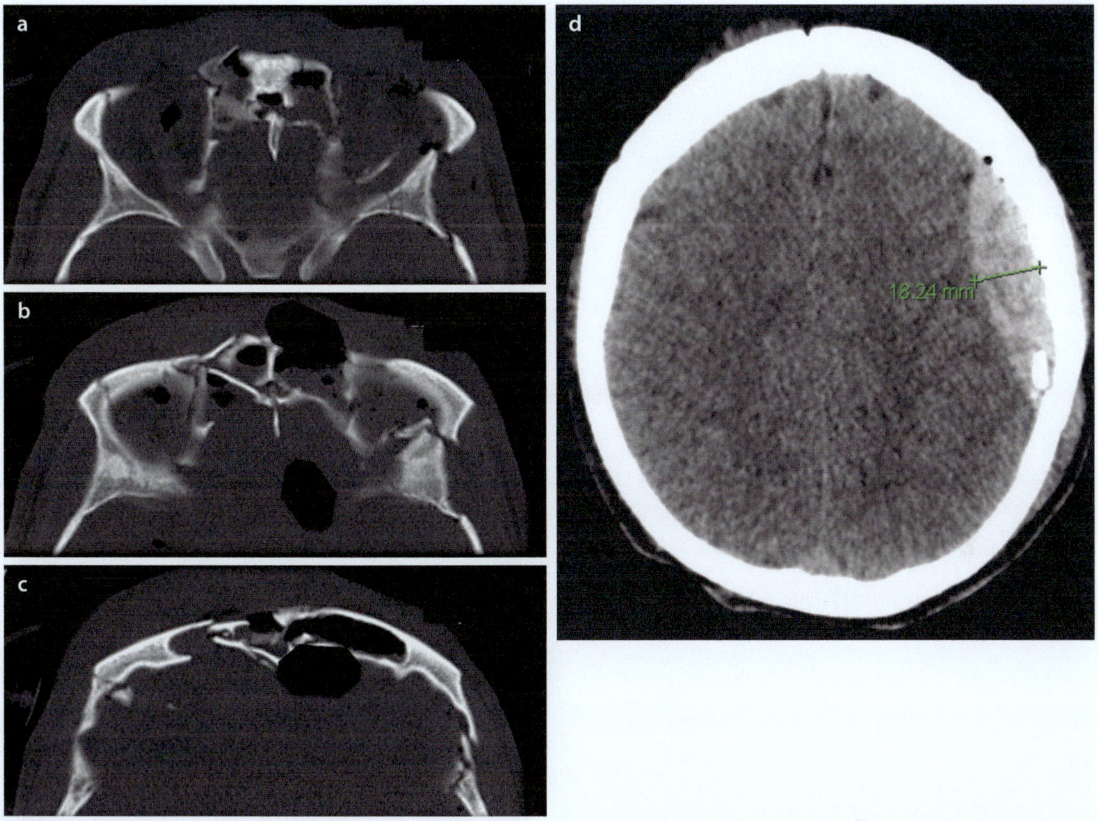

Fig. 4.10 Complex frontobasal injury after a drop from 2 m height with multiple fractures of both orbits **a**, **b**, the frontal sinuses **c** and the frontal convexity of the skull with a left-sided frontolateral epidural haematoma **d**. CT scan with bone window **a**, **b**, **c** and brain window **d**

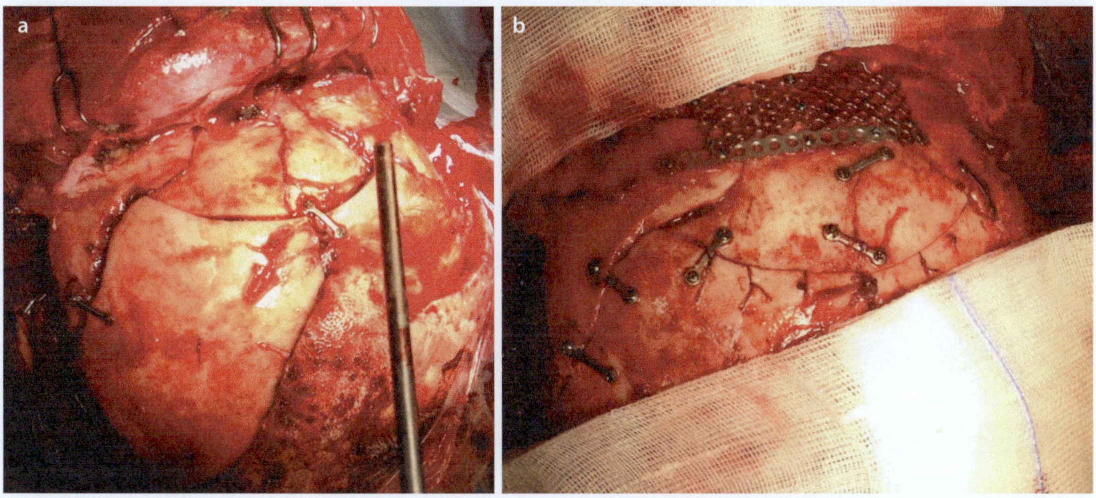

Fig. 4.11 Patient from previous figure. Intraoperative photograph before **a** and after **b** osteosynthetic reconstruction of the complex frontobasal injuries and evacuation of the epidural haematoma. Reconstruction of the frontal convexity with mini-plates and of the anterior wall of the frontal sinus with titanium mesh **b**

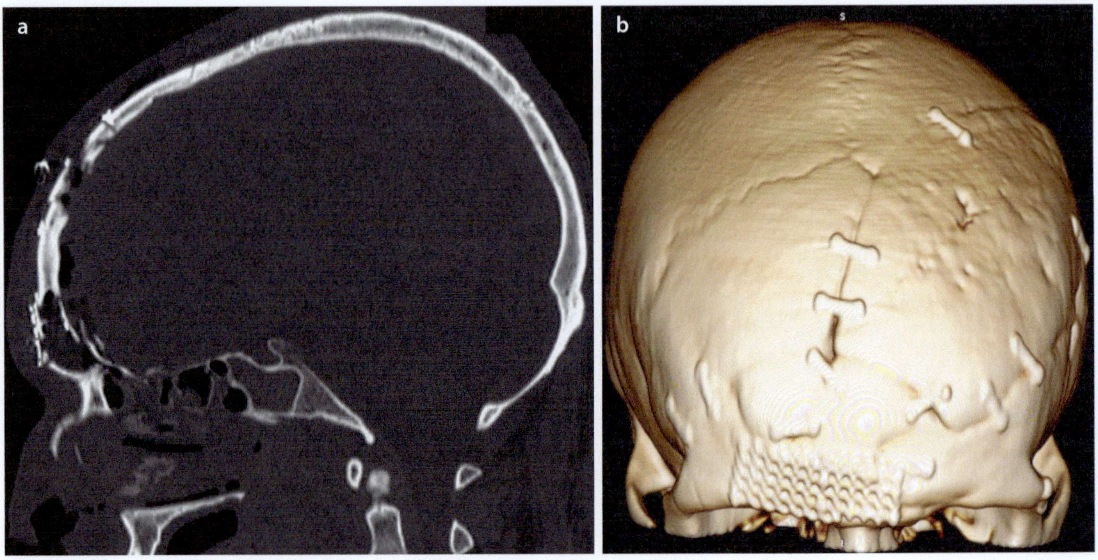

■ **Fig. 4.12** Patient from ■ Figs. 4.11 and 4.12. Postoperative result after reconstruction of the anterior and posterior walls of the frontal sinuses **a** and the frontal convexity **b**. CT scan with bone window **a** and 3D volume rendering **b**

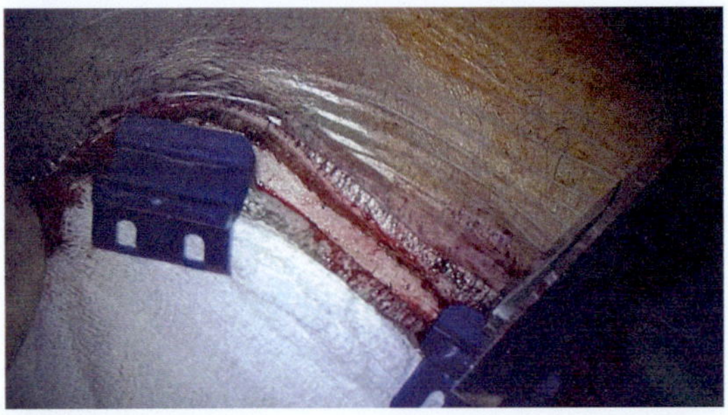

■ **Fig. 4.13** Bifrontal skin incision with the use of LeRoy clips for haemostasis

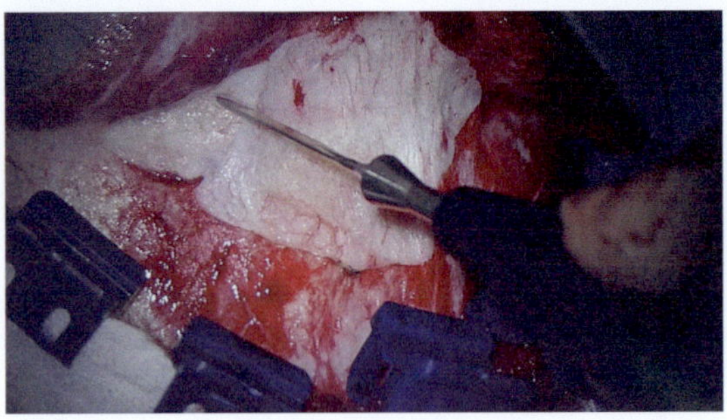

■ **Fig. 4.14** Retraction of the galea and dissection of the pericranial flap with the monopolar

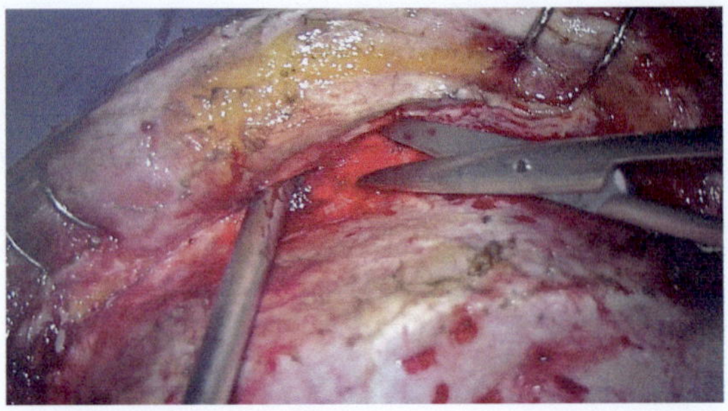

■ **Fig. 4.15** Final dissection of the pericranial flap in the supraorbital region

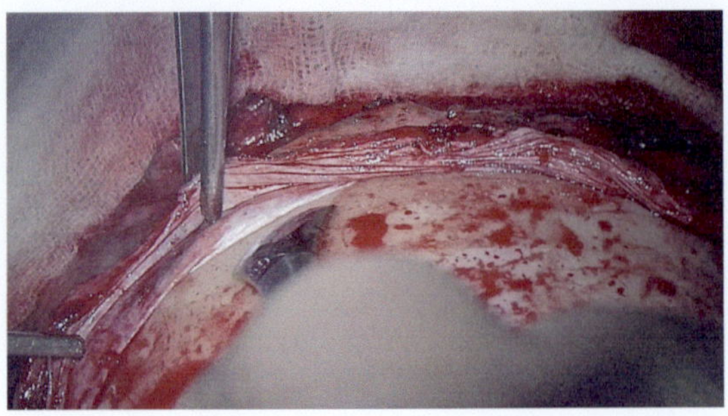

■ **Fig. 4.16** Dissection of the periosteum from the skull

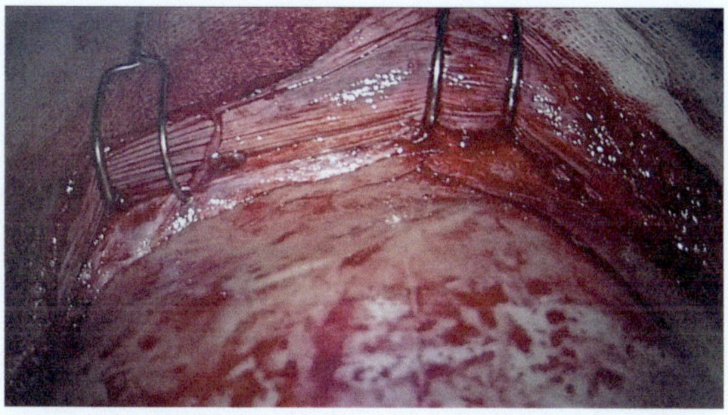

Fig. 4.17 Retraction of the pericranial flap with self-retracting hooks. A supraorbital fracture line can be seen on the right side

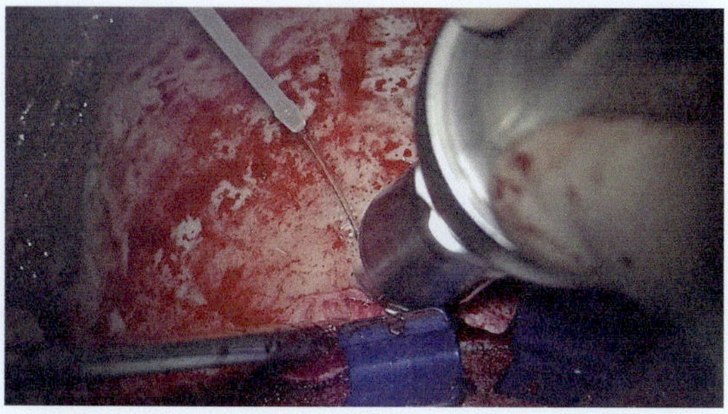

Fig. 4.18 Placement of a burr hole in the midline just above the superior sagittal sinus

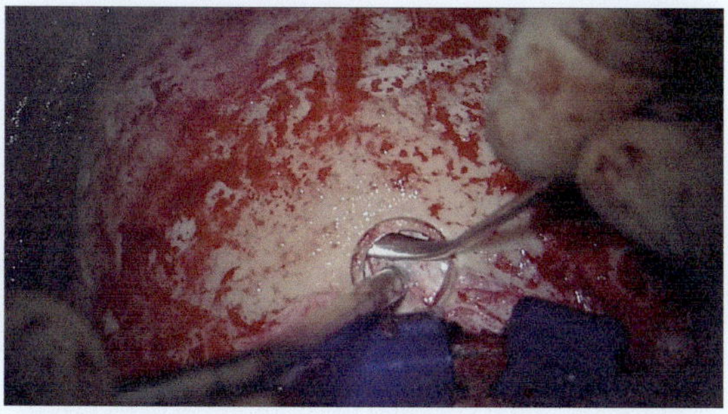

Fig. 4.19 Desiccation of the dura starting from the burr hole in preparation for the craniotome to avoid injury of the dura and/or the superior sagittal sinus

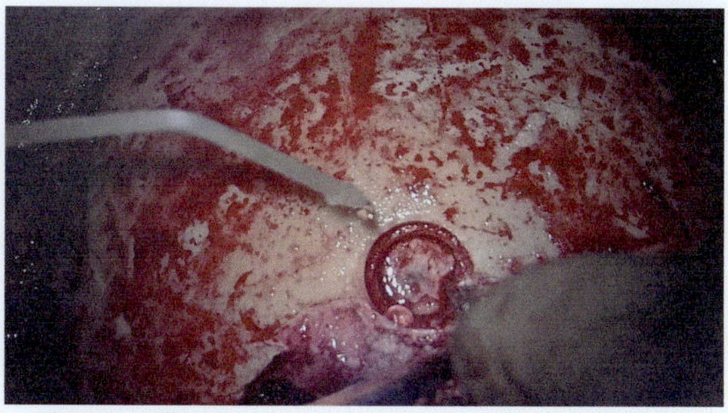

Fig. 4.20 Starting of the craniotomy

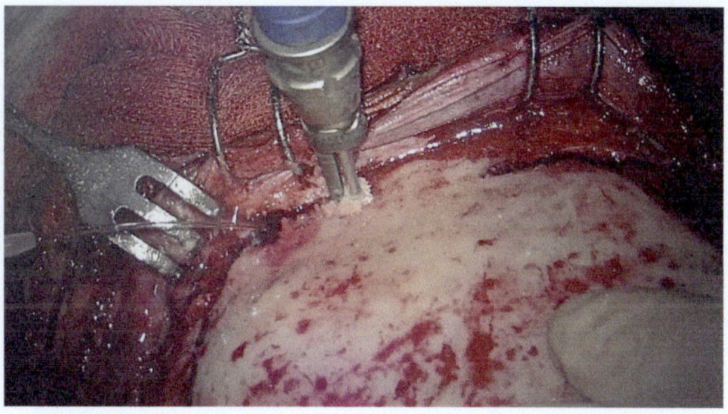

Fig. 4.21 Completion of the craniotomy just above the nasion

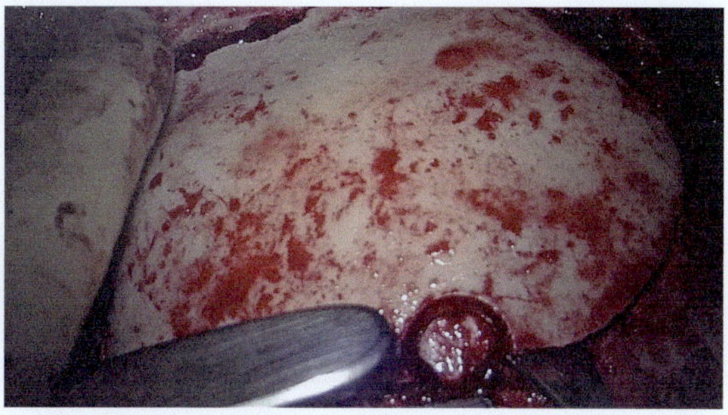

Fig. 4.22 Elevation of the bone flap

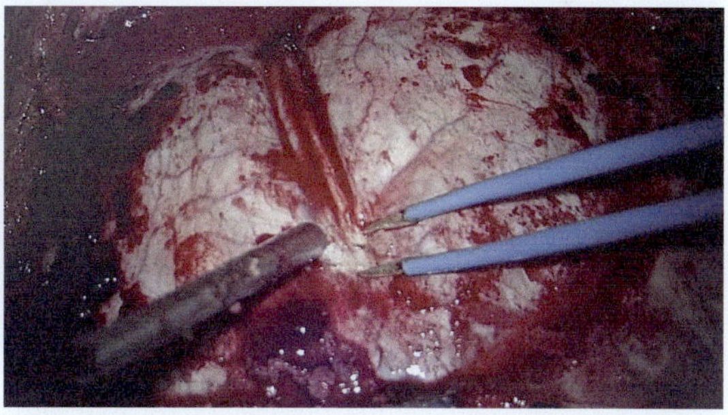

Fig. 4.23 Dural exposure after elevating the bone flap

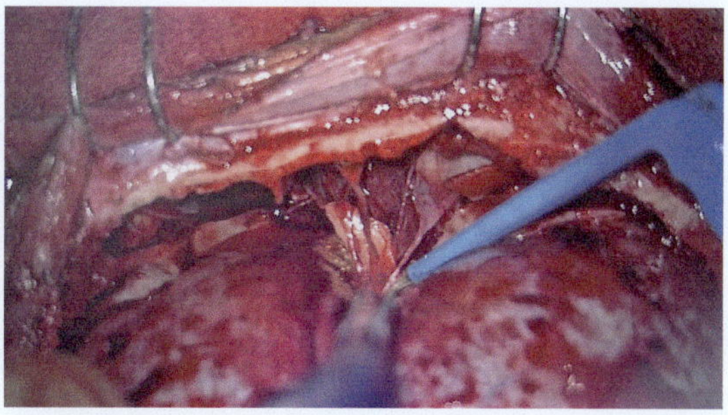

Fig. 4.24 Removal of a fragment of the posterior wall of the frontal sinus

4

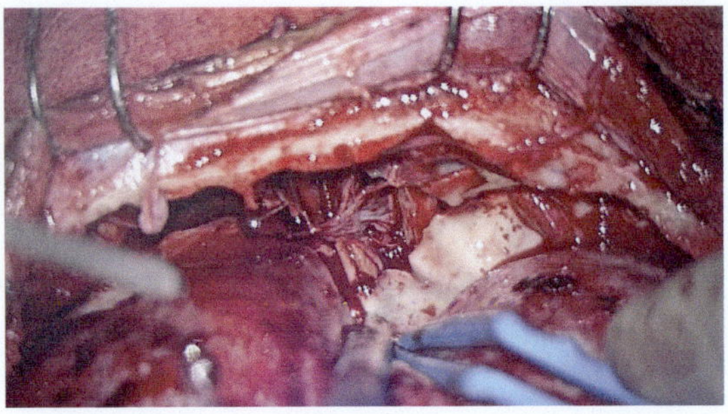

Fig. 4.25 Retraction of the right frontal lobe and inspection of the right orbital roof

tailored piece of titanium mesh that presses the flap against the bone and fastened to the orbital roofs and the planum sphenoidale with screws (Fig. 4.29). This technique provides a safe and efficient seal to the anterior skull base. Finally, the dura covering the frontal lobes is inspected, and any dural tears are closed by covering them with TachoSil™.

If there is a relatively small and lateralised injury, it is possible to modify the surgical intervention to a one-sided craniotomy with selective closure of the defect (Fig. 4.30).

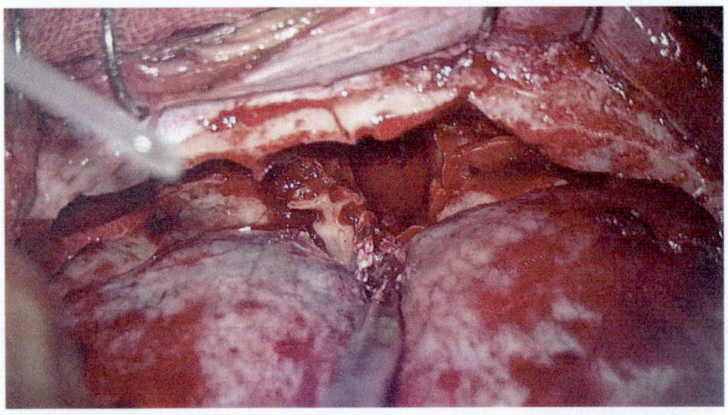

Fig. 4.26 Exposure of a heavy injury of the anterior skull base

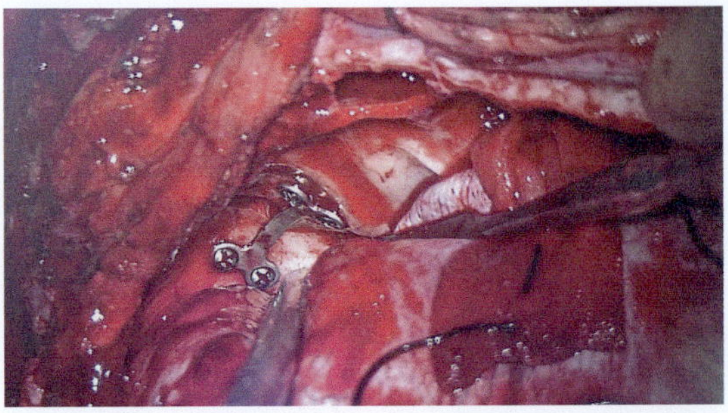

Fig. 4.28 Fixation of the left orbital roof (lateral side)

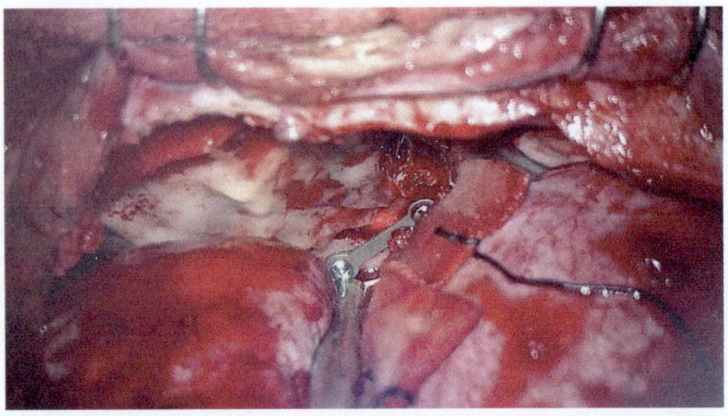

Fig. 4.27 Refixation of the loose left orbital roof with a titanium plate (medial side)

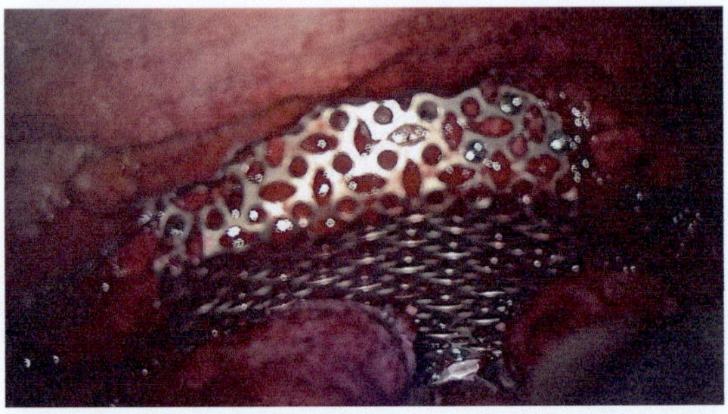

Fig. 4.29 After covering the frontobasal defect with the pericranial flap the anterior skull base is reconstructed with titanium mesh

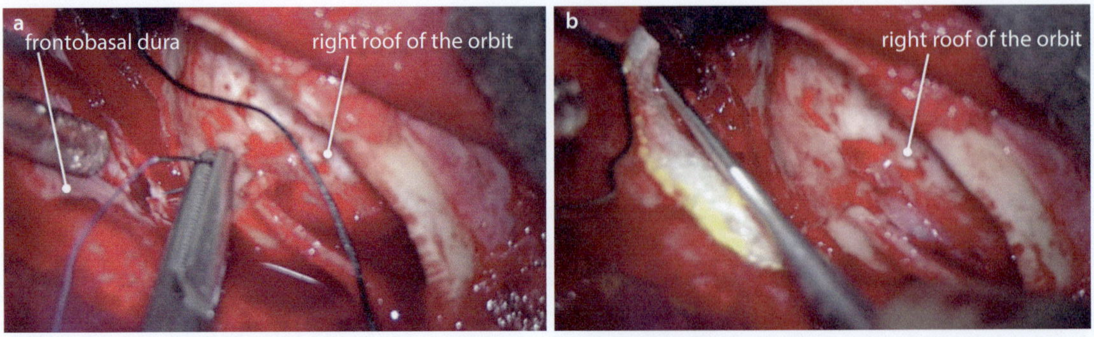

Fig. 4.30 Circumscribed lateralised frontobasal injury on the right side. Therefore, used a lateralised frontal craniotomy for focussed surgical treatment of the defect. Suturing the dural injury **a**. Additional sealing of the dura with TachoSil **b**

4.2 Injuries to the Middle Fossa

4.2.1 General Information

A fracture of the base of the middle fossa has a potential risk to form an epidural haematoma within a few hours due to a rupture of the middle meningeal artery. In cases of an epidural haematoma, an immediate emergency surgery for evacuation is indicated.

Fractures of the petrous bone are evidence of a massive force during the trauma because the petrous bony pyramid is one of the most stable osseous structures in the human body. Besides injuries to the inner ear and the facial nerve, there is also a risk for laterobasal CSF fistula.

If the trauma includes the sella region which is located just medial to the middle fossa, it is crucial to check the CT scan for injuries to the internal carotid artery (usually confirmed on a CT angiogram) because dissections of the intima layer or carotid-cavernous fistulas carry high morbidity.

4.2.2 Clinical Signs

Injuries of the middle fossa, the sella region or the lateral skull base are often asymptomatic and are primarily diagnosed on the initial trauma CT scan.

Possible clinical signs of fractures of the petrous bone are:

- Postauricular haematoma
- CSF leak from the ear (in case of ruptured eardrum) or from the nose (through the Eustachian tube)
- Meningitis if CSF leak persists
- Hearing impairment, dead ear or vertigo due to an injury of the inner ear
- Facial nerve palsy (more frequent in transverse than in longitudinal fractures of the petrous bone)

The severity of a facial nerve palsy is classified using the House and Brackmann scale, which has therapeutic and clinical relevance (◘ Table 4.2).

◘ Table 4.2 House-Brackmann facial nerve grading system [9, 14]

Grade	Function	At rest	Motion		
			Forehead	Eye	Mouth
I: Normal	Normal facial function in all areas	Normal	Normal	Normal	Normal
II: Mild dysfunction	Slight weakness noticeable on close inspection; may have very slight synkinesis	Normal symmetry and tone	Moderate to good function	Complete closure with minimum effort	Slight asymmetry
III: Moderate dysfunction	Obvious but not disfiguring difference between two sides; noticeable but not severe synkinesis, contracture, and/or hemifacial spasm	Normal symmetry and tone	Slight to moderate movement	Complete closure with effort	Slightly weak with maximum effort
IV: Moderately severe dysfunction	Obvious weakness and/or disfiguring asymmetry	Normal symmetry and tone	None	Incomplete closure	Asymmetric with maximum effort
V: Severe dysfunction	Only barely perceptible motion	Asymmetry	None	Incomplete closure	Sight movement
VI: Total paralysis	No movement	Loss of tone	None	None	None

Fractures of the base of the middle fossa with symptomatic injury of the greater petrosal nerve are very rare. It leads to disorders of the secretion of the lacrimal glands and the mucosa of the nasopharynx which are of variable clinical relevance.

Injuries in the sella region and/or of the cavernous sinus can cause damage of the cranial nerves III, IV and VI causing ophthalmoplegia or strabismus. A special kind of injury is the carotid-cavernous fistula. In this case, the trauma causes an arteriovenous shunt between the internal carotid artery and the cavernous sinus leading to congestion of the episcleral veins.

Typical clinical signs are:

- Chemosis
- Pulsating exophthalmos
- Loss of vision
- Ophthalmoplegia with diplopia
- Bruit over the globe

Severe fractures of the middle fossa may cause bleeding from the fracture itself or from a ruptured middle meningeal artery leading to an epidural haematoma. This is often asymptomatic during the first hour(s) after trauma but secondarily leads to a loss of consciousness after an interval of normal lucidity. In cases of a rapid development of an epidural haematoma, an ipsilateral dilated pupil may develop due to herniation of the temporal lobe and consecutive pressure on the oculomotor nerve. This is an acute life-threatening situation and an indication for emergency surgical intervention.

4.2.3 Investigations

Typical findings are thin fracture lines of the skull base in the bone window CT scan (Fig. 4.31). If there are additional injuries of the thorax, abdomen or extremities requiring further sedation and ventilation, a clinical neurological evaluation will not be possible. Thus, it is necessary to perform a control CT scan after 6 h to exclude a fracture-associated epidural haematoma.

In cases of clinical signs of facial nerve palsy a referral to the ENT service for an EMG of the facial nerve is necessary to assess the severity of the nerve injury. The EMG findings will guide the decision for further intervention. Furthermore, it is useful to perform an audiogram to diagnose any related damage of the inner ear.

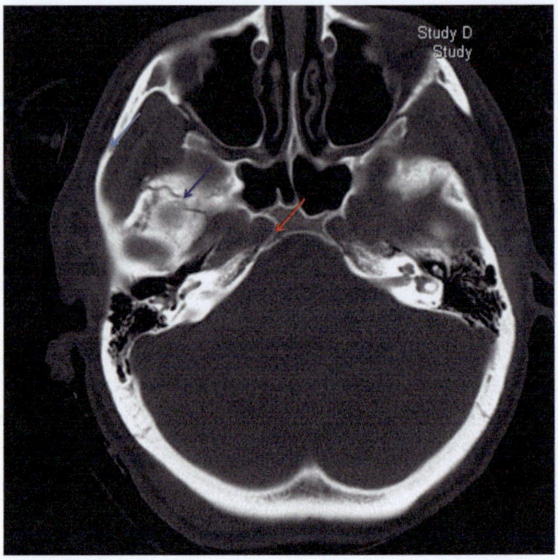

Fig. 4.31 Fracture of the right temporal skull base (*dark blue arrow*) involving the carotid canal medially (*red arrow*) and with a fracture of the zygomatic arch laterally (*light blue arrow*). CT scan bone windows

If there are fracture lines into the carotid canal on the initial CT scan, it is crucial to perform a CT angiogram to exclude a dissection of the internal carotid artery.

In cases of clinical signs of a carotid-cavernous fistula, a conventional angiogram of cerebral blood vessels is indicated with the view to provide treatment via stenting and/or coil embolisation within the same angiographic session if required.

4.2.4 Therapeutic Options

Emergency surgical evacuation is indicated in cases of a space-occupying epidural haematoma with clinical and radiological signs of uncal herniation. The standard therapy is a temporal craniotomy with evacuation of the haematoma, application of dural tack-up sutures and insertion of an epidural drain for 2 days.

Nevertheless, in most cases of fractures of the temporal skull base, treatment remains conservative. Surgery is indicated in cases of a CSF leak from the ear or the nose (see above). The surgery is performed by ENT surgeons (transmastoid approach) or neurosurgeons (subtemporal approach) depending on the location and extent of the laterobasal injury.

If an immediate posttraumatic facial nerve palsy is present with confirmed acute denervation

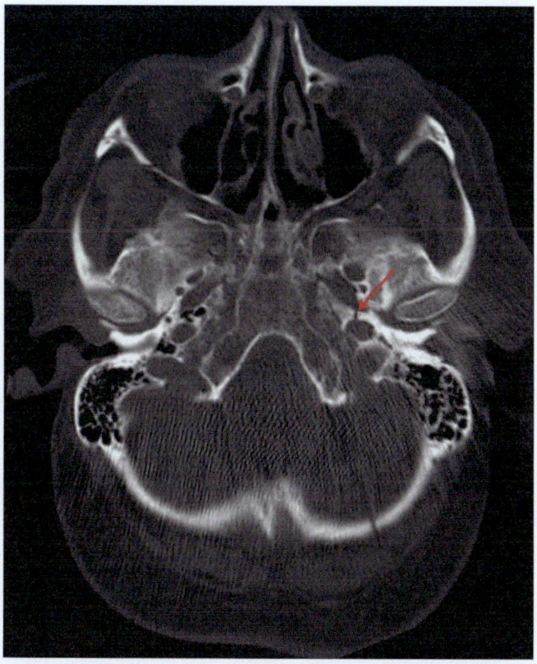

Fig. 4.32 Fracture of the left lateral skull base involving the carotid canal (*arrow*). CT scan in bone window

on EMG, a surgical decompression of the facial nerve by an ENT surgeon is indicated. Besides a decompression alone, it can be necessary to perform an anastomosis with or without a nerve transplant or a hypoglossofacial anastomosis.

In cases of a laterobasal fracture involving the carotid canal (Fig. 4.32) with evidence of intimal injury of the internal carotid artery (see above), an intravenous heparin infusion should be commenced.

4.3 Injuries of the Posterior Fossa

4.3.1 General Information

An epidural haematoma is the most threatening condition following a fracture in the posterior fossa that may cause mass effect on the cerebellum and brainstem with consecutive loss of consciousness. In such a case, emergency surgery is indicated via a suboccipital craniotomy and evacuation of the epidural haematoma. The surgeon needs to be aware that an epidural haematoma in the posterior fossa may arise from a tear of the dural venous sinus.

Fractures involving the occipital condyles combined with fractures of the atlas or axis may result in instability of the craniocervical junction, which influences the surgical treatment options (see ► Sect. 4.4).

4.3.2 Clinical Signs

Posterior fossa fractures without dislocation and without injury to the cerebellum or brainstem are asymptomatic in most cases and are diagnosed radiologically. In cases of severe injuries, these clinical signs may occur:

- Persisting occipital headaches or nuchal pain
- Nausea and vertigo
- Primary loss of consciousness in cases of brainstem contusions
- Secondary loss of consciousness in cases of an epidural haematoma
- Ataxia, dysmetria, disorders of coordination and other cerebellar symptoms following contusions of the cerebellum
- Dysphagia and abnormal coughing reflex after injury of the 9th and 10th cranial nerve

4.3.3 Investigations

A CT scan during the initial trauma check will demonstrate skull fractures and may reveal an epidural haematoma. In cases of injuries involving the craniocervical junction, it is necessary to perform a CT angiogram to rule out injury to the vertebral arteries. If it is not possible to rule out such an injury, an angiogram of the vertebral arteries may be required.

Fractures crossing the transverse or the sigmoid sinus can lead to an injury to their lumen leading to sinus thrombosis and venous obstruction. A thrombosis can be diagnosed on a CT or MR angiogram with imaging of the venous phase, and the diagnosis holds significant relevance to treatment (see below).

4.3.4 Therapeutic Options

Most cases of fractures of the posterior skull base are treated conservatively, especially if the fracture is not dislocated (Fig. 4.33). As discussed above, it may be necessary to repeat the cranial CT scan after 6 h to exclude an epidural haematoma if the patient is sedated and ventilated allowing only a

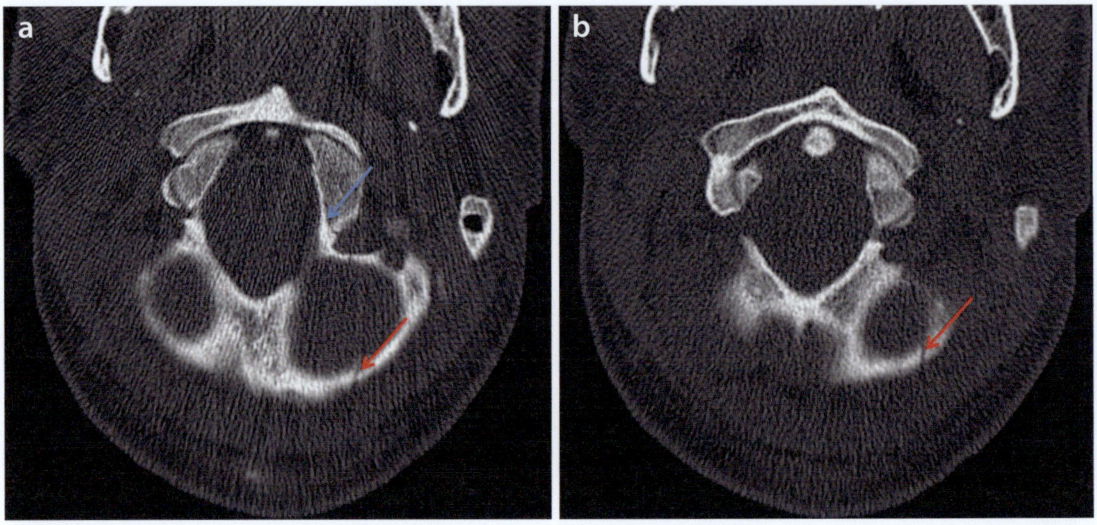

Fig. 4.33 Fracture of the suboccipital skull base on the left side (*red arrows*) with involvement of the occipital condyle (*blue arrow*). CT scan, bone window

limited neurological assessment. Epidural haematomas with a thickness more than the thickness of the skull should be evacuated immediately, especially when associated with clinical or radiological deterioration.

If there is radiological evidence of a fracture-associated thrombosis of a dural venous sinus, an intravenous heparin infusion is indicated to avoid a venous infarction of the brain. Thrombosis in this region significantly affects the drainage of the superior sagittal and straight sinus.

4.4 Injuries of the Craniocervical Junction

4.4.1 General Information

The craniocervical junction is the bony, vascular and neural interface between the skull base and the spine. Thus, injuries to the craniocervical junction with consecutive instability and dislocation are potentially life-threatening. In general, there are injuries of bony and/or ligamentous structures.

Fractures in this region affect the occipital condyles as well as the first and second vertebrae (the atlas and axis). Ligamentous injuries mainly affect the alar ligaments, the transverse ligament of the atlas and the apical ligament of the dens as well as the capsules of the atlanto-occipital joint and the atlanto-axial joint.

Fractures of the atlas are classified using Gehweiler's scale. Type I and II are isolated fractures of the anterior and posterior arch of the atlas, respectively. Type III is a combined fracture of the anterior and posterior arch of the atlas (also known as a Jefferson's fracture), which is a very unstable condition because there is always an additional ligamentous injury (Fig. 4.34). The rare type IV and V fractures are fractures of the lateral masses and the transverse processes, respectively (Bühren 2013).

Fractures of the dens of the axis are classified using the Anderson and D'Alonso grading. A fracture of the tip of the dens (type I) is associated with a tear out of the alar ligaments and is classified as stable. The most frequent fracture, type II (more than 60% of cases), goes through the base of the dens and is considered unstable. A type III fracture involves the corpus axis and is also unstable.

Fractures through the roots of the vertebral arch of the axis are classified using the Effendi grading: no dislocation (type I), dislocation of more than 3 mm (type II) and complete luxation of the second against the third vertebra with catching of the facet joints (type III) (Bühren 2013).

Any unstable biomechanical injury is an indication for surgery (see below). Through the years, newer imaging modalities (CT, MRI, angiogram) and more advanced surgical techniques have helped to provide individually adapted operative solutions that have replaced the protracted immobilising procedures of the past.

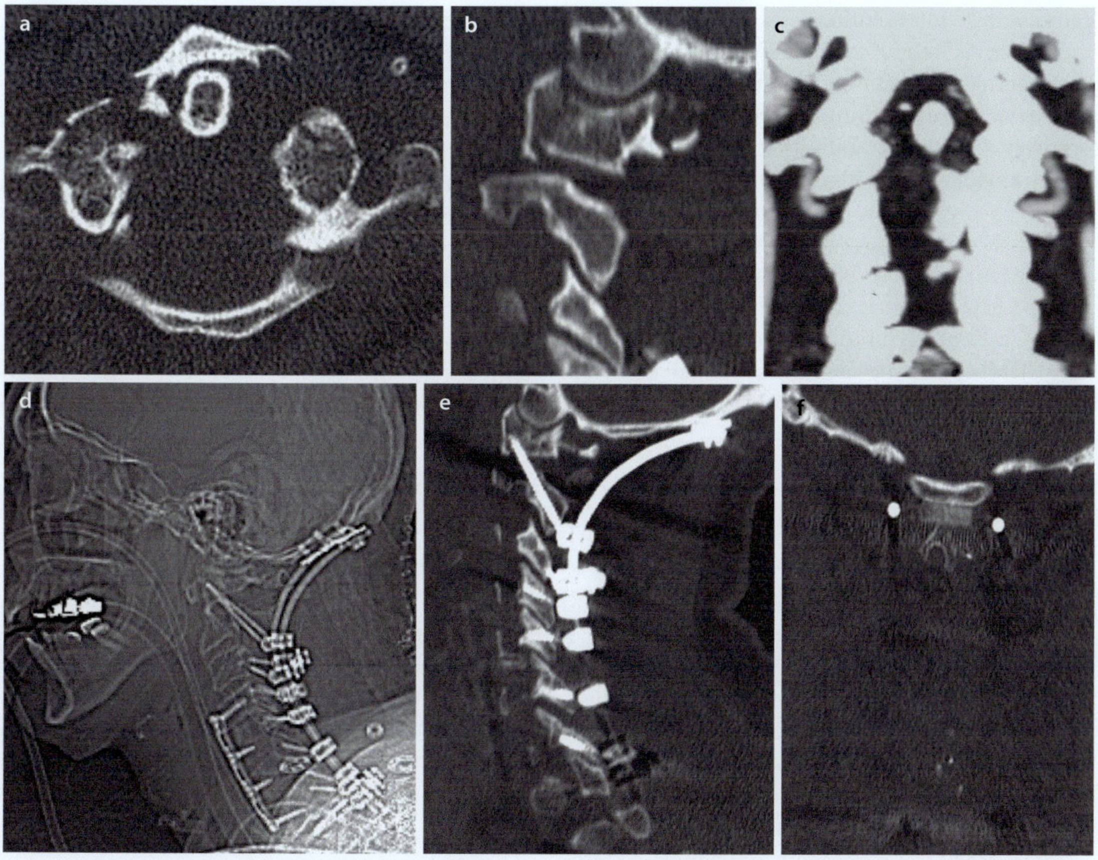

Fig. 4.34 Multiple fractures of the atlas with involvement of lateral masses on both sides (Gehweiler type III and IV), CT with bone window, axial **a** and sagittal plane **b**. Preoperative CT angiogram for the visualisation of the vertebral arteries **c**. Postoperative visualisation of the whole dorsoventral instrumentation in a case of complex injury and instability of the cervical spine, CT topography **d**. Transarticular screwing of C1 and C2 as well as an occipital plate fixation and lateral mass fusion of the cervical spine caudally, sagittal CT scan in bone window **e**. Alloplastic bone graft implant between the vertebral arches of C1 and C2 for improved bony fusion, coronal CT scan in bone window **f**

4.4.2 Clinical Signs

In most cases, injuries of the craniocervical junction are diagnosed radiologically during the trauma workup CT scan because the patient requires sedation and ventilation due to the severity of injuries.

Awake patients report persisting neck pain due to osseoligamentous injury. Neurological deficits are rare because the spinal canal is relatively wide at the level of the craniocervical junction.

If instability and dislocation lead to compression of the spinal cord or the medulla oblongata, these injuries usually have a fatal outcome.

4.4.3 Investigations

The initial CT scan shows fractures and dislocations at the craniocervical junction. If there is a complex injury, an MRI should be considered to diagnose ligamentous injuries, ruptures of intervertebral discs of the cervical spine or fracture-associated spinal epidural haematomas.

By performing a CT angiogram, ideally during the initial trauma scan, a dissection of the vertebral arteries should be excluded. If the CT angiogram leaves any doubt, a conventional angiogram is required to confirm the diagnosis and to indicate anticoagulation therapy or radiological intervention. Furthermore, a CT angiogram is helpful to visualise the course of the vertebral arteries at the craniocervical junction and detect a high-riding vertebral artery preoperatively if surgical stabilisation is indicated [3]. If there is evidence of a high-riding vertebral artery, there is a higher risk of intraoperative injury to this vessel during surgery, with higher risk using transarticular screw placement to C1/C2 than with pedicle screws at C2 [16].

In cases of asymptomatic injuries, the degree of instability can be assessed by a lateral functional X-ray examination to plan the further treatment of the patient.

4.4.4 Therapeutic Options

During the emergency treatment, the neck and cervical spine is immobilised safely by using a Stiffneck™ orthosis (Laerdal, Puchheim, Germany). If instability of the craniocervical junction is diagnosed, the orthosis must be left on until surgical stabilisation. If the injury is considered stable, conservative treatment may be continued with a soft collar (Param GmbH, Hamburg, Germany).

Because of improvements in diagnostic methods and surgical treatment options over the last decade, the use of the halo-vest brace for the treatment of instabilities of the craniocervical junction has decreased.

In cases of proven instability, the best option in a patient in good medical condition is always an osteosynthetic stabilisation that aims to restabilise the spine, improve neurological deficits and treat potential deformities.

Isolated and therefore stable fractures of the vertebral arch of the atlas (Gehweiler type I and II) and fractures of the apex of the dens (type I by Anderson and D'Alonzo) are treated conservatively by a soft orthosis. Type II fractures of the dens of the axis can be surgically treated by a classical dens screw osteosynthesis if there is no evidence of osteoporosis.

In all other cases, there are a variety of anterior and posterior fusion techniques for the surgical treatment of unstable fractures of C1 and C2 [10]. For complex, multisegmental and highly unstable injuries, the occipitocervical fusion with transarticular screwing of C1 and C2 is the safest method (◘ Fig. 4.34).

4.4.5 Surgical Technique for the Occipitocervical Fusion

Firstly, the lateral mass screws need to be placed, beginning from C3 and then moving caudally. The number of levels depends on the extension of the cervical spine's injury. The transarticular screw fusion of C1/C2 starts at the caudal portion of the facets of C2.

The trajectory of the drilling is relatively steep in a cranial direction. The trajectory is checked with lateral fluoroscopy. The correct trajectory in the coronal plane is verified with a dissector that is placed into the joint space of C1/C2. After the drill has gone through the C2 vertebra, it needs to be verified through contact with the dissector; otherwise there will be a lateral or medial bias. In this case, the direction of the drilling needs to be corrected. If the joint space is reached correctly, the drilling can be continued into the lateral mass of C1. This step is also checked with lateral fluoroscopy. After fixation of the occipital plate, the fusion can be completed by placing the connecting rods into the polyaxial screw heads and fixing them into position (◘ Fig. 4.34).

References

1. Bernal-Sprekelsen M, Rioja E, Enseñat J, Enriquez K, Viscovich L, Agredo-Lemos FE, Alobid I. Management of anterior skull base defect depending on its size and location. Biomed Res Int. 2014;2014:346873. https://doi.org/10.1155/2014/346873. Epub 2014 May 7.
2. Biron VL, Gross M, Broad R, Seikaly H, Wright ED. Radial forearm free flap with titanium mesh sandwich reconstruction in complex anterior skull base defects. J Craniofac Surg. 2012;23(6):1763–5.
3. Peng CW, Chou BT, Bendo JA, Spivak JM. Vertebral artery injury in cervical spine surgery: anatomical considerations, management, and preventive measures. Spine J. 2009;9:70–6.
4. Chin D, Harvey RJ. Endoscopic reconstruction of frontal, cribiform and ethmoid skull base defects. Adv Otorhinolaryngol. 2013;74:104–18.
5. Eloy JA, Patel SK, Shukla PA, Smith ML, Choudhry OJ, Liu JK. Triple-layer reconstruction technique for large cribriform defects after endoscopic endonasal resection of anterior skull base tumors. Int Forum Allergy Rhinol. 2013;3(3):204–11.
6. Giovannetti F, Ruggeri A, Buonaccorsi S, Pichierri A, Valentini V. Endoscopic endonasal approaches for cerebrospinal fluid leaks repair. J Craniofac Surg. 2013;24(2):548–53.
7. Hausamen JE, Schmidseder R Beteiligung der vorderen Schädelbasis bei Frakturen des Mittelgesichts.

In: Schuchardt K (editor) Fortschr Kiefer GesichtsChir, Bd XIX. Stuttgart/New York: Thieme; 1975. p. 134–6.
8. Hausamen JE, Machtens E, Reuther J, Eufinger H, Kübler A, Schliephake H. Mund-, Kiefer- und Gesichtschirurgie. Operationslehre und –atlas. Berlin Heidelberg: Springer; 2012. p. 240–1.
9. House JW, Brackmann DE. Facial nerve grading system. Otolaryngol Head Neck Surg. 1985;93:146–7.
10. Josten C. Halswirbelsäule. In: Bühren B, Josten C, editors. Chirurgie der verletzten Wirbelsäule. Berlin Heidelberg: Springer; 2013. p. 137–74.
11. König SA, Ranguis S, Gramlich V, Spetzger U. Reconstruction of the anterior skull base after major trauma or extensive tumour resection. Acta Neurochir. 2015;157:139–44.
12. Mielke D, Mayfrank L, Psychogios MN, Rohde V. The anterior interhemispheric approach – a safe and effective approach to anterior skull base lesions. Acta Neurochir. 2014;156(4):689–96.
13. Oberascher G. Diagnostik der Rhinoliquorrhoe. Eur Arch Otorhinolaryngol Suppl. 1993;1:485–92.
14. Reiß M. Facharztwissen HNO-Heilkunde. Berlin Heidelberg: Springer; 2009. p. 910–4.
15. Wolf G, Greistorfer K, Stammberger H. Der endoskopische Nachweis von Liquorfisteln mittels der Floureszeintechnik. Ein Erfahrungsbericht über 925 Fälle. Laryngorhinootologie. 1997;76(10):588–94.
16. Yeom JS, Buchowski JM, Kim HJ, Chang BS, Lee CK, Riew KD. Risk of vertebral artery injury: comparison between C1-C2 transarticular and C2 pedicle screws. Spine J. 2013;13(7):775–85.

Tumors of the Skull Base

The original version of this chapter was revised. An erratum to this chapter can be found at https://doi.org/10.1007/978-3-319-64018-1_9

Electronic Supplementary Material The online version of this chapter (https://doi.org/10.1007/978-3-319-64018-1_5) contains supplementary material, which is available to authorized users.

A. König, U. Spetzger (eds.), *Surgery of the Skull Base*,
https://doi.org/10.1007/978-3-319-64018-1_5

5

Editor's Comment
Uwe Spetzger

The big chapter about tumors of the skull base demonstrates the different aspects and neurosurgical techniques by renowned and very experienced skull base surgeons in a compact form. Due to the consecutive illustration with corresponding intraoperative photographic images, every single step of even complex surgical procedures can be reproduced and understood underlining the didactic value of the book. By means of the different tumor entities, the different surgical approaches including their advantages and disadvantages are demonstrated. The surgical and further strategies are explained from a practical point of view by using selected clinical cases as examples.

Due to the large surgical expertise of Uta Schick from Münster, the chapter about skull base-related gliomas of the optic pathway and the hypothalamus was integrated right after the chapter about skull base meningiomas.

The team of Copenhagen University neurosurgery and in particular Kåre Fugleholm and Lars Poulsgaard describe the neurosurgical treatment of acoustic neuromas including different surgical approaches as well as complication management including reconstruction procedures of the facial nerve in detail.

The group of Pierre Roche from Marseille gives a comprehensive overview of the therapy of skull base chordomas in which the focus is on the didactic explanation of microsurgical anatomy and different approaches to the clivus.

By means of seven selected clinical cases, the complexity and individualization of approach planning for microsurgical resection of craniopharyngiomas are demonstrated by Torstein Meling from Oslo. In this chapter, surgical and modern alternative therapeutic options are explained in detail.

The huge surgical expertise of Takanori Fukushima and the skull base group from Raleigh demonstrates the microsurgical treatment of epidermoids and dermoids. Due to the extraordinary high number of cases, the results in terms of recurrence rates and complication rates and especially the strategies for avoiding surgically induced complications are of high interest.

Another chapter by this group deals with glomus jugulare tumors of the skull base. Their surgical treatment belongs to the most difficult procedures at the skull base being associated with the highest complication rates. Here, microsurgical approaches to the craniocervical junction and special strategies for avoiding complications are described in a unique way.

Like the Copenhagen group that uses the four-hand technique for the surgery of acoustic neuromas, also for the complex surgery of glomus jugulare tumors, the four-hand technique is recommended by the authors which points to the fact that the assistant or second surgeon, respectively, plays a much more important role than in other neurosurgical procedures.

The detailed chapter about pituitary adenomas which was written by the group of Nick Thomas from London delivers a comprehensive overview of the classification of the different pituitary tumors including a comparison of endoscopic versus microsurgical technique and points onto alternative treatment options.

The last chapter illustrates the multidisciplinary therapy of skull base metastases where surgical treatment always has to be considered as just one part of a comprehensive neuro-oncological concept.

5.1 Meningiomas of the Skull Base

U. Schick and H. Borghei-Razavi

Meningioma is considered the most primary intracranial neoplasm, representing 14.3–19.0% of all intracranial tumors. Approximately one-third of meningiomas are classified as typical skull base meningioma, subsuming tumors that we are going to describe in this chapter.

The skull base is an area with multiple neural structures as well as brain-supplying adjacent arteries and veins. Meningiomas growing on or within the skull can thus be very challenging for the neurosurgeon. Therefore, complete tumor removal without injury of the neural or vascular structures is not always possible. Surgery in this area, especially around the optic nerve and also in the petroclival region, is risky and tricky.

The surgeon must be familiar with the normal anatomical variations and surgical anatomy of the skull base to understand the pathological variations caused by these lesions and to manage them properly.

5.1.1 Optic Nerve Sheath Meningioma (ONSM)

General Information

ONSMs represent 1–2% of all meningiomas, 1.7% of all orbital tumors, and approximately 35% of all intrinsic tumors of the optic nerve.

Classical primary ONSM arises from the meningothelial cap cells of the arachnoids surrounding the intraorbital optic nerve and may extend along the optic canal intracranially. Secondary ONSM extends from the planum sphenoidale into the subdural or subarachnoid spaces surrounding the nerve within the optic canal and ultimately within the orbit. ONSM occurs predominantly in middle-aged women.

Classification

Our classification system [1] based on tumor location and extent is provided to clarify the possible manifestations of ONSM (◘ Fig. 5.1).

Type I is located purely intraorbitally. Type Ia is restricted to a flat extension around the optic nerve. Type Ib is manifested as a large bulbiform mass, growing concentrically around the optic nerve with marked proptosis. Type Ic shows exophytic tumor growth upon the optic nerve (◘ Fig. 5.2).

Type II is located intraorbitally with extension through the optic canal or superior orbital fissure. Type IIa manifests as an intraorbital tumor with tumor growth through the optic canal. Type IIb involves the orbital apex and the superior orbital fissure and sometimes even infiltrates the cavernous sinus.

Type III is located intraorbitally along the whole length of the optic nerve to the globe (not only within the apex) with large intracranial tumor extension (more than 1 cm). Type IIIa extends to the chiasm. Type IIIb involves the

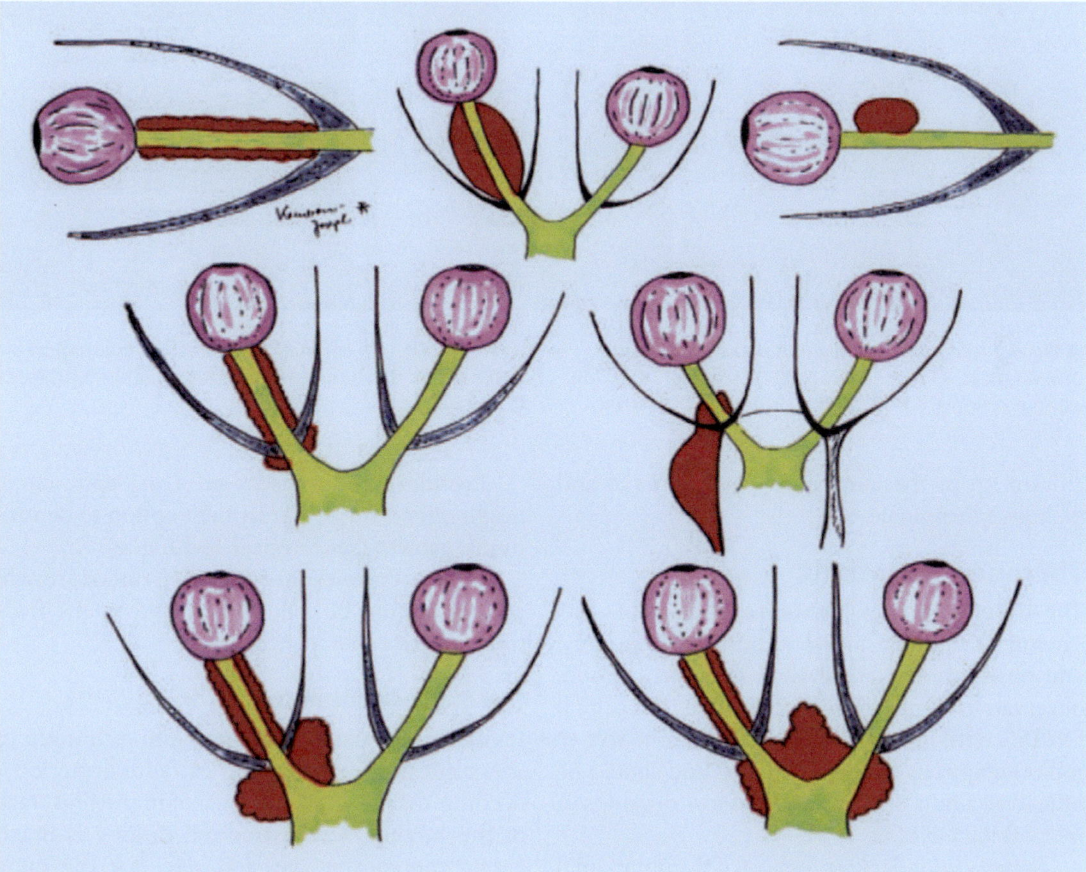

◘ **Fig. 5.1** Drawings of different types and subtypes of ONSMs according to their location. For more description of each type, please refer to the text. *Upper*: Type I, purely intraorbital lesions. Type Ia is a flat tumor extension around the optic nerve (one patient, *left*). Type Ib is widespread; it presents as a large bulbiform mass around the optic nerve (*center*). Type Ic is an exophytic tumor on the optic nerve (*right*). *Center*: Type II, intraorbital ONSMs with extension through the optic canal or superior orbital fissure. Type IIa represents an intraorbital tumor with growth through the optic canal (*left*), and Type IIb represents tumors of the apex, superior orbital fissure, or cavernous sinus (*right*). *Lower*: Type III, intraorbital lesions with widespread intracranial tumor extension. Type IIIa ONSMs are intraorbital with intracranial extension to the chiasm (*left*), and Type IIIb lesions are intraorbital with widespread intracranial extension to the chiasm, contralateral optic nerve, and planum sphenoidale (*right*) (Schick et al. [1] with permission)

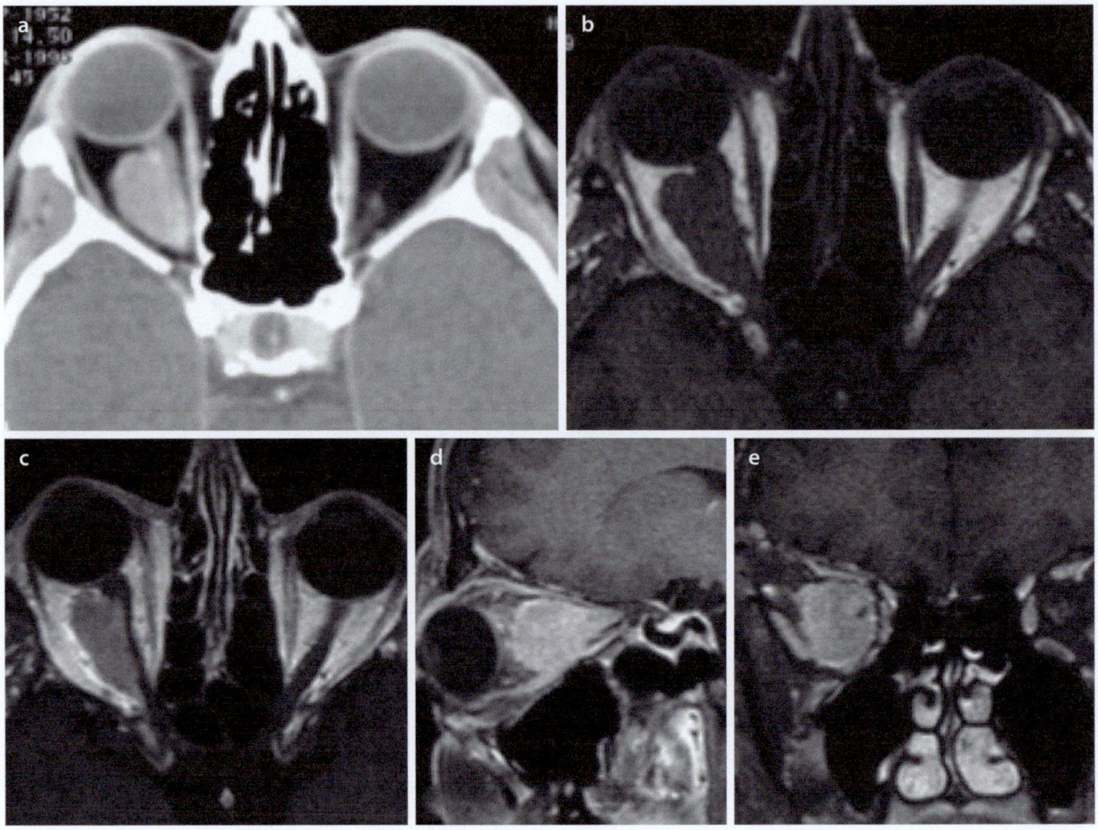

Fig. 5.2 Preoperative imaging of the right-sided ONSM Type Ic. **a** Preoperative axial CT scan, **b** T1 axial MRI without contrast, **c** T1 axial with contrast, **d** T1 sagittal with contrast, **e** T1 coronal fat suppressed. The surgical approach for this tumor would be lateral orbitotomy (see Fig. 5.3)

chiasm up to the contralateral optic nerve and planum sphenoidale.

Therapeutic Options

The loss of vision in ONSMs is a question of time. Treatment options can be radiotherapy, surgery, and observation. If the visual function is good, observation alone can be employed in intraorbital ONSMs until progression is apparent. The role of radiotherapy has to be reevaluated and should be offered to adults once mild vision loss develops in intraorbital ONSMs.

Surgery with decompression of the optic canal and intracranial tumor resection is still favored for tumors with intracanalicular and intracranial extension [2].

Tumors with exophytic intraorbital mass are amenable to be excised via a lateral orbitotomy (Figs. 5.2 and 5.3).

Prechiasmatic transection of the optic nerve might offer a surgical treatment option to control tumor growth (see Surgical Technique).

In cases of residual or recurrent tumor growth, surgery should be followed by stereotactic fractionated radiotherapy (SFRT).

Surgical Technique

In the last years, we changed our technique of decompression, performing extradural pterional decompression of the optic canal in the first stage of the surgery. This extradural drilling is much easier, more extensive, and safer for the optic nerve, avoiding any damage to the optic nerve. The second step remained intradural with tumor removal (Fig. 5.4).

In tumors without intracranial extension, an extradural pterional approach was favored with sphenoid ridge drilling, posterior orbitotomy,

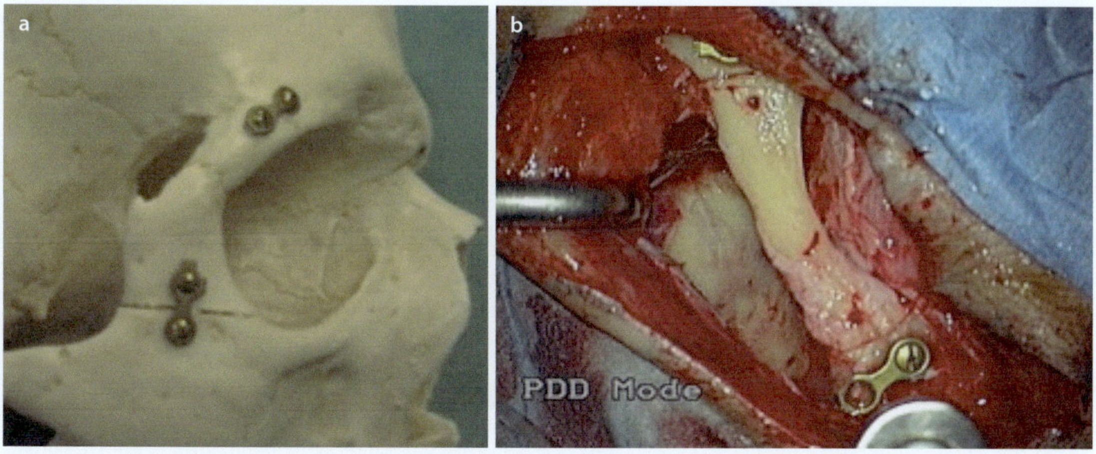

Fig. 5.3 Area of removing the lateral orbital rim for lateral orbitotomy. **a** Schematic view, **b** intraoperative view

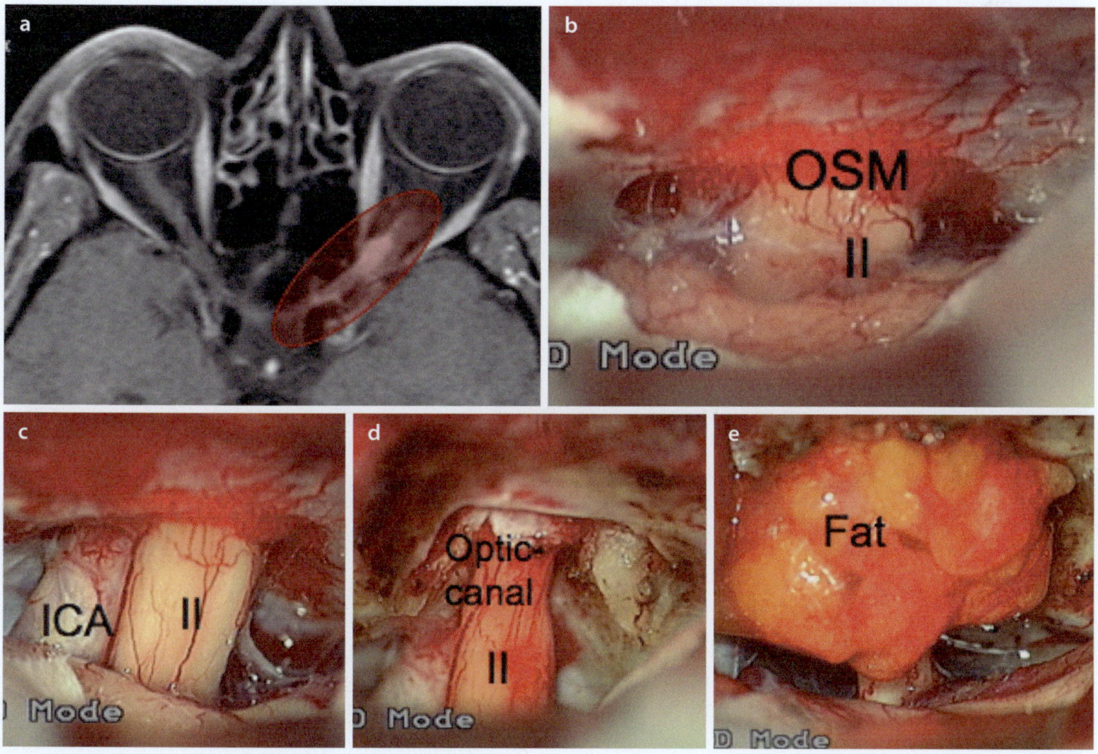

Fig. 5.4 **a** T1 axial MRI scan with contrast of the left-sided ONSM Type II. **b** Intraoperative view before tumor removal, **c** after opening the arachnoid layer, **d** after extradural optic nerve decompression and intradural removal of the intracranial tumor, **e** covering the drilled optic canal with autologous fat (*OSM* optic sheath meningioma, *II* optic nerve, *ICA* internal carotid artery)

decompression of the superior orbital fissure, and unroofing of the optic canal.

As we have explained above, for tumors with exophytic laterally located intraorbital mass, we prefer the lateral orbitotomy approach (Figs. 5.2 and 5.3).

In blind patients with disfiguring painful proptosis, a prechiasmatic transection of the optic

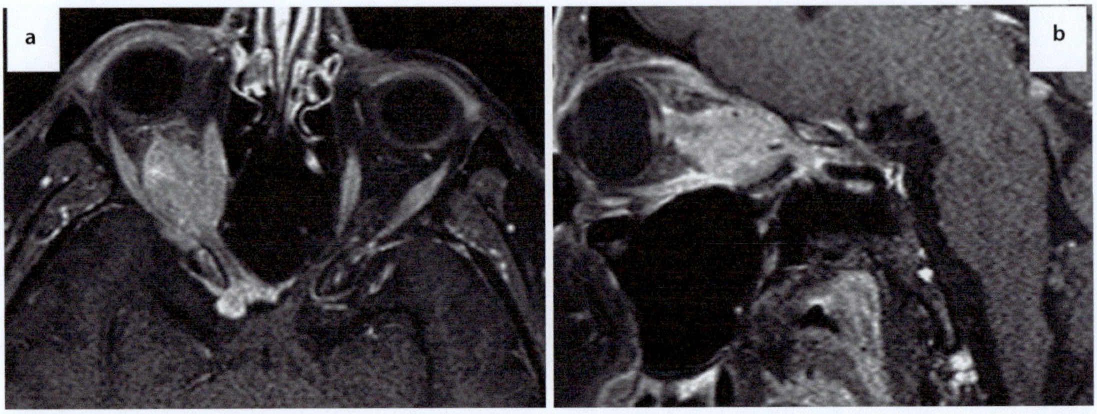

Fig. 5.5 T1-weighted MRI scan showing a homogenously contrast-enhancing ONSM (*right*) growing from the orbit through the optic canal to the chiasm. The chiasm itself is still tumor-free. **a** Axial view, **b** sagittal view

nerve was performed intradurally, and the intraorbital part of the tumor was removed as well [3]. The intraorbital optic nerve was transected just behind the globe and deep in the apex and also intradurally 2–3 mm anterior to the chiasm. Tumor freedom of chiasm in preoperative magnetic resonance imaging (MRI) with contrast is the most important criterion for this surgical method (Fig. 5.5).

Summary

Our classification system differentiates the intraorbital, intracanalicular or intrafissural, and intraorbital and intracranial types of ONSMs.

Surgery with decompression of the optic canal and intracranial tumor resection is favored for tumors with intracanalicular and intracranial extension.

5.1.2 Tuberculum Sellae and Planum Sphenoidale Meningioma

General Information

Approximately 25% of the anterior skull base meningiomas originated from tuberculum sellae and planum sphenoidale. Women are affected three times more often than men. The disease is diagnosed in the fourth or fifth decade. The tumor originates from the tuberculum sellae, chiasmatic sulcus, limbus sphenoidale, and diaphragma sellae. Tuberculum sellae meningiomas very commonly extend into both optic canals—a problem that is underestimated in published reports. The new classification system introduced recently by Sekhar et al. has considered also the extension of the tumor into optic canals [4] (Fig. 5.6a–c). These tumors tend to displace the optic chiasm posteriorly and the optic nerves laterally and superiorly.

Clinical Signs and Symptoms

Visual loss in one eye with optic atrophy is the initial and most common symptom. In most patients, visual loss has an insidious onset, and the course is progressive. It may, however, be acute or fluctuating. Monocular blindness may be present in half of the patients before surgery. Incongruity and asymmetry of the visual field defect are common findings.

Diagnostics

Preoperative ophthalmological examination should consist of testing the patients' visual acuity, fundoscopy, and Goldmann perimetry for visual field defects.

Oculomotor function should be evaluated preoperatively along with other neurological functions. Endocrinological tests (adrenal, thyroid, and gonadal axes, specific gravity of the urine, and fluid balance) should be done preoperatively and at 1 week and 3 months postoperatively.

All patients should be evaluated by computed tomography (CT) and MRI with and without contrast (Fig. 5.7). In many cases, high-resolution CT shows the hyperostosis of the planum sphenoidale and tuberculum sellae or calcification within the tumor. Both T1- and T2-weighted MRI should be done in three planes to analyze the relation to vascular and neighboring structures and the evaluation of tumor extension to both optic canals.

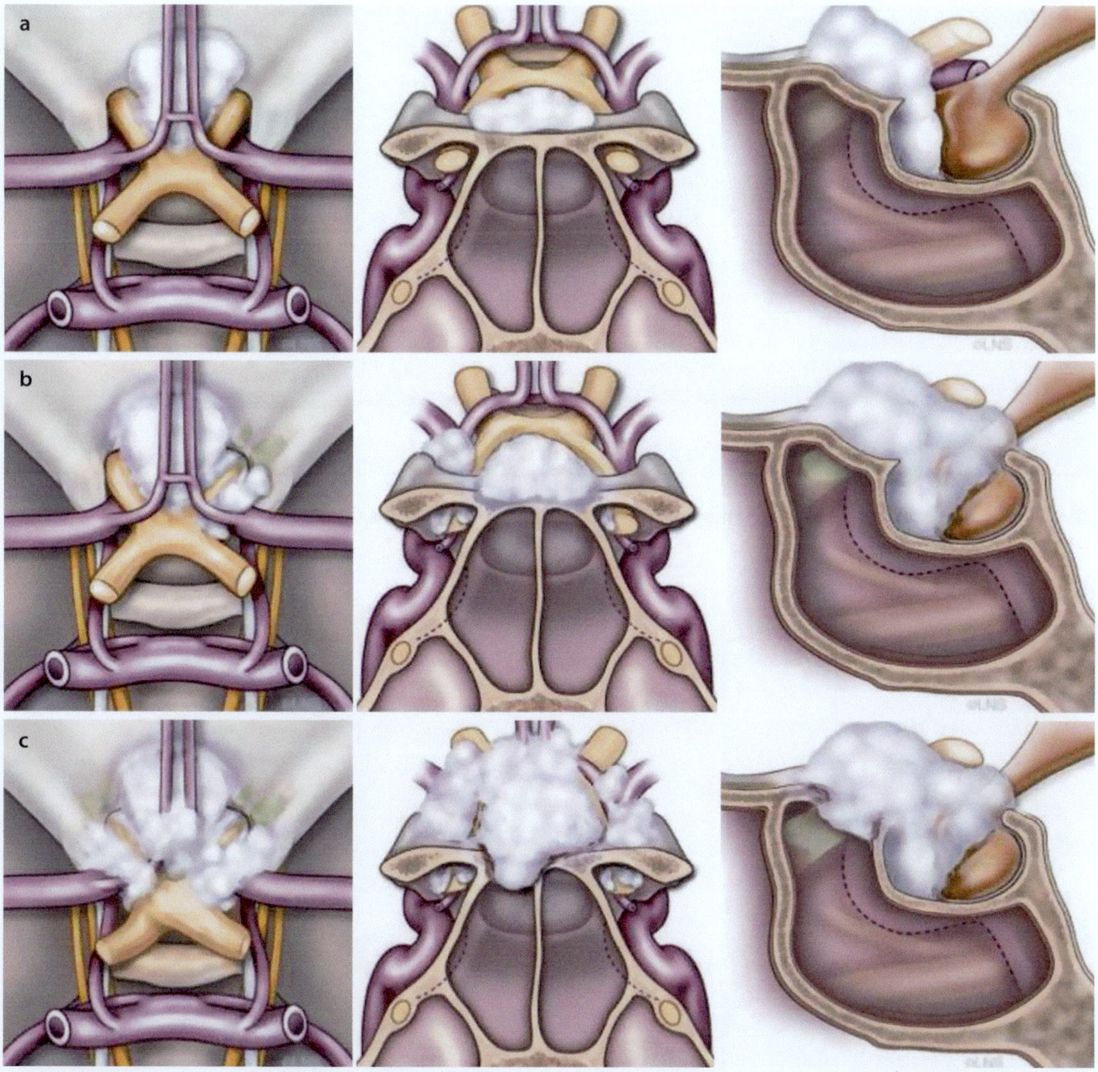

Fig. 5.6 Illustrations showing the new classification system for planum sphenoidale and tuberculum sellae meningiomas. **a** (Class I): Showing a <2 cm tumor, with no extension into the optic canal and no ICA or ACA encasement. **b** (Class II): Showing a >4 cm tumor, with >5 mm extension into the right optic canal, and >180° encasement of the right ICA. **c** (Class III): Showing a >4 cm tumor, with >5 mm extension into both optic canals, >180° encasement of bilateral ICAs or ACAs, and bone invasion with extension into the sphenoid (Mortazavi et al. [4] with permission)

The enlargement of the optic canal should be evaluated in preoperative CT scan with bone window.

Therapeutic Options

For the time being, we believe that the role of microsurgical decompression is still the best choice of treatment providing optimal tumor management and visual recovery.

The indications for endoscopic approaches are tumors smaller than 2 cm situated on the midline with no extension into the optic canal and no vessels encased in tumor.

This method has the major drawback of having very high rates of cerebrospinal fluid (CSF) fistulas (up to 30% depends on the center's experience).

Surgical Technique

We prefer the approach to these tumors through a unilateral frontotemporal, on the side of visual deterioration. In bilateral involvement, the right side is preferred [5].

In some special cases with asymmetric ipsilateral tumor growth under the optic chiasm, we

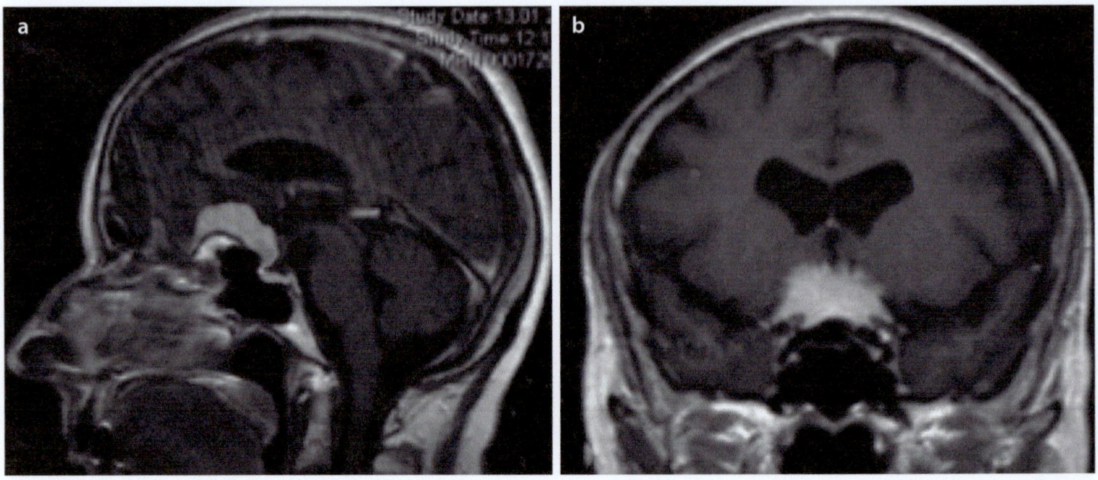

Fig. 5.7 Post-contrast T1-weighted magnetic resonance imaging showing a tuberculum sellae meningioma. **a** Sagittal view, **b** coronal view

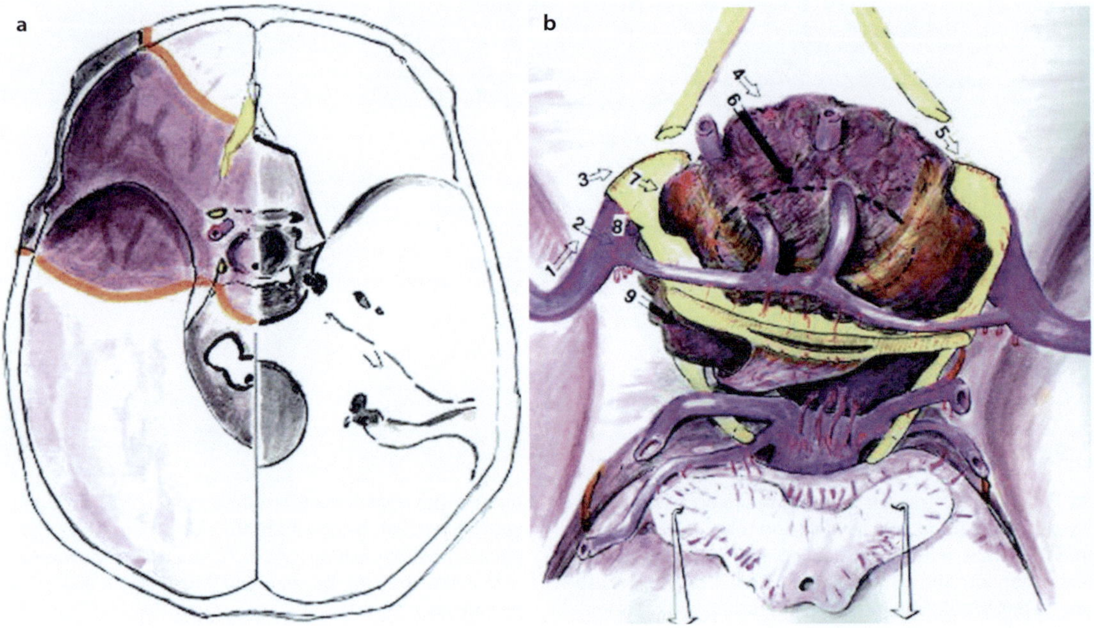

Fig. 5.8 **a** Schematic drawing of the target areas visible through a pterional approach (intradural structures left sided and bony structures right sided). **b** Anatomical sketch of the tuberculum sellae meningioma with adjacent structures (the brain stem and its vessels are retracted). Surgical steps: (*1*) identification of the M1 segment, (*2*) internal carotid artery bifurcation, (*3*) ipsilateral optic nerve and optic canal, (*4*) interruption of the blood supply and debulking, (*5*) contralateral optic nerve, (*6*) dissection from the skull base along the interoptic fold, (*7*) dissection of the arachnoidal plane from the ipsilateral optic nerve, (*8*) dissection from the A1 segment and (*9*) from the chiasm (see also the detailed description of steps in the text) (Schick et al. [5] with permission)

prefer to approach the tumor from the contralateral side for better visualization of the tumor.

The drainage of CSF is done by opening the basal cisterns. Sylvian fissure is routinely opened, and the M1 segment of the middle cerebral artery is exposed (Fig. 5.8, Step 1). The internal carotid artery (ICA) is identified (Step 2), and this leads to the exposure of the ipsilateral optic nerve (Step 3), which might be covered by the tumor. The anterior tumor capsule is opened, and the basal blood supply is interrupted by lifting the tumor and coagulating the feeding arteries (Step 4).

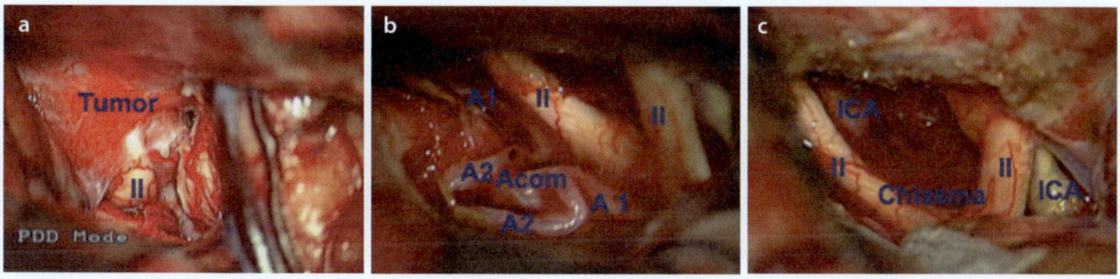

Fig. 5.9 Intraoperative view of the tumor presented in Fig. 5.2. **a** Tumor exposure, **b** complete tumor removal with exposure of the ACOM, A1 and A2. **c** Changing the microscope view and patient's position to expose both the optic nerve and ICA (pay attention that with 30° head rotation in pterional approach, the contralateral ICA seems to be medial to the contralateral optic nerve) (*ACOM* anterior communicating artery, *ICA* internal carotid artery, *II* optic nerve)

The tumor is further debulked to reduce its volume until the contralateral optic nerve became visible (Step 5). The tumor located medial to the ipsilateral optic nerve is then removed from the skull base (Step 6).

This step was followed by the dissection of the arachnoidal plane from the ipsilateral optic nerve (Step 7). After interruption of the basal blood supply, the tumor became soft and thus could easily be detached from the arachnoid plane of the gyrus rectus, the A1 segment of the anterior cerebral artery (ACA), or the anterior communicating artery. Finally, the tumor is removed from the A1 segment (Step 8) and the chiasm (Step 9) (Figs. 5.8 and 5.9). The protection of the optic and chiasmatic blood supply is extremely important to preserve vision.

Particularly, the small vessels from the carotid artery to the optic nerve have to remain in their arachnoidal layer and should not be occluded. In cases of hyperostotic planum sphenoidale, the basal dura was excised, and the bone was drilled away. The defect was covered with fat, TachoSil (absorbable fibrin sealant patch), and fibrin glue.

In optic canal involvement, the first 3–5 mm of the optic canal, which is fibrous, is opened. The bony roof is drilled away if there is further tumor extension. The ophthalmic artery below the optic nerve is exposed and preserved. If necessary, the optic nerve sheath is opened until the annulus of Zinn is reached and the tumor around the optic nerve is carefully removed. In contrast to ONSMs, the tumor mass in the optic canal in tuberculum sellae meningiomas can easily be dissected from the optic nerve.

Summary

In the majority of patients with tuberculum sellae meningiomas, total resection may be achieved through a unilateral pterional approach with minimal complications.

5.1.3 Sphenoid Wing, Clinoidal, and Tentorial Fold (TF) Meningiomas

General Information

Sphenoid wing meningiomas account for more than 20% of all intracranial meningiomas. Sphenoid wing and clinoidal meningiomas are classified based on their origin along the sphenoid wing as clinoidal, middle, and lateral sphenoid wing lesions. The more medially located clinoidal meningiomas represent a distinct clinicoanatomic entity, and historically, the resection of these lesions has been associated with significant morbidity and mortality and advances in cranial base surgery.

Al-Mefty classified clinoidal meningiomas into three categories based on the anatomic site of origin and degree of surgical difficulty: Type I, with severe adherence to the carotid; Type II, with the presence of an interfacing arachnoid plane between the tumor and the carotid artery; and Type III, originate at the optic foramen and extend into the optic canal and at the tip of the anterior clinoid process.

Clinical Signs and Symptoms

Visual disturbance is present in the majority of patients, ranging from slight decrease of vision and partial field defect to complete loss of vision. Other symptoms, in the order of frequency, included seizure, headache, anosmia, cognitive deficit, diplopia, dizziness, proptosis, and gait disturbance. Anosmia and cognitive defects are mainly present in tumors of giant sizes, extending into multiple regions.

Diagnostics

Preoperative MRI with and without contrast and magnetic resonance angiogram (with time-of-flight sequence) is used to determine the tumor location, size, and involvement of surrounding structures. These structures mainly included the ICA, ACA, optic canal and nerves, and the surrounding brain tissue.

5

Preoperative CT scan with thin slices (1 mm, multislice CT) is very useful to clarify the bone involvement (hyperostosis) and also the involvement of the optic canal and planning the surgical strategy.

Surgical Procedure and Technique

Nowadays, we do not recommend the cranio-orbital zygomatic approach for the resection of clinoidal or any type of sphenoid wing meningiomas. Although this provides the surgeon with a low-based approach, multiple avenues of dissection and minimal brain retraction are, however, very destructive and time consuming. We believe that a pterional approach with wide opening of the dura toward the basis provides a suitable corridor to remove different types of clinoidal and sphenoid wing meningiomas. Intraoperative visual-evoked potential (VEP) is the new routine monitoring technique that we use during the operation around the optic nerve (◘ Fig. 5.10).

To achieve the optimal visual outcome in microsurgically resected meningiomas involving the optic nerve, wide bony extradural decompression of the optic canal with or without anterior clinoidectomy [6] (180–270° optic nerve decompression depends on the clinoid process anatomy and involvement) might be advocated (◘ Fig. 5.11, ◘ Video 5.1).

It can be performed in different stages of operation depending on the tumor size and intraoperative bleeding from the tumor.

This procedure increases the maneuverability of the optic nerve and carotid artery at their intradural entries. Moreover, it reduces dramatically the intradural bleeding from the tumor during removal (extradural devascularization).

◘ Figure 5.12 shows the preoperative MRI of the patient with large left-sided medial sphenoid wing meningioma with extension to the TF (◘ Fig. 5.12a–c).

We prefer to do the surgical approach via a unilateral frontotemporal craniotomy.

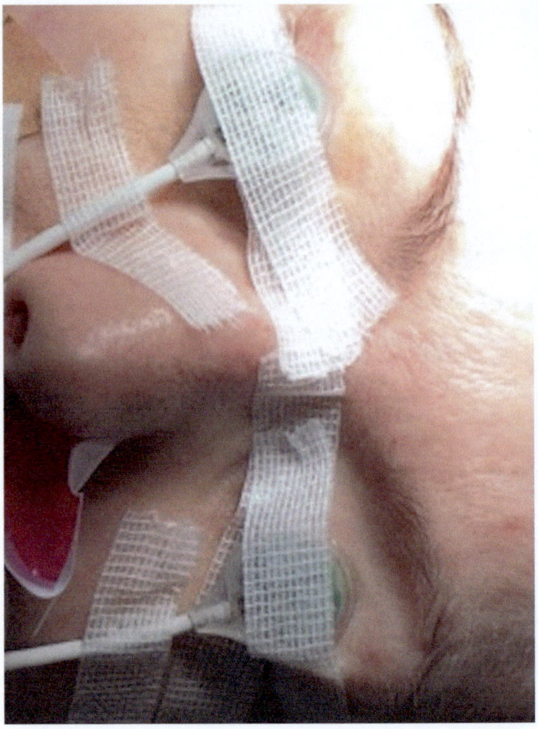

◘ **Fig. 5.10** Intraoperative use of VEP during microsurgery of meningioma around the optic nerve

Craniotomy is extended to the middle of the orbital rim and 1 cm above the margin.

After opening the dura, the Sylvian fissure is frequently split by the tumor.

The first step (plane) is the coagulation of the tumor origin on the dura of the medial sphenoid wing (dura of the skull base). This step is very important, as it results in tumor devascularization and softness.

We usually start the coagulation of the tumor origin from the temporal skull base. The coagulation of the tumor from the dura at the base should be continued until encased carotid artery and optic nerve appear. The direction of bipolar coagulation should be toward the tumor and away from the vital structures. Water irrigation is very important to avoid heat injury to these structures. If it is not easy to find the optic nerve, it is useful to follow the olfactory nerve backward until it crosses the optic nerve.

Intraoperative Doppler sonography is very useful in many difficult cases to find the encased carotid artery. After the identification of the optic nerve and carotid artery, oculomotor nerve should be identified at its entrance to the cavernous sinus (oculomotor cistern, ◘ Fig. 5.13a).

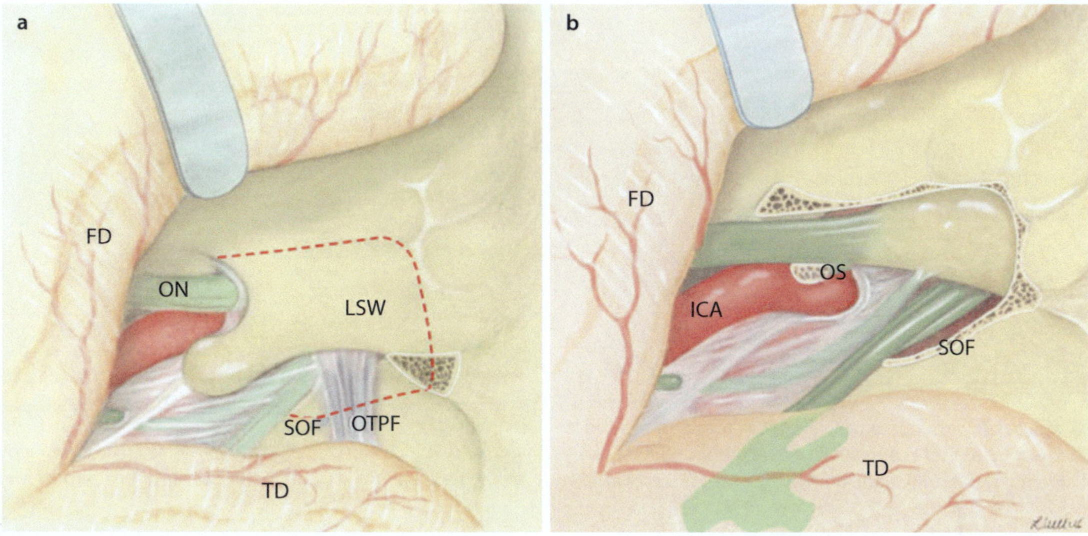

Fig. 5.11 **a** Illustrative anatomy centered on the anterior clinoid process and surroundings; intracranial view from dorsolateral to anteromedial. The angle between anterior and middle cranial fossae has been flattened to allow a drawing of the neurovascular structures rather side by side and not, as in reality, hidden by each other. The dura mater of the skull base resected: *OC* optic canal, *ACP* anterior clinoid process, *SOF* superior orbital fissure, *LSW* lesser sphenoid wing, *OTPF* orbitotemporal periosteal fold, *FD* frontal dura, *TD* temporal dura. **b** Illustrative anatomy after resection of ACP and opening of the SOF, as well as transection of OTPF. This drawing shows the amount of bone that is drilled during the stepwise procedures as described. This technique not only affords access to the distal dural ring of the ICA near the optic strut but also facilitates a wide decompression of the SOF and the OC. *OS* optic strut (*right side*) (Lehmberg et al. [6], Springer)

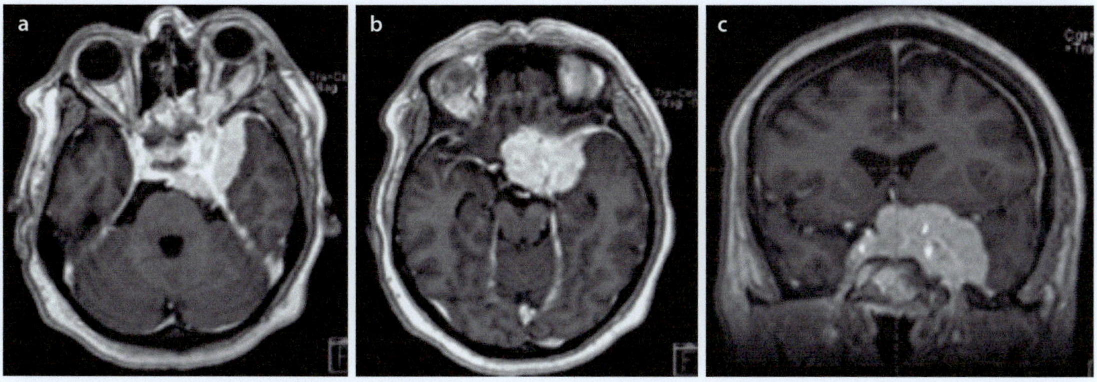

Fig. 5.12 Preoperative MRI of the patient with large left-sided medial sphenoid wing meningioma with extension to the tentorial fold. **a**, **b** Axial view, **c** coronal view

The second step (plane) is the coagulation and shrinkage of the tumor capsule. The M2 segment of the medial cerebral artery should be also identified. Following this segment (M2) to the proximal is very helpful in the final identification of the M1 segment and carotid bifurcation. Now, the tumor should be debulked with the CUSA (cavitron ultrasonic surgical aspirator). In this step, the following maneuvers should be continued over and over: coagulation and shrinkage of tumor capsule, pushing the capsule to the tumor cavity, and debulking with CUSA.

The third step (plane) is the tumor removal around the carotid artery and optic nerve and finally carotid bifurcation and A1 (Fig. 5.13b).

If the tumor extended to the tentorial notch (see the discussion in the following part), the fourth step should be the identification of the trochlear nerve toward tentorial notch and the removal of the tumor in this part (Fig. 5.13c).

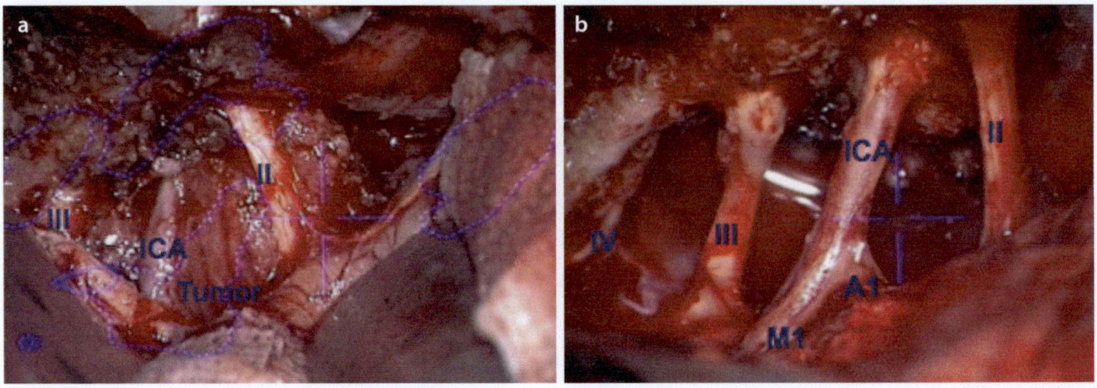

Fig. 5.13 Intraoperative view of the tumor presented in Fig. 5.12: **a** After coagulation of the tumor origin and partial removal (Step 1 in text). **b** After total tumor removal with identification of cranial nerves II–IV and ICA bifurcation (Step 4 in text). The course of cranial nerve IV should be identified before removal of the tumor extension into the tentorial fold

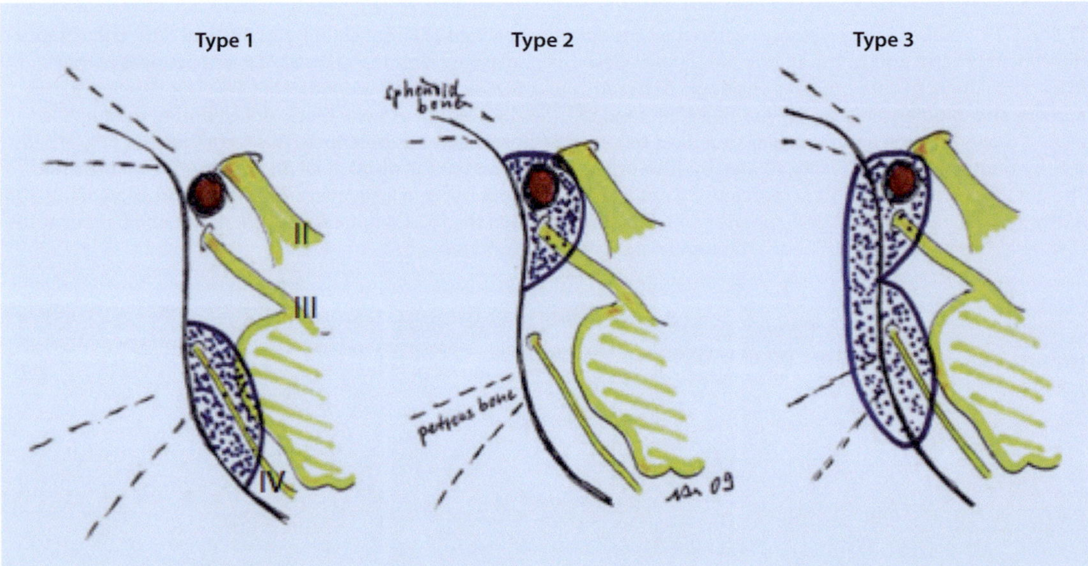

Fig. 5.14 TFM (tentorial fold meningioma) classification: Type I, TF meningiomas with origin in the dorsal portion of TF; Type II, with extension into the anterior portion of the middle fossa; and Type III, a combination of Types I and II (*II* optic nerve, *III* oculomotor nerve, *IV* trochlear nerve) (Hashemi et al. [7], Springer)

In clinoid process meningioma or small medial sphenoid wing meningioma with the involvement of the optic canal, we prefer to perform extradural pterional decompression of the optic nerve in the first stage of operation before opening the dura.

TFM (Tentorial Fold Meningioma): A Unique Entity

From a surgical perspective, TFM or medial sphenoid wing meningiomas with extension to the TF are a unique entity of tumors. They involve the supratentorial and infratentorial space and often are in close contact to the cavernous sinus, cranial nerves, and mesencephalon. Complete resection is challenging and can be hazardous. Surgical outcome is related to a topographical classification.

We classified this tumor according to tumor extension in three different types: Type I (TFMs with compression of the brain stem), Type II (with extension into the anterior portion of middle fossa), and Type III (a combination of Types I and II; Fig. 5.14).

Surgical Technique

In the majority of patients with TFMs, total resection can be achieved through a pterional (for Type II), subtemporal (for Type I), or combined (for Type III) approaches but with a high rate of permanent morbidity.

In the first step, the trochlear nerve that is usually covered by the tumor should be identified and preserved below the tentorial edge. In some cases, elevation of the tentorium with a suture is very helpful to identify the trochlear nerve below the TF.

In cases in which it is difficult to find the oculomotor nerve, following the fourth nerve to the anterior is useful to find it. In cases with tumor extension below the tentorium (Type III), after the identification of the trochlear nerve, the tentorial dura behind the dural entrance of the trochlear nerve is divided in the direction to the petrous apex to remove the infratentorial part of the tumor. After complete tumor removal, the abducens nerve can be identified at the entrance of Dorello's canal.

Summary

Due to the close proximity to important neurovascular structures, sphenoid wing meningiomas, especially medial sphenoid wing meningioma, with the involvement of the clinoid process and optic nerve require special surgical attention and technique to achieve the highest level of safety with maximal extent of resection.

We should always keep in mind that the primary surgical goals and principles include at first the preservation of the quality of life followed by the preservation of neurological functions. Nevertheless, the resection should be performed as radical as possible to gain a good tumor control. Radiotherapy should be offered as an effective alternative treatment in recurrent tumors.

5.1.4 Sphenoorbital en Plaque Meningiomas

General Information

Meningiomas en plaque (sphenoorbital meningiomas) constitute approximately 4% of all meningiomas. These are complex tumors involving the sphenoid wing, orbit, and cavernous sinus, which make their complete resection difficult or impossible. Sphenoidal hyperostosis that results in incomplete resection makes these tumors prone to high rates of recurrence postoperatively.

We believe that the surgical treatment of sphenoorbital en plaque meningiomas is safe and effective: in our series of more than 100 patients, a low morbidity rate was recorded and visual function improved in approximately two-thirds of the patients.

Clinical Findings

The duration of symptoms is usually long because of the minimal discomfort that is produced. Proptosis is the initial and most common symptom followed by cosmetic deformity with no neurological deficits. Finally, marked hyperostosis of the sphenoid bone and diffuse tumor invasion lead to cranial neuropathies caused by foraminal encroachment. The most common cranial nerve deficit is optic neuropathy.

Surgical Technique

For this type of meningioma, pterional approach has been well described in the literature.

For the use of CT scan-guided cranioplasty (CAD implant), we use always a special gauge as a guide for pterional craniotomy (◘ Fig. 5.15).

The *first step* of the tumor surgery is purely extradural bony decompression. The hyperostotic bone is drilled away until the normal shape of the bone (compared with the contralateral side) is remodeled. Craniotomy is usually extended to the middle of the orbital rim, and the dura mater is dissected from the sphenoid bone. The first steps

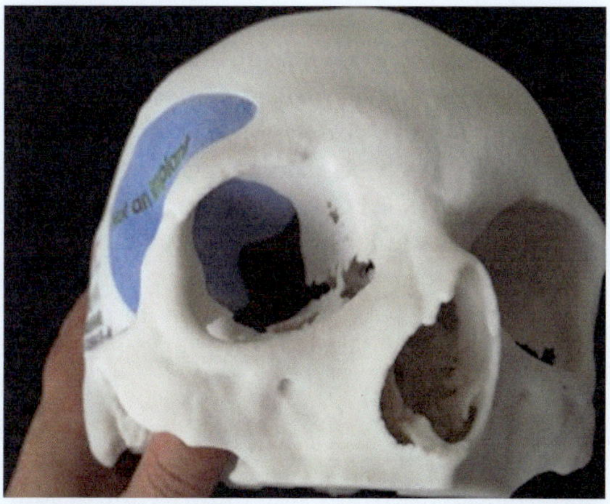

◘ **Fig. 5.15** Reconstruction of the sphenoid wing, lateral orbital wall, and orbital roof using individual preordered CT scan-guided cranioplasty (CAD implant, Biomet)

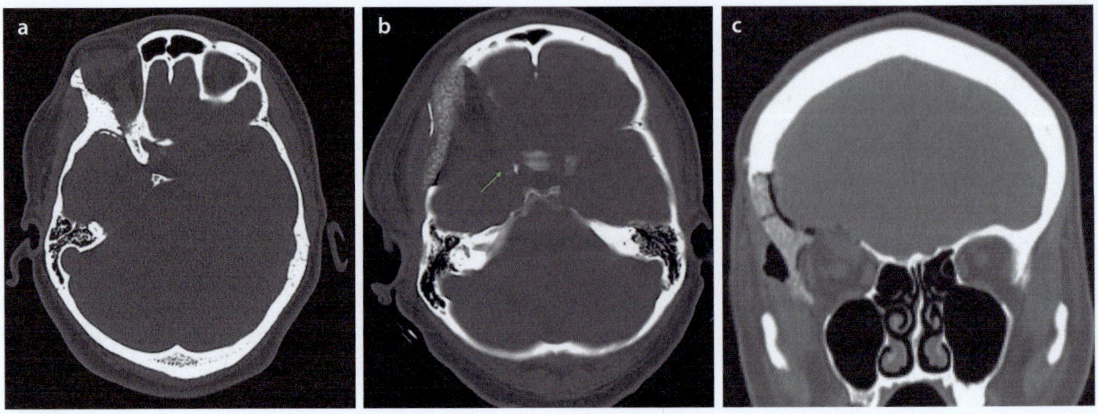

Fig. 5.16 **a** Preoperative CT scan of a patient with right-sided huge sphenoorbital meningioma with involvement of the right optic canal. **b** Postoperative CT scan (axial view) after extradural tumor drilling and anterior clinoidectomy (*arrow* shows a removed part of clinoid process) followed by intradural tumor removal and reconstruction of the orbital roof. **c** Coronal view

of the operation are entirely extradural and involve drilling the lesser wing of the sphenoid bone down to the superior orbital fissure and the bone of the lateral orbital wall down to the foramen rotundum until the beginning of the inferior orbital fissure is exposed.

Then, a partial anterior clinoidectomy is performed (Fig. 5.16a, b), and the optic canal is unroofed extradurally whenever tumor involvement is present. Do not open the periorbita at this stage.

The *second step* is the resection of the tumor intradurally, and it is somehow easy. The basal dura is excised as far as possible up to the superior orbital fissure and the optic canal. A small portion of the dura should be remained to be used for duraplasty later.

The *third step* is the reconstruction of the dura. The dura is tightly closed with audiomesh (collagen bioimplant), TachoSil (fibrin sealant patch) inside and outside, and autologous fat.

The *fourth step* is opening the periorbita in the case of tumor infiltration of intraorbital structures. After opening the periorbita, the lateral periorbital tumor is dissected from the beginning of the superior orbital fissure and intraorbitally to the superior rectus and levator muscles or the lateral rectus muscle. In cases in which there is an infiltration of the ocular muscles, only the exophytic tumor is removed and the muscles are not resected. The periorbita is closed only with the insertion of audiomesh upon the opened part (it should not be closed tightly to let the exophthalmus come back to the normal position postoperatively) [8].

The *last step* is the reconstruction of the sphenoid wing, lateral orbital wall, and orbital roof using individual preordered CT scan-guided cranioplasty (CAD implant, Biomet; Figs. 5.15 and 5.16 b, c). This new method of reconstruction results in acceptable functional and cosmetic outcomes.

Summary

The goals of surgery are acceptable cosmetic and functional results with tumor control and minimal morbidity.

The aggressive resection of tumor-invaded structures in the cavernous sinus, superior orbital fissure, or orbital apex is not recommended because of the attendant serious risk of morbidity. In case of tumor progression in this part, radiation should be considered. Surgery should be performed as early and as radically as possible to obviate future recurrence. Radiotherapy remains an alternative for recurrences or subtotal resections.

5.1.5 Petroclival Meningiomas

General Information

Basal posterior fossa meningiomas can be classified into the clival, petroclival, sphenopetroclival, foramen magnum, and cerebellopontine (CP) angle types depending on the zone of adherence. The tumors known as petroclival meningiomas can be broadly defined as those attached to the lateral sites along the petroclival borderline where the sphenoid, petrous, and occipital bones meet.

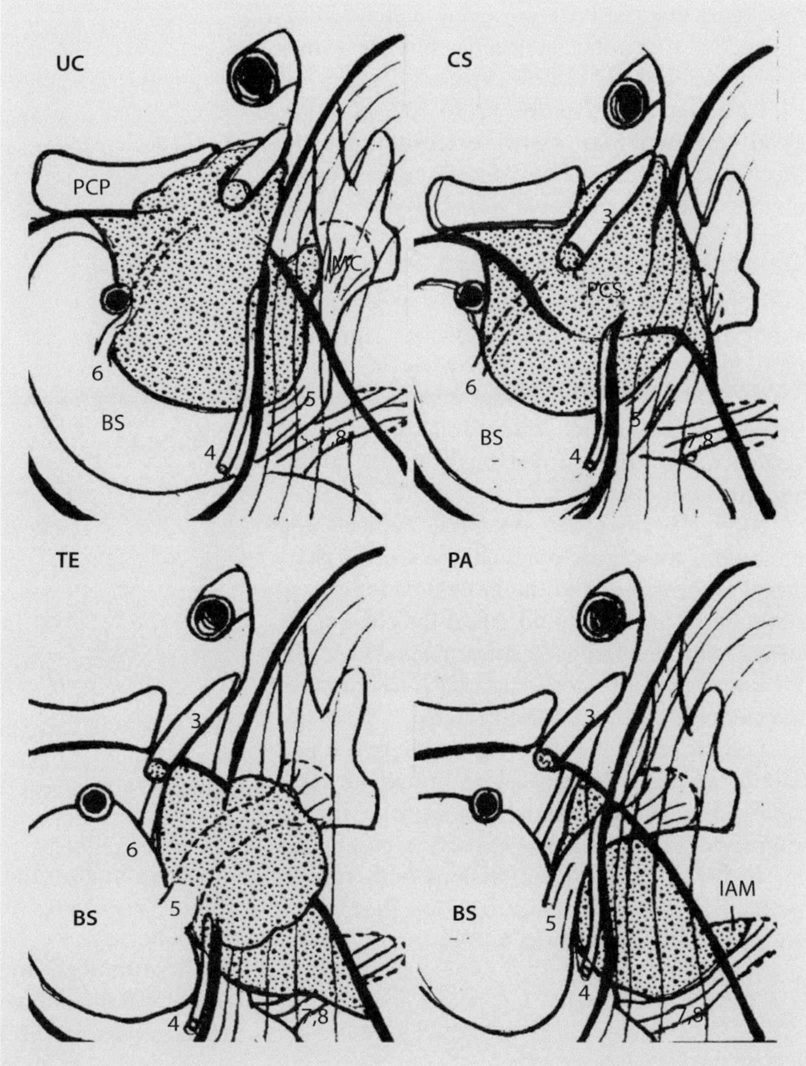

■ **Fig. 5.17** Four subtypes of petroclival meningioma: *upper left*, the upper clivus (*UC*) type; *upper right*, the cavernous sinus (*CS*) type; *lower left*, the tentorium (*TE*) type; *lower right*, the petrous apex (*PA*) type. The shaded regions indicate tumors. The numbers indicate cranial nerves. *PCP* posterior clinoid process, *PCS* posterior cavernous sinus, *IAM* internal auditory meatus, *BS* brain stem, *MC* Meckel's cave (Ichimura et al. [10])

Petroclival tumors are located in an anatomically complicated area containing the dural folds, venous sinuses, and cranial nerves III–VIII. Therefore, a small anatomical variation in the zone of origin presents different clinical features and choice of surgical approaches that can influence the outcome [9, 14].

Kawase et al. preliminarily classified petroclival meningiomas into four subtypes based on MRI and surgical observations (■ Fig. 5.17). This classification is useful to predict the relation between the tumor and the cranial nerves based on symptoms and images.

Clinical Manifestations

As we discussed above, petroclival meningiomas can be classified into four subtypes (UC, CS, TE, and PA; for abbreviations, see the description of ■ Fig. 5.17) based on their origin. The clinical signs of petroclival meningiomas are cranial nerve III–VIII deficits and signs associated with the brain stem and cerebellar compression.

The characteristic symptom of the UC type is ataxia caused by the direct compression of the brain stem or cerebellar peduncle. The primary goal of surgery is brain stem decompression in lifesaving situations.

Extraocular paresis was significantly noted in the CS type. This is because the abducens nerve is fixed intradurally in the inferomedial triangle of the cavernous sinus from the point of dural penetration to Dorello's canal.

The TE type did not have any characteristic clinical symptoms other than trigeminal neuropathy. Regarding the PA type, many patients complained of trigeminal neuralgia, but the tumor rarely extends into Meckel's cave.

Based on the literature, up to 70% of petroclival meningiomas show extension to the Meckel's cave. The rate of extension differs based on the tumor type, as explained above.

Controversies in Approach Selection

In the literature, there is a great deal of discussion about the merits of using Kawase's approach (anterior petrosal approach) vis-à-vis the retrosigmoid (RS) approach with suprameatal extension (RISA: retrosigmoid intradural suprameatal approach) for tumors involving both the middle and posterior fossa.

Although there are potential benefits and limitations with each approach, the specific characters of the tumor and the individual functional status of the patient should reflect the goals of the surgery and the proposed surgical approach. The RS approach is a powerful approach to lesions of the CP angle and ventral brain stem.

Lesions involving the trigeminal porus and Meckel's cave can be approached through Kawase's approach or a suprameatal extension of the RS approach [11]. Kawase's approach is best suited for accessing middle fossa lesions with smaller petroclival components located above the internal auditory canal (IAC; ◘ Fig. 5.18).

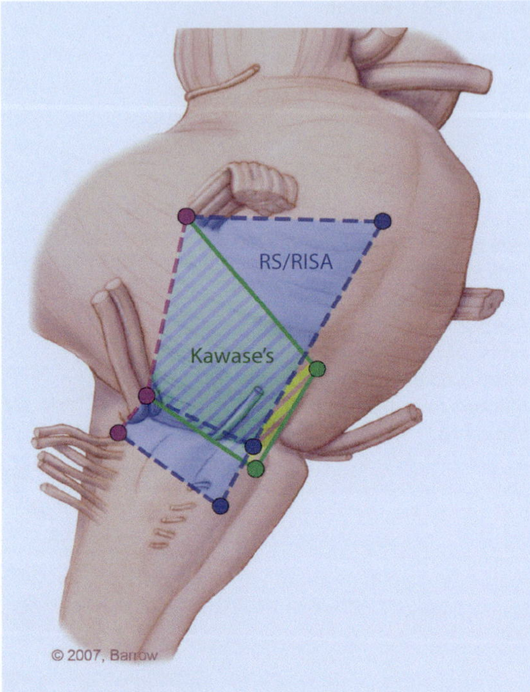

◘ **Fig. 5.18** Schematic representation of calculated areas for the RS/RISA (*blue*) and Kawase's (*green*) approaches (Chang et al. [11])

Surgical Technique

Extended RS Approach

Under general anesthesia and with intraoperative electrophysiological neuromonitoring (somatosensory evoked potential, electromyography of cranial nerves VI–XII) and using intraoperative transesophageal echocardiography (TEE) for the early detection of the air emboli, the patient is positioned in a semisitting position (with the head rotated away from the surgical site). An area approximately two fingerbreadths posterior to the mastoid is identified for the incision.

After standard RS craniotomy, the dura is opened parallel to the sinuses. After drainage of CSF from the cisterna magna, the CP angle with the IAC and its cranial nerves VII–VIII, the suprameatal tubercle, the petrosal vein, cranial nerve V, and the lower cranial nerves are identified and exposed.

Depending on the origin, petroclival meningiomas can change the normal anatomy of the cranial nerves.

These tumors' origins are mostly anterior to the V–IX cranial nerves. There are three corridors to access the tumor ventral to the cranial nerves.

The *first corridor* is above the V cranial nerve. We use always this corridor as a first window to attack the tumor because of the resistance of the trigeminal nerve to manipulation. Here, if the suprameatal tubercle is large and on the way to the tumor, it will be drilled away (◘ Fig. 5.19). In this stage, the tumor should be internally debulked, reduced in its petroclival component, and bimanually dissected from the surrounding neurovascular structures to obtain brain stem decompression.

The *second corridor* is the window between cranial nerve V and VII–VIII complex. Special attention should be given to the facial nerve because it is the most common nerve in danger during the RS approach. In some cases, the basilar artery is encased by the tumor, and it is not easy to dissect the tumor from its perforators. Finally, after tumor resection in this corridor, abducens

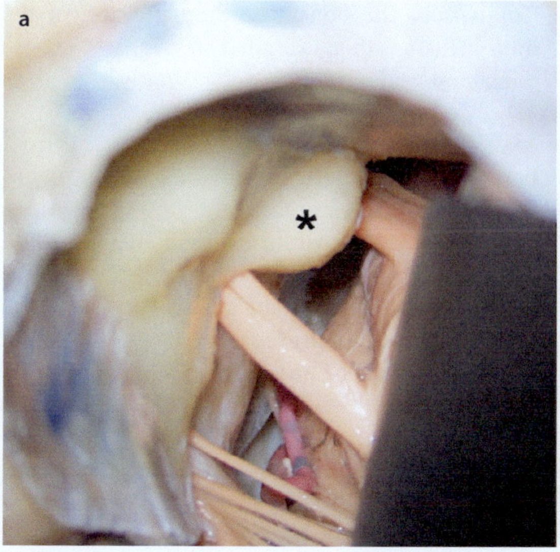

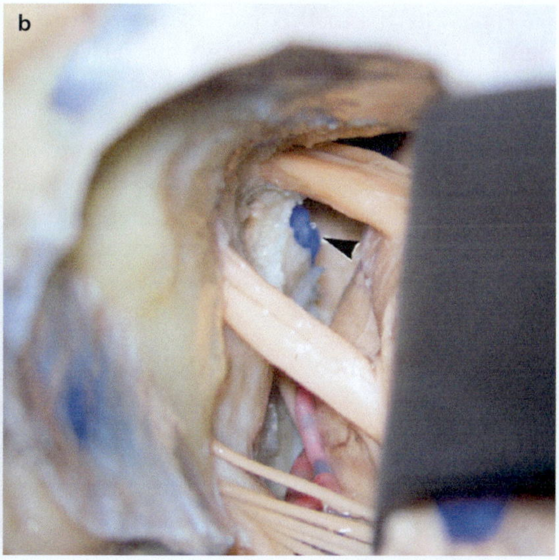

Fig. 5.19 **a** Photograph showing a large suprameatal tubercle (*) seen through the RS approach. **b** The tubercle has been removed via the RISA approach. In this exposure, Dandy's vein (superior petrosal vein Type III which emptied into the superior petrosal sinus) was sacrificed (*arrowhead*) (Chang et al. [11])

nerve will be identified ventrally at the entrance of Dorello's canal.

In cases with caudal extension, the *third corridor* will be the window between cranial nerve VII–VIII complex and the caudal cranial nerves. In tumor removal ventral to the cranial nerves, our invented-angle microbipolar forceps are very helpful as a multipurpose instrument because the forceps could be used for cutting, coagulation, and grasping of the tumor ventral to and also between cranial nerves V and IX [9, 12, 14].

In the case of supratentorial tumor components (middle fossa extension), the tentorium could be cut at the lower part (1–2 cm) toward the petrous ridge under the visualization and protection of cranial nerve IV to remove the tumor portion in the middle fossa. The removal of the tumor in the middle fossa opens a corridor up to the oculomotor nerve at the entrance of the cavernous sinus.

Nevertheless, in most of the cases, the tumor opens a way from posterior fossa to the middle fossa, and there is no need to open the tentorium.

In all of the cases, superior petrosal vein and other bridging veins should be identified and protected to prevent venous infarction [13].

As we have discussed above, in meningiomas with extension to Meckel's cave, we prefer to remove the tumor via middle fossa extradural anterior petrosectomy (Kawase's approach).

In cases with the involvement of the brain stem (edematous brain stem in MRI T2 sequence), a small part of the tumor should remain on the brain stem. It can guarantee a more suitable functional outcome for the patient.

Anterior Petrosal Approach

To access the posterior fossa from middle fossa in Kawase's approach, the dura of the middle fossa should be peeled from the skull base until the petrous ridge is identified. The middle meningeal artery should be interrupted after coagulation to allow the manipulation beside the foramen spinosum. The greater superficial petrosal nerve (GSPN) is the most reliable superficial landmark on the middle cranial fossa for drilling of the petrous apex (Kawase's triangle) in the extradural anterior transpetrosal approach (ATPA). It is the lateral border of Kawase's triangle [9, 14].

The GSPN should be clearly recognized before drilling at Kawase's triangle to avoid the risk of injury to the facial nerve and ICA (Fig. 5.20).

The eminencia arcuata is the posterior border of Kawase's triangle, and it must be preserved if hearing is to be preserved. The anterior border of Kawase's triangle is trigeminal impression (bony impression of Gasserian ganglion).

After drilling the anterior part of the petrous bone, the dura of the posterior fossa is exposed

(◘ Fig. 5.21a, b). In this part of the approach, dural incisions are made above and below the superior petrosal sinus. At this point, a double Weck clip or ligature is applied to close the superior petrosal sinus, and cuts are made toward an edge of the TE, behind the entrance point of the trochlear nerve, to preserve it. The bilateral retraction of the tentorial leaflets with sutures allows for the visualization of the posterior fossa and anterior part of the pons. The dura incision of the middle fossa is then extended anteriorly to expose the lateral wall of the CS.

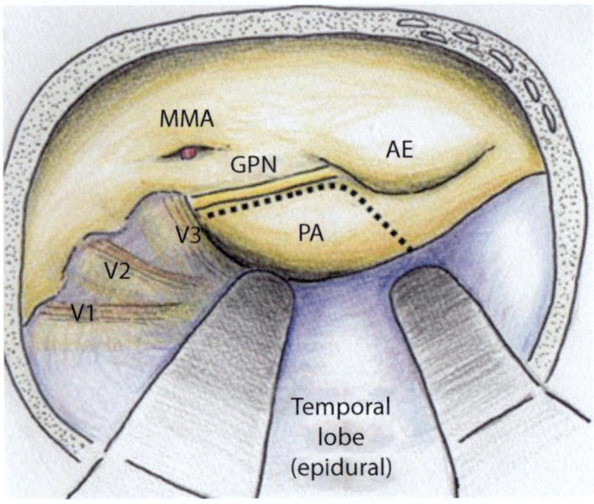

◘ **Fig. 5.20** Schema of the standard ATPA (anterior transpetrosal approach). The standard ATPA is a fundamentally epidural procedure to expose the petrous apex. The middle meningeal artery is coagulated and cut. The GPN (greater petrosal nerve) is dissected in the interdural layer. *AE* arcuate eminence, *GPN* greater petrosal nerve, *MMA* middle meningeal artery, *PA* petrous apex, *V1* ophthalmic nerve, *V2* maxillary nerve, *V3* mandibular nerve. *Dotted line* is the lateral border of anterior petrosectomy (Ichimura et al. [10], Springer)

Summary

Petroclival meningiomas are located in an anatomically complex area containing dural folds, venous sinuses, and cranial nerves IV–XII. Therefore, even very small anatomical variations in the zone of origin can influence the outcome and present drastically different clinical features and choices of surgical approach.

The conclusions about the appropriate surgical approach are thus the particular aspects of the case.

5.1.6 Foramen Magnum Meningiomas

General Information

Foramen magnum meningiomas are divided into two main types: craniospinal (originating intracranially and extending downward) and spinocranial (originating in the upper spinal canal and extending intracranially).

Ventral foramen magnum meningiomas originate from the basal groove in the lower third of the clivus, anterior to the medulla, and project inferiorly toward the foramen magnum (◘ Fig. 5.22a, b). Spinocranial meningiomas, which originate from the upper cervical area, are usually posterior or posterolateral to the spinal

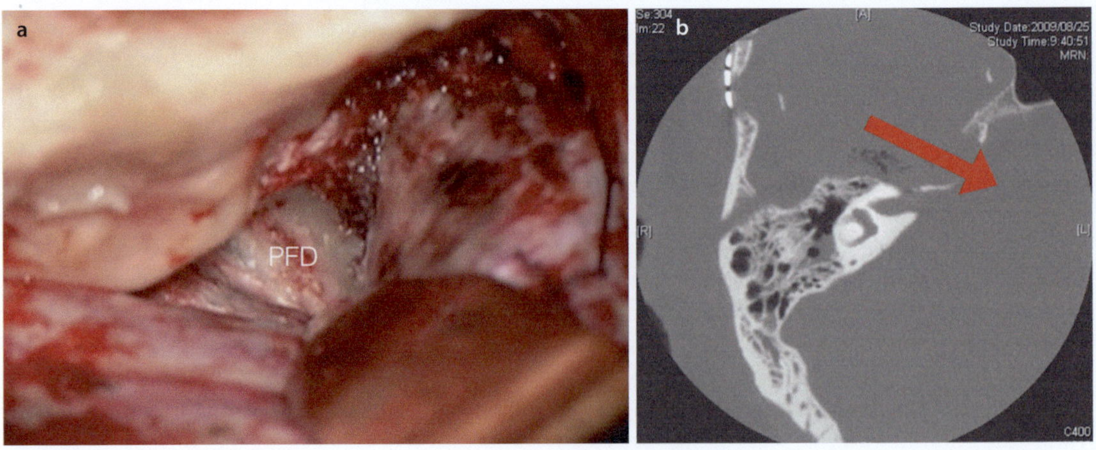

◘ **Fig. 5.21** **a** Exposure of the posterior fossa dura (*PFD*) after anterior petrosectomy. **b** Postoperative axial CT scan of the patient after removing a large right-sided petroclival meningioma via Kawase's approach. The *red arrow* shows the corridor of access from the middle fossa to posterior fossa after anterior petrosectomy

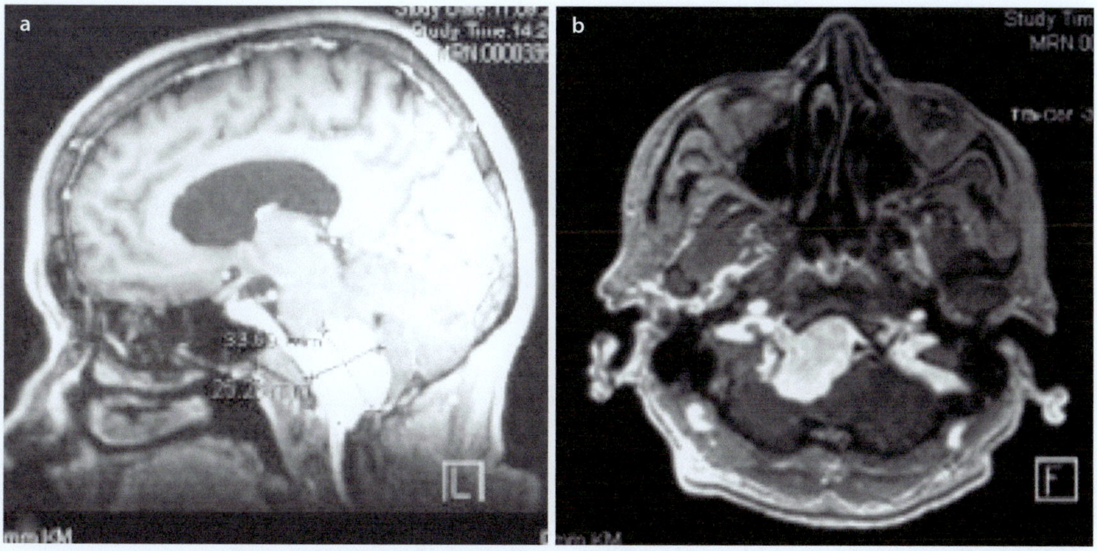

Fig. 5.22 Preoperative MRI of the patient with right-sided ventral foramen magnum meningiomas. **a** Sagittal view, **b** axial view

cord and project superiorly into the cerebellomedullary cistern.

Clinical Signs and Symptoms

Patients with lesions in this location may present with unusual symptoms and are often misdiagnosed. Cervical pain (usually unilateral), motor and sensory deficits (especially involving the upper extremities and, in later stages, progressing to spastic quadriplegia), and cold, clumsy hands with intrinsic hand atrophy constitute the well-documented clinical triad that identifies foramen magnum meningiomas.

Surgical Technique

Lateral or posterior foramen magnum meningiomas can be resected using a standard inferior suboccipital approach. However, in ventral foramen magnum meningiomas, because of the involvement of the lower cranial nerves and vertebrobasilar artery complex and significant brain stem compression, we prefer resection of these tumors using the transcondylar approach.

For the transcondylar approach, we prefer the semisitting position with intraoperative monitoring of the caudal cranial nerves and using intraoperative TEE for the early detection of the air emboli.

The incision that we prefer is the modified hockey stick, although the linear incision could be also another favorable option. The incision starts at the tip of the ipsilateral mastoid, continues above the superior nuchal line, and then curves to the midline and down to the level of C3 (Fig. 5.23a). Such type of incision provides enough space for C1–C2 navigated transpedicular screw fixation if complete condylar resection happened during this approach.

The skin flap is then elevated. The preservation of a muscle «cuff» at the level of the superior nuchal line is helpful for the correct approximation of the musculature at the end of the procedure and in the prevention of a CSF leak. After the exposure of the C1, the posterior arch of C1 is followed laterally to the sulcus arteriosus, which marks the medial limit of the vertebral artery. The skeletonization of the vertebral artery is not anymore recommended, and it should be enough to see or palpate the pulsation of the artery [15].

After the position of the sulcus arteriosus and the vertebral artery is identified, the ipsilateral posterior arch of the atlas is removed, either with the footplate of a high-speed drill or with rongeurs. In semisitting position, it is very crucial to use bone wax at the remained part of C1 to stop any bleeding from the spongy bone and to prevent air entrance to the venous plexus followed by air emboli.

The lip of the foramen magnum is then identified, and a small craniotomy is performed with the aid of a high-speed drill or

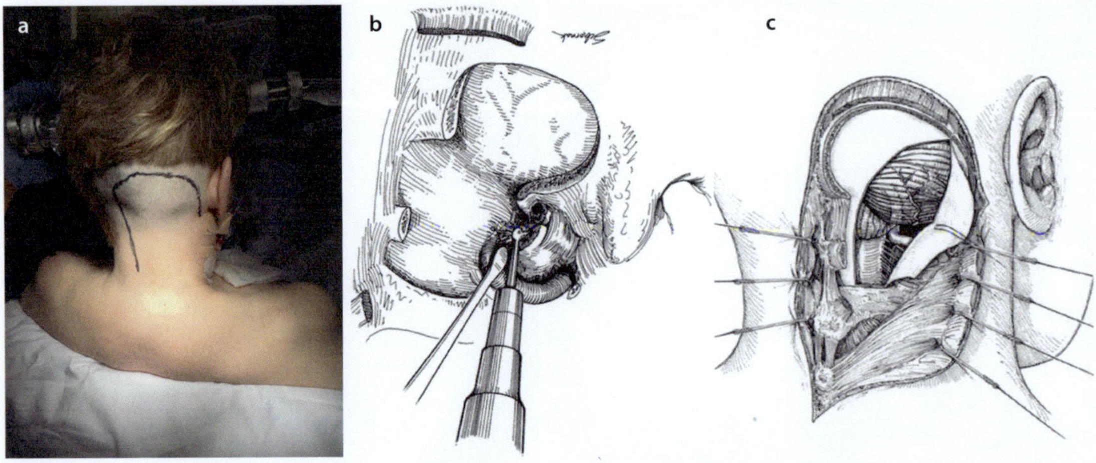

Fig. 5.23 **a** Modified hockey stick incision for right transcondylar approach in semisitting position. **b** Partial condylectomy after removing the C1, before opening the dura (pay attention to oblique dural entrance of vertebral artery). **c** Exposure of a ventral foramen magnum anatomy (*schematic view*) through the right transcondylar approach after opening the dura

craniotome. The next key step is the drilling of the condyle (Fig. 5.23b). Although debate exists regarding how much condyle needs to be drilled, we usually let the lesion dictate how much removal of the condyle is necessary. In our opinion, after drilling more than half of the condyle, the C0–C2 fusion surgery should be mandatory.

We usually open the dura in a curvilinear fashion with special attention to the vertebral artery oblique entrance to the dura (Fig. 5.23b). After the dura is opened, the exposure obtained encompasses the lower cranial nerves to C2 (Fig. 5.23c). A superior extension of this basic approach allows the surgeon to follow lesions up to the internal auditory meatus.

There are two corridors of attack to the tumor in this approach. The first corridor is above the intradural part of vertebral artery, and the second corridor is below it. Special attention should be given to the loop of the hypoglossal nerve curving over the vertebral artery. Figure 5.24 shows the exposure of a ventral foramen magnum meningioma through the transcondylar approach.

In some situations, it is necessary to sacrifice the C1 nerve root to expand the exposure. We usually use local anesthetic for the accessory nerve to prevent the firing of the trapezius muscle during the gentle nerve's manipulation.

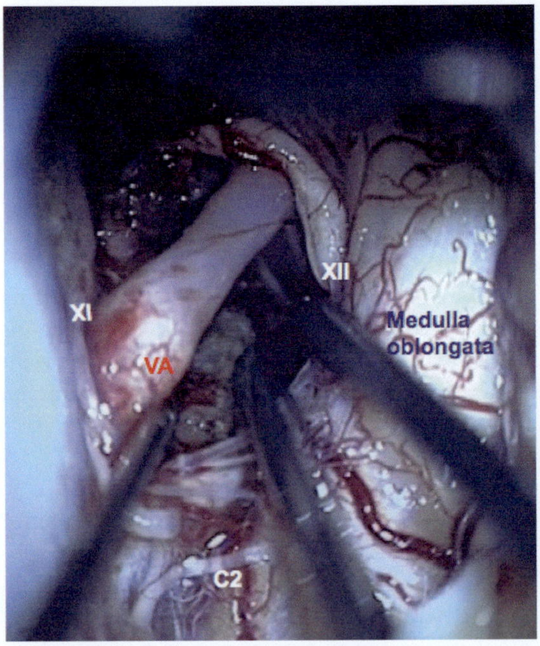

Fig. 5.24 Intraoperative view of the far lateral approach to the left-sided ventral foramen magnum meningioma (*VA* vertebral artery, *XI* accessory nerve, *XII* hypoglossal nerve, *C2* second cervical nerve)

Summary

Advances in microsurgical techniques, neurological anesthetic management, and skull base approaches have led to improved results of foramen magnum meningiomas. The far lateral approach allows a tangential, unobstructed view of the lateroventral cervicomedullary area and can be applied effectively to manage ventral foramen magnum meningiomas.

5.2 Optic Pathway and Hypothalamus Gliomas

H. Borghei-Razavi and U. Schick

5.2.1 General Information

Optic pathway (OPG) and hypothalamus gliomas encompass a spectrum of findings ranging from lesions confined to the optic nerve only, lesions affecting the optic chiasm and hypothalamus, and to lesions with diffuse involvement of a large part of the optic pathway and neighboring structures. The origin of globular tumors in a suprasellar location may be indistinguishable; they can originate from either the chiasm or the hypothalamus because there are no discernible anatomic borders between these two structures.

As a relatively uncommon cause of vision loss in children, they affect young children more than adolescents or adults.

The majority (59–70%) of patients with optic pathway gliomas present before age 10 and another 20–22% by age 20. These are relatively rare tumors, but they comprise 5% of all brain tumors in children and 25–30% of all brain tumors in children less than 5 years old.

The incidence of neurofibromatosis Type I (von Recklinghausen's disease) among patients with optic gliomas is 10–70% (mean, 25%). Fifteen percent of patients with neurofibromatosis Type I have optic gliomas. OPGs associated with neurofibromatosis Type I (NF1) generally have an even more favorable course [16].

The majority of pediatric low-grade astrocytomas in the optic/chiasmatic region are typical *pilocytic astrocytoma* [17]. The rest of them (10%) may be other gliomas such as fibrillary pilomyxoid astrocytoma (grade 2 WHO).

Adult patients with OPG can be divided into two groups: adult patients with tumors diagnosed in childhood and adult patients diagnosed during adulthood [18].

Orbital optic glioma without involving the chiasm is a special entity in glioma surgery that can be cured with a suitable treatment plan.

5.2.2 Clinical Findings

The presentation of optic pathway glioma depends on the location of the tumor within the visual pathway. Generally, involvement of the optic tracts and other postchiasmal structures at tumor diagnosis is associated with a higher probability of visual acuity loss [19].

Optic nerve gliomas which comprise approximately 25% of optic gliomas typically present with slow, painless, unilateral visual loss, optic disc swelling or atrophy, proptosis, or strabismus. Rarely, patients with optic nerve gliomas may develop a central retinal vein occlusion, iris rubeosis with neovascular glaucoma, or ocular ischemic syndrome (◘ Fig. 5.25).

Chiasmal gliomas typically present with slow bilateral visual loss, optic disc swelling or atrophy, strabismus, or variable visual field defects (◘ Fig. 5.26).

Hypothalamic gliomas may be signified by precocious puberty and diencephalic syndrome (Russell's syndrome) consisting of emaciation, euphoria, hyperkinesis, or hydrocephalus. It can also be manifested with obesity.

Tumors of hypothalamic origin may not cause visual symptoms. Suprasellar gliomas extending into the third ventricle often cause obstructive hydrocephalus (◘ Fig. 5.27).

The diagnosis of OPHG is often delayed, and these tumors can be quite large at discovery.

5.2.3 Investigations

Magnetic resonance imaging (MRI) is superior to computerized tomography in the evaluation of the canalicular, chiasmal, and optic tract/hypothalamic extent of the glioma. Cyst formation in or around the solid tumor may be present.

Optic nerve gliomas show bulb-shaped intraorbital enlargement of the optic nerve with extension of the tumor to the apex, which results in a tortuous course and often kinking appearance (◘ Fig. 5.25).

Chiasmal hypothalamic gliomas appear as an enlargement of the chiasm or as a suprasellar mass, occasionally with a cystic component. The lesions are isointense or hypointense on T1-weighted images and hyperintense on T2-weighted images

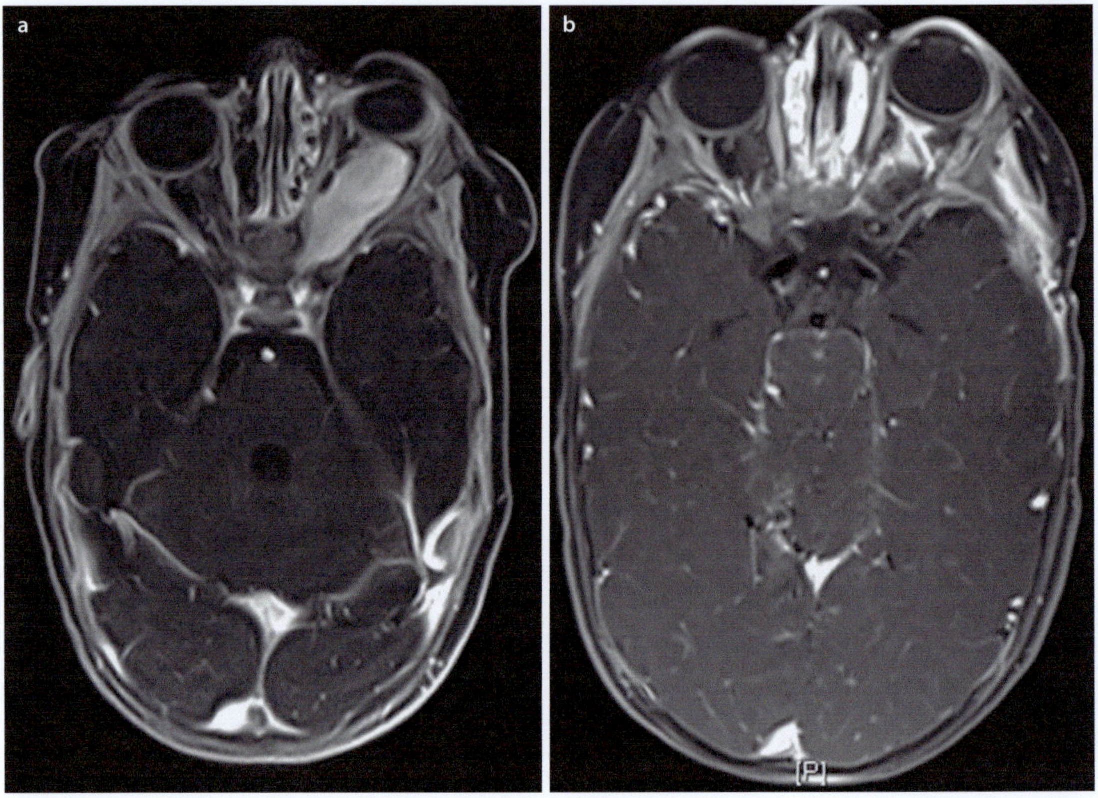

Fig. 5.25 **a** Preoperative axial MRI with contrast of the 6-month-old baby shows tumor growth from the orbit into the optic canal and further tumor extension into the intracranial space affecting the ipsilateral optic nerve, but not having infiltrated the chiasm. **b** Postoperative axial MRI with contrast of this case shows complete removal of the tumor and the optic nerve via prechiasmatic and extradural transection

and may be enhanced with gadolinium. The MRI appearance is almost pathognomonic (Figs. 5.26 and 5.27).

The *differential diagnosis* of children with suprasellar gliomas includes craniopharyngioma, pituitary adenoma, germ cell tumor, and hypothalamic hamartoma.

Differentiating between optic nerve neoplasm and inflammation may be difficult.

5.2.4 Therapeutic Options

Treatment should be considered when there is documented clinical worsening manifested by visual loss or radiographic progression indicated by tumor enlargement.

When the patient has symptoms or the tumor is progressing, or both, treatment is necessary. Although radical tumor resection is ideal, because of the anatomic structures present around the tumor, aggressive surgery would compromise visual, neurological, and endocrine functions. Therefore, total resection is not possible without risk of complications [21].

Chemotherapy

Chemotherapy has been frequently the primary mode of treatment of symptomatic children over the past two decades as a result of the significant latent morbidity associated with RT. At present, many clinicians consider chemotherapy to be the first-line treatment in children because of fewer side effects compared to RT [20]. In children younger than 3 years, it is usually the only adjuvant treatment because intellectual and other functions are relatively well preserved.

The SIOP LGG 2004 study applied stringent criteria for diagnostic work-up, guidelines for surgical procedures, and clear indications to start nonsurgical therapy, offering an individualized sequence of treatment modalities according to established guidelines for subgroups defined by

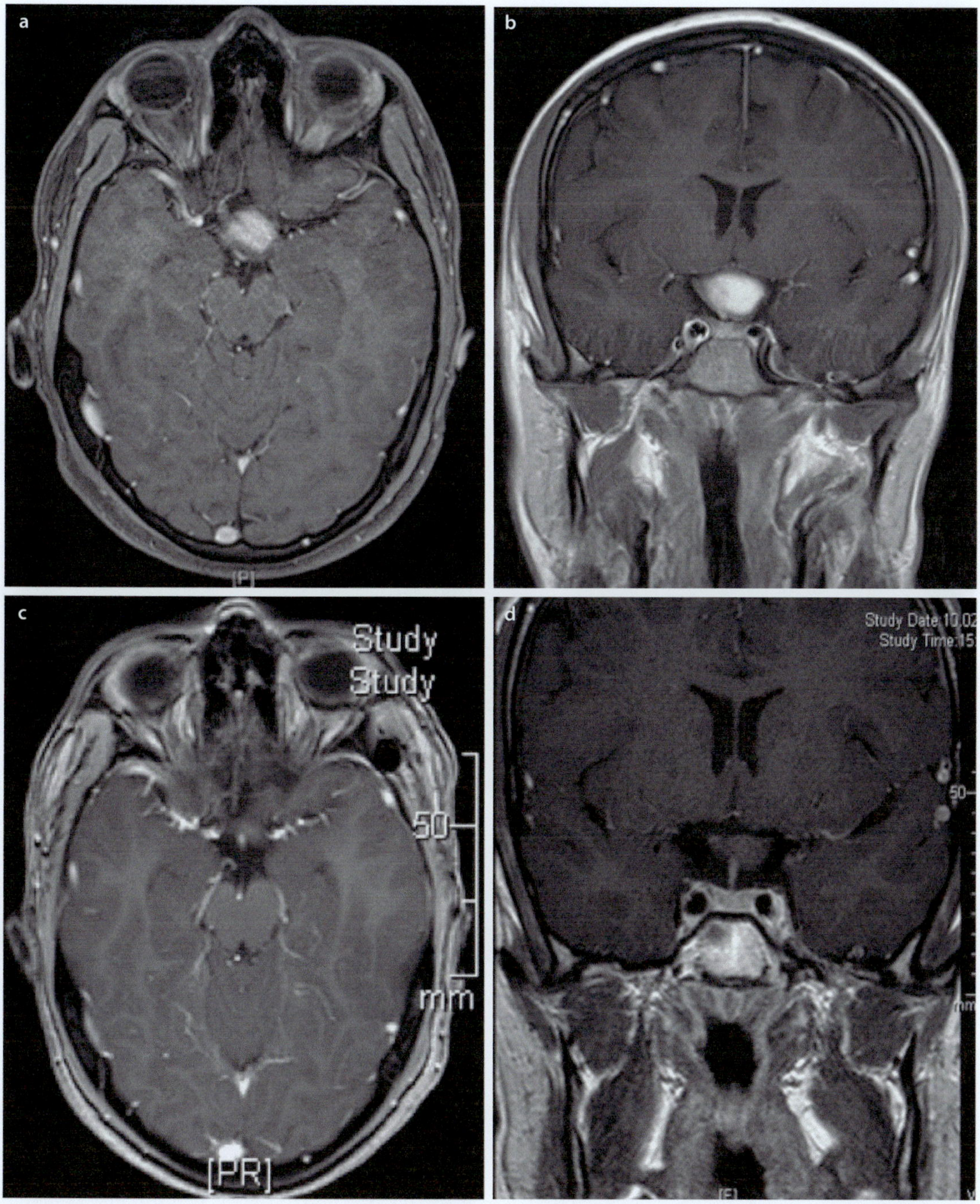

Fig. 5.26 Preoperative MRI of the 14-year-old patient with chiasmal glioma, axial **a** and coronal **b**. Postoperative 1-year follow-up MRI after tumor biopsy and radiotherapy, axial **c**, coronal **d**

the tumor location and the presence or absence of neurofibromatosis NF1. The published protocol of this European study can be used as a guideline for chemotherapy of different children with optic LGG (siop-lgg.cineca.org).

Radiation Therapy (RT)

Older children and those with progressive disease during chemotherapy or with relapse after the completion of chemotherapy are treated with RT [22] (Fig. 5.26).

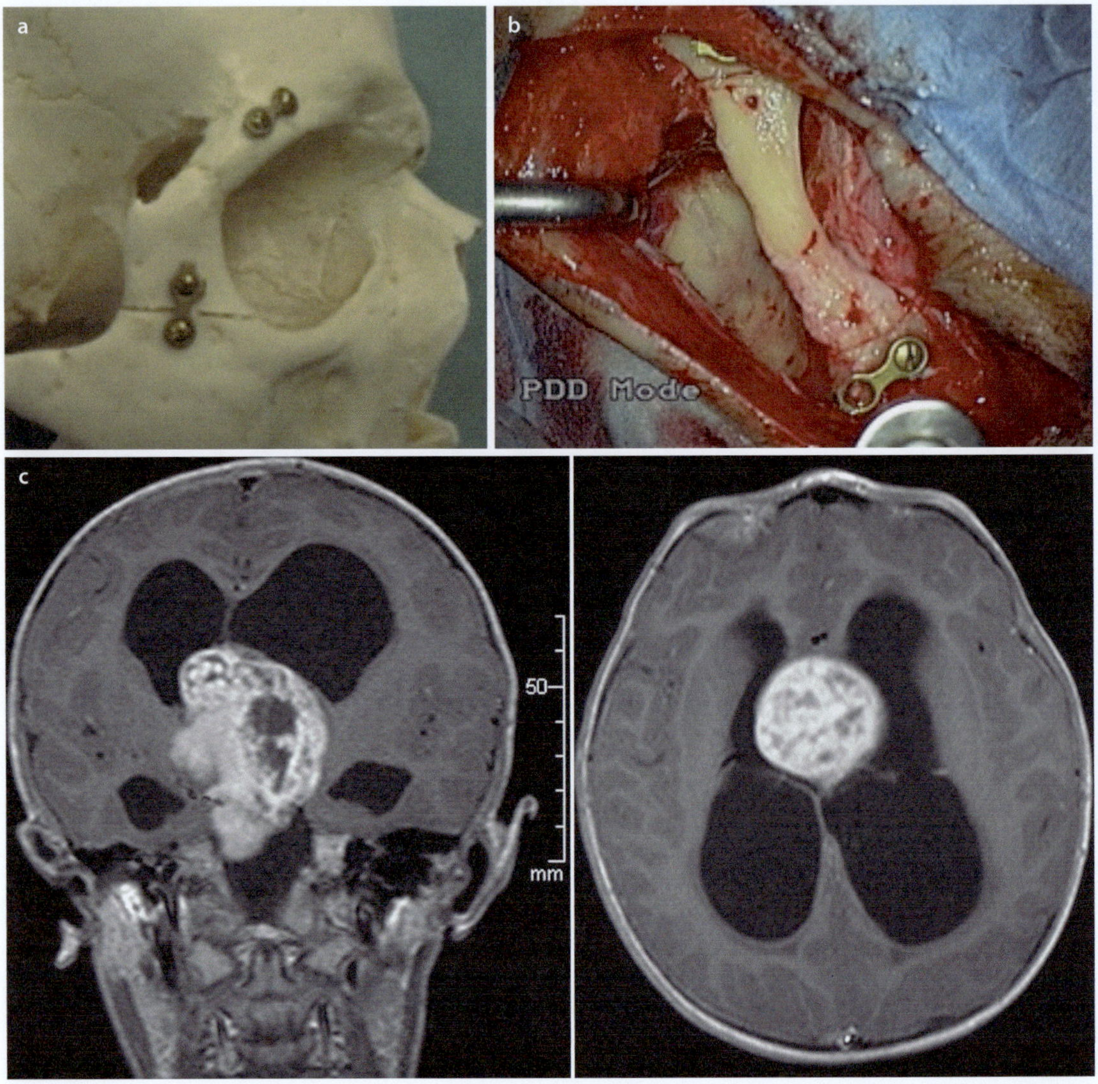

Fig. 5.27 Preoperative coronal **a**, axial **b**, and sagittal **c** MRI of the 1-year-old baby with diffuse hypothalamic suprasellar glioma

5.2.5 Surgical Treatment

Optic Nerve Glioma Without Involvement of the Chiasm

As explained previously, orbital glioma without involvement of the chiasm and contralateral eye (Fig. 5.25) is a special entity in optic glioma that can be cured with suitable planning. In the literature, only 5–10% of optic nerve gliomas recur in the chiasm after «complete» intraorbital excision. In *blind patients* with *ipsilateral proptosis* and who are in *pain* without involving the chiasm, gross total tumor removal with prechiasmatic transection of the optic nerve could be achieved.

No recurrence in our series emphasizes that performing prechiasmatic transection in highly selected cases of optic nerve glioma might offer a further treatment option to avoid tumor growth toward the chiasm without any adjuvant therapy.

Our selected approach is pterional intra- and extradural with the opportunity to resect the infiltrated optic nerve (Fig. 5.28) and transection of the nerve 2–3 mm behind the globe extradurally and 2–3 mm prechiasmatic intradurally and complete removal of the affected intracanalicular part of the optic nerve in between (Figs. 5.29 and 5.30—see also surgical approaches).

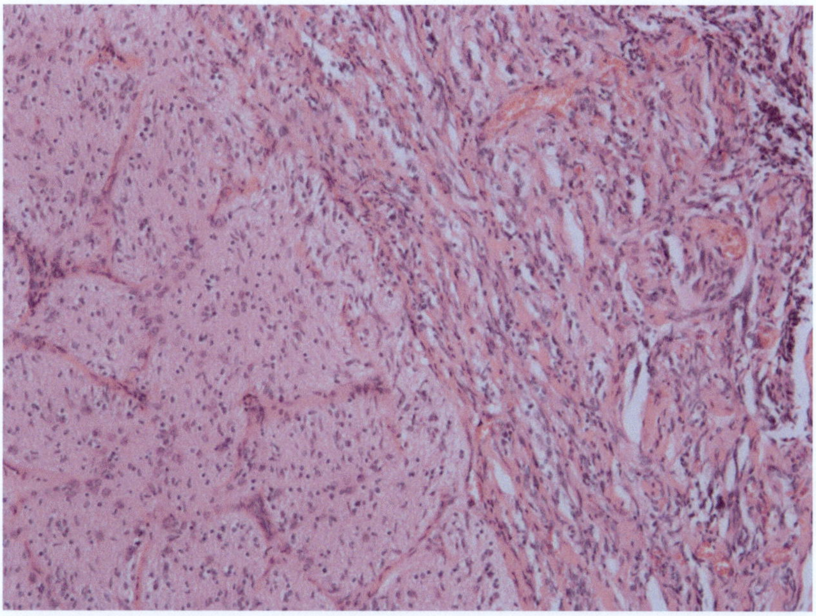

Fig. 5.28 Pathology of case in Fig. 5.25: Diffuse astrocytoma infiltrating the optic nerve (*left*) and meninges (*right*). Hematoxylin and eosin

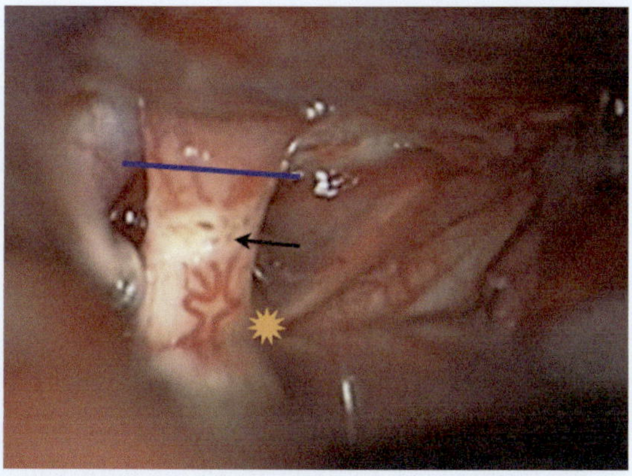

Fig. 5.29 Intradural exposure of the left optic nerve and chiasm in Fig. 5.25 emphasize the freedom of chiasm (*yellow star* shows the chiasm, *blue line* shows the border of the tumor in prechiasmatic region, *black arrow* shows the exact place of transection anterior to the chiasm and posterior to the tumor border)

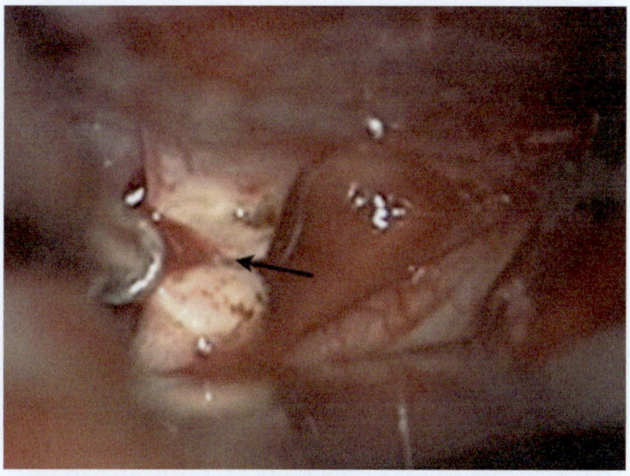

Fig. 5.30 Beginning the tumor removal by left prechiasmatic transection of the optic nerve intradurally (follow *black arrow* from Fig. 5.30 to Fig. 5.29—see also Video 5.2)

Chiasmal Hypothalamic Tumors

Although incomplete surgical resection has not been shown to affect survival, the benefits of surgery include histologic verification, cytoreduction to allow increased sensitivity to adjuvant therapy, and restoration of CSF circulation (Figs. 5.26 and 5.27).

Injury to the hypothalamus may lead to hypothalamic *obesity*, memory loss, electrolyte imbalance, or behavioral changes. Manipulation of arterial vessels may lead to ischemic injury and result in a cerebrovascular event.

The suitable surgical approach for debulking depends on the direction of maximal tumor extension [23]. Adjuvant therapy should be used based on the above discussion.

Approximately 50% of patients with suprasellar astrocytoma have obstructive hydrocephalus, which can be treated with a shunt. Because of obstruction at the interventricular foramen or anterior third ventricle, fenestration of the septum pellucidum or bilateral shunts is needed.

Diffuse Optic Pathway Gliomas

Surgical resection is not feasible for gliomas diffusely involving the optic pathway, including the optic chiasm, tracts, and radiations and the brain stem. These structures are treated nonsurgically with chemotherapy or RT, or both.

Obstructive hydrocephalus should be treated with a shunt.

Surgical Approaches

Combined Pterional Intra- and Extradural Approach

To perform a combined intra- and extradural approach, following a pterional craniotomy, first, the superior orbital fissure is exposed extradurally, and a partial anterior clinoidectomy is performed.

As a next step, the optic canal and the orbit are opened by drilling carefully the lateral and medial sides of the optic canal as well as the roof and the lateral wall of the orbit itself, finally allowing exploration of the optic nerve and the periorbita.

In particular, with respect to cosmetic outcome, special attention is paid to leaving the supraorbital rim intact. By a midline incision, the periorbita is opened, and the intraorbital part of the tumor-infiltrated optic nerve could be displayed and finally resected.

To achieve a vast tumor resection, the optic nerve needs to be transected extradurally behind the bulb with 2–3 mm distance from the bulb to preserve the integrity of the eyeball.

After removing the tumor-infiltrated optic nerve inside the orbit (intraorbital–intraconal part), the intracanalicular part of the tumor should be removed.

The affected part of the optic nerve at the apex should not be transected directly because of the risk of injury to the superior branch of the oculomotor nerve. The tumor should be gently pulled out in the apex and the optic canal underneath the nerve.

Next, the dura should be opened. After gentle retraction of the frontal lobe, the tumor-infiltrated nerve could be exposed, and tumor masses are removed by preserving all adjacent vascular and nervous structures with special attention paid to the ophthalmic artery before nerve transection.

By performing a prechiasmatic transection of the optic nerve, a complete removal of the tumor-infiltrated nerve can be achieved (◘ Figs. 5.28, 5.29, and 5.30; ◘ Video 5.2).

The dura is later closed tightly. To prevent a cerebrospinal fluid (CSF) leak extradurally, the optic canal should be closed by fat, TachoSil, and fibrin glue.

Finally, the periorbita should be closed by fat, fibrin glue, audiomesh, and autologous resected bone of the orbital roof without using any foreign bodies such as small plate or screws in children.

Lateral Orbitotomy

Lateral orbitotomy provides excellent exposure of the lateral compartment of the orbit and can be used for well-defined periorbital and intraconal tumors located lateral, dorsal, and basal to the optic nerve. The skin incision begins superiorly and laterally in the eyebrow and is carried posteriorly along the zygomatic bone. Then the temporalis fascia is incised, beginning at the midportion of the frontozygomatic bone. Transection of the optic nerve in the apex is also possible by this approach.

Supraorbital Approach

Supraorbital craniotomy can be carried out using a keyhole-sized burr hole plus a small craniotomy. The tumor can be removed after decompression of the optic nerve via removal of the optic canal roof and anterior clinoid process and then intradurally.

Anterior Interhemispheric Transcallosal Approach

For resection of tumors with suprasellar extension or intraventricular tumors, an anterior interhemispheric transcallosal approach is used to gain direct access to the third ventricle. The fornix needs to be protected on both sides. One can separate the upper portion of the hypothalamic glioma from the lateral wall (thalamus), but the inferior portion below the hypothalamic sulcus tends to blend into the hypothalamus. Only the exophytic portion and central core of the tumor are amenable to removal (◘ Fig. 5.31).

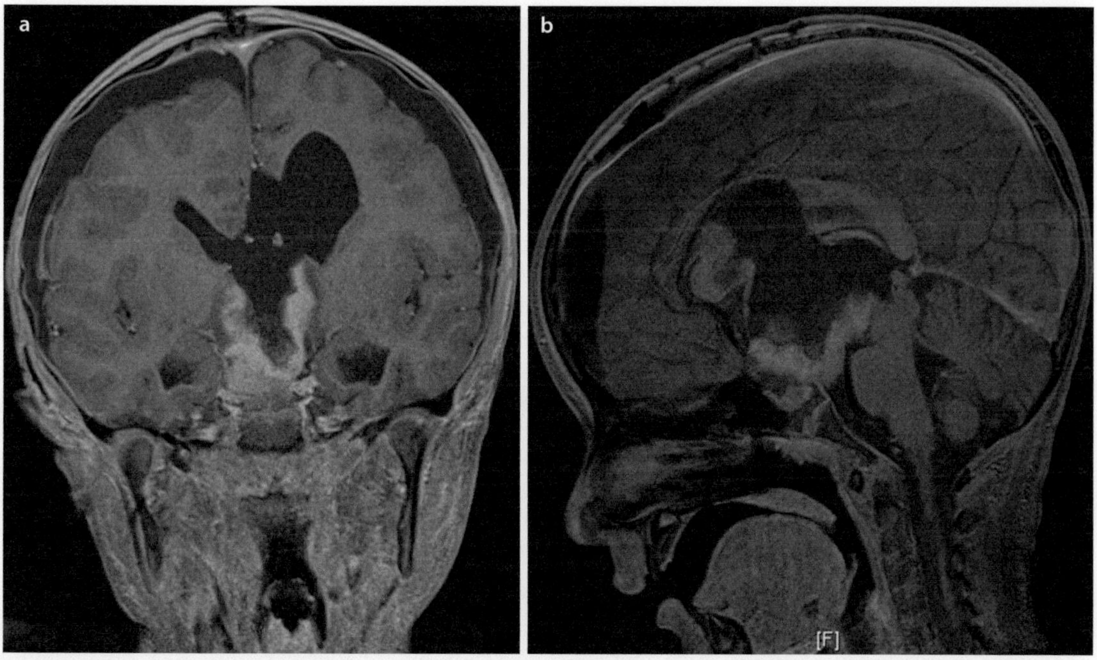

■ **Fig. 5.31** Postoperative MRI of the patient presented in ■ Fig. 5.29 after tumor debulking via interhemispheric transcallosal approach, coronal **a** and sagittal **b**

5.3 Acoustic Neuromas

K. Fugleholm

Acoustic neuroma (AN) aka vestibular schwannoma or acoustic neuroma is a benign sporadic tumor or a manifestation of neurofibromatosis Type 2 (NF2) with bilateral ANs. After pituitary adenoma, it is by far the most common skull base tumor with a current incidence in Denmark of more than 22 per million per year [71]. The current management modalities for AN are watchful waiting, microsurgery, stereotactic irradiation, or biological therapy.

The development of acoustic neuroma surgery has paved the way for posterolateral skull base surgery in general, and AN constitutes a separate entity in the skull base surgery specialty. A patient with an AN often presents with minor symptoms, making treatment prophylactic to a more severe deterioration of health, which may or may not happen after an uncertain period of time. Surgical treatment of AN is a complex undertaking with a potential for added severe and lasting disability, and the importance of a centralized team-based approach in order to deploy adequate advantage of experience cannot be overstated [35]. The present text will focus on the practical aspects of AN surgery, from preoperative work-up to surgery.

5.3.1 Classification of AN

AN is classified according to size, location, mass effect, structure, histology, and degree of removal. In 2003 it was agreed that the size of an AN should be reported as the largest extrameatal diameter [46]. A subdivision into intracanalicular (no extension beyond porus), small, medium-sized, large, and giant AN is often used, but there is unfortunately no consensus about the size distribution for each class. Others have suggested various classifications, of which the Koos grading according to mass effect [48] has been used frequently before the consensus paper in 2003. AN can be lateral or less frequently medial [77]. The structure of an AN can be described as cystic or solid. The grade of removal of AN has been suggested (Kanzaki) to be reported as either total, near total (less than 2% left), partial (less than 5% left), or subtotal (more than 5% left). AN is benign and contains various amounts of histologically distinct areas (Antoni A/ Antoni B), but primary malignant AN (◘ Fig. 5.42, [34]) and malignant transformation of AN [27] have been reported. Malignant AN is classified as malignant peripheral nerve sheath tumor (MPNST) and belongs in the sarcoma group.

5.3.2 Strategy for Management of AN

Sporadic AN

◘ Figure 5.32 suggests pathways to select patients for surgery. The management strategies have been changing toward a more conservative management during the past decades [33]. There is limited evidence base for optimal choice of management, and it seems that all patients with small to medium tumors experience high rates of tumor control and excellent facial nerve outcomes regardless of treatment modality and that patient-related factors are the drivers of quality of life, rather than treatment modality [32]. Treatment of AN is not only influenced by medical evidence and preferences of doctors and patients but also by local tradition, health economy, and infrastructure. Hence, the best management option for a specific patient, given the individual circumstances, may be outside the outlined pathways in ◘ Fig. 5.32, where the assumption is unlimited and safe access to all treatment modalities.

AN Associated with NF2

In terms of decision-making and surgical technique, the bilateral and sometimes multiple ANs in NF2 patients represent a difficult and

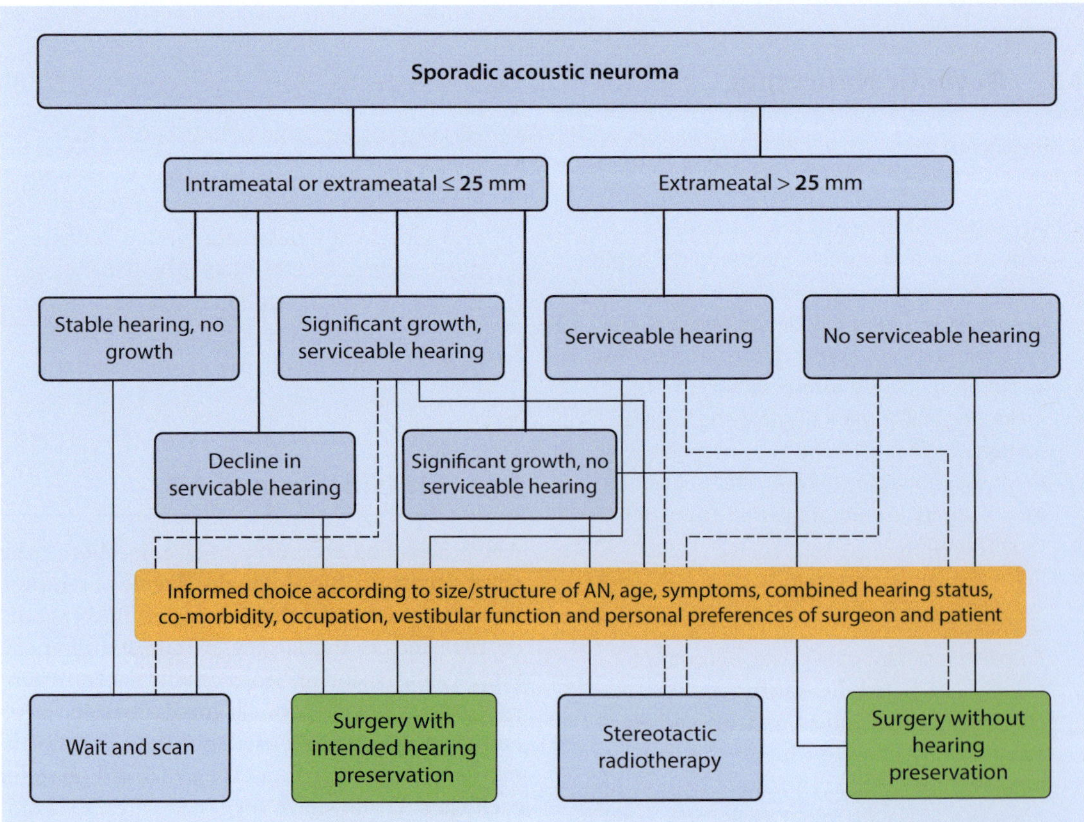

◘ **Fig. 5.32** Suggested patient selection shown as a flowchart. Full lines show likely pathways; *dotted lines* show unusual pathways. Few patients with AN >25 mm are followed with wait and scan, but this is still the exception and is not shown

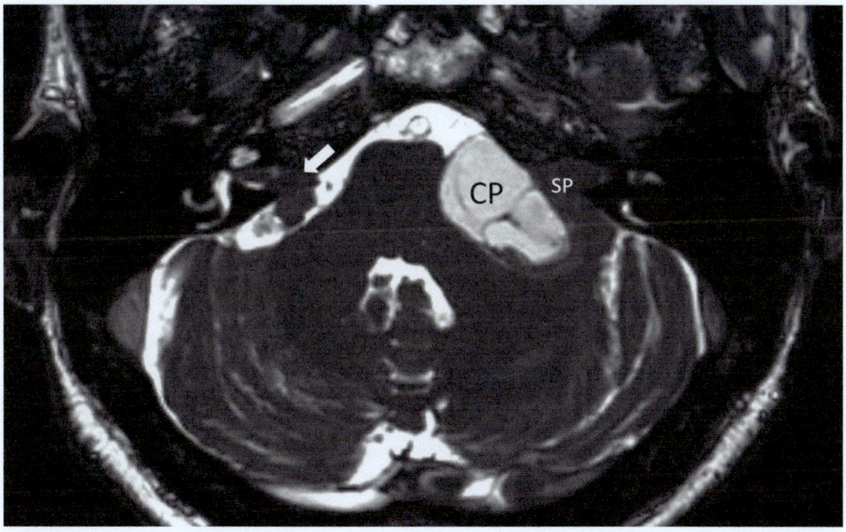

Fig. 5.33 T2 axial MRI of an NF2 patient with a small AN on the right side (*white arrow*) and a large partly cystic (*CP*), partly solid (*SP*) AN on the left side. This patient had normal hearing on both sides but enlargement of the cystic AN on serial imaging. A selective decompression of the cystic AN was carried out with a retrosigmoid approach without any loss of hearing

more complex challenge compared to sporadic AN. Radiation therapy is less effective in NF2 [62], whereas biological therapy (bevacizumab) represents a further alternative to surgery [59]. There is a high lifetime risk of complete deafness regardless of management strategy. NF2 patients often have other benign tumors, such as schwannomas arising from other cranial nerves, meningiomas, and peripheral schwannomas, contributing to the burden of the disease. Due to the complexity of the disease, multidisciplinary centralized care has been introduced in some countries [39]. The strategy regarding surgery is more conservative than with sporadic AN, and when surgery is performed, it may be less aggressive and always balanced against the chance of hearing preservation. Surgery may have decompression of the meatus or tumor with possible release of the cochlear nerve as the only goal (Fig. 5.33). Severe brain stem compression is a typical absolute indication for surgery, but any chance of hearing preservation should still be pursued, and cochlear implant [50, 75] or brain stem implant [52] is an option to be considered for hearing restoration. Patients under the age of 30 with unilateral symptomatic AN should be genetically tested for NF2 mutations prior to the choice of treatment strategy as they have a significant risk of NF2 and development of a contralateral AN [40].

Hydrocephalus Associated with AN

More than 10% of patients with AN have associated hydrocephalus at presentation. In the vast majority of AN patients presenting with hydrocephalus, this condition is relieved by surgical removal of the AN, and this should therefore be performed before any treatment of the hydrocephalus, unless the hydrocephalus is presenting as an emergency [41]. In cases where surgery is not the optimal management strategy, treatment should follow current general guidelines for treatment of hydrocephalus. If indicated, a ventricular–peritoneal shunt should be placed on the contralateral side.

5.3.3 Preoperative Management

Outpatient Assessment and Counsel ing

Imaging will invariably be available at the time of referral to the AN surgeon. After assessing the MRI, the history and neurological examination are the next important steps toward the pretreatment evaluation. Individual counseling is mandatory and rightly expected by patients at the first encounter. Factors such as AN size, age, overall hearing status, comorbidity, occupation, and life philosophy should be recorded and integrated in the decision-making toward informed consent for the chosen treatment strategy. If surgery is chosen as the preferred treatment strategy (Fig. 5.32), there is still a decision to make regarding the approach (Fig. 5.34).

Neuroradiological Investigations

MRI is the standard imaging modality for preoperative assessment of AN. Ideally, the MRI includes axial T1, axial T2, and axial, coronal, and

Approach	Indications and advantages	Disadvantages	Positioning	Incision
Translabyrinthine	All sizes of AN, where hearing preservation is not an issue.	Loss of hearing, restricted access anterior to meatus, complex anatomy.	Supine, head turned 60 degrees away	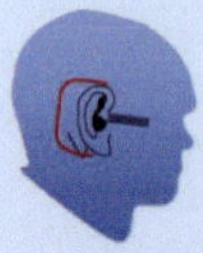
Retrosigmoid	All sizes of AN and for meatal decompression in NF2. Simplest approach.	Cerebellar retraction for large tumors, late contact to facial nerve, postoperative headache.	Prone, head turned 45 degrees	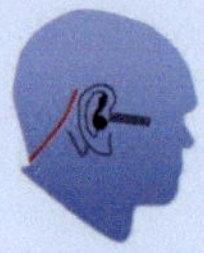
Presigmoid	Intended hearing preservation in small AN without extension to fundus.	Restricted space, no access to fundus, few series published.	Supine, head turned 80 degrees away	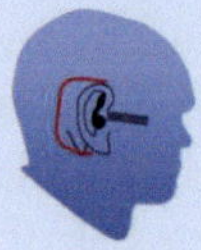
Subtemporal (middle fossa)	Small AN, all extradural except meatus, small risk of CSF leak, suitable for meatal decompression in NF2.	Temporal lobe retraction. Restricted access to posterior fossa, complex anatomy.	Supine head turned 60 degrees away	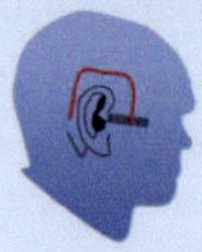
Endoscopic (retrosigmoid)	Small to medium sized AN with intended hearing preservation.	New method, not fully established, endoscopic experience needed.	Semi-sitting, head rotation away	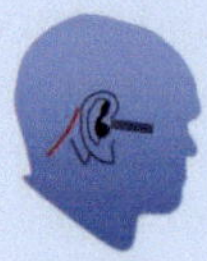

Fig. 5.34 Surgical approaches for the resection of acoustic neuromas

sagittal T1 with intravenous contrast, as well as a 3D CISS/FIESTA axial sequence (Fig. 5.35). This selection of sequences is far from always provided by the referring doctor. With an optimal high Tesla MRI and a 3D CISS/FIESTA axial sequence, nerves and vessels are seen in the meatus (Fig. 5.35), and it is sometimes possible to assess the likely course of the cranial nerves around a small- or medium-sized AN. Recently, MRI tractography has been employed with some success to track the course of the meatal nerves in relation to large ANs [74].

The appearance of an extrameatal AN on MRI is typical (Fig. 5.36), and the diagnosis is fairly easy to the trained eye. An AN appears as a rounded solid or cystic contrast-enhancing pro-

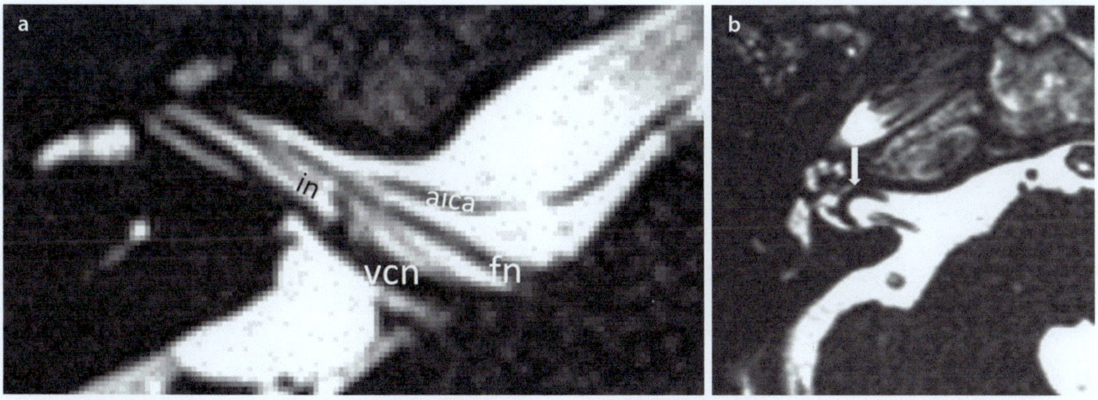

Fig. 5.35 FIESTA T2 axial MRI of the normal meatus on the right side with vestibulocochlear nerve (*vcn*), facial nerve (*fn*), loop of anterior inferior cerebellar artery (*aica*), and intermedius nerve (*in*). Loop of anterior inferior cerebellar artery (*white arrow*) deep in the right meatus, as an incidental finding

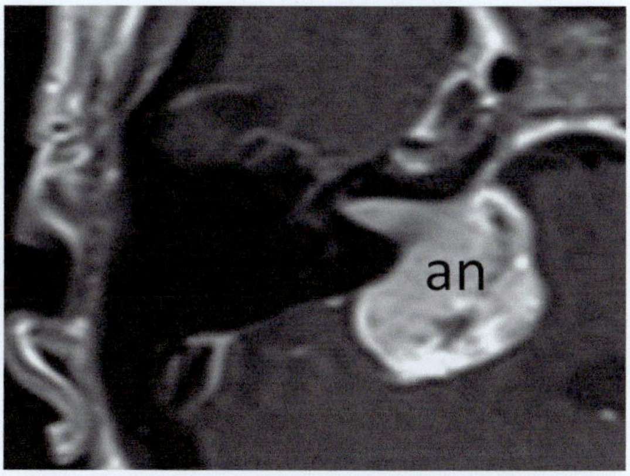

Fig. 5.36 Axial T1 MRI with gadolinium showing a typical extrameatal AN (*an*) without cystic elements. The small areas without contrast enhancement may represent degenerative change corresponding to the histological Antoni B areas. This should not be confused with cystic elements

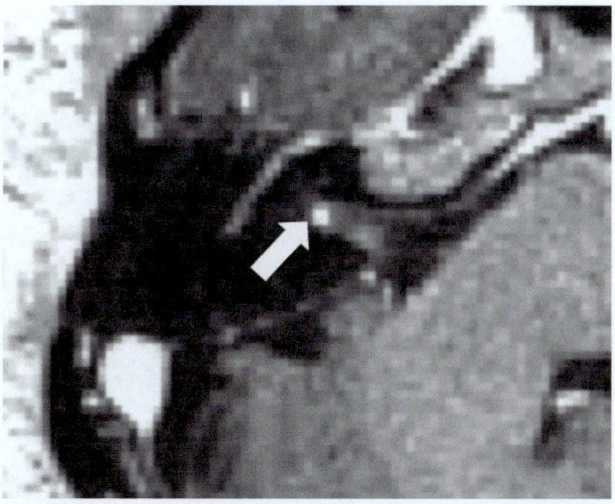

Fig. 5.37 Axial T1 MRI with gadolinium showing a small enhancement (*white arrow*) representing a small AN in the fundus of the right meatus. This type of enhancement can also represent a loop of the anterior inferior cerebellar artery (Fig. 5.35) or an inflammatory lesion of one of the nerves in the meatus

cess with the «center of gravity» corresponding to the meatus, and usually involvement of this. Very small intrameatal ANs appear as enhancing nodules (Fig. 5.37) in sharp contrast to the appearance of a giant AN (Fig. 5.38). Before growing extrameatal, the intrameatal AN often fills the meatus (Fig. 5.33, right meatus). Extrameatal ANs have a mushroomlike appearance on axial and coronal images due to the involvement of the meatus and frequently a significant meatal expansion compared to the contralateral side.

A computer tomography (CT) scan will rarely be available at the time of referral. A thin slice CT scan of the skull base provides a detailed information about the bony anatomy and is still a standard preoperative investigation in some practices. It is true that the position of semicircular canals, jugular bulb, and emissary veins may influence the choice of surgical approach, but this can also be assessed on a state-of-the-art MRI scan (see above). As a CT scan provides little additional information to MRI, involves a large dose of radiation, and may delay assessment and treatment, this investigation is no longer a standard in the preoperative work-up but may be added depending on the available resources and the AN surgeon's preference.

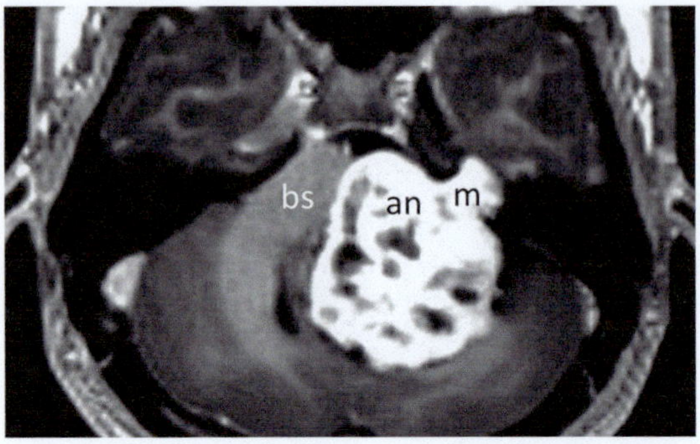

Fig. 5.38 Axial T1 MRI with gadolinium showing a giant AN (*an*) on the left side with a large expansion of the meatus. This patient had a marginal facial palsy preoperatively, and it was not possible to preserve the facial nerve or find the proximal end on the brain stem (*bs*). The patient had a facial–hypoglossal end-to-side anastomosis (▶ Chap. 20) and ended up with House–Brackmann grade 3 function

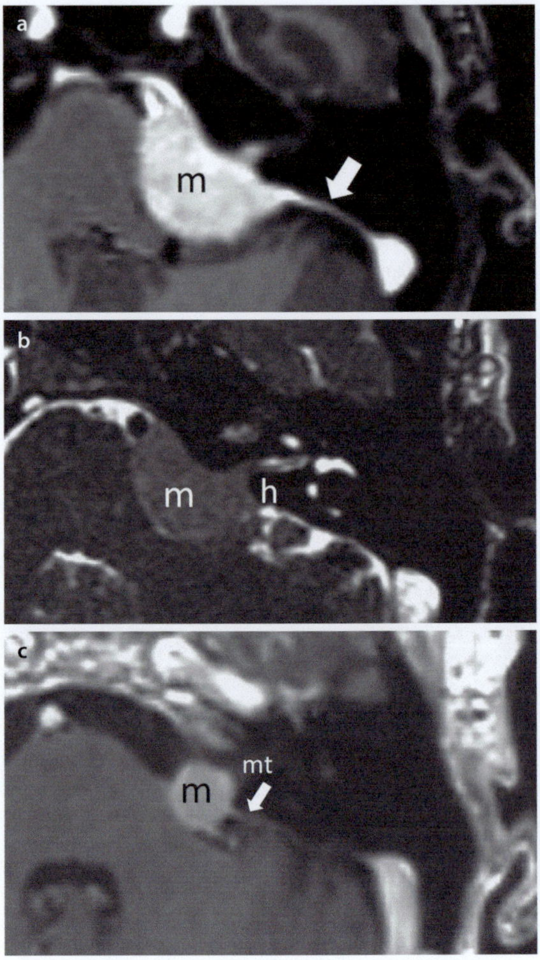

Fig. 5.39 Axial T1 MRI with gadolinium showing typical meningioma (*m*) centered on the left meatus and growing into this. Enhancement of the adjacent dura (*white arrow*) forming a dural «tail» is typical for a meningioma, but not for an AN. The same meningioma (*m*) as in AN but with T2 axial MRI showing a hyperostosis (*h*) of the petrous bone around the porus and a narrowing of the meatus. Hyperostosis is typical for meningioma, especially at the point of insertion, but it is not seen with AN. Axial T1 with gadolinium showing a nodular meningioma at the left meatus (*m*). There is no tumor in the meatus (*mt*), which can also be the case with AN, and there is only a vague dural «tail» (*white arrow*)

Angiography is not needed for differential diagnosis or preoperative assessment. Angiography is used for assessment and embolization of glomus tumors, but these tumors share few characteristics with AN on MRI. Angiography and possible endovascular embolization should as an exception be considered in the rare event of AN in children, where the rich vascularization may pose a significant and even life-threatening surgical risk [60].

Differential Diagnosis

Few patients are diagnosed with AN by the AN surgeon. The first assessment of an AN patient is therefore that of the clinical information, and MRI images are included in the referral. It is at this stage that suspicion of a possible differential pathology should be raised, as additional imaging and information may be needed to increase diagnostic accuracy before seeing the patient. With the benefit of combined clinical and MRI information available after assessment of the patient, the diagnosis of AN is so characteristic that radiotherapy is routinely offered as treatment for a growing AN, without biopsy. Having noted that, even experienced skull base surgeons and neuroradiologists can sometimes be surprised by the pathology.

All the lesions mimicking AN on MRI may cause cochlear, facial, and/or vestibular nerve dysfunction. It is noteworthy that AN on a rare occasion can originate distal to the meatus, from the cochlea or vestibule [72]. Differential diagnoses include other benign tumors, malignant tumors, infectious disease, inflammatory disease, or a vascular lesion. Meningioma arising from the petrous meninges (Fig. 5.39) can mimic AN and is often referred to as AN. Wide contact with the petrous bone, frequent hyperostosis at the insertion point, and a dural «tail» usually distinguish this pathology from AN. Large schwannomas arising from the lower cranial nerves (Fig. 5.40) do not involve the meatus, but the jugular foramen, and will have a lower center of gravity. Often the patient

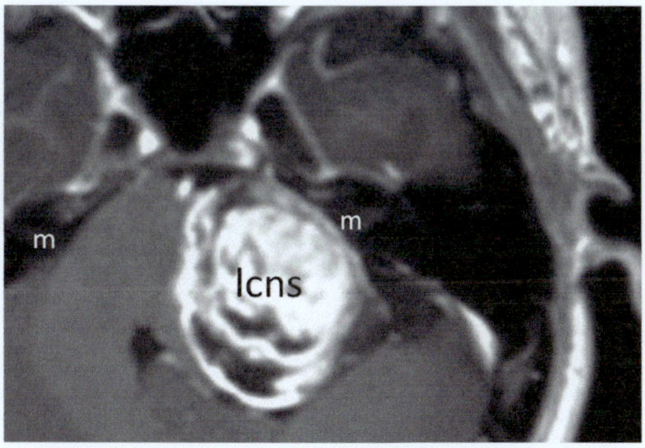

Fig. 5.40 Axial T1 MRI with gadolinium showing a large left-sided lower cranial nerve schwannoma (*lcns*) which may at a quick glance be confused with an AN. In this case, the tumor is not entering the meatus (*m*), which should raise the suspicion that it is not an AN

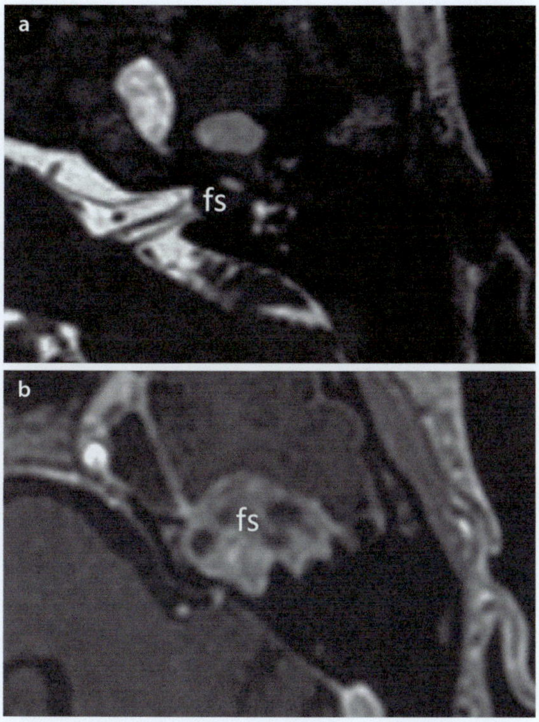

Fig. 5.41 FIESTA T2 axial MRI showing a space-occupying lesion in the left meatus. This is a facial schwannoma. Axial T1 MRI with gadolinium showing that the same facial schwannoma has a much larger component coming from the geniculate ganglion and growing above the petrous bone. This is not seen with an AN

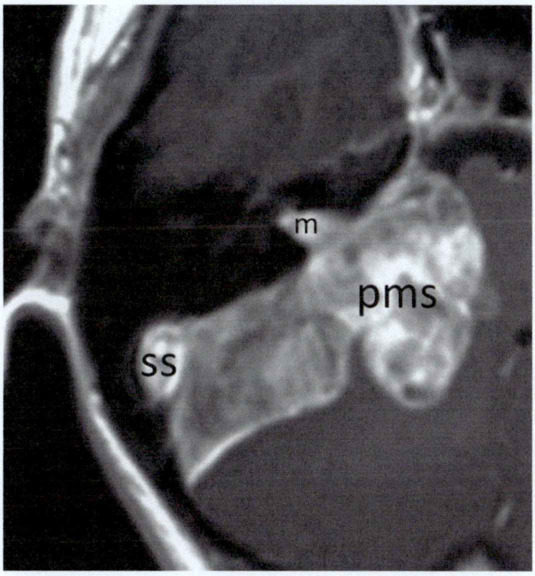

Fig. 5.42 Axial T1 MRI with gadolinium showing a primary malignant schwannoma (*PMS*) or malignant peripheral nerve sheath tumor on the right side. The tumor is filling the meatus (*m*), and the anterior part has the configuration of a regular AN, whereas the posterior part seems to have broken through the capsule and is expanding all the way back to the sigmoid sinus (*ss*). This young patient had two operations, radiotherapy and chemotherapy, but sadly died a few years after presentation despite aggressive therapy

has symptoms or signs of lower cranial nerve deficits. Moreover, even giant ANs rarely invade the jugular foramen. Schwannomas of the facial nerve (Fig. 5.41) are sometimes intrameatal, but arising near the geniculate ganglion, and cause bony erosion. Facial palsy is the typical presentation, as opposed to AN, where complaints of facial weakness are the exception. Very infrequently tumors arising from the medial structures, such as the cerebellum or the choroid plexus, involve the meatus, and hence hemangioblastoma, plexus papilloma, or even pilocytic astrocytoma may masquerade as AN. Small spots of enhancement in the meatus (Fig. 5.37) may represent inflammatory or infectious lesions, especially in the presence of cranial nerve deficits disproportionate to the size of the lesion, and will often disappear on serial imaging. Enhancing lesions representing a malignant disease and involving the meatus may be primary (Fig. 5.42) or secondary (Fig. 5.43). The pattern and time course of cranial nerve involvement should raise the suspicion of an aggressive disease. The anterior inferior cerebellar artery sometimes forms a loop into the meatus (Fig. 5.35), and this also causes meatal enhancement on MRI. Vascular pathology is otherwise rare but an anterior inferior cerebellar artery aneurysm in the meatus can be an unpleasant surprise when operating for an AN [42, 58].

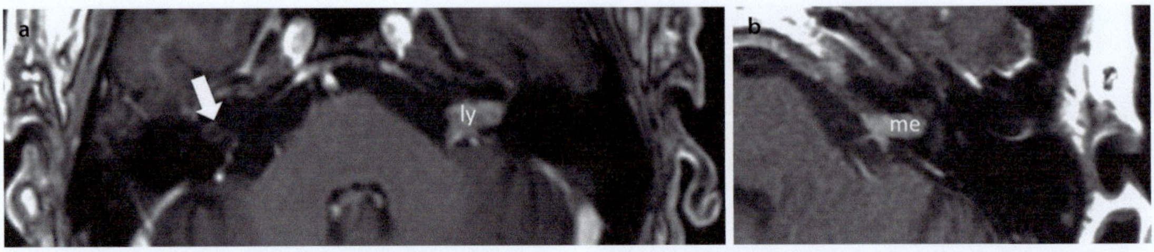

Fig. 5.43 Axial T1 MRI with gadolinium showing B-cell lymphoma (*ly*) in the left meatus. He presented with hearing loss and facial palsy. It turned out that there was bilateral meatal involvement, as indicated by the faint enhancement (*white arrow*) on the right side. A biopsy was obtained via left retrosigmoid approach, and the patient was cured by hematological treatment. Axial T1 MRI with gadolinium showing a left-sided meatal metastasis (*me*) from a known breast carcinoma. The patient had a left retrosigmoid approach for biopsy and radiotherapy and did well for some years. She died from multiple metastases

Audiological and Vestibular Tests

Hearing status on both sides should be assessed by pure-tone audiogram and speech discrimination test. Which combination the hearing level and speech discrimination is serviceable is a matter of constant debate among AN surgeons, but patients quite often have a sensible opinion as well, if they are asked. Hearing is important, not only for the choice of treatment modality but also for the choice of surgical approach. Vestibular function tests will help to predict the immediate postoperative course in terms of nausea, vomiting, and vertigo. Postoperatively the patient must rely on the opposite vestibular apparatus, and the status of this may help predict the degree of vertigo and balance problems in the long term, something which is more important to AN patients than previously acknowledged [32].

Blood Analyses

Surgery of large or giant ANs can from time to time lead to major blood loss and a need for blood transfusion. Therefore, the blood type should be determined prior to surgery. A match is rarely necessary, unless the patient has atypical antibodies. No further blood analysis is needed for otherwise healthy patients without history or clinical signs of coagulopathy. Patients on anticoagulation or antiplatelet therapy and patients who take dietary supplements with anticoagulative effect, such as fish oil, should pause this prior to surgery, except when there is an absolute indication, for example, due to a stent or a mechanical heart valve. In such cases, the anticoagulation treatment must be bridged with heparin around the time of surgery.

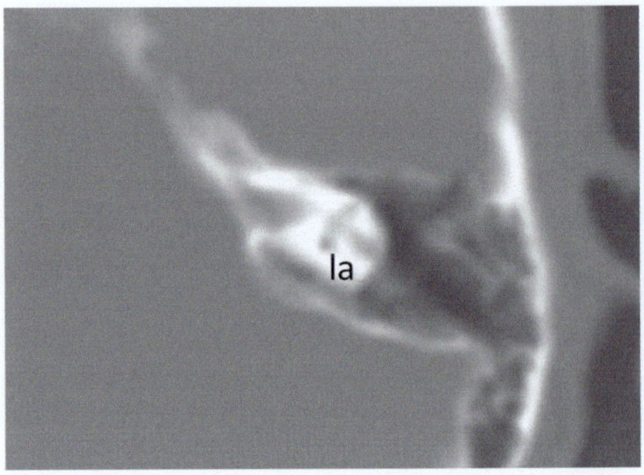

Fig. 5.44 Bone window axial CT showing an almost fully pneumatized mastoid process with the labyrinth (*la*) standing out as a dense block of the bone. In this situation, the mastoidectomy is easy, but the facial nerve may be suspended in an air cell, making the opening of the fallopian canal and identification of the nerve dangerous, if this anatomical variant is not suspected

Other Preoperative Considerations

Once it has been decided to operate, there are still details that can help foreseeing problems during surgery.

It is of value to note the dominance of the ipsilateral sigmoid sinus, to know whether it can be sacrificed if accidentally damaged.

A well-pneumatized mastoid process (Fig. 5.44) makes the mastoidectomy easy, but beware of the possible suspension of the fallopian canal and facial nerve in air cells.

Extensive bony erosion of the meatus makes the last part of the bony exposure more challenging and predicts trouble during the facial nerve dissection, especially at the porus edge.

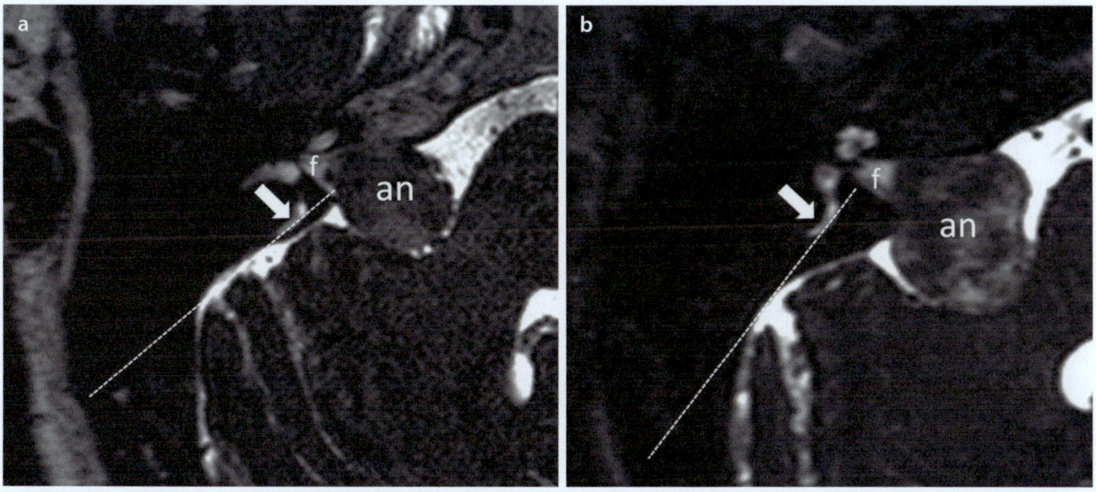

Fig. 5.45 FIESTA T2 axial MRI showing an AN (*an*) in a patient with an almost normal hearing and no tumor in the fundus (*f*). The anatomy is not favorable for a retrosigmoid or presigmoid approach, as the posterior semicircular canal (*white arrow*) is in the way. The dotted line shows the limited access to the fundus. FIESTA T2 axial MRI showing an AN (*an*) in another similar patient with an almost normal hearing and no tumor in the fundus (*f*). The anatomy here is favorable for a retrosigmoid or presigmoid approach, as the posterior semicircular canal (*white arrow*) is not in the way. The *dotted line* shows sufficient access to the fundus

The position of the posterior semicircular canal can limit the access to the fundus in the retrosigmoid approach (Fig. 5.45).

High position of the jugular bulb may deter some surgeons from the translabyrinthine approach, but in reality, this may also be a problem when opening the meatus from the retrosigmoid approach. Although a high bulb can reduce access, it is possible to remove even large ANs via the translabyrinthine approach, when the bulb is «egg shelled» and pushed aside [61].

A very «tight» posterior fossa in a young patient may warrant a preoperative lumbar spinal drain for early and safe CSF release.

5.3.4 Operative Setup, Technique, Approaches, and Tumor Excision

Intraoperative Neuromonitoring

Facial nerve monitoring [38] by facial electromyography (EMG) has improved facial nerve outcome after AN surgery. It can be set up by the surgeon with little extra effort and cost, and no AN should be removed without facial nerve monitoring, if there is a functioning facial nerve. A two-channel EMG with free running recording from the orbicularis oris and orbicularis oculi muscles is sufficient in most cases, but in the rare case of a preoperative partial facial palsy, four-channel recording is useful to increase the sensitivity. Continuous monitoring by either facial motor evoked potentials [51] or facial nerve root exit zone-elicited compound muscle action potential (FREMAP) is a new method offering a possible additional protection of the facial nerve at the cost of extra equipment and specialist staff in theaters.

Cochlear nerve monitoring in hearing preservation surgery can be performed by auditory evoked potentials (AEP), but this is not very useful due to the long delay arising from the necessary 500–2000 times averaging of the potential. A much better feedback can be obtained from continuous, direct, auditory evoked dorsal cochlear nucleus action potentials (AEDNAP). At the cost of additional equipment and specialist staff, this method may well prove to increase the quality of intraoperative decision-making as well as the chance of hearing preservation.

For giant AN, additional monitoring of the lower cranial nerves, of the trigeminal motor nerve, and of the abducens nerve by EMG, and continuous motor/sensory evoked potentials, can be used. This is probably reducing the risk of postoperative cranial nerve and brain stem problems, although this has not been investigated thoroughly.

Microsurgical Technique in AN Sur gery

For centuries, craftsmen have traveled the world to pick up new inspiration and knowledge of their trade. In a similar way, each surgeon will develop his own preference regarding techniques, instruments, and equipment, and in this process, it is advisable to visit other skull base surgeons. Seeking inspiration from others and sharing experience are still important elements in the way the specialty is taken forward and developed.

The microsurgical technique used in AN surgery is similar to the technique used for other skull base tumors but perhaps with more uniform strategies and phases. There are clear similarities to mine clearing. With 100% attention to the task, quick advancement can be made through safe corridors, whereas the surgeon(s) must reduce the pace when hidden «mines» are anticipated close by. At the tumor removal stage of the operation, the nerve stimulator becomes a mine seeker. Without a sufficient experience and a detailed knowledge of the pathological anatomy, the operation will progress very slowly due to lack of confidence and unnecessary caution. Surgeons' fatigue will then be inevitable, posing a further risk of complications. After a long operation and complete excision, the facial nerve is not safe until the wound is closed, as I was taught by Glenn Neil-Dwyer, my first AN master and mentor.

There are different opinions regarding the use of cutting burrs or diamond burrs. The truth is probably that you should use the instruments that you are familiar with and which are safe. Cutting burrs are very fast and produce little heat. Cutting burrs are more sensitive to unstable bearings in the attachment, which will make the burr jump. This is dangerous. Diamond burrs are slower and produce more heat, which is also dangerous. Diamond burrs are more accurate and do not jump. Many surgeons start out with cutting burrs and change to diamond burrs when close to the facial nerve or the meatus.

It is not possible to learn microsurgical technique or AN surgery by reading a book. The technique is best developed through a combination of studies of anatomy and surgery books (e.g., [57, 78]) and Internet-based anatomy/surgical video resources, work in the anatomy lab, microscope training, and most importantly surgical assistance to experienced AN surgeons.

Retraction

The need for retraction depends on the size of the AN, the CSF release, the approach, the age of the patient, the anatomical variations, and the surgical setup. Retractorless surgery should become the standard [49], and when using the four-hand technique (see below), fixed retraction is unnecessary for any of the approaches, perhaps with the exception of extradural retraction for the subtemporal approach. If fixed retraction is used, the risk of cerebellar ischemia and retraction-related cerebellar dysfunction is high [24].

Four-Hand Technique for AN Surgery

Acoustic neuroma surgery spans the classical territories of neurosurgical and otological surgery and is also known as neurotological surgery. Starting with House and Hitzelberger [44], a long tradition of collaboration between surgeons of the two specialties has evolved, especially for the translabyrinthine approach. For the larger tumors, the approach is typically performed in the morning by the otological surgeon and the tumor resection carried out in the afternoon by the neurosurgeon, although many variations of collaboration exist. For the retrosigmoid approach, the sequence could be the reverse, or the procedure may be done by one surgeon altogether. Instead of two senior surgeons working after each other in a serial fashion, the four-hand technique allows two senior surgeons to work in parallel (◘ Fig. 5.46). Such a concept has already been adopted for endoscopic surgery for some time and works equally well for skull base surgery in our setting. The technique requires a good and respectful relationship between the surgeons and a microscope allowing both surgeons to have equal access and visual depth.

Ideally each surgeon is able to book his own patients and remains responsible for the patient before and after surgery. The surgeon in charge of the patient takes the lead during the operation by performing the drilling, supported by the other surgeon. The advantages of the four-hand technique are that both surgeons are able to perform the entire procedure, that the operating time can be shortened significantly with less risk of surgeon fatigue and complications from prolonged unchanged position of the patient on the operating table, that fixed retraction can be avoided, that the intraoperative decision-making is improved, that there is a build-in continuous learning

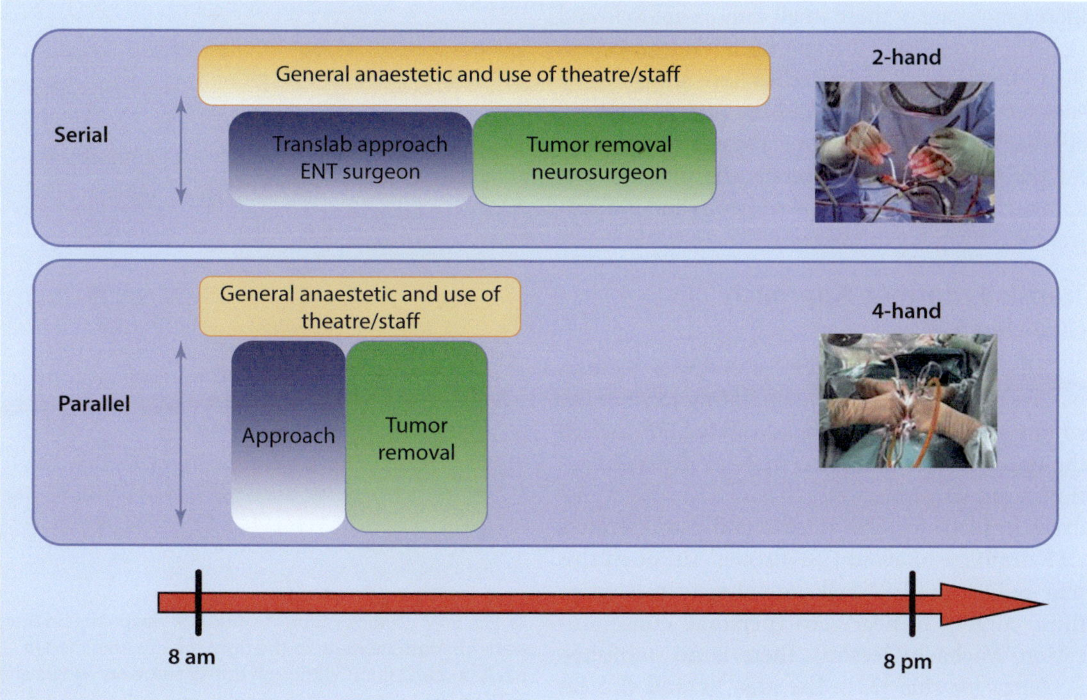

Fig. 5.46 Schematic representation of the difference in organization and use of resources between serial and parallel (four-hand technique) collaboration between two senior skull base surgeons. Time axis (*red arrow*). The area of each square under the yellow bars represents the effort of one surgeon

process, that both surgeons can deal effectively with the whole range of complications, and that the surgeons can replace each other as the surgeon in charge of the patient postoperatively, when needed. It is difficult to see any drawbacks of this method. The question of who is finally responsible for the care of the patient has to be clearly defined, and both surgeons have to be present on the operating day, but this is not different from other setups, where the two surgeons are involved in a serial rather than parallel fashion.

Intraoperative Decision-Making

A few decades ago, complete excision of an AN was the only acceptable result for some AN surgeons, regardless of functional outcome. Now, subtotal or near total excision with preservation of function may be the only acceptable result for the patient. Hence, the relentless pursue of complete tumor removal, continuing long into the night, has given way to a less rigid and more patient-oriented practice. How old is the patient? Is the cochlear nerve or the facial nerve preservation the real challenge in this case? When do we stop? These are among the questions considered or discussed intraoperatively. Tumor resection may be ended several times, and every time, after reconsideration, a small opening may allow further progress, on some occasions leading to a total excision and preservation of the facial nerve after all. Retrospective analysis shows that remnants of AN carry a low re-treatment risk [36, 43, 68] and that remnants are less likely to grow than untreated AN [76]. Acoustic neuroma remnants rarely transform into malignant tumors, whether irradiated or not [27]. Refinements of intraoperative monitoring are likely to allow the surgeon(s) to go closer to the edge and leave a smaller tumor remnant behind, when complete excision with preservation of function is not achievable. This is important as the re-treatment rate is related to the size of the tumor remnant [54, 76].

Approaches

The translabyrinthine and retrosigmoid approaches remain the workhorses for AN surgery (Fig. 5.34). Very few AN surgeons use the other approaches routinely, and if they do, it is primarily for small ANs. The subtemporal approach is best for small ANs with intended hearing preservation, and as an increasing share of these small tumors are followed rather than removed, this approach is now used less than previously. No approaches have shown to be superior to the translabyrinthine or retrosigmoid approaches for larger tumors. The exact indication for the translabyrinthine versus the retrosigmoid approach varies between AN surgeons and is a subject for continuing discussions.

Translabyrinthine Approach (◘ Video 5.3)

The patient is in general anesthesia without paralysis and placed on the operating table in the supine position with the head rotated 60° toward the opposite side and fixed in 3- or 4-point fixation. Some surgeons prefer to have a lumbar spinal drain in place for CSF release and postoperative CSF drainage to avoid CSF fistula. Although this may reduce the CSF leak rate after translabyrinthine surgery to near zero (personal communication, Michael Gleeson), there is no published evidence for this [37]. The area behind the ear is shaved, and a curved incision is marked from the mastoid tip to 1 cm above the attachment of the pinna (◘ Fig. 5.34). The incision line is infiltrated with local anesthetic. The facial electrodes, ground electrode, and reference electrode are placed, and the monitoring system is tested. An incision for harvesting of the fat graft is marked and infiltrated with local anesthetic at the lower part of the abdomen lateral to the midline. The patient is strapped to the table across the chest to allow tilting of the table during surgery. For a large or giant AN, it may be wise to secure access to a sural nerve branch graft from the lateral aspect of the foot, just in case (▶ Sect. 5.3.6). Washing and draping is done in a standard fashion, and the microscope is adjusted and draped.

The translabyrinthine approach should be tailored to the size and position of the AN. Intracanalicular disease can often be managed without mobilization of the sigmoid sinus, whereas large or giant tumors require more mobilization of adjacent structures, sometimes including division of the superior petrosal sinus and the tentorium.

The skin incision is taken to the fascia/pericranium, and the skin flap is dissected separately and turned forward. About 5 mm inside the skin incision, the fascia/pericranium is incised and turned forward with exposure of the bone. ◘ Figure 5.47 shows the «mind map» (some would say «mine map») of the translabyrinthine approach. By memorizing the sequence of landmarks before surgery, the rather complex approach soon becomes familiar, as the landmarks become waypoints on the route to the meatus. The bony exposure stops where the spine of Henle (◘ Fig. 5.47a) marks the edge of the external meatus (◘ Fig. 5.47b). The fascia/pericranial flap is turned forward and retracted together with the skin flap.

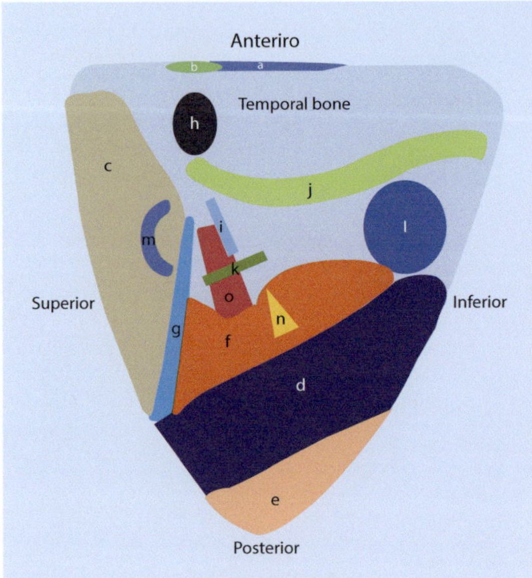

◘ **Fig. 5.47** «Mind map» of landmark waypoints on the translabyrinthine route to the right meatus, depicted in a schematic fashion. Although not all surgeons progress in the same sequence, it is useful to memorize the landmarks. For the experienced AN surgeon, this becomes a subconscious routine, and the focus can then be on the individual anatomy of the patient. Letters: **a** external auditory meatus, **b** spine of Henle, **c** temporal dura, **d** sigmoid sinus, **e** retrosigmoid posterior fossa dura, **f** presigmoid posterior fossa dura, **g** superior petrosal sinus, **h** mastoid antrum, **i** lateral semicircular canal, **j** fallopian canal with descending facial nerve, **k** posterior semicircular canal, **l** jugular bulb, **m** superior semicircular canal, **n** endolymphatic duct, **o** internal acoustic meatus

The triangular area defined by the temporal dura (◘ Fig. 5.47c), the external meatus, and the sigmoid sinus (◘ Fig. 5.47d) is drilled away, and the temporal dura and the sigmoid sinus are exposed. The temporal dura can be quite vascular, and a postoperative extradural hematoma is a risk if this bleeding is arterial and not managed effectively. Pneumatization of the mastoid process (◘ Fig. 5.44) may make this part very easy and quick but can also pose a higher risk during facial nerve exposure as the fallopian canal and descend-

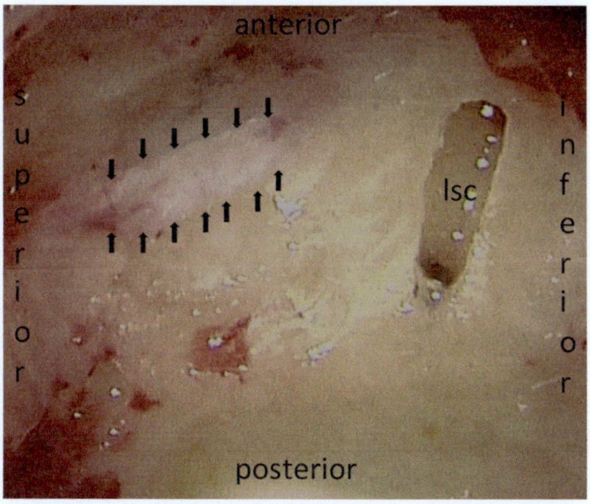

■ **Fig. 5.48** Intraoperative photo showing the identification of the facial nerve (*black arrows*) in the fallopian canal on the right side. The lateral semicircular canal (*lsc*) is an important landmark found posteroinferiorly to the facial nerve at the same depth, as illustrated. The facial nerve is still covered by a thin window of the bone

ing part of the facial nerve can then be suspended in an air cell. It is important to expose a few mm of the posterior fossa dura (■ Fig. 5.47e) behind the sigmoid sinus to allow dynamic retraction during tumor excision. During the exposure of the sigmoid sinus, the emissary vein(s) may lead to profuse bleeding. The veins(s), large or small, can be pushed toward the sinus, backward out of their canal, with repeated application of bone wax on a thin dissector. The vein is then appearing as a small hose when the bone has been removed and can then be safely coagulated. Lesions of the sigmoid sinus are not unusual and can be dealt with by a piece of muscle or Spongostan and a 4-0 resorbable suture. The presigmoid dura (■ Fig. 5.47f) and superior petrosal sinus (■ Fig. 5.47g) can then be identified. The antrum (■ Fig. 5.47h) is found at a vertical line directly underneath the spine of Henle. As a positive identification of the antrum, the short process of the incus is seen protruding from the middle ear cavity. Further bone is removed at the posterior aspect to identify the dense bone of the labyrinth (■ Fig. 5.44), without getting near the fallopian canal. There is no need to identify the digastric groove for this approach.

The microscope is introduced, and the pace is now slowed down significantly. The lateral semicircular canal (■ Figs. 5.47i and 5.48) is an important landmark for the descending facial nerve in the fallopian canal (■ Fig. 5.47j). While exposing the labyrinth, either the posterior (■ Fig. 5.47k) or lateral (■ Fig. 5.47j) semicircular canal is encountered first. Careful drilling lateral to the lateral semicircular canal will show a white–gray color change and tiny blood vessels as a warning before the nerve is exposed (■ Fig. 5.48). Even with a thin bony cover, the nerve can be identified with the nerve stimulator on a high stimulus current such as 0.3 mA. The canal is opened just enough to get a reliable EMG response, which is then used as a reference when needed during the rest of the procedure. A long latency, low amplitude, polyphasic response, already at this stage, is a warning of a very thin facial nerve on the tumor and a difficult high-risk nerve dissection. A sharp bone edge is shaped along the fallopian canal for a safe identification before further drilling is performed. The next structure to look for is the jugular bulb (■ Fig. 5.47l), which will show as a rounded darkening of the bone at the lower aspect of the exposure. The superior semicircular canal (■ Fig. 5.47m) is removed toward the temporal dura. The endolymphatic duct (■ Fig. 5.47n) will appear at further dissection between the temporal bone and the posterior fossa dura anterior to the sigmoid sinus. The dural component of this can be pulled out of the bony canal or transected. It is now important to expose the meatus at the central part, not at the fundus, where the risk of facial nerve damage is higher. The bone is gradually removed above and below the meatus to get at least 180° opening of the meatus. Whether the fundus needs to be opened depends on the extension of the tumor. When the bony crest between the upper and lower vestibular nerves (Bill's bar) can be identified with a blunt micro hook, sufficient fundus exposure has been achieved. It is the removal of the bone superior to the meatus that carries the highest risk of facial nerve damage.

The dura is opened in a linear fashion from the sigmoid sinus to the meatus. The facial nerve position in the medial part of the meatus is examined with the nerve stimulator. The CSF is released by a careful mobilization of the tumor capsule with a dissector at the inferior aspect toward the cisterna magna. It is now time for tumor excision (see below).

Retrosigmoid (Suboccipital) Approach (■ Video 5.4)

The patient is in general anesthesia without paralysis and placed on the operating table in the prone position with the head rotated 30°

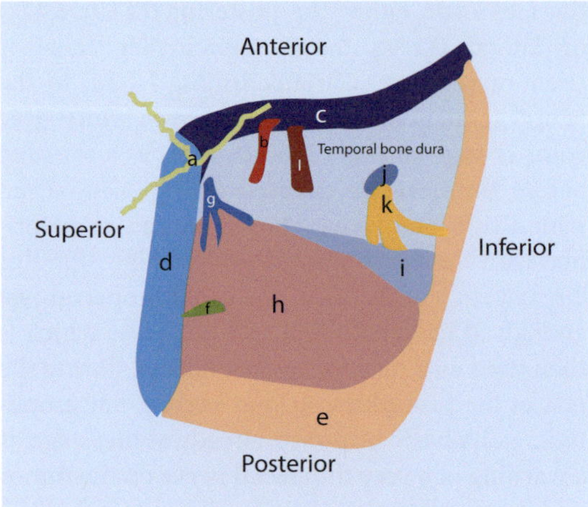

Fig. 5.49 «Mind map» of landmark waypoints on the retrosigmoid (suboccipital) route to the right meatus, depicted in a schematic fashion. Letters: **a** asterion, **b** emissary vein, **c** sigmoid sinus, **d** transverse sinus, **e** posterior fossa dura after opening and retraction, **f** bridging the vein between the cerebellum and the tent, **g** petrosal sinus, **h** right cerebellar hemisphere, **i** brain stem, **j** jugular foramen, **k** lower cranial nerves, **l** internal acoustic meatus

toward the same side and fixed in 3- or 4-point fixation. Some surgeons prefer the sitting position or park-bench position for this approach. The area behind the ear is shaved, and a straight oblique incision is marked from 3 cm above the asterion (Fig. 5.49a) to the spinous process of C2 (Fig. 5.34). The incision line is infiltrated with local anesthetic. The facial electrodes, ground electrode, and reference electrode are placed, and the system is tested. If needed, electrodes and sound applicator for cochlear nerve monitoring are mounted and tested. Washing and draping is done in a standard fashion, and the microscope is adjusted and draped. The skin is incised straight to the bone starting above the asterion (Fig. 5.49a), and the muscles are then divided to expose the posterior fossa bone toward the foramen magnum. Self-retaining retractors are placed. A groove is drilled along the sigmoid sinus to expose the dura just medial to the sinus. Exposed air cells are sealed with bone wax. The emissary vein(s) (Fig. 5.49b) will be encountered at this stage and can be managed by pushing bone wax repeatedly into their bony canal. In this way, the vein is dissected backward out of the canal and can be coagulated on the sigmoid sinus (Fig. 5.49c) when the bone is removed. The groove should go as far as the transition between the sigmoid and transverse sinuses (Fig. 5.49d). From this point, a craniotomy can be performed with the craniotomy attachment, avoiding a lesion to the transverse sinus. The craniotomy should be 3–4 cm wide and reach close to the foramen magnum, to allow CSF release. It is important to expose the entire medial edge of the sigmoid sinus to reduce cerebellar retraction during tumor removal. From this point, the remaining part of the approach is intradural, and as large AN will be encountered before the meatus is opened, some preliminary tumor resection may be needed to allow a space for opening of the meatus. The dura (Fig. 5.49e) is opened along the sigmoid sinus in a curved fashion with a distance of 5 mm to the sinus to allow watertight closure. Avoid cruciate or t-shaped incisions as these are very difficult to close watertight. The microscope is introduced. By carefully passing a brain retractor, sliding between the dura and cerebellum, toward the foramen magnum, it is possible to open the cisterna magna with a blunt hook and get CSF release. This is a critical step, and with larger tumors, further progress is almost impossible without this maneuver. When CSF is released, there may be tension and tear of a posterior bridging vein (Fig. 5.49e) entering the tent, or tear of the petrosal vein (Fig. 5.49f), situated with significant variations somewhat deeper in the angle between the tent and the petrosal dura. The vein passing from the cerebellum to the tent posteriorly can be identified and divided, whereas the petrosal vein should be preserved when possible [47]. The cerebellum (Fig. 5.49h) is displaced posteriorly, and the brain stem (Fig. 5.49i) comes into view. The jugular foramen (Fig. 5.49j) is identified with the lower cranial nerves (Fig. 5.49k). For hearing preservation, the meatus (Fig. 5.49l) is now opened from behind, 180°. While drilling, the cerebellum is best protected by large pieces of Spongostan, which will not be caught in the drill. The posterior semicircular canal (Fig. 5.45) will be the limitation of the meatal opening, and access to the fundus is not always possible. If this is the case, the fundus can be assessed with the aid of an endoscope at the end of tumor excision (see below).

Subtemporal (Middle Fossa) Approach

The patient is in general anesthesia without paralysis and placed on the operating table in the supine position with the head rotated 60° toward the opposite side and fixed in 3- or 4-point fixa-

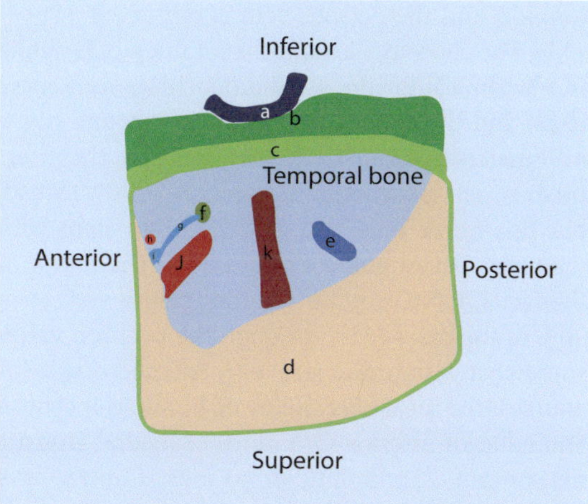

Fig. 5.50 «Mind map» of landmark waypoints on the subtemporal (middle fossa) route to the right meatus, depicted in a schematic fashion. Letters: **a** top of the pinna, **b** theca externa of the temporal bone, **c** craniotomy edge, **d** temporal dura, retracted, **e** arcuate eminence covering the superior semicircular canal, **f** facial hiatus, **g** greater superficial petrosal nerve (GSPN), **h** foramen spinosum (with middle meningeal artery divided), **i** foramen ovale, **j** petrous segment of the internal carotid artery, **k** internal acoustic meatus

tion. The area above the ear is shaved, and a curved incision is marked from the zygomatic arch to the top of the mastoid process, centered above the top of the pinna (Figs. 5.34 and 5.50a). The incision line is infiltrated with local anesthetic. The facial electrodes, ground electrode, and reference electrode are placed, and the system is tested. If needed, electrodes and sound applicator for cochlear nerve monitoring are mounted and tested. Washing and draping is done in a standard fashion, and the microscope is adjusted and draped. The skin is opened and reflected downward as a separate flap. Then the temporal muscle fascia is incised, and the temporal muscle is reflected forward in order to preserve its nerve and blood supply. A small burr hole is placed at the root of the zygomatic process (Fig. 5.50b) and a small craniotomy performed, with two-thirds anterior and one-third posterior to the external meatus. Opening of mastoid air should be avoided, if possible, as this increases the risk of postoperative CSF rhinorrhea. After leveling the inferior edge (Fig. 5.50c) of the craniotomy with the anterior surface of the petrous bone, extradural dissection is started. Extradural retraction of the temporal dura (Fig. 5.50d) is needed. As there is no direct temporal lobe contact, the impact of retraction is less, and gradual increase of the retraction will displace CSF and compensate for the lack of open CSF release. Custom-made retractor systems fixed on the craniotomy edge exist for the subtemporal approach, but retractors fixed to the head fixation system can also be used. Although fixed retraction should generally be avoided in skull base surgery, this may be the exception, even when using the four-hand technique. Landmarks on the petrous bone are the arcuate eminence (Fig. 5.50e), hiatus facialis (Fig. 5.50f), greater superior petrosal nerve (GSPN, Fig. 5.50g), foramen spinosum (Fig. 5.50h) with the middle meningeal artery, and foramen ovale (Fig. 5.50i). Watch out, as the facial nerve at the geniculate ganglion, the superior semicircular canal at the arcuate eminence, and the carotid artery (Fig. 5.50j) at the GSPN may be dehiscent. If the superior semicircular canal is opened or dehiscent, keep the suction away from the opening and seal it with a small piece of fascia or pericranium. After the extradural dissection, the landmarks are as outlined in Fig. 5.50. The internal meatus (Fig. 5.50j) is found at a line approximately 60° from the GSPN or, if measuring the angle between the arcuate eminence and the GSPN, at the junction between two-thirds and one-third measured from the GSPN. With the tip of a spatula locked at the petrous ridge, the inner part of the meatus should be identified and opened first. This part of the meatus is up to 10 mm below the surface of the bone, as opposed to the thin bone covering the fundus and geniculate ganglion at the lateral aspect. The meatus is then opened 180° backward toward the fundus. Due to the position right under the dura, the facial nerve is at high risk, especially from heat produced by the drill. Is it important not to open the cochlea just anterolateral to the fundus and posteromedial to the carotid artery and GSPN? The middle ear cavity is just lateral to the superior semicircular canal and should not be opened either, due to the risk of CSF leak. The dura is opened very carefully, as the facial nerve is not protected by the vestibular nerves, as it is in the posterior fossa approaches. The dissection and removal of the tumor in the meatus follow the same principles as with other approaches. The approach can be extended by transection of the superior petrosal sinus and the tentorium, but this will only give a slightly better exposure of the posterior fossa, and the subtemporal approach is not advisable for large ANs. Tumor excision then follows (see below).

Retrolabyrinthine Presigmoid Approach

This approach is performed with the same steps as in the translabyrinthine approach but without the labyrinthectomy. The labyrinth is blue lined. Access is narrow, and good exposure of the retrosigmoid dura is required, allowing retraction of the sigmoid sinus. This technique can be used for small or intracanalicular AN not extending to the fundus. The technique has also been demonstrated for endoscope-assisted removal of large AN [45].

Retrosigmoid Fully Endoscopic Approach

While many surgeons have used the endoscope to assist AN surgery, this procedure is new and at the pioneering stage, with few publications of results [65–67]. The patient is in general anesthesia and placed in the supine semisitting position with the head rotated 60° to the opposite side. The approach corresponds to that used for microvascular decompression of the trigeminal nerve, and the landmarks correspond to those used for the retrosigmoid approach. The details of the endoscopic procedure are described in [65].

Tumor Excision

After dural opening, CSF release, and identification of the facial nerve in the meatus, stepwise central debulking followed by dissection of capsule is the standard way forward. For small tumors, the vestibulocochlear and facial nerve can be identified early at the brain stem, and tumor dissection is then fairly straight forward in terms of surgical anatomy but still sometimes time consuming. In large tumors, it is extremely important to find and keep the plane between the arachnoid membrane and tumor capsule. After stimulation of the capsule, the initial debulking at the dorsal aspect of the tumor may be done with rongeurs, followed by ultrasonic aspirator. Low suction on the aspirator reduces the risk of breaching the capsule with damage to nerves, vessels, and brain stem. If in doubt, the stimulator can be used at increasing stimulation strength to judge the thickness of capsule between aspirator and facial nerve. The cerebellum, lower cranial nerves, trigeminal nerve, and brain stem are successively dissected free and covered by cottonoids, and the petrous vein is preserved, if possible. The choroid plexus at the foramen of Luschka is a landmark for the vestibulocochlear root entry zone, and the facial root exit zone is found a few millimeters anterior to this. In between, the intermedius nerve can often be seen as a thin thread, but this nerve may also exit the brain stem with the facial or vestibulocochlear nerve. The course of the facial nerve is on the anterior tumor surface in 90% of the cases [63], although the position varies somewhat with tumor size [64]. An anterosuperior course is the most likely followed by anterior central and anterior inferior. One-third of medial acoustic neuromas [77] with little or no meatal tumor have a split facial nerve [73] compared to only 2% when the tumor is reaching the fundus [73]. More than 3% may have a dorsal course of the facial nerve over the tumor surface, and this variant is associated with less complete tumor removal and a higher retreatment rate compared to anterior courses of the nerve [56]. The facial nerve can be trapped between cystic elements of an AN, but a true intratumoral location of the facial nerve is fortunately rare.

The steps and progression of the tumor removal vary between surgeons. Some prefer an early dissection at the meatus, whereas others find the facial nerve at the brain stem first. The facial nerve can make a significant loop on the anterior aspect of the tumor. The most difficult place to get the right plane between the facial nerve and the tumor is at the porus edge, and here, the best approach is from proximal to distal, if the space allows. When dissection is carried out from proximal to distal, the remaining tumor may end up being attached only to the facial nerve. This happens more often with medium-sized AN and carries a high risk of facial nerve damage by displacement. If the facial nerve is torn or transected and without continuity, the connection between the proximal and distal ends must be restored immediately in the same surgical session. There are very few good reasons to postpone this to a second stage surgery. The remaining AN is removed, and the ends are approximated directly or connected with a sural or greater auricular nerve graft (► Sect. 5.3.6).

If a nerve block occurs during tumor excision, this might disappear after a few minutes, and the EMG signal then comes back. If the nerve is structurally intact and nerve block remains despite technical integrity of the facial nerve monitor, additional «safe» tumor may be removed before stopping surgery. The process of facial nerve dissection requires dexterity, patience, and stamina, and it is sometimes utterly painstaking. Here it is worth remembering that «just a few more moments of your time may save a lifetime of misery for your patient» (said by Professor Ugo Fisch to his fellow Michael Gleeson in 1985).

Hemostasis

Intracranial postoperative hematoma is a life-threatening complication to AN surgery (◘ Fig. 5.51). It is easy to control bleeding when removing small- to medium-sized AN, whereas large and giant AN can have a rich blood supply in combination with involvement of «native» vessels on the tumor capsule and pose a much bigger challenge. The blood supply to the AN comes from the anterior inferior cerebellar artery, mainly from the porus edge, and as this is also a difficult location to oversee, angled bipolar forceps may be needed to obtain hemostasis here. To keep the progress during dissection of the tumor capsule, venous bleeding is sometimes best dealt with in a temporary fashion by a hemostatic agent such as Spongostan or Surgicel and cottonoids. After tumor removal, these sites then represent multiple «bombs,» with potential vigorous bleeding when the cottonoids are removed. The hemostasis' work is often carried out at the end of a long operation, and the surgeon has to resist the temptation to accept a little oozing. At this point, application of further hemostatic agents such as Flowseal may help, if the exact location of the remaining bleed cannot be identified. Even when the rinsing water is crystal clear, a postoperative hematoma may form, for example, from a small artery, which has come out of spasm after closure. The risk of postoperative hematoma, and the sometimes sinister consequences of not identifying this at an early stage, warrants overnight recovery in an intensive care setting.

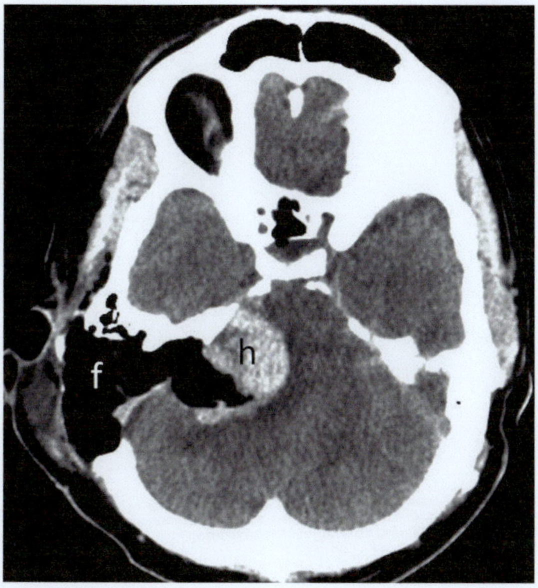

◘ **Fig. 5.51** Axial CT scan showing a postoperative hematoma (h) after translabyrinthine approach and total removal of a large AN on the right side. The hematoma was evacuated acutely and the patient recovered with some ataxia. Fat graft (f)

Closure

The dura cannot be closed in a watertight fashion in the translabyrinthine, presigmoid, and subtemporal approaches, whereas this is usually possible for retrosigmoid approach whether endoscopic or not. It is important to seal all air cells opened on the way in. There may not be obvious air cells when the meatus is drilled open in the retrosigmoid approach, but this should be checked, as this is a common site for CSF fistula. After suturing as much of the dural opening as possible, the abdominal fat is used to obliterate the dead space left in the translabyrinthine and presigmoid approaches. Fat, fascia, or muscle or a combination of this can be used to seal the antrum and middle ear. Care should be taken not to damage the chorda tympani, if the incus is removed. Fibrin or artificial sealant can be applied to reinforce the closure. Bone cement or bone chips collected during the mastoidectomy are also used to various extents for this purpose. The soft tissues should always be closed in two layers with the fascia acting as an internal compression of the fat graft, if this is used. Finally, a tight head bandage is applied.

5.3.5 Complications of AN Surgery

The mortality from AN surgery is less than 1%, and of the general surgical complications, postoperative hematoma is responsible for two-thirds of the mortality [70].

The risk of complications is related to tumor size. Facial palsy, CSF leak, trigeminal and lower cranial nerve deficits, wound infection/dehiscence, vertigo, and ataxia are other complications. The special management of facial nerve injuries is covered in the following chapter.

5.3.6 Management of Facial Nerve Complications in Skull Base Surgery

Characteristics and Time Course of Deficits After Facial Nerve Lesions in Skull Base Surgery

Facial nerve damage is a relatively common complication following lateral skull base surgery. Focus is usually on the weakness of the face, but a number of other complaints can be related to facial nerve lesions intracranially or in the base of the skull. In addition to facial weakness, patients may also complain of ipsilateral symptoms relating to tear production, salivation, taste, sensation in the outer ear canal as well as ear pain, dryness in the nose, and less often hyperacusis. ◘ Figures 5.52 and 5.53 show a schematic overview of the function of nerve fibers carried in the facial nerve and the likely deficits resulting from facial nerve lesions at different levels from the brain stem to the stylomastoid foramen. Surgical lesions distal to the stylomastoid foramen, related to skull base surgery,

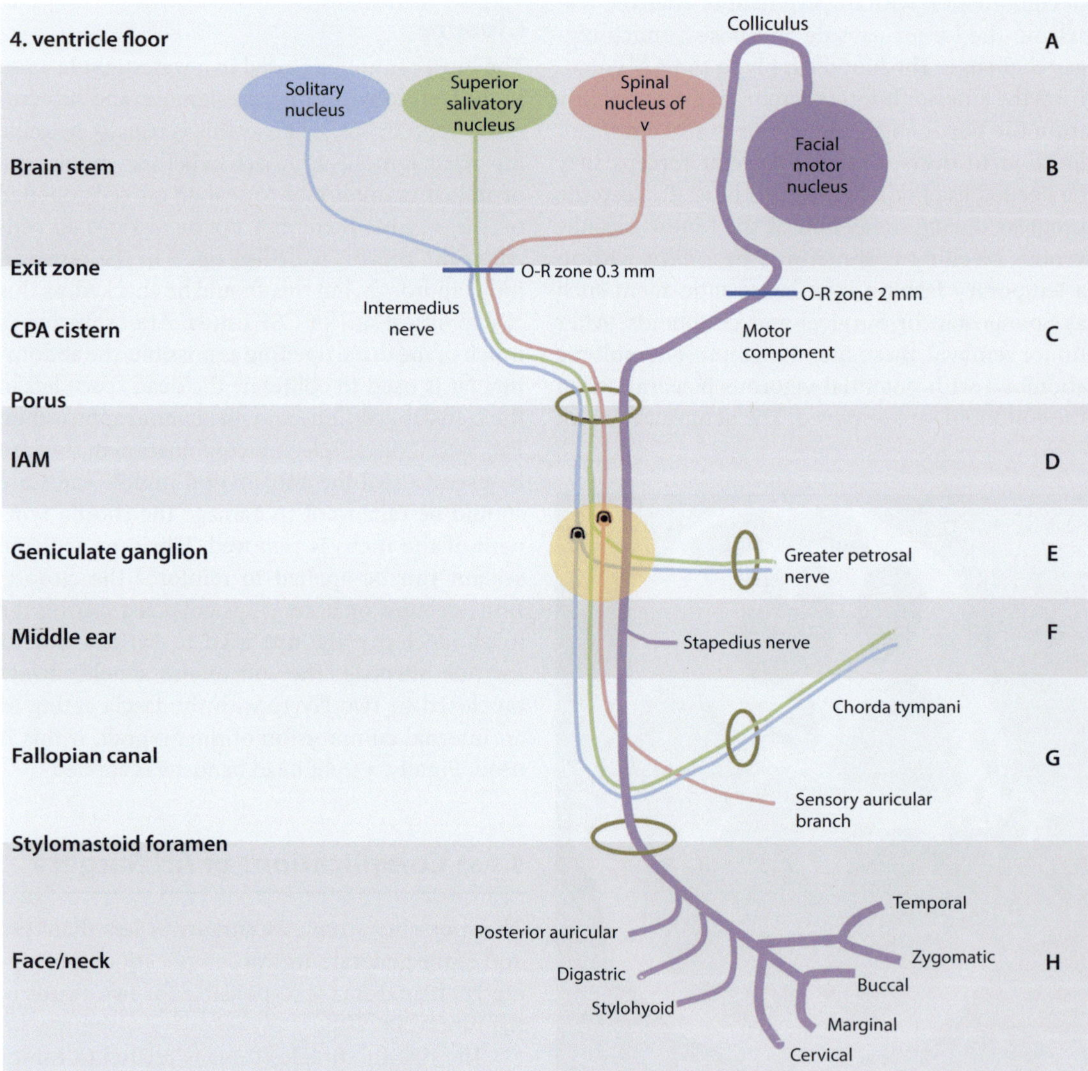

◘ **Fig. 5.52** Schematic outline of the facial nerve and its branches at different anatomical levels. Note that the facial nerve carries fibers from the intermedius nerve. This nerve leaves the brain stem together with the eighth nerve or between the facial nerve proper and the eighth nerve. The Obersteiner–Redlich (O–R) zone is the zone of transition between central and peripheral myelin and hence the level from which regeneration of axons is possible. The capital letters A–H refer to ◘ Fig. 5.53

Component	Function	Complaint	A	B	C	D	E	F	G	H
Facial nerve proper	Motor fibres for the face and neck mimical muscles	Weakness of the face, incomplete eye closure								
Greater Petrosal Nerve (GSPN)	Taste fibres from palate and presynaptic parasympathetic fibres to the lacrimal gland and mucosa in nose and sinuses via the pterygopalatine ganglion.	Changes in tear production, dryness of nose and sinuses, changes in taste on the palate			*					
Stapedius nerve	Motor fibres for the stapedius muscle	Sounds perceived as very loud (hyperacusis)			*					
Chorda Tympani	Taste fibres from anterior 2/3 of tongue and presynaptic parasympathetic fibres to the subm andibular and sublingual glands via the submandibular ganglion	Changes in taste on the tongue, changes in formation of saliva (~50% on same side)			*					
Sensory auricular branch	Sensory fibres from outer ear canal and part of the outer ear.	Sensory loss or neuralgic pain in outer ear canal.			*					

Fig. 5.53 Components and functions of the facial nerve. Typical complaints after damage and likely involvement (*dark gray*) after damage at different levels (*A–H*) depicted in Fig. 5.52. * The intermedius nerve is often damaged in its cisternal course if the facial nerve is damaged at the same level, for example, during removal of a large acoustic neuroma

are primarily lesions to the frontal branch, which can be seen after an orbitozygomatic approach. These lesions can be avoided [69].

When the facial nerve is transected at a certain level, immediate deficits will follow, but an acute facial paralysis will not present in the same fashion in all patients. Depending on the age of the patient and the status of the muscles, the resting tone in the face after complete denervation may be enough for sufficient eye closure, at least for some days after the lesion, and in some patients for much longer. In other patients, eye closure is a problem from the outset. With the facial nerve damaged, but in continuity, the clinical picture may range from paralysis to a discrete paresis with a variety of deficits related to the functions carried by the intermedius nerve (Fig. 5.53). Function may then return over a period of weeks (no axonal loss) to months (axonal loss) depending on the nature of the lesion.

Even with a normal facial nerve function the day after surgery, some patients will experience a delayed reaction with a significant facial palsy. This usually occurs within the first weeks after surgery, and in the absence of postoperative infection or hematoma, the patient should be reassured that function will return to near normal. A short course of high-dose steroids has been suggested in this situation, but this is not based on a strong evidence.

Identification of Facial Nerve Problems During Surgery

The motor function of the facial nerve can be monitored intraoperatively (▶ Sect. 5.3), and this should be done in all lateral skull base surgery, where manipulation of the facial nerve is likely. Loss of the electromyography (EMG) response during surgery can happen due to physical damage to the nerve, due to heat from the bipolar coagulation or drill, or due to ischemia. If the nerve is not divided, a conduction block may only be temporary, and in that case, the EMG response may sometimes recover after a while [55]. There is currently no method of intraoperative monitoring of the functions carried via the intermedius nerve.

Intraoperative monitoring of brain stem function by auditory evoked potentials and sensory evoked potentials may reveal damage to the brain stem. Although there is some variation in the blood supply to the pons, lesions affecting the facial nucleus are most likely due to occlusion of the anterior inferior cerebellar artery or the pontine perforators from the basilar artery.

Same Stage Management of Intraoperative Facial Nerve Lesions

Loosing facial nerve continuity during a skull base procedure is unnerving, but failure to repair the nerve in the same procedure, if possible, is unreasonable. If a surgeon is skilled enough to perform complex lateral skull base surgery, he or she should also know the simple technique on how to repair a complete facial nerve lesion.

Direct End-to-End Anastomosis

In a situation where the continuity of the facial nerve is lost during surgery of a benign pathology, the best recovery of function will result from a direct end-to-end anastomosis. This is often possible in acoustic neuroma surgery, where the nerve may be elongated by the tumor, allowing the ends to reach after complete tumor resection. There is very little peri- or epineurium in the cisternal segment of the nerve, so suture is not a good option if the lesion is at this segment. Instead, the ends should be adapted on the dura or a piece of Gelfoam, and the position then is secured by fibrin glue, which is sufficient to resist the forces applied by change of the head position during postoperative mobilization. Postoperative function is likely to return to House–Brackmann grade (HB) 2–3, with a good resting tone. If the ends do not reach each other without tension, an interpositional nerve graft is needed.

Interpositional Nerve Graft

The donor nerve for an interpositional nerve graft should match the size of the facial nerve. The great auricular nerve runs superficial to the sternomastoid muscle and is easily available with a minor extension of the original incision in most lateral skull base approaches. Sensation over the parotid gland, over the mastoid process, and on the ear will be lost. A good alternative is one of the terminal branches of the sural nerve, which can be harvested with very little morbidity just distal to the lateral malleolus, and has a diameter similar to the cisternal segment of the facial nerve. If a longer graft is needed, the sural nerve is the best choice, as only 3–4 cm can be harvested from the great auricular nerve as opposed to 20 cm from the sural nerve. A third option is an allograft [31], which works well for shorter nerve gaps but is currently quite costly and not readily available in all parts of the world. After end-to-end adaptation, the anastomosis is secured with fibrin glue if the lesion is intracranial. If the distal anastomosis is extracranial, two 7-0 nylon sutures secure the anastomosis here. It is important to reverse the nerve graft distal to proximal to avoid that regenerating axons are misdirected by small nerve branches along the course of the graft.

Second Stage Management of Intraoperative Facial Nerve Lesions

In a few patients, the facial nerve function is permanently lost due to complications of a skull base procedure. This may, despite loss of the EMG response during surgery, not be clear from the outset, as some hope for facial nerve recovery will exist when the facial nerve is left in anatomical continuity. When the facial nerve is obviously lost during surgery and there is for some reason no possibility of the same stage repair, or when no facial nerve recovery has happened after 6 months, a nerve transfer is usually the best option for reanimation of the face. This is hopefully not a routine situation in a skull base practice, and it is therefore advisable to seek help from, for example, peripheral nerve surgeons or plastic and reconstructive surgeons. If more than 18 months have passed since the lesion, the facial nerve and muscles are atrophied and unlikely to allow any recovery from a nerve transfer. In that situation, a cross facial nerve transfer to a free vascularized gracilis muscle graft or static procedures are the only options to restore symmetry and alleviate some of the problems experienced with facial nerve paralysis [29].

Hypoglossal-Facial Anastomosis

In this procedure, motor fibers from the hypoglossal nerve are directed into the facial nerve by means of an extracranial anastomosis between the two nerves. A side-to-end technique with or without interpositional nerve graft preserves function of the tongue and is now the gold standard ([25, 53], ◘ Fig. 5.54). Restoration of the tone and symmetry at rest (HB 3) is the most significant result, whereas few patients regain any social function, such as a spontaneous smile, although this has been seen, especially in young patients.

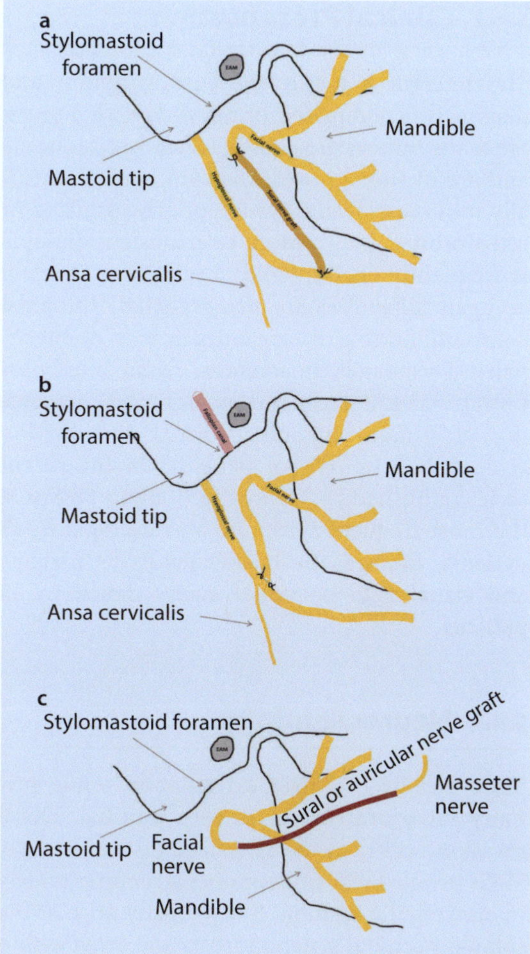

Fig. 5.54 Schematic drawings showing the principles of facial reanimation by hypoglossal–facial and masseteric–facial nerve transfers. **a** Hypoglossal–facial transfer with interpositional graft (sural or auricular donor nerve) and end-to-side connection to hypoglossal nerve. **b** Intratemporal transposition and direct end-to-side connection to hypoglossal nerve. **c** Masseteric to facial transfer with interpositional graft (sural or auricular donor nerve) and end-to-end connection to the masseter nerve

Masseteric-Facial Anastomosis

This procedure is gaining popularity and is probably the gold standard of the future. Results are now reported from a large series of patients [28, 30]. In this procedure, the masseter nerve is transected as proximal as possible and connected end to end to the facial nerve by means of a nerve graft (Fig. 5.54). To lose the function of the masseter muscle on one side is bearable. Resting tone in the face is restored after the hypoglossal–facial anastomosis, but it seems that activation of the face is easier by clinching the teeth than by moving the tongue, and more patients regain some social function.

Cross Facial Nerve Transfer to Free Vascularized Gracilis Muscle Graft

This procedure works best for younger patients and is usually carried out by plastic and reconstructive surgeons. A sural nerve graft is anastomosed to the zygomatic branch of the contralateral facial nerve and tunneled subcutaneously to the paralyzed side. Time is allowed for regeneration of axons through the sural nerve graft, and a free vascularized gracilis muscle graft is then placed and allowed to be innervated by the axons from the opposite side. This provides some improvement, but the results are inferior to hypoglossal or masseter nerve transfers to the facial nerve.

Static Procedures and Muscle Transfer

A range of static procedures can help restore passive symmetry and eye closure [29]. These techniques include implantation of fascial slings, implantation of a gold weight in the upper eyelid, and partial tarsorrhaphy. In some situations, a transfer of the temporal muscle may restore some function.

Postoperative Care of Patients with Facial Palsy

In case of a partial palsy, facial exercises may improve function to some degree, but time is the most important factor in recovery. A range of specific techniques for facial exercises has been described, but there is currently little evidence for the effect [26]. Active facial exercises in the absence of any facial muscle function on the affected side are only going to increase the difference between the two sides, which will if anything worsen the cosmetic appearance. Passive exercise and massage should be used until reinnervation takes place. There is currently no good evidence for or against transcutaneous muscle stimulation to avoid atrophy while waiting for reinnervation. As some patients with facial nerve palsy also have reduced tear production and in addition with anesthesia of the cornea (due to a concomitant trigeminal lesion), focus on postoperative eye care is important to avoid corneal abrasions and reduced vision. Patients should have neutral eye drops and will often need an occlusive bandage at night.

5.4 Chordomas

L. Troude, O. Soumare, A. Melot, and P.-H. Roche

Chordomas involve the central skull base in 30% of cases. This rare and locally malignant tumor has challenged the standard of care and has fascinated the skull base surgeons for decades. Uncertainty remains about the biological behavior, prognosis factors, and better treatment. Still some tumors will be cured with a single-session surgical procedure, while other patients will experience multiple regrowth and untreatable chordomas whatever we do. The role of adjunctive radiation therapy (RT), the technique to use, and the timing of RT are still under debate. Recent advances in skull base surgical techniques and refinement of endoscopic practice have brought new tools to offer a better radical resection than in the past. The goal of this chapter is to describe the different subtypes of skull base chordomas (SBCs) and to clarify the role and results of the microsurgical resection in the management of SBCs. We will exclude from our purpose the chordomas arising from the craniocervical junction and upper cervical spine.

5.4.1 General Considerations

Chordomas arise from the rest of vestigial notochordal cells. They represent 1–4% of primary bone tumors. SBCs represent 0.2% of all intracranial tumors and 6% of skull base tumors. Their incidence rate is about 0.08 per 100,000 patient-years. This incidence is twofold greater in males and fivefold greater incidence in the Caucasian population [81]. Chordoma families are rare. The tumor is rare before the age of 40. Peak incidence is in the fourth to seventh decade, and median age at the time of diagnosis is 60 years (range 3–95 years). About one-third of chordomas involve the clivus and spheno-occipital region (spheno-occipital synchondrosis). Luschka was probably the first to identify a jellylike tumor mass at the level of the clivus in 1856, but the link with notochord was originally understood by Ribbert in 1894. Cushing was the first to report a case of SBCs successfully removed in 1909.

5.4.2 Clinical Presentation

The interval between the first symptom and diagnosis is comprised of a few days to 3 years. Since the tumors are mainly located extradurally and are of slow growth, the symptoms are usually minimal. Headaches are poorly localized or retro-orbital. Intermittent or persistent diplopia is frequently encountered. Swallowing problem and gait difficulties are also reported. The most common finding on examination is abducens palsy. Dysphagia, hoarseness, facial numbness (30%), and gait ataxia are less common, depending of tumor location. Normal examination is described in 20% of patients. In the recent series published by George [89] about 58 SBCs, the most frequent symptom was diplopia in 43 patients, followed by headaches in 19 patients and visual field or visual acuity deficit in 15 patients.

5.4.3 Neuroradiology

SBCs usually originate extradurally, while primary intradural origin is very unusual. Dural invasion occurs at the late stage of their course. SBCs invade local and regional structures widely in an irregular fashion. SBCs mostly arise at the spheno-occipital synchondrosis and grow within the clival bone in the majority of cases. Parasellar area is involved in 60%, foramen magnum in 25%, CPA in 25%, infratemporal fossa in 10%, and parapharyngeal and/or retropharyngeal space in 10%. SBCs may remain focal and well circumscribed but display usually an aggressive pattern with regional and multifocal invasion. Seeding in the operative route has been reported in up to 7% of cases and metastasis in 7–12% of cases, particularly to the lungs, lymph nodes, and bones.

A careful neuroradiological work-up is required before treatment (◘ Fig. 5.55). There is a lack of reliable radiological finding that makes the distinction between chordomas and chondrosarcomas on CT scan and MRI. CT scan shows a well-circumscribed but invasive, lytic soft tissue lesion. The mass usually contains large calcifications and bone sequestra. CT is very useful to evaluate the bony extension. MRI is the single best imaging modality. SBCs display a homogenous hypointense T1 and bright hyperintense

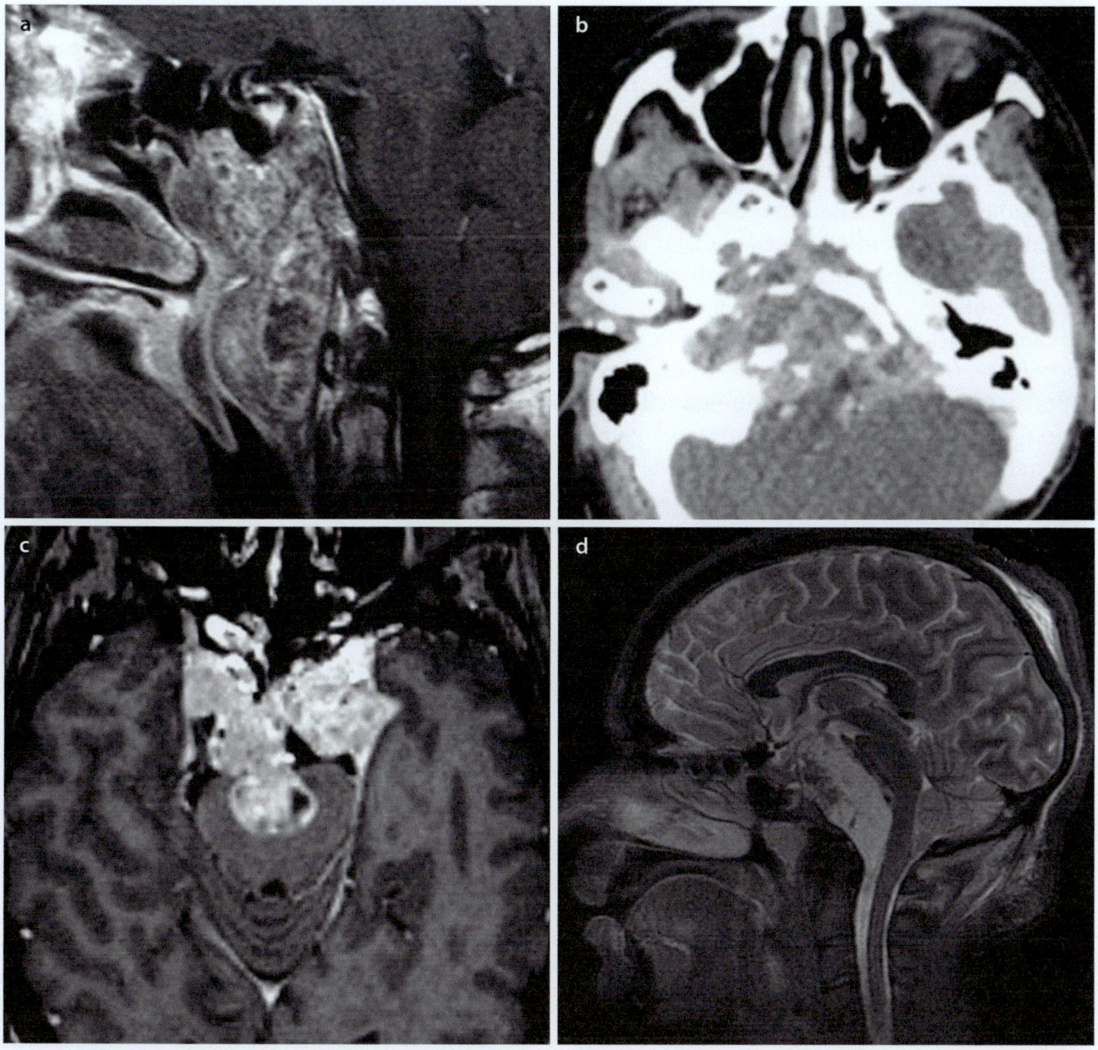

Fig. 5.55 Imaging of various presentations of skull base chordomas according to their origin. Chordomas usually originate extradurally **a** and **b**. Sagittal contrast-enhanced T1-weighted magnetic resonance imaging (MRI) shows a heterogeneous enhancement linked to a variable calcified content **a**. Non-enhanced CT scan **b** reveals a slightly hyperdense mass which contains large calcifications and bone sequestra. Dural invasion may occur at the late stage of tumor growth **c**. Remnants of the notochord may be found in the intradural clival area; thus, purely intradural chordomas can be described **d**—T2-weighted MRI

T2 signal. They are enhanced moderately and heterogeneously after contrast injection. The mass is polylobulated, and major vascular structures are displaced or encased in up to 80% of cases. Abnormal vascularity is generally absent on angiography, but angiography can be done to assess the vascularization of the brain if an arterial bypass and balloon occlusion test are considered. Preoperative embolization is worthless in the management of SBCs. SBCs should be differentiated from the ecchordosis physaliphora first described by Luschka and from benign notochordal cell tumors. Both are slow-growing tumor mass and can be assimilated to notochordal hamartomas.

5.4.4 Pathology

SBCs are grayish tumors and firm to gelatinous in consistency. They include foci of calcification and bone sequestra. Histologically they contain physaliphorous cells, which are large, vacuolated, and mucus-containing cells organized in a lobular pattern [95]. These cells express an immunoreactivity for EMA, cytokeratin, and rarely S-100 proteins. Brachyury has been more recently described as a powerful marker of chordomas, and co-expression of cytokeratin and brachyury by tumor cells reaches 100% specificity. Three histopathological variants are recognized: classic, chondroid, and dedifferentiated chordomas [82]. The distinctive prognosis value of these variants is not established. About 10% of chordomas show histologic features of malignancy. Chromosome aberrations (hypodiploid or near-diploid karyotypes) are described in 62% of tumor cell karyotypes. Chromosome 1 monosomy and gain of chromosome 7 are frequent chromosomal abnormalities. Genome analysis indicates losses on 1p (50%), while most frequent gains are on 7q in 75%. Linkage analysis showed defect of 1p36.13 in 85% of cases. Candidate genes in this region are well-identified tumor suppressor genes. A p53 deregulation is frequently observed.

5

5.4.5 Treatment

Conservative management or simple biopsy is not an option [88]. Historical reports indicate that in the absence of treatment, the tumor growth leading to death was the rule within 6 months to 2 years. Current treatment options rest mostly on level-4 and very limited level-3 evidence. It is recommended to manage the patients in multidisciplinary teams.

Surgical Treatment

Aggressive surgical resection is the standard of care for SBCs. The first shot should be optimal. We learn from the results of major series that repeated surgery is associated with worst prognosis in terms of progression-free survival (PFS), overall survival (OS), and morbidity [99]. For the last decade, the trend is to select endoscopic approaches considering the midline location and the extradural growth for most of these tumors. However, each surgical strategy is associated with proper limitations and complications.

A variety of open skull base techniques have been developed through lateral transpetrosal corridors but also transfacially and subfrontally. These approaches mainly proceed with a lateral-to-medial or superior-to-inferior trajectory via an extensive amount of bone resection. They expose the patient to some degree of brain retraction before and after dura opening and cranial nerve manipulation. The most illustrative technique is the subtemporal–preauricular infratemporal fossa approach [98]. This procedure exposes the two upper thirds of the clivus and petrous apex, cavernous sinus, and infratemporal fossa through an extended corridor. Less invasive are a variety of transpetrosal routes named epidural anterior petrosectomy or combined petrosectomy which are more dedicated to petrous apex and intradural petroclival area with limited control of the clivus. During these lateral approaches, at risk structures are the neuro-otological content inside the petrous bone, the brain stem and temporal lobe, the intradural cranial nerves, and the basilar artery including its branches and perforators. In the situation of repeated surgery for recurrent chordomas, particularly the ones that have been already irradiated, the scar tissues and the adhesion of the tumor to critical structures may complicate seriously the resection. In these same patients, reconstructions and closure may be technically challenging with a high risk of CSF leaks and meningitis.

Extended endonasal approaches are ventral, midline approaches that pass through the ethmoid and sphenoid sinuses [87]. They are very logical to reach and to fully expose extradural midline chordomas, taking advantage of natural anatomic corridors (sinuses and nasal cavities). The endoscope offers an access to the parasellar extension of chordomas inside the cavernous sinus and Meckel's cave. Here, there is a need to perform an ethmoidectomy and translocate the carotid siphon medially to reach the lateral compartment. Technical variants are also required to reach the infratemporal fossa. The petrous apex is also under control, but while the tumor spreads toward the internal auditory canal and cerebellopontine angle, manipulation of the tumor becomes hazardous. In this latter situation, planning an additional transpetrosal procedure should be anticipated. Another limitation is the access to the compartment of the tumor that involves the carotid artery bifurcation and even more laterally which means that a combined endoscopic and transcranial strategy should be considered.

From an endoscopic endonasal perspective, the clivus is divided into superior clivus, middle clivus, and inferior clivus:

- Superior clivus also called sellar clivus and formed by the dorsum sellae is limited superolaterally by the posterior clinoid processes,

inferomedially by the sellar floor, and inferolaterally by cranial nerve VI through Dorello's canal just below the level of the floor of the sella and medial to the paraclival segment of the internal carotid artery (ICA) located laterally.
- Middle clivus, also named the sphenoidal clivus, extends vertically, from the sellar floor superomedially and Dorello's canal superolaterally at the uppermost aspect of the petroclival fissure and the level where the ICA enters the cavernous sinus to the floor of the sphenoid sinus corresponding to the roof of the choana. The middle clivus is limited laterally by the paraclival ICA and petroclival fissure and inferolaterally by the lacerum segment of the ICA, the foramen lacerum above the fibrous attachments of the Eustachian tube, and the parapharyngeal muscles. The Vidian nerve is a key landmark as it runs within the Vidian canal through the pterygoid body just below the sphenoid body toward the lateral portion of the foramen lacerum.
- Inferior clivus extends from the roof of the choana corresponding to the floor of the sphenoid sinus to the foramen magnum and is termed the nasopharyngeal clivus. The inferior clivus is limited laterally by the Eustachian tubes and more laterally by the parapharyngeal segment of the ICA.

The binostril-expanded endoscopic four-hand (surgical team including ideally an otorhinolaryngologist and a neurosurgeon) transclival approach is the endoscopic endonasal approach required for skull base chordoma resection. For the purpose of this surgical procedure-dedicated tools as neuronavigation using MR and angioMR imaging with CT, monitoring of cranial nerves in addition to brain stem and somatosensory evoked potentials, high-speed and low-profile extendable drill, surgical Doppler ultrasonography with microprobe, endonasal bipolar forceps, and low-profile ultrasonic aspirator is substantial.

First of all, if dural penetration is suspected, before opening the anterior midline wide corridor to the clivus, a posterior mucosal nasoseptal flap pediculated on the sphenopalatine artery is realized and kept in place in the oropharynx through the choana, unilaterally or bilaterally depending on the predictable size of the oteo-dural skull base defect to be reconstructed.

The widened endoscopic endonasal transclival approach requires the following steps: removal of the middle turbinate in one chosen nostril, outfracturation and lateral luxation of the middle turbinate in the other side, resection of the posterior portion of the nasal septum, large anterior sphenoidotomy, and removal of all the septa within the sphenoid sinus to allow identification of all the bone landmarks. These septa resections have to be realized up to their attachments such as to the opticocarotid recess paying attention not to damage the optic nerve or the ICA.

At this stage, the sphenoidal clivus (middle clivus) is exposed from the level of the floor of the sella turcica down to that of the sphenoid sinus corresponding to the roof of the choana.

Surgical endoscopic endonasal access to the sellar clivus (superior transclival approach) may require a pituitary gland superior transposition, extradurally, interdurally, or intradurally, with preservation of the stalk, to reach the dorsum sellae and the posterior clinoid processes.

To gain access to the nasopharyngeal clivus (inferior clivus), one must strip the nasopharyngeal fascia and completely remove the vomer and the floor of the sphenoidal sinus until the Vidian nerves are identified laterally exposing inferiorly the clivus up to the level of the Eustachian tubes.

A critical technical point when removing chordomas localized at the junction of the superior and middle clivus is to avoid damaging the abducens nerve when passing through Dorello's canal and crossing the inferior side of Grüber's ligament. The method consists of removing the bone and periosteal dura surrounding the superomedial attachment of Grüber's ligament to posterior clinoid process and upper clivus in the interdural space, following its course inferolaterally to petrous apex until identification of the abducens nerve at their intersection point.

Extension of SBCs in the suprasellar suprachiasmatic area and the anterior cranial fossa across the anterosuperior aspect of the pituitary fossa requires the transtuberculum–transplanum module, which is limited laterally, from posterior to anterior, by medial opto-carotid recesses which are landmarks of the optic nerves in the optic canals and paraclinoid segments of the ICA, optic nerve prominences, and lamina papyracea (medial wall of orbits). It consists of completing the anterior rostral exposure by performing a posterior ethmoidectomy until identification of the posterior ethmoidal arteries anteriorly and leaving the rostral attachments of the nasal septum to the ethmoid roof thus to minimize the risk of damaging the olfactory nerve endings. Once this has been done, the tuberculum sellae and the planum sphenoidale are removed in a posteroanterior direction.

In the midline, rostro-caudally, there is no limitation of the endoscopic endonasal transclival approach from the frontal sinuses to the craniovertebral junction.

When addressing extension of SBCs lateral to the parasellar and paraclival ICA (cavernous sinus, lateral recess of the sphenoid sinus, Meckel's cave, middle cranial fossa) or at the level of petrous bone, above or under the horizontal ICA, the basic transpterygoid route is required using the maxillary sinus as a working corridor which can be widened if needed to get access to the most lateral aspect of the posterior wall of the maxillary sinus and the infratemporal fossa. This is performed in a stepwise manner, starting with a wide midmeatal antrostomy (uncinectomy added to the previously completed middle turbinectomy) followed by a medial maxillectomy and extending to an ipsilateral anteromedial maxillotomy. Once this wide nasomaxillary window is opened, the posterior wall of the maxillary sinus and the ascending process of the palatine bone are removed to expose the pterygopalatine fossa. The content of the pterygopalatine fossa is then mobilized laterally once the sphenopalatine artery and posterior nasal branch have been coagulated and transected. The Vidian canal is exposed just lateral to the junction of the sphenoid floor with the base of the medial pterygoid plate and drilled, following the Vidian artery posteriorly as an inferolateral landmark for the anterior genu of the ICA. Once the anterior genu has been isolated, then the bone surrounding the horizontal segment can be removed proceeding the drilling in a caudal to rostral trajectory from the inferior margin of the medial pterygoid plate to flush its plane to the middle cranial fossa and foramen rotundum. The bone around the maxillary nerve is removed until it disappears into the dura mater of the middle fossa drilling away the bone located between the foramen rotundum and the Vidian canal toward the junction of the horizontal petrous segment of the ICA and its anterior genu giving access under the ICA horizontal petrous segment to the petroclival synchondrosis. The ICA is then followed superiorly from the genu, and the bony carotid parasellar prominence is removed exposing the quadrangular space which is bounded by the parasellar ICA medially, the maxillary nerve laterally, the horizontal petrous ICA inferiorly, and the abducens nerve superiorly. Removing the bone surrounding the ICA allows lateralization to gain access to the medial petrous apex. The quadrangular space gives access to Meckel's cave and middle cranial fossa. Passing above cranial nerve VI gives access to the superior portion of the cavernous sinus. Caudally the dissection can be pursued laterally identifying the lateral pterygoid plate which is drilled rostrally to flush its plane to the middle cranial fossa and foramen ovale opening the access to the posteromedial part of the infratemporal fossa.

Lateral spreading of the tumor from the inferior clivus and foramen magnum, to the level of hypoglossal canal within the occipital condyle, and to the jugular foramen may require in addition to the transpterygoid corridor a resection of the Eustachian tube enlarging the route laterally until the limit of the parapharyngeal ICA.

At the end of an endoscopic endonasal transclival procedure, when the dura has been violated, obtaining a watertight closure to prevent CSF leak is mandatory. The osteo-dural skull base defect repairing can be realized in five steps, first, filling the intradural dead space and reestablishing an arachnoidal tissue barrier using a thin layer of fibrin glue and then covering the dural aperture using a single layer of dural substitute positioned extradurally. Once this has been achieved, overlapping and embedding the extradural space with resorbable semirigid material shaped to conform to the bony defect and drag the dural substitute extradurally in an overlay mode, therefore, the vascularized pediculated nasoseptal mucosal flap is placed over the reconstruction of the clivus to support it and, finally, packing of the sphenoid cavity using abdominal fat to fill it and hold the reconstruction in place.

Table 5.1 displays the results of a series that included 20 patients and more operated via selected transcranial skull base approaches or EEAs. It seems difficult to conclude for the superiority of one approach than the other. In a recent review done by Komotar et al. [91] about clival SBC, a higher rate of GTR in the EEA group than in the transcranial group, lesser cranial nerve deficits, and no difference in CSF leak percentages was shown. But an attempt to compare complication

Table 5.1 Operative outcomes and complications in open versus endoscopic resection of clival chordomas

Technique	Autors	Nb	Previous Surg (%)	Mean Age	Gross Tot. Resect. (%)	Near Tot. Resect. (%)	Partial. Resect, (%)	Mean FU	1 yr PFS (%)	5 yrs PFS (%)	lyr OS (%)	5 yrs OS (%)	CSF Leak (%)	Men-ingiti dis (%)	CN palsy (%)
Transcranial approaches	Colli and Al-Mefty [85]	53	28	41	45	28	26	46	80	51	-	86	5	1	22
	Samii et al. [97]	37	–	38	49	50		63	78	18	-	65	5	5	12
	Takahashi et al. [101]	32	–	41	15		17	36	50	29	92	92	7	7	20
	Wu et al. [103]	79	22	36	11	51	17	64	81	53	87	68	–	–	25
	Sen et al. [99]	45	27	41	58	42		60	–	48	–	75	20	15	95
	Di Maio et al. [86]	95	55	42	71	29		38	80	56	90	74	6		25
	Komotar et al. [91] *Review*	639	33	43	48	48	4	59	66–80	69	–	66	7	6	24
Endoscopic endonasal approach	Stippler et al. [100]	20	40		45	20	35	13	65 during FU		95 during FU		25	0	5
	Koutourousiou et al. [93]	60	42	41	67	25	8	14	67 during FU		90 during FU		20	3	7
	Chibbaro et al. [84]	54	40	49	65	17	18	34	78 during FU		96 during FU		8	14	0
	[91]Review	127	33	44	61	27	12	18	83 during FU		95 during FU		5	1	1

Legends: *CN* cranial nerve, *CSF* cerebrospinal fluid, *FU* follow-up, *PFS* progression-free survival, *OS* overall survival rates and oncological results in both groups looks inadequate: The retrospective design of reports, the lack of controlled studies, the interferences of redo surgery, and the heterogeneity of postoperative RT regimen are serious limitations. Moreover, the authors of this review stressed that approaches targeted different tumors in terms of location with more cavernous sinus invasion in the group of EEA and more petrosal and intradural invasion in the open group [91]. Shorter follow-up in the EEA group is another significant limitation.

Indications for the selection of approaches incorporate the following parameters: The origin and extension of the SBC, as shown on the initial radiological work-up, is of paramount importance. The general condition and neurological status of the patient and history of previous surgeries are also considered. Petrous apex and petroclival location without moderate invasion of the bony clivus deserves lateral skull base approaches, while midclivus tumors are eligible for extended endoscopic approaches particularly when the intradural extension is reduced or absent. There are tumors that require combined approaches and that should be individually discussed by an expert skull base team who is trained to the full panel of techniques.

5.4.6 Radiation Therapy

In SBCS, postoperative radiation therapy is quite uniformly adopted as an adjuvant treatment. There are radiobiological and topographic arguments to favor proton therapy or combined proton and photon therapy versus conventional radiation therapy in SBCs. Reported by [94], the 3-year local control rate was 69.2% (+/-6.0%) for SBCs. The majority of treatment failures are due to dose limitations. The most frequent complications are visual decline (5%) and endocrine abnormalities (20%). Temporal lobe or brain stem radiation injuries are also reported (10%). Radiosurgery gives promising results (60% of 3-year PFS) with low rates of complications [92]. Long-term results are expected. To be effective, the treatment should be delivered on a residual tumor volume that does not exceed 30 cm^{3}. Carbon ion irradiation is another option still confidential with recently published results [102] in a large group of 155 SBC patients.

Table 5.2 indicates the main published series that included at least 20 patients in different RT protocols. Five- and ten-year PFS and OS are shown. Complications are also reported. For the reasons that were expressed about the surgical series, there is no clue about the standard of care to adopt with RT. The theoretical advantage of Bragg peak effect for the use of protons is counterbalanced by the limitations of available machines. Radiosurgery takes benefit of its extremely targeted treatment and few side effects but is limited on focal tumors and the need to precisely identify the limits of what should be treated which is challenging for locoregional tumors like chordomas. New RT techniques are emerging and will be evaluated with substantial delay.

To summarize, analysis of the literature provides heterogeneous statistics about oncological results in terms of progression-free survival (PFS) neither for overall survival (OS), due to the recruitment bias of the different centers. The SEER program of the National Cancer Institute [83] provided data on a large cohort of SBCs who underwent the whole panel of treatments. Five-year survival for the 1975–1984, 1985–1994, and 1995–2004 cohort was 48.5%, 73.0%, and 80.7%, respectively, with improved survival in the more recent cohorts ($P < 0.01$).

5.4.7 Prediction of Prognosis

Biological factors are probably the most important factors to consider for the prognosis of chordomas. Recent immunohistochemical studies and molecular biology suggest that two loci, 1p36 and 7q33, are associated with chordoma progression and recurrence. Increased p53 levels are associated with decreased survival levels. Changes in the relative expression of the cadherin–catenin complex reflect chordoma aggressiveness. High levels of transforming growth factor alpha and basic fibroblast growth factor expression are linked to higher rates of recurrence. Strong fibronectin expression may also be a marker of aggressiveness.

Initial Karnofsky Performance Scale, lack of intradural invasion, focal extension, and initial management in a center of reference are parameters that influence tumor control and overall survival of SBCs. While it has not been clearly shown with SBCSs, radical resection provides a positive impact on survival of SBCs, as reported by Sen et al. [99] about a series of 71 clival chordomas.

Table 5.2 Studies and patient characteristics in published series of patients with clival chordoma treated with radiation therapy

Autors	Technique	Nb	Mean age	Prior RT (%)	Prior surg (94)	Mean FU	Median target Vol. (cc)	Median margin dose (Gy/CGE)	5 yrs PFS (%)	5 yrs OS (%)	Complica-tion (%)
Amichetti et al. [79] *Review*	PBRT	416	38	–	–	46	–	66–83	69	80	5–17
Yasuda et al. [104]	PBRT	30	45	45	30	46	–	68, 9	70	83	3
Amichetti et al. [79] *Review*	Carbon	206	46	–	–	38	–	48–30	64	80	20
Amichetti et al.[79]	RT	191	44	–	–	65	–	52, 7	36	36	0–5
Amichetti et al. [79] *Review*	FSRT	45	37	–	–	27	56 (17–215)	66, 6	50	82	2
Amichetti et al. [79] *Review*	GKS	109	37	–	–	56	21.1 (0.4–129)	15.4	56	75	0–33
Kano et al. [90]	GKS	71	45	20	58	62	7, 1 (0, 9–109)	15	66	80	8
Sahgal et al. [96]	IMRT	24	46	0	24	36	14.5 (1.70–85.60)	76	65	86	33

Legends: *CGE* cobalt gray equivalent, *CN* cranial nerve, *CSF* cerebrospinal fluid, *FSRT* fractionated stereotactic radiation therapy, *FU* follow-up, *GKS* Gamma Knife surgery, *Gy* gray, *IMRT* intensity-modulated RT, *PFS* progression-free survival, *OS* overall survival, *PBRT* proton beam RT

5.4.8 Conclusions and Perspective

Chordomas are challenging skull base neoplasms. In spite of benign histology, they are locally malignant and display a significant trend to regrow locally. Radical resection is the first stair standard of care, but true GTR is not the rule. Optimal tailored surgery using the arsenal of cranial base techniques is the most validated first-line treatment. Since SBCs are mostly midline extradural tumors, the role of neuroendoscopy (EEA) is increasing logically. There is still room available for lateral transpetrosal approaches for the larger tumors that extend laterally and intradurally. Both techniques should be masterized by referring centers who should concentrate on the cases. Postoperative radiation of the remnant chordoma and tumor bed is recommended using various modalities, including charged particles and radiosurgery. The appropriate identification of the postoperative target is the prerequisite to achieve an effective radiation treatment. More than the extent of resection, tumor biology appears to be the major prognosis factor. Its understanding will provide new therapeutic targets for molecular agents since conventional chemotherapy has no effect. However, the scarcity of preclinical models (human chordoma cell lines, xenograft) capable of testing in vivo responses to new therapies hampers the development of new medical strategies. The identification of the PI3K/AKT/mTOR pathway dysfunction in chordomas has been demonstrated and is now under investigation for trials using inhibitors of this molecular target [80]. There is a need to organize registers dedicated to these rare tumors and to launch prospective randomized studies to assess the benefit of adjuvant treatments including targeted therapies.

5.5 Craniopharyngiomas

T. R. Meling

Craniopharyngiomas are quite rare, slow-growing, extra-axial, benign, partly cystic epithelial tumors of the sellar region. Symptoms frequently develop insidiously and are caused by compression of the pituitary, hypothalamus, third ventricle, and optic pathways. Radical surgery is challenging and may cause severe morbidity. Treatment of craniopharyngeomas remains somewhat controversial, and the two main options attempt at gross total resection or planned limited surgery followed by radiotherapy. There is a plethora of surgical approaches, none of which are universally superior to the others but are useful in our armamentarium to tailor a case-specific approach.

5.5.1 General Information

Etiology

A craniopharyngioma is a slow-growing, extra-axial lesion that can be defined as a benign, partly cystic epithelial tumor of the sellar region presumably derived from remnant epithelium of this hypophyseal–pharyngeal duct and/or Rathke's cleft [150]. Consequently, craniopharyngiomas have intimate relationships with the circle of Willis, third ventricle, hypothalamus, optic pathways, and pituitary stalk. The arterial supply of a craniopharyngioma is usually from the anterior cerebral arteries (ACAs) and anterior communicating artery (ACOM) or from the internal carotid arteries (ICAs) and posterior communicating arteries (PCOMs).

Epidemiology

The annual incidence of craniopharyngioma in North America is 0.13 per 100,000 with an equal sex distribution [108]. The diagnosis is more common in the pediatric group as 30–50% of all cases become apparent in childhood and adolescence. Craniopharyngiomas are rare in children younger than 2 years of age and are most often diagnosed in children aged 5–14 years. They constitute 4% of all childhood intracranial tumors [150], and craniopharyngiomas are the most common tumor in the sellar region in children.

Differential Diagnosis

There are several lesions in the sellar and suprasellar region to consider as differential diagnosis (▫ Table 5.3).

Table 5.3 Differential diagnosis

Cystic lesions	Rathke's cleft cyst, dermoid and epidermoid cyst, and arachnoid cyst
Solid tumors	Pituitary adenoma, germinoma, hypothalamic hamartoma, hypothalamic–optic pathway glioma, PNET, metastasis, and meningioma
Inflammatory lesions	Langerhans cell histiocytosis, lymphocytic hypophysitis/infundibulitis, suprasellar abscess, sarcoidosis, and tuberculosis
Vascular lesions	Carotid–cavernous fistula, cavernous sinus hemangioma, and giant suprasellar carotid aneurysm

Prognosis

The overall survival rate varies, but in large series, up to 93% of patients had a 10-year recurrence-free survival and 96% overall 10-year survival [141, 159]. The most significant factor associated with craniopharyngioma recurrence is the extent of surgical resection [151, 158, 159], with lesions greater than 5 cm in diameter carrying a markedly worse prognosis [152, 159]. However, there is an excess mortality after treatment for a craniopharyngioma that is especially marked in patients with childhood-onset disease and among women [144].

Tumor Classification

Craniopharyngiomas can be classified according to histological appearance, imaging appearance, and location.

Histology

Craniopharyngioma is classified into two histological types, namely, adamantinomatous and papillary [150].

Adamantinomatous Type

Histologically, the classical craniopharyngioma contains nests of basaloid and stellate epithelial cells that resemble the dental ameloblastic organ and are also seen in a rare bone called adamantinoma [150].

Another distinctive feature of the adamantinomatous variant is scattered nodules of «wet» keratin that frequently calcify, leading to calcifications of the tumor. Furthermore, portions of this keratinous debris elicit an intense inflammatory and foreign body giant cell reaction responsible for the adhesions between the tumor and the surrounding tissues.

Adamantinomatous craniopharyngiomas are predominantly cystic or cystic–solid. The cysts are filled with a brownish, lipid- and cholesterol-rich viscous fluid resembling a machine oil.

The adamantinomatous subtype occurs at all ages, from the fetal and newborn period to late senescence, but is most frequent in children and adolescents [150]. The incidence is bimodal, being highest in childhood and adolescence, but with a second peak around 40–60 years of age [150].

Papillary Type

The papillary craniopharyngioma variant contains only squamous epithelium without any adamantinomatous component. It is predominantly a solid tumor and has a low propensity for cyst formation and calcification [150].

These tumors lack the cholesterol deposits and the turbid cyst fluid and also carry a more favorable prognosis. They do not form keratin nodules and hence have less perifocal inflammation and adhesions.

In contrast to the adamantinomatous type, the papillary craniopharyngioma is rarely seen in children and occurs almost exclusively in adults, and its peak incidence is between 50 and 70 years of age [150].

Grading

Although histologically benign, craniopharyngiomas can be biologically quite aggressive tumors. They tend to surround and adhere to vital structures such as the pituitary gland and stalk, the hypothalamus, the optic pathways, and the vessels of circle of Willis. There is often a marked gliosis in the adjacent brain structures secondary to a strong inflammatory reaction, making the tumor especially adherent to these structures and hinders attempts at complete resection.

Imaging

Craniopharyngiomas can be classified according to their imaging appearance. The tumors can be primarily cystic, solid, or mixed. Furthermore,

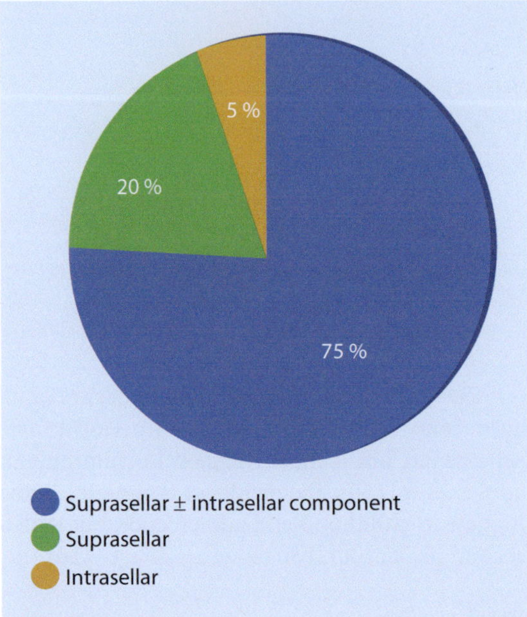

Fig. 5.56

calcification, a hallmark of a craniopharyngioma, is seen in up to 90% of the cases [116].

Location

We can classify craniopharyngiomas according to their location, be it relative to the pituitary stalk, sella turcica, optic chiasm, or diaphragma sellae.

These tumors have different growth patterns depending on wherefrom along the craniopharyngeal duct they arise. Tumors arising from the proximal portion may be restricted to the ventricular region, whereas those that arise from the middle portion grow into the suprasellar spaces and/or extend into the third ventricle, and those from the distal portion grow intrasellarly with or without a suprasellar extension.

We can classify craniopharyngiomas according to their location relative to the sella turcica (Fig. 5.56). According to this scheme, approximately three quarters are suprasellar with an intrasellar component. Approximately one in five is purely suprasellar, whereas one in twenty is purely intrasellar [143].

We can also classify craniopharyngiomas according to their location relative to the optic chiasm (Fig. 5.57). According to Hoffman, tumors are either (a) sellar, i.e., subchiasmatic and confined to the sella or protruding only a short distance above the diaphragm; (b) prechiasmatic, i.e., growing forward and pushing the optic chiasm and anterior cerebral arteries superior and posterior; (c) retrochiasmatic, i.e., growing posteriorly into the third ventricle and displacing the optic chiasm anteriorly; or (d) giant craniopharyngioma with varying growth patterns and (e) Tumor predominantly in the third ventricle [124].

Wang et al. proposed a classification of that emphasizes the relationship to the diaphragma sellae [157]. The craniopharyngiomas are dichotomized into (i) subdiaphragmatic or (ii) supradiaphragmatic tumors. Subdiaphragmatic lesions can have either an intact or a disrupted diaphragma sellae. Subdiaphragmatic tumors with an intact diaphragm will push and distend the diaphragm, thereby maintaining a «capsule» that prevents adhesions between the tumor and the optic chiasm and anterior cerebral vessels. In contrast, subdiaphragmatic lesions with a disrupted diaphragm will acquire an «hourglass» configuration as it grows through the aperture into the suprasellar space with the diaphragm forming a waistband. These lesions extend retrochiasmatically, and continued growth results in anterior displacement of the optic pathways; adhesions to superior neural elements, particularly the hypothalamus; and growth into the third ventricle through its thin floor. Supradiaphragmatic lesions have no intrasellar component. They grow posteriorly in the retrochiasmatic direction as well as laterally into adjacent CSF cisterns. Supradiaphragmatic lesions often adhere to adjacent neural structures including the hypothalamus, optic nerves, chiasm and tracts, floor of the third ventricle, and lower cranial nerves. These lesions also have a propensity to erode through the thin floor of the third ventricle causing hydrocephalus.

5.5.2 Clinical Signs and Symptoms

Craniopharyngiomas are typically slow-growing tumors, and consequently, symptoms frequently develop insidiously. They are often detected only after the tumors attain a diameter of about 3 cm, and duration between onset of symptoms and diagnosis is usually around 6 months but can be up to many years [125, 126].

The clinical presentation of craniopharyngiomas is a direct result of their location and growth pattern but is nevertheless non-specific. They compress the optic pathways, infiltrate the

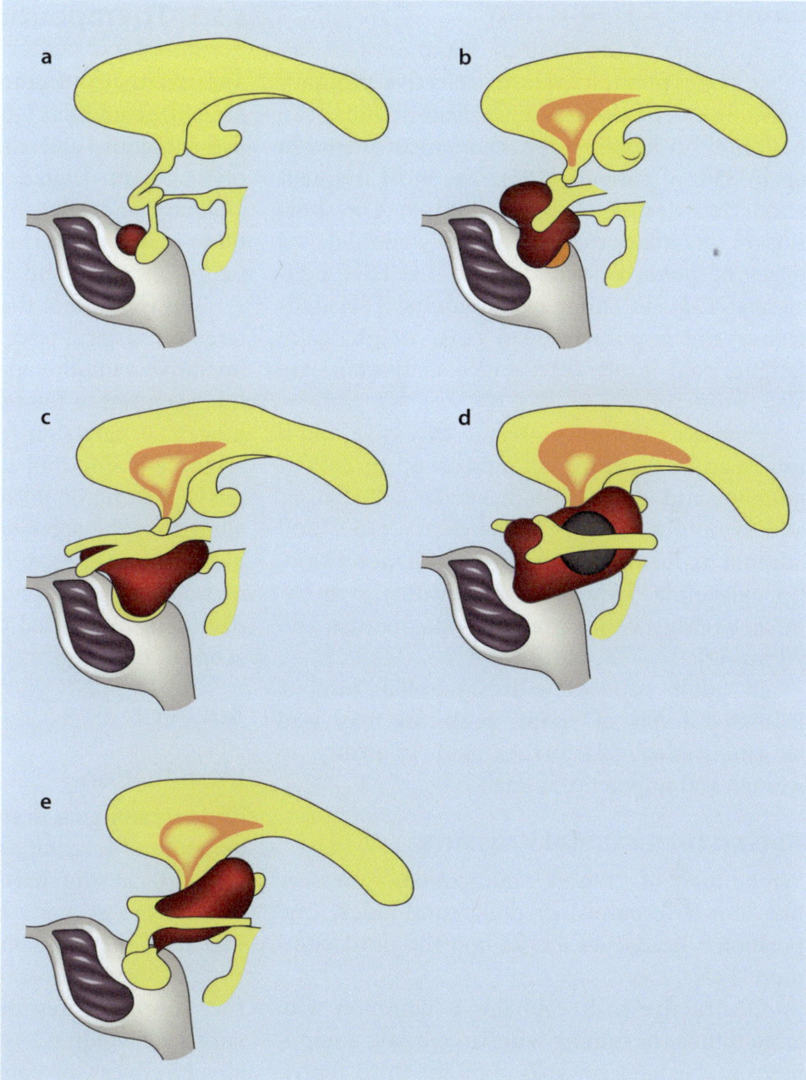

Fig. 5.57 Location of craniopharyngiomas relative to the optic chiasm. **a** Sellar, i.e., subchiasmatic and confined to the sella or protruding only a short distance above the diaphragm. **b** Prechiasmatic, i.e., growing forward and pushing the optic chiasm and anterior cerebral arteries superior and posterior. **c** Retrochiasmatic, i.e., growing posteriorly into the third ventricle and displacing the optic chiasm anteriorly. **d** Giant craniopharyngiomas with varying growth patterns. **e** Tumor predominantly in the third ventricle

hypothalamus, and can extend into the third ventricle, leading to visual disturbances, hypothalamic–pituitary dysfunctions and hydrocephalus, or combinations thereof.

Interestingly, children and adults may have dissimilar clinical presentations. Children present more often with endocrine dysfunction, progressive visual loss, symptoms of raised intracranial pressure, and papilledema, whereas adults more uniformly have visual impairment.

Lastly, there is a relationship between the anatomical location of the craniopharyngioma and the clinical presentation in that a prechiasmal location typically results in findings of optic atrophy (e.g., progressive decline of visual acuity, constriction of visual fields), a retrochiasmal location is associated with hydrocephalus with signs of increased intracranial pressure (e.g., papilledema, horizontal double vision), and, lastly, an intrasellar craniopharyngioma usually manifests as headache and/or endocrinopathy.

Visual Disturbance

Compression of the anterior visual pathways can cause decreased visual acuity, visual field deficits (commonly bitemporal hemianopia), and optic disc swelling or atrophy. Visual disturbances are present in two-thirds of the adults [147] but are often reversible after surgery. The smaller children are less aware of optic pathway dysfunction and often present after the visual damage becomes irreversible [105].

Endocrine Dysfunction

Compression of the pituitary gland or stalk can cause panhypopituitarism or selective pituitary hormone deficiencies, and dysfunctions can be found on baseline endocrine assessments in up to 85% of patients [153]. The most frequent endocrine dysfunctions in children are short stature secondary to GH deficiency and delayed onset of puberty secondary to LH/FSH deficiency [153]. In children and adults, TSH deficiency and hypothyroidism (e.g., weight gain, fatigue, cold intolerance, and constipation) are also common.

5

Diabetes insipidus (e.g., excessive fluid intake and urination) is found in up to 20% of patients, and almost 25% have associated signs and symptoms of ACTH deficiency [153] and adrenal failure (e.g., orthostatic hypotension, hypoglycemia, hyperkalemia, cardiac arrhythmias, lethargy, confusion, anorexia, nausea, and vomiting).

In adult patients with intrasellar tumors, increased levels of serum prolactin may lead to amenorrhea/galactorrhea and infertility in women and impotence in men.

Raised Intracranial Pressure

Symptoms of raised intracranial pressure like slowly progressive, dull, continuous, and positional headaches are among the most common [131].

Obstructive hydrocephalus is common with large tumors or tumors with large cystic components that extend upwards to fill the third ventricle. The level of obstruction is often the foramina of Monro, and therefore it is commonly seen with retrochiasmatic tumors.

Clinical signs like papilledema are particularly alarming and associated with reduced visual acuity and color perception.

Neuropsychological Dysfunction

Large tumors can cause symptoms and signs like impairment of executive functions, psychomotor retardation, emotional immaturity, apathy, and personality changes due to compression of orbitofrontal cortex [137], and hydrocephalus can lead to altered memory and mentation. Apathy, incontinence, and hypersomnia have also been described [145].

5.5.3 Therapeutic Options

The treatment of craniopharyngiomas is multifaceted, given their location, their diverse clinical presentations, and the potential complications of treatment. Hence, the treatment is multidisciplinary and often involves neurosurgery, ophthalmology, endocrinology, pediatric oncology/neuro-oncology, and radiation oncology.

The traditional therapeutic approach is centered on surgical resection, with or without postoperative radiotherapy. Complete excision with total removal of the tumor is associated with the longest progression-free survival. However, as multiple endocrinopathies and eating disorders are very common postoperatively [125, 126, 155], alternative therapies aimed at minimizing the surgical morbidity have been developed. Treatment of postoperative hypopituitarism, hypothalamic disorders, and visual disturbances is beyond the scope of this chapter.

Surgery

Introduction

The primary goal in the treatment of craniopharyngiomas is complete removal of the tumor without causing harm. However, our surgical aggressiveness must be tempered by the facts that craniopharyngiomas are benign lesions with a 92% 35-year overall survival rate [143] and that morbidity resulting from poorly executed surgery, including hyperphagia and morbid obesity, blindness, or panhypopituitarism, will have severe, lifelong implications for the quality of life of the patient [154]. Subtotal resection followed by adjuvant radiotherapy produces good results, with 5-year progression-free survivals of 70% reported in the recent literature [113]. A trend toward less radical surgical approaches has been observed, accompanied by a reduced rate of severe hypothalamic lesions [127]. On the other hand, surgery is the only possibility for a cure, and in reality, the only chance for a cure is the first operation, and incomplete removal more often than not leads to multiple surgical procedures which also negatively impact the quality of life [128].

The way I approach this preoperatively is to carefully review the MRI images to make an

Table 5.4 Preoperative work-up

CT scanning	CT caput reveals the tumor cysts and calcifications. Calcifications are seen in 90% of the pediatric craniopharyngiomas and in 40% of the adults 3D CT of the skull base demonstrates any bony involvement, including expansion of the sella turcica and erosions of the dorsum sellae/clinoid processes CT angiography will delineate the relationships between the tumor and vascular structures, particularly in the internal carotid artery and its branches and the anterior circulation vessels
MR imaging	The signal intensity on MRI is often highly heterogeneous, as it depends on the protein content of the cysts and the calcifications of the solid tumor T1-weighted images in the axial, sagittal, and coronal planes delineate tumor margins with relationships to pituitary, pituitary stalk, optic chiasm and tracts, hypothalamus, and third ventricle. 1 mm fine cuts give detailed information about relationships between the tumor and adjacent neural structures T1-weighted with contrast improve detection of nodular tumor components and delineation of the cyst walls T2-weighted images demonstrate cystic components, typically hyperintense, and can delineate cyst and cyst wall from ventricle. Craniopharyngioma cysts are typically hypointense on T1 and often hyperintense on T2, but cysts that are hyperintense on T1 are likely to contain blood degradation products, high protein concentration, or both MR angiography might be a useful tool to assess the perilesional arterial anatomy
Neuroendocrine testing	Serum levels of cortisol, ACTH, prolactin, TFTs (FT4 and TSH), insulin-like growth factor 1 (IGF-1), growth hormone, LH, FSH, testosterone in men, and estradiol in women Diabetes insipidus (DI) must be ruled out by taking a history of urinary output and thirst and measuring sodium and osmolality in serum and urine
Neuro-ophthalmic assessments	Visual acuity, visual fields (preferably Goldmann perimetry), and ocular paresis must be undertaken Ishihara color plates are effective means of screening the patient's color vision

educated guess as to whether the tumors have a favorable or unfavorable scenario with respect to complete resectability. If we have a favorable scenario (e.g., tumor size <3 cm, subdiaphragmatic location with intact diaphragma sellae), plan A will be complete removal with the option of converting to a plan B with subtotal resection if the intraoperative findings are such that the risks of serious morbidity outweigh the benefit of a complete removal. If we have an unfavorable scenario (e.g., not involving the hypothalamus, tumor size >6 cm, supradiaphragmatic location with complete engulfment of the pituitary stalk in a child with normal or near-normal endocrinological function), plan A will be an incomplete removal with the option of converting to a plan B with complete resection if the intraoperative findings turn out to be more favorable than anticipated. If complete removal is not possible, the goal should be maximal safe decompression of the optic chiasm and the ventricular system, to gain enough distance (3 mm) between the residual tumor and the critical structures to allow for a safer radiosurgery.

Preoperative Work-Up

Radiology

A thorough imaging work-up includes CT scanning, MRI with and without gadolinium in three planes, and MR angiography. This neuroimaging provides critical information about the tumor's consistency, vascularity, and its relationship to the surrounding structures (Table 5.4). Furthermore, preoperative peritumoral edema in T2-weighted/FLAIR images is associated with a postoperative hypothalamic syndrome [140].

Preoperative Medical Management

Good medical management of the craniopharyngioma patient is crucial to the overall outcome. In addition to undergoing extensive preoperative endocrinological investigations (Table 5.8), specific attention must also be paid to the intraoperative and postoperative endocrinological status of the patient.

Diabetes insipidus (DI) occurs preoperatively in 6–38% and must be ruled out or confirmed (Table 5.8).

Unless the tumor is small, all craniopharyngioma patients are presumed to be deficient in ACTH and supplemented with corticosteroids preoperatively. Hypocortisolism is potentially lethal, and dexamethasone is mandatory for patients presenting with adrenal dysfunction. In addition, steroids are also indicated if a perifocal vasogenic edema is present around the tumor.

Ophthalmology

Neuro-ophthalmic assessment is important both pre- and postoperatively (Table 5.4).

Approaches

Surgery for craniopharyngiomas is challenging because as these tumors enlarge, they may elevate and infiltrate the optic chiasm as well as the hypothalamic region. Occasionally, they extend into the pituitary fossa or posteriorly to the ventral pons, and rarely, they invade the basal ganglia or the brain parenchyma. Craniopharyngiomas may also encase or displace vessels that form the circle of Willis. Usually, the ICAs and PCOMs are displaced laterally, the ACOM and ACAs are displaced anteriorly, and the basilar artery (BA) is displaced posteriorly.

No surgical approach is without inherent limitations. Hence, there is a plethora of different approaches to craniopharyngiomas [146], and none of which are universally superior to the others but are useful in our armamentarium to tailor a case-specific approach. However, for the sake of clarity, we can divide them into transcranial and transsphenoidal approaches (Table 5.5).

When choosing an approach, the different growth patterns are of importance (Fig. 5.57). Although large suprasellar craniopharyngiomas may be resected through an extended transsphenoidal approach, a transcranial approach is often necessary when the predominant tumor component is suprasellar. Conversely, if the predominant portion of the tumor is intrasellar, the approach is usually transsphenoidal as the suprasellar component often can be delivered into the sella and evacuated.

Transcranial Approaches

In the transcranial approaches, a craniotomy and dura opening will expose the intradural tumor component (Table 5.5). Intradurally, different surgical corridors can be used for the resection of the craniopharyngioma (Table 5.6).

Transnasal Approaches

In the endoscopic transnasal, transsphenoidal approach, generous removal of the contents of the nasal cavity and sphenoid sinus is required (Table 5.9) to expose the sella turcica. The endoscope offers a superior light and a direct visualization, and many of the critical neurovascular structures will be medial to the tumor, reducing the risk of accidental injury to these structures [117, 130]. In the extended endoscopic approach (EEA), the tuberculum sellae, planum sphenoidale, and/or dorsum sellae are removed to increase the exposure.

Choice of Surgical Approach

The choice of surgical approach is generally based on the location and size of the tumor (Fig. 5.57) but also factoring in patient age, degree of endocrine deficiencies at presentation, and tumor consistency.

Sometimes the decision is easy. In purely subdiaphragmatic tumors, be it with or without a suprasellar extension, we use the endoscopic transnasal–transsphenoidal technique (Case 1). Conversely, in a purely intraventricular tumor, we use a unilateral, frontal, interhemispheric, transcallosal approach (Case 2).

More often than not, the decision is not this straightforward. If a large calcified tumor component is located in a deep sella turcica with a largely cystic supradiaphragmatic extension through a disrupted diaphragm, we tend to favor an endoscopic transnasal–transsphenoidal approach since complete removal then is very difficult via a craniotomy, be it a transsylvian or a subfrontal approach (Case 3). However, in very small children, the transnasal approach can be very limited, and the sphenoid sinus may not even be pneumatized yet. Furthermore, in patients with a preexisting hydrocephalus, especially those that carry an increased risk of postoperative CSF leaks like high BMI, pulmonary hypertension, or sleep apnea, a craniotomy offers a much lower CSF leak rate.

In a supradiaphragmatic, extraventricular craniopharyngioma, the surgical approach is subfrontal (Case 4) or transsylvian via a frontotemporal craniotomy (Case 5). The endoscopic

Table 5.5 Overview of the most commonly used approaches for craniopharyngioma resection

Frontotemporal (pterional) craniotomy	Description	The pterional or frontotemporal craniotomy is the standard craniotomy for a transsylvian approach to suprasellar lesions [152]
	Strengths	It offers good visualization of the optic nerves and optic chiasm, and the surrounding structures after the Sylvian fissure have been opened widely As it is our workhorse, the normal locations of critical structures are very familiar, something which is of critical importance when a craniopharyngioma has completely displaced and/or encased them
	Limitations	The pterional craniotomy raises a very large bone flap, often at least 4.0×6.0 cm Lends a restricted view of tumor components that have grown high up into the third ventricle, often necessitating the use of retractors and/or an endoscope in large craniopharyngiomas Visualization of the sella is limited, especially medial to the ipsilateral ICA and optic nerve. This is of critical importance when the solid part of a craniopharyngioma is located in a deep sella turcica Resection of the intrasellar component is medial to the ipsilateral optic nerve, which can lead to accidental nerve injury Resection of a subchiasmatic tumor component is medial to the ipsilateral ICA and PCOM, which can lead to accidental injury to these vessels
Lateral supraorbital (LSO) craniotomy	*Description*	A smaller variant of the pterional approach is the lateral supraorbital craniotomy. The craniotomy is essentially a 2.5×3.0 cm in the supraorbital region The intradural trajectory is slightly more medial and subfrontal than via a pterional–transsylvian approach, but the difference between trajectories is small when in the central skull base region The skin incision can be either the standard curvilinear incision behind the hairline ad modum Hernesniemi or a smaller 5 cm eyebrow incision that starts from just medial to the supraorbital nerve ad modum Perneczky
	Strengths	The advantages of this approach are a shorter skin incision that is hidden by the eyebrow, preservation of the frontal branch of the facial nerve and the superior temporal artery (STA), shorter scar and improved cosmetic appearance vis-a-vis a pterional approach, less brain exposure, less brain retraction, and a shorter time to open and close the craniotomy As with the pterional craniotomy, the normal locations of critical structures are very familiar, something which is of critical importance when the tumor has displaced and/or encased them As with the unilateral frontal craniotomy, the LSO provides a direct and short route to lesions that lie anterior to the optic chiasm. The temporalis muscle requires very little elevation
	Limitations	The general limitations of this approach are a steeper learning curve, a more restricted space with less room to maneuver and mobilize critical structures, the need for frequent microscope repositioning for optimal illumination and focus, and, lastly, the skin incision may leave a visible scar in the eyebrow if not performed well The more specific limitations for craniopharyngioma surgery are similar to that of the pterional approach but even more so for visualization of a tumor component in the third ventricle, often necessitating the use of retractors or an endoscope Visualization of the sella may be even more limited than in a pterional approach because of the orbital dome. This leads to a restricted view of a solid part of a craniopharyngioma located deep in the sella turcica, necessitating the use of an endoscope Lastly, resection of an intrasellar component is medial to the ipsilateral optic nerve, which can lead to accidental nerve injury, and resection of a subchiasmatic tumor component is medial to the ipsilateral ICA and PCOM, which can lead to accidental injury to these vessels

(continued)

Table 5.5 (continued)

Frontotemporal orbitozygomatic (FTOZ) craniotomy	*Description*	In the transcranial approaches, a craniotomy and dura opening will expose the intradural tumor component. Intradurally, different surgical corridors can be used for the resection of the craniopharyngioma (Table 5.6) The frontotemporal orbitozygomatic (FTOZ) craniotomy is a skull base variant of the pterional craniotomy that includes osteotomies in the orbital rim and zygoma
	Strengths	It provides an improved working area in the central skull base area It lowers the line of sight to the superior aspects of the tumor if it grows way up into the third ventricle, leading to less frontal lobe retraction in order to visualize the operative site
	Limitations	Unless the tumor is high into the third ventricle, the FTOZ does not offer any significant advantages over the two abovementioned approaches This approach carries a higher rate of temporal muscle atrophy than with a pterional craniotomy. Postoperative atrophy of the temporalis muscle may be a consequence of direct injury to muscle fibers by improper dissection or excessive retraction, ischemia from interruption of the primary arterial supply, or denervation There is a higher rate of frontal sinus breaches and violation of the frontal and/or other paranasal sinuses is a source of harmful complications There is also a higher rate of TMJ discomfort than with a pterional craniotomy Cosmetic defects may arise due to inaccurate repositioning of the bone flap Lastly, enophthalmus and pulsatile exophthalmus have been described
Mini-orbitofrontal (MOF) craniotomy	*Description*	A smaller variant of the FTOZ approach is the mini-orbitofrontal (MOF) craniotomy with a transpalpebral skin incision in the natural skin crease of the upper eyelid The craniotomy is essentially a 2.5 × 3.0 cm in the supraorbital region, similar to the LSO, but includes removal of parts of the superior orbital rim and roof, as well as the lateral orbital wall
	Strengths	By removing the superior orbital rim and parts of the orbital roof, the orbital contents can be mobilized downward, allowing a much lower line of sight to the superior aspects of a tumor high in the third ventricle than the pterional or LSO can offer. Removal of the lateral orbital wall further increases the superior reach Like a unilateral frontal craniotomy, the MOF provides a direct and short route to lesions that lie anterior to the optic chiasm The cosmesis is excellent. Whereas both ciliary and supraciliary incisions involve a cut across the frontalis muscle that can result in eyebrow asymmetry, the skin incision here is very short and hidden in the palpebral crease Similar to an LSO via an eyebrow incision, the MOF preserves the frontal branch of the facial nerve and the STA, affords an improved cosmetic appearance vis-a-vis a pterional or FTOZ craniotomy, has much less brain exposure and brain retraction, and is very quick to open and close Lastly, the temporalis muscle requires very little elevation
	Limitations	Like for the LSO, the general limitations of this approach are a steeper learning curve, a more restricted space with less room to maneuver and mobilize critical structures, the need for frequent microscope repositioning for optimal illumination and focus, and, lastly, the need to learn the skin incision from an oculoplastic surgeon to perform it well The more specific limitations for craniopharyngioma surgery are similar to that of the pterional approach like suboptimal visualization of the tumor components deep in the sella turcica and that any resection of intrasellar components is medial to the ipsilateral optic nerve, which can lead to accidental nerve injury, and resection of a subchiasmatic tumor component is medial to the ipsilateral ICA and PCOM, which can lead to accidental vessel injury

Table 5.5 (continued)

Subfrontal approach	*Description*	In the classical subfrontal approaches, a craniotomy is performed in the anterior half of the frontal bone, either to the midline (unilateral) or crossing the midline (bilateral), and allows for a translamina terminalis approach to a third ventricle craniopharyngioma These approaches are well tested and can be very useful for lesions located in the anterior cranial fossa and in the supra- and parasellar area. In experienced hands, the approach is a safe and reliable procedure that gives excellent access to the main neurovascular structures of the central skull base region The extent and direction of tumor growth determines if the unilateral or the bilateral subfrontal approach should be used
	Strengths	Provides a direct and short route to lesions that lie anterior to the optic chiasm A bifrontal craniotomy allows trajectories to the sellar and parasellar region either subfrontally or interhemispherically The temporalis muscle does not require elevation
	Limitations	Requires a bicoronal skin incision The unilateral approach carries a higher rate of frontal sinus breaches than the pterional craniotomy, and for the bifrontal craniotomy, the frontal sinus is always entered and requires a cranialization The bifrontal approach puts both olfactory nerves at risk Visualization of the sella turcica is limited, even with drilling of the tuberculum sellae. This is of critical importance in patients where a prefixed chiasm restricts access to the sella. Therefore, accurate preoperative neuroradiological assessment for optimum surgical planning is crucial
Interhemispheric approach	*Description*	An interhemispheric, transcallosal approach is necessary when the tumor is entirely within the third ventricle (Fig. 5.57e) In the classical interhemispheric approach, a unilateral craniotomy is performed in the posterior part of the frontal bone. The craniotomy is placed two-thirds in front and one-third behind the coronal suture, perhaps just crossing the midline slightly to allow for some lateral retraction of the superior sagittal sinus and falx cerebri The interhemispheric fissure is opened, and the corpus callosum is incised 15 mm between the pericallosal arteries to gain access to either the ipsilateral lateral ventricle or the velum interpositum If the transventricular route is chosen, the third ventricle is entered either through the lateral ventricle via the foramina of Monro or via a transchoroidal, sub-plexus, fornix-sparing approach. The transforaminal approach is most appropriate when the foramen is expanded, and the craniopharyngioma cyst located within the third ventricle can be decompressed and delivered into the foramen If the midline approach is chosen, the velum interpositum is entered and the third ventricle is entered via a transcallosal–interseptal–interforniceal approach [161]. However, the velum interpositum is usually narrow and poorly defined anatomically, and because bilateral forniceal injury can cause severe memory deficits, this approach is often reserved for cases in which there is either a cavum septum pellucidum or significant mass effect that has anatomically separated the fornices
	Strengths	The interhemispheric, transcallosal approach provides a direct route to lesions that lie entirely within the third ventricle The small sectioning of the callosum leads to minimal long-term consequences and avoids transgression of the cerebral cortex
	Limitations	The surgical corridor is very long and narrow It is a technically demanding approach, and extra care must be taken to avoid damaging the medial draining veins to prevent venous infarction The approach carries a risk of injury to one (transventricular) or both (interforniceal) fornices with subsequent potential for memory disturbances The transforaminal approach is only appropriate when foramen of Monro is expanded The optic chiasm, optics tracts, and pituitary stalk cannot be identified, if at all, until the very end of the resection

(continued)

Table 5.5 (continued)

Transcortical approach	*Description*	In the transcortical approach, the craniotomy is usually centered on the coronal suture, midway between the stephanion and bregma. The dura mater is opened, and the middle frontal gyrus or sulcus is dissected, and the lateral ventricle is entered Transcortical approaches are only suited for cases where the craniopharyngioma has caused ventricular enlargement and have large cystic components in the lateral ventricle(s) or as part of combined approaches in dealing with a more complex morphology
	Strengths	The transcortical approach provides a direct route to tumor cysts that lie in the lateral ventricle(s) and to the lesion that lie entirely within the third ventricle through an enlarged foramen of Monro
	Limitations	The surgical corridor is very long and narrow The sectioning of the cerebral cortex may lead to seizures The approach carries a risk of injury to the ipsilateral fornix with a potential memory disturbance The transforaminal approach is only appropriate when foramen of Monro is expanded The optic chiasm, optics tracts, and pituitary stalk cannot be identified, if at all, until the very end of the resection The sellar and parasellar region is not visualized
Transsphenoidal approach	*Description*	Successful endoscopic, transnasal, transsphenoidal resection of a craniopharyngioma requires a generous removal of the contents of the nasal cavity, sphenoid sinus, and sellar contents. When predominantly in the sella, these tumors erode the bony floor and enlarge the sella Adequate suprasellar decompression occurs when the arachnoid membrane that surrounds the tumor descends into the operative field, and CSF leakage occurs intraoperatively when the arachnoid is disrupted
	Strengths	Visualization of the sella turcica is very good, and this is of critical importance when the solid part of a craniopharyngioma is located deep in the sella Resection of the intrasellar component and of the subchiasmatic tumor component is caudal to the optic nerves and medial to the oculomotor nerves, reducing the risk of accidental injury to these structures [117, 130] The endoscope offers a superior light and a direct visualization. Endoscopes with angles of 30 or 45° allow for visualization of both lateral tumor extensions and tumor components that have extended into the third ventricle [117]
	Limitations	The main limitation of an extended endonasal approach is the extremely high CSF leak rate (15–25%) compared to a transcranial approach even in the most experienced hands [111, 130, 135], and these CSF leaks lead to a very high rate of postoperative meningitis Other general limitations of this approach are a steeper learning curve, a longer working distance with reduced microsurgical precision, the very extensive removal of normal anatomical structures in the nasal cavity with potential postoperative nasal complications, a much more restricted workspace with less room to maneuver and mobilize critical structures, the need for harvesting a large mucosal–septal flap for dural closure, and the need for postoperative nasal packings Although an angled endoscope allows for visualization of very lateral tumor extensions, there are often no instruments that can reach the tumour, leaving us sometimes in a situation where «what you see is not what you get» Resection of the suprachiasmatic tumor component is cranial to the optic chiasm, which can lead to accidental nerve injury Lastly, the control of vascular structures is inferior to some of the abovementioned craniotomies as both the ICAs and PCOMs with their branches lie lateral and behind the subchiasmatic tumor components

Table 5.6 Intradural surgical corridors

Corridor	Where	Area exposed
The subchiasmatic corridor	Between the optic nerves and below the optic chiasm	Tumor tissue in the subchiasmatic area The corridor can be widened by drilling the tuberculum sellae
The opticocarotid corridor	Between the optic nerve and internal carotid artery	Tumor tissue with parasellar extension The corridor can be widened by an extradural anterior clinoidectomy and opening of the distal dural ring to lateralize the ICA
The oculomotor–carotid triangle	Between the internal carotid artery and oculomotor nerve	Tumor tissue with far lateral extension in the cavernous sinus The corridor can be widened by opening the oculomotor cistern to lateralize the oculomotor nerve
The translamina terminalis corridor	Above the optic chiasm and through the lamina terminalis	Tumor tissue that extends into the third ventricle

transnasal–transsphenoidal approach can also be used in these cases, but we favor the craniotomy because of the extremely low CSF leak rate.

In a supradiaphragmatic craniopharyngioma with an intraventricular extension, our preferred surgical approach is subfrontal via a mini-orbitofrontal (MOF) craniotomy (Case 6).

Lastly, in very large tumors and in tumors with wide lateral extensions, we also prefer the FTOZ craniotomy, which also allows for a generous access to both a subfrontal and transsylvian approach (Case 7).

Postoperative Care

Intraoperative use of mannitol should be minimized in order to optimize fluid management in the patient. Diabetes insipidus (DI), reported to be present in 50–90% postoperatively [111, 112, 135, 138, 161], is a potentially fatal complication. Fluid balance and electrolyte status should be carefully monitored postoperatively. Low-dose substitution should be given if needed.

All patients with craniopharyngiomas are given perioperative steroids to avoid hypocortisolism.

We do not use anticonvulsant medication routinely as the risk of postoperative seizures is quite low when the electrolyte levels are well controlled.

Cyst Drainage

For predominantly cystic craniopharyngiomas, intracavitary therapy remains an option. By inserting a catheter into the cyst and connecting it to an Ommaya reservoir, repeated cyst aspirations can be performed to lower the pressure and relieve symptoms [118, 149].

The Ommaya reservoir can also be used for instillations of various agents into the cyst to induce scarring of the wall, thereby decreasing the volume of cystic craniopharyngiomas or reducing cyst recurrences. Agents include substances like radioactive yttrium (^{90}Y) [156], phosphorus (^{32}P) ([106, 122, 132], or iodine (^{125}I) [107] and holmium-166–chitosan complex [119], the chemotherapeutic agent bleomycin [110, 133, 142], and chemotherapy with interferon alpha [109, 115].

Radiation Therapy

The high morbidity associated with radical resection of some craniopharyngiomas has led to the development of alternative treatment strategies aimed at minimizing the surgical morbidity. As craniopharyngiomas are radiosensitive, radiation therapy (RT) has now become an important adjunct in the management protocol of patients, and RT is often used whenever total resection is not achieved surgically, intended or not. Patients who have undergone subtotal resections should be considered for RT, and patients fare better if they undergo RT early, rather than at tumor regrowth.

The fundamental principle of radiotherapy is that of selective ionization of the tumor tissue, by means of high-energy beams of radiation. Ions and free radicals are formed from the intracellular water or from the biological materials and produce irreparable damage to DNA, proteins, and lipids, resulting in the cell death.

Fractionated Radiotherapy

In fractionated RT, currently the mode most frequently used for craniopharyngiomas, an external megavoltage photon beam (X-ray) is used to deliver a total dose of 54 Gy [139]. The tumor is irradiated with a high radiation dose while at the same time increasing normal tissue tolerance by fractionation of the total dose.

Stereotactic Radiosurgery

In stereotactic radiosurgery (SRS), a Gamma Knife from Elekta uses the convergence of multiple beams of gamma rays generated from 201 radioactive cobalt sources to achieve a highly focused radiation in a single dose to the target volume.

SRS for craniopharyngiomas is effective [134], but despite the high precision, some radiation is delivered beyond the confines of the target volume, and important perifocal structures, particularly the optic chiasm, are at risk [121]. Consequently, the radiation must be given so that the dose to the chiasm does not exceed 10 cGy, while the tumor itself receives a maximal dose of 19–2 Gy. Thus, if a tumor is in too close proximity to the optic pathway (2–3 mm), Gamma Knife is generally not recommended. Furthermore, Gamma Knife treatment is not very effective for predominantly cystic tumors.

Linear Accelerator-Based Therapies

Linear accelerators (LINACs) produce megavoltage photon beams (X-ray) and can also deliver a highly focused radiation dose. Examples include the Novalis Shaped Beam Radiosurgery system from Brainlab [123], the Trilogy from Varian, and the CyberKnife from Accuray [129].

Whereas the Gamma Knife has 201 radioactive cobalt sources arrayed in the helmet to deliver a variety of treatment angles, on a LINAC, the gantry (the emission head) moves in space to change delivery angles. A stereotactic frame restricts the patient's head movement while the machine can move the patient and/or the gantry in space to change the delivery point.

The diameter of the energy beam leaving the emission head can be adjusted to the size of the lesion by means of multileaf collimators that consist of a number of metal leaflets that can be moved dynamically during treatment in order to shape the radiation beam to conform to the mass to be ablated. The latest generation LINAC is capable of achieving extremely narrow beam geometries, such as 0.15–0.3 mm.

The restrictions mentioned for the Gamma Knife also apply for LINACs with respect to proximity of critical neurovascular structures. In recent years, however, intensity-modulated radiation therapy (IMRT) techniques make the radiation dose to conform more precisely to the three-dimensional shape of the tumor by modulating (i.e., controlling) the intensity of the radiation beam in multiple small volumes, thereby allowing higher radiation doses to be focused on the tumor while minimizing the dose to surrounding normal critical structures like the optic chiasm.

Proton Beam Therapy

In proton beam therapy (PBT), protons are produced by a medical cyclotron and subsequently accelerated in successive travels through a circular, evacuated conduit using powerful magnets, until they reach sufficient energy. The protons are then released toward the target volume in the patient's body. Due to a phenomenon called Bragg's peak, most of the protons' energy is deposited within a limited distance, sparing the tissue beyond this range (and to some extent also tissue inside this range) from the effects of the radiation.

This gives PBT advantages over other forms of radiation, as this property of protons allows for conformal dose distributions to be created around even very irregular-shaped targets and for higher doses to targets surrounded by radiation-sensitive structures such as the optic chiasm or brain stem [114, 136, 148].

Chemotherapy

Apart from the abovementioned use of intracavitary bleomycin in giant cystic craniopharyngiomas, attempts at using systemic chemotherapy in the treatment of craniopharyngiomas have not been successful [120].

Biologic Therapy

The craniopharyngioma cyst fluid has elevated levels of several inflammatory cytokines like

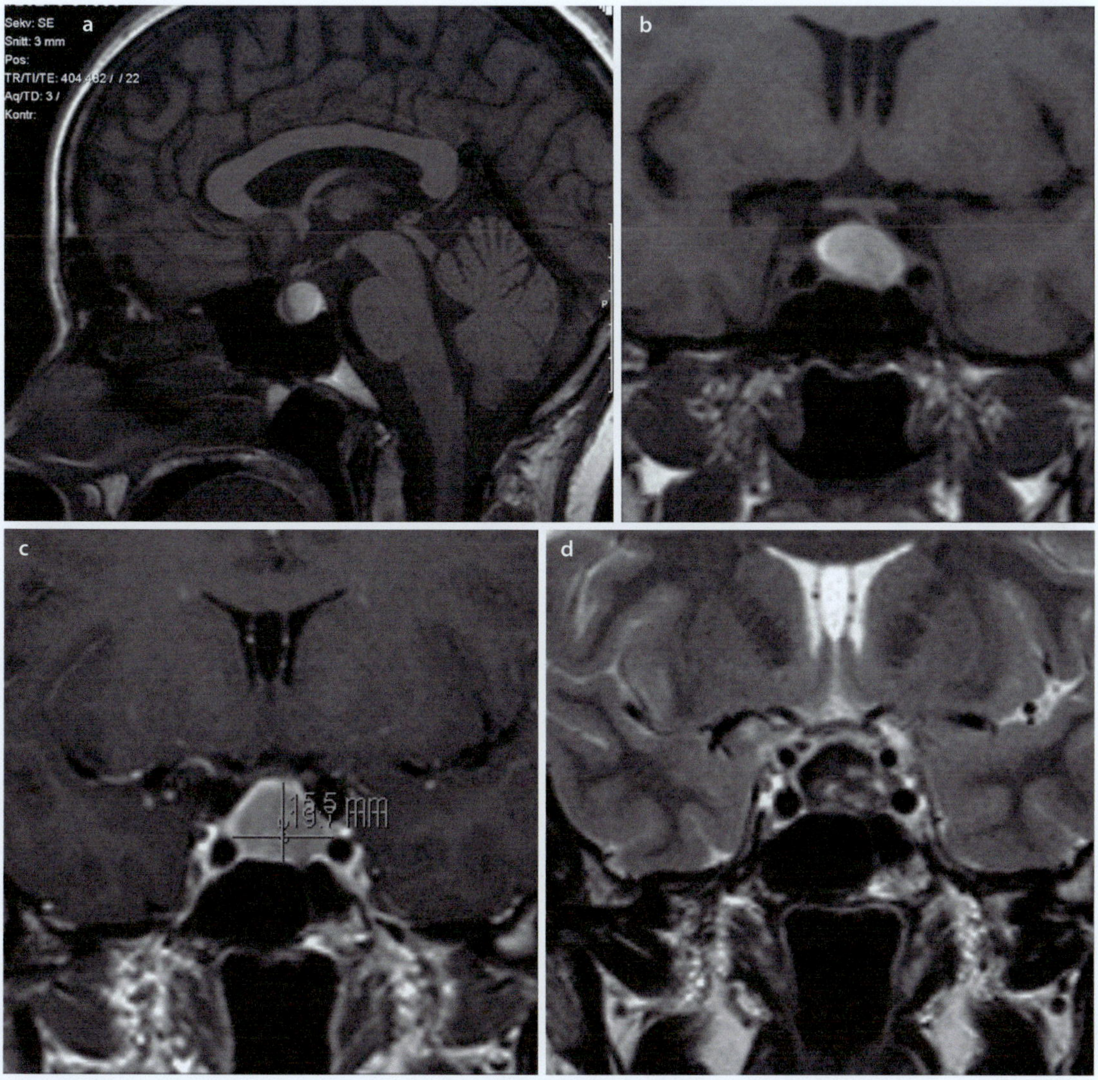

Fig. 5.58

interleukin 1alpha and tumor necrosis factor-alpha levels, and in smaller studies, interferon alpha-2a has shown a positive therapeutic effect on progressive or recurrent craniopharyngiomas [160].

5.5.4 Cases

Case 1: Transsphenoidal Approach

Hx

A 35-year-old woman presented with elevated serum prolactin and mild bitemporal deficits on Goldmann perimetry.

Dx

MR showed a 20 mm purely intrasellar craniopharyngioma, partly cystic and partly solid (Fig. 5.58).

Sx

Because of the purely intrasellar location, the patient underwent a standard transnasal, biportal, transsphenoidal complete excision of an adamantinomatous craniopharyngioma (Fig. 5.5).

F/O

She had an uneventful recovery and her visual field cuts are complete resolved, although she was left with a partial hypopituitarism postoperatively. After 6 years of follow-up, there are no signs of recurrence.

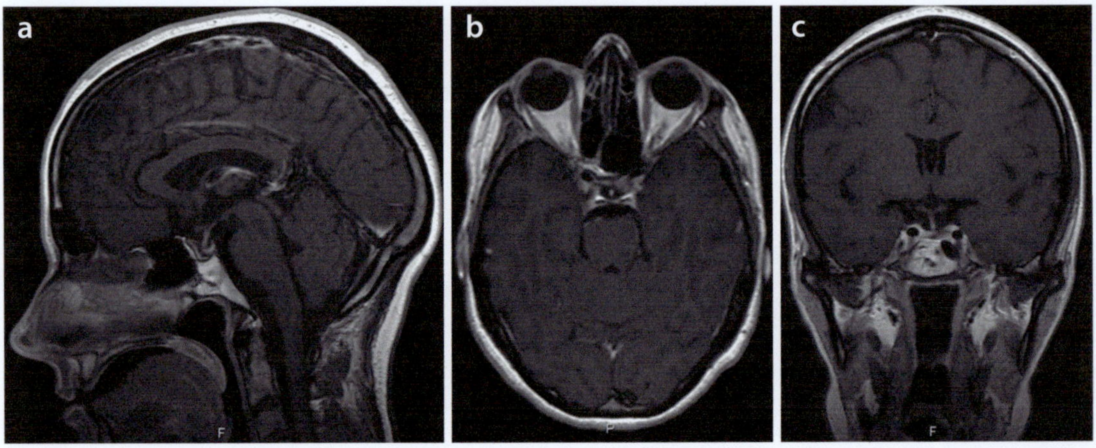

Fig. 5.59

Case 2: Interhemispheric, Transcallosal Approach

Hx

A 20-year-old woman presented with headaches, anorexia, lower-quadrant hemianopia, and short-term memory disturbances. Her endocrinological status was normal apart from an elevated serum prolactin.

Dx

MR showed a 29 mm large solid craniopharyngioma located purely in the third ventricle causing a moderate obstructive hydrocephalus (Fig. 5.60).

Sx

The patient underwent a standard right-sided unilateral frontal 3 × 4 cm craniotomy for an interhemispheric, transcallosal, transforaminal approach for this adamantinomatous craniopharyngioma. The ipsilateral fornix, optic chiasm, hypothalamus, and pituitary stalk were anatomically preserved, and we were able to obtain a complete excision of the tumor (Fig. 5.61).

F/O

She had an uneventful recovery, but she had a slight right-sided temporal visual field defect postoperatively. She had a transient DI that resolved after a few months and has a normal quality of life without medication. After 1 year of follow-up, there are no signs of recurrence.

Case 3: Extended Endonasal Approach

Hx

An 8-year-old girl presented with headaches, severe growth retardation, and panhypopituitarism without any visual pathway disturbances.

Dx

MR showed a 29 mm large craniopharyngioma, partly cystic and partly solid and calcified, extending sub- and retrochiasmatically from the sella turcica to the third ventricle causing an obstructive hydrocephalus, as well as engaging the ACOM complex and the basilar apex complex (Fig. 5.62).

Sx

Despite her young age and narrow nasal spaces, we felt that the deep sella turcica with its heavily calcified tumor would be difficult to clear out completely via a craniotomy. Hence, we opted for an extended endonasal approach and achieved a complete excision of this adamantinomatous craniopharyngioma (Fig. 5.63).

F/O

She had no new-onset visual field cuts, and her preoperative panhypopituitarism did not resolve. Regretfully, she developed a postoperative CSF leak, probably due to the insipient hydrocephalus and had to undergo implantation of a ventriculoperitoneal shunt. After 7 years of follow-up, there are no signs of recurrence.

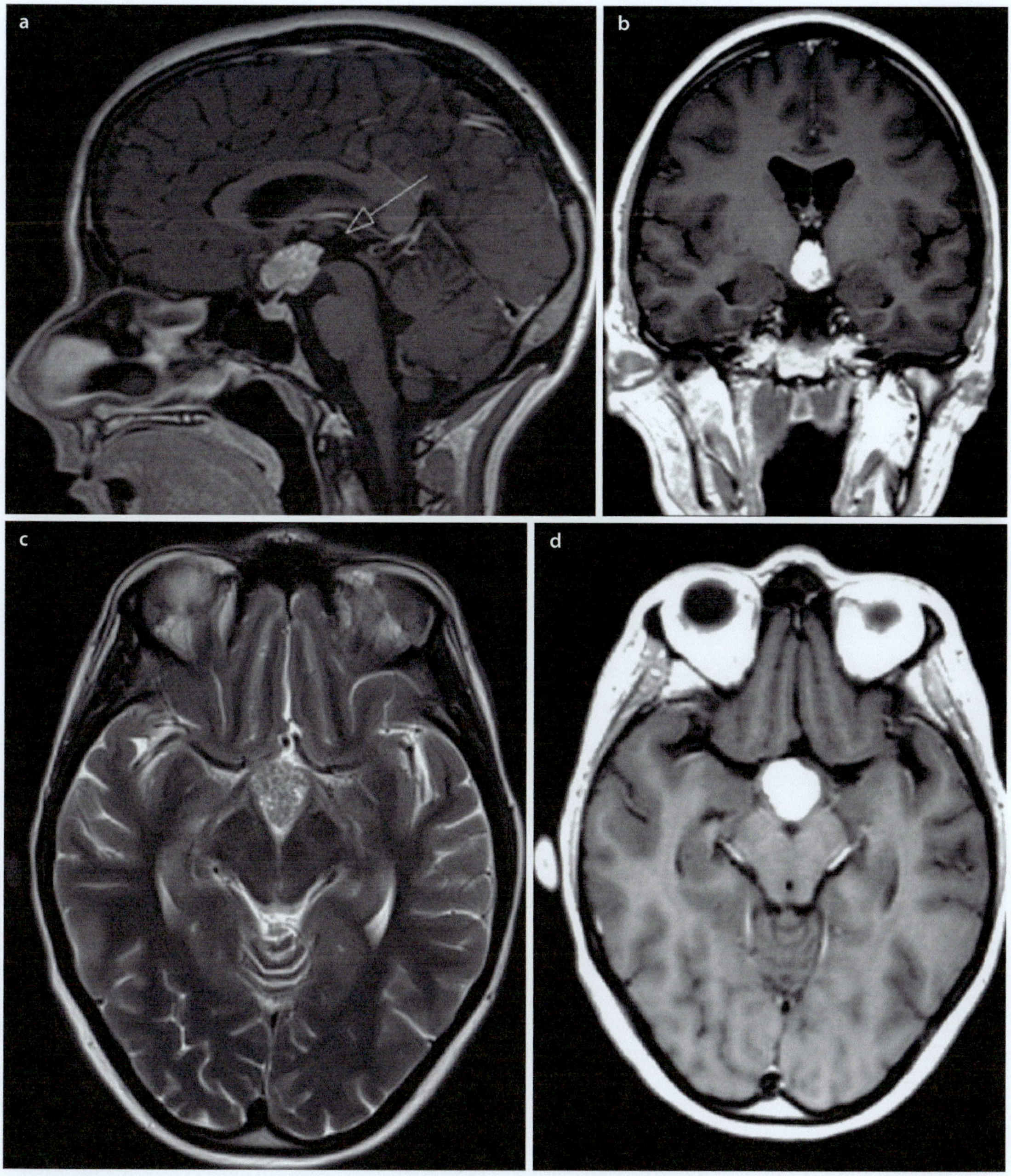

Fig. 5.60

Case 4: Unilateral Frontal Craniotomy

Hx

A 17-year-old man presented with headaches and severe visual losses. His visual acuity was 0.05 on the right side and only perception of hand motion on the left side. Endocrinological status was panhypopituitarism.

Dx

MR showed a 51 mm large craniopharyngioma extending sub- and retrochiasmatically from the sella turcica into the third ventricle causing an

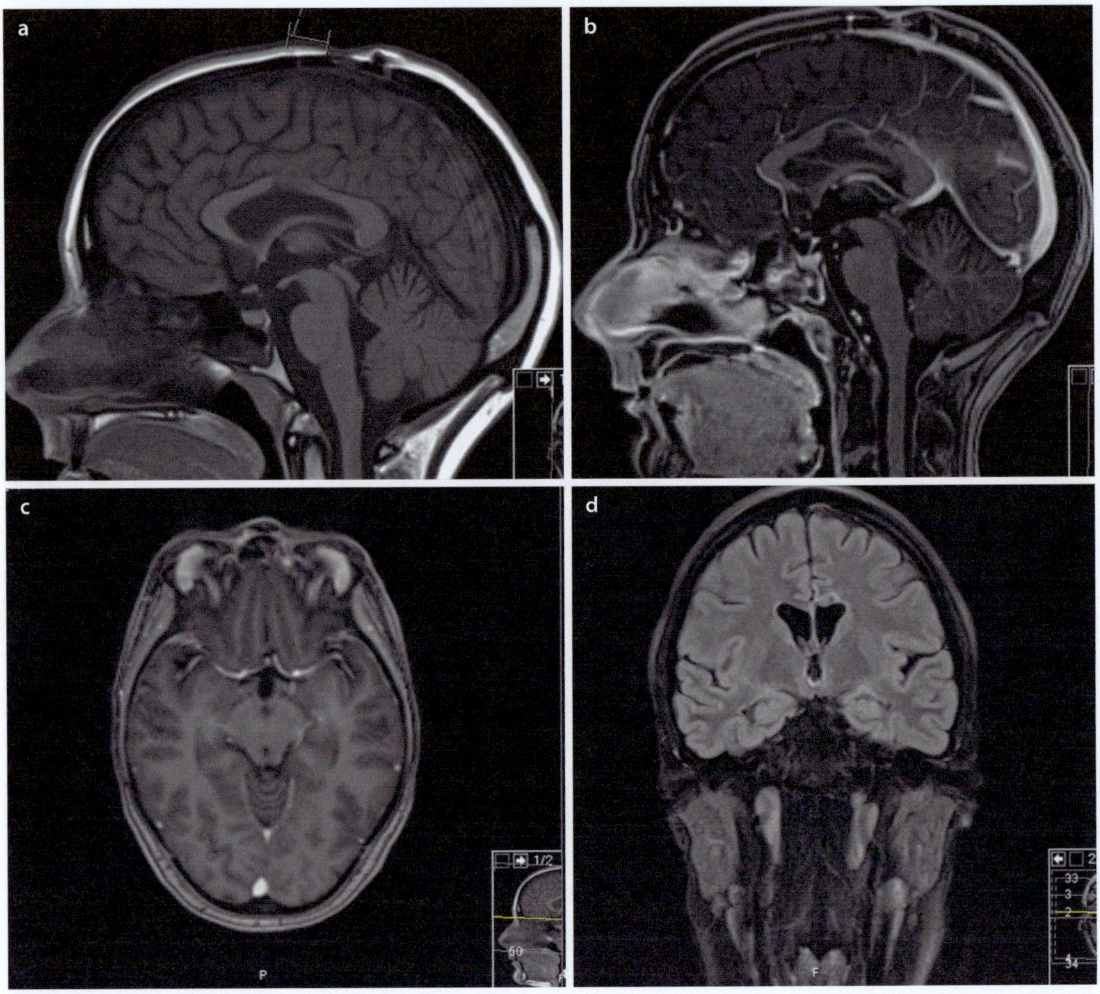

Fig. 5.61

obstructive hydrocephalus, as well as engaging the ACOM complex and the basilar apex complex (Fig. 5.64).

Sx

The patient underwent a standard right-sided unilateral craniotomy for a subfrontal translaminal approach for this adamantinomatous craniopharyngioma. Due to firm adhesions to the walls of the hypothalamus, the resection was near total, deliberately leaving a small remnant in the anterior third ventricle (Fig. 5.65).

F/O

Postoperatively the patient had panhypopituitarism and no improvement of his vision, but the hydrocephalus resolved. He underwent Gamma Knife therapy to his residual tumor shortly after surgery, but subsequently developed a cystic regrowth 6 years later (Fig. 5.66).

The patient underwent an extended endonasal approach for a complete excision (Fig. 5.67). Regretfully, he developed a postoperative CSF leak, probably due to an incipient hydrocephalus and weakening of the dura by the previous radiation therapy. He had to undergo a new craniotomy to repair this leak, but after 6 years of follow-up, there are no signs of recurrence.

Case 5: Frontotemporal Craniotomy

Hx

A 37-year-old woman presented with headaches and bitemporal hemianopia, but her endocrinological status was normal.

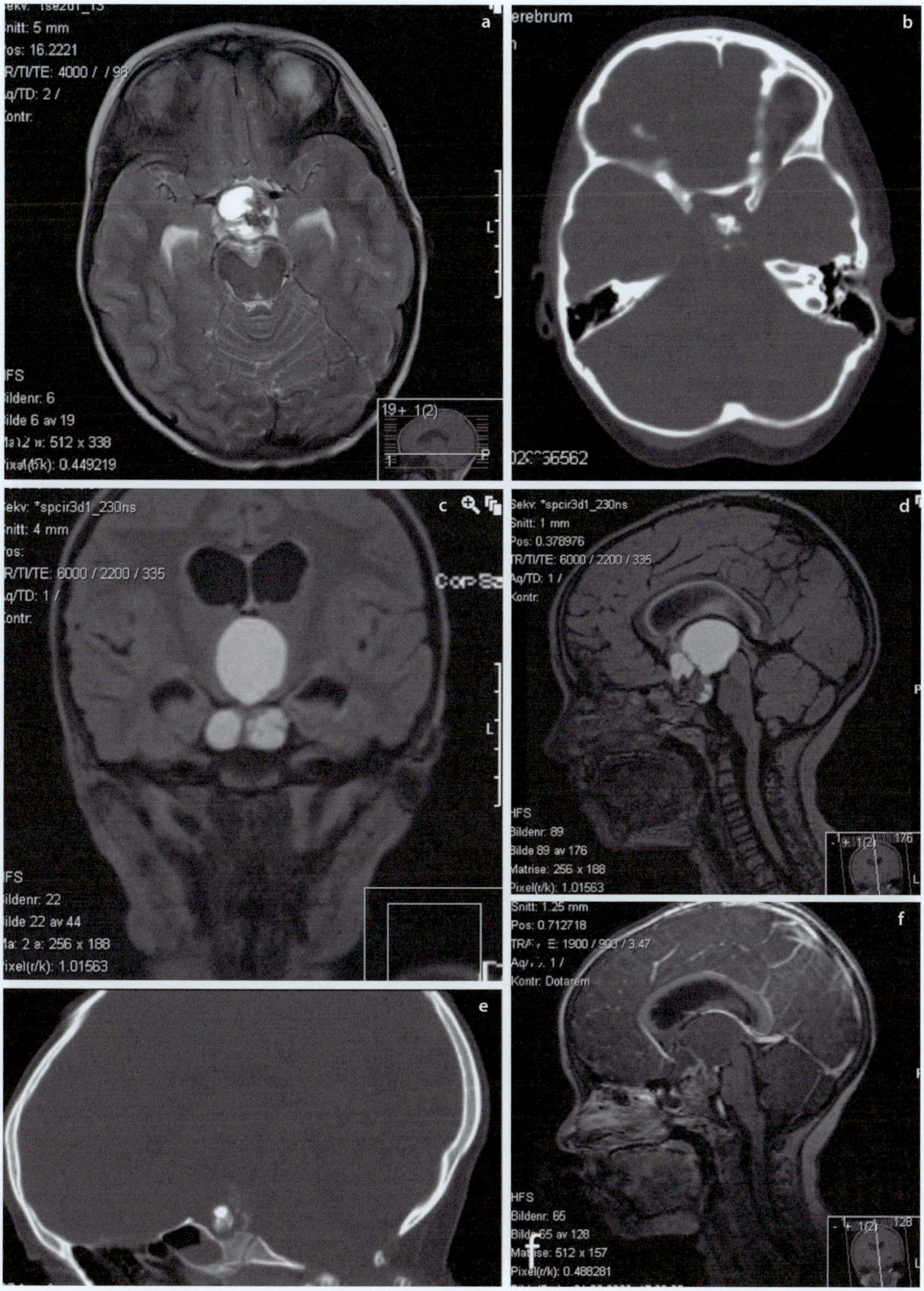
a
nitt: 5 mm
os: 16.2221
Aq/TD: 2 /
Kontr:
HFS
ildenr: 6
ilde 6 av 19
ixel(r/k): 0.449219
b
erebrum
c
ekv: *spcir3d1_230ns
nitt: 4 mm
R/TI/TE: 6000 / 2200 / 335
q/TD: 1 /
ontr:
FS
ildenr: 22
ilde 22 av 44
ixel(r/k): 1.01563
d
Sekv: *spcir3d1_230ns
Snitt: 1 mm
Pos: 0.378976
TR/TI/TE: 6000 / 2200 / 335
Aq/TD: 1 /
Kontr:
HFS
Bildenr: 89
Bilde 89 av 176
Matrise: 256 x 188
Pixel(r/k): 1.01563
e
f
Snitt: 1.25 mm
Pos: 0.712718
Kontr: Dotarem
HFS
Bildenr: 65
Pixel(r/k): 0.488281

Fig. 5.62

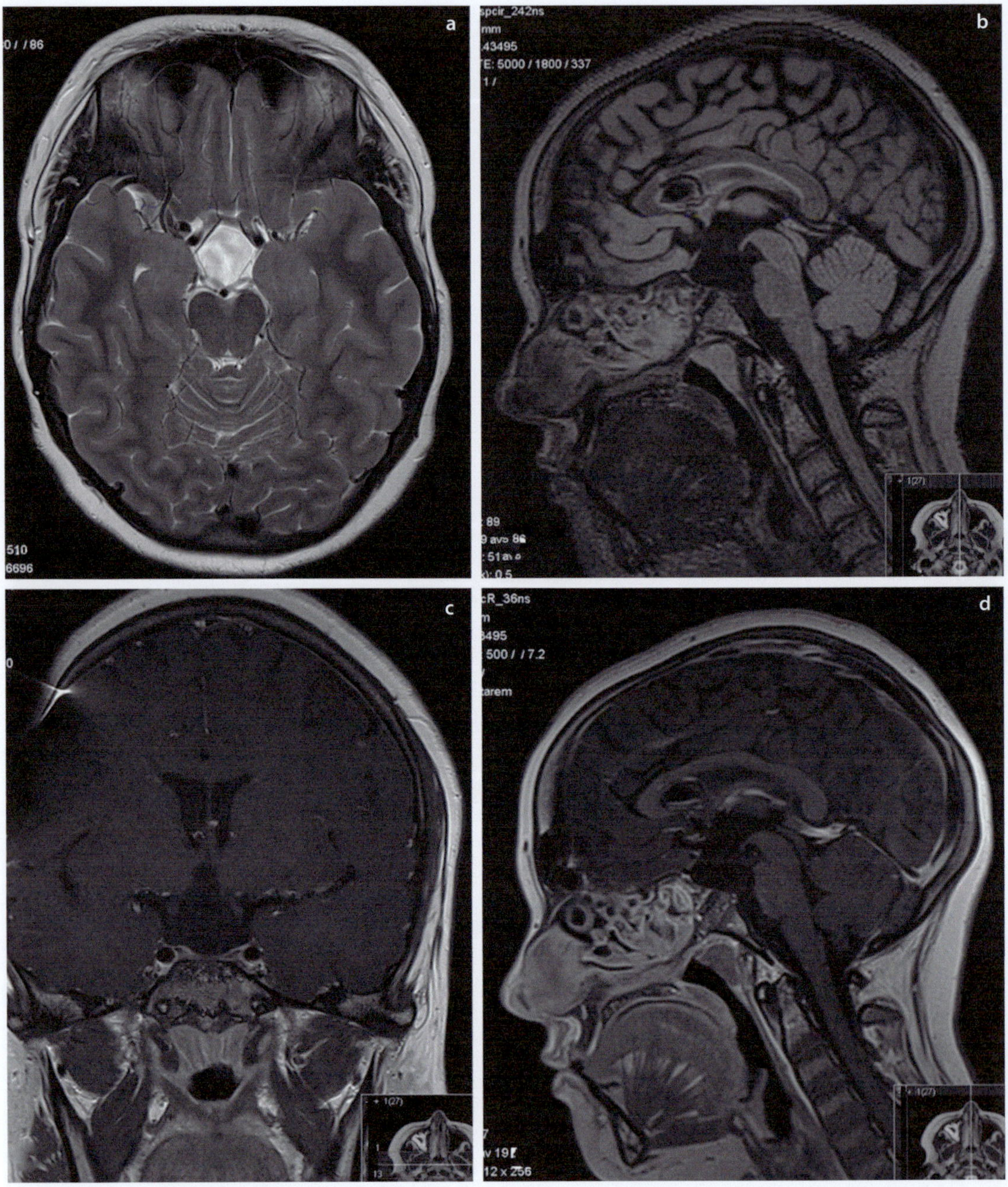

Fig. 5.63

Dx

MR showed a 20 mm large predominantly cystic supradiaphragmatic lesion on the pituitary stalk compressing the optic chiasm (Fig. 5.68).

Sx

The patient underwent a right-sided frontotemporal craniotomy for a transsylvian approach. The pituitary stalk, which was very firm and completely invaded by an adamantinomatous craniopharyngioma, was cut to obtain a complete excision of the tumor (Fig. 5.69).

F/O

She had an uneventful recovery and her visual field cuts are complete resolved, although she was

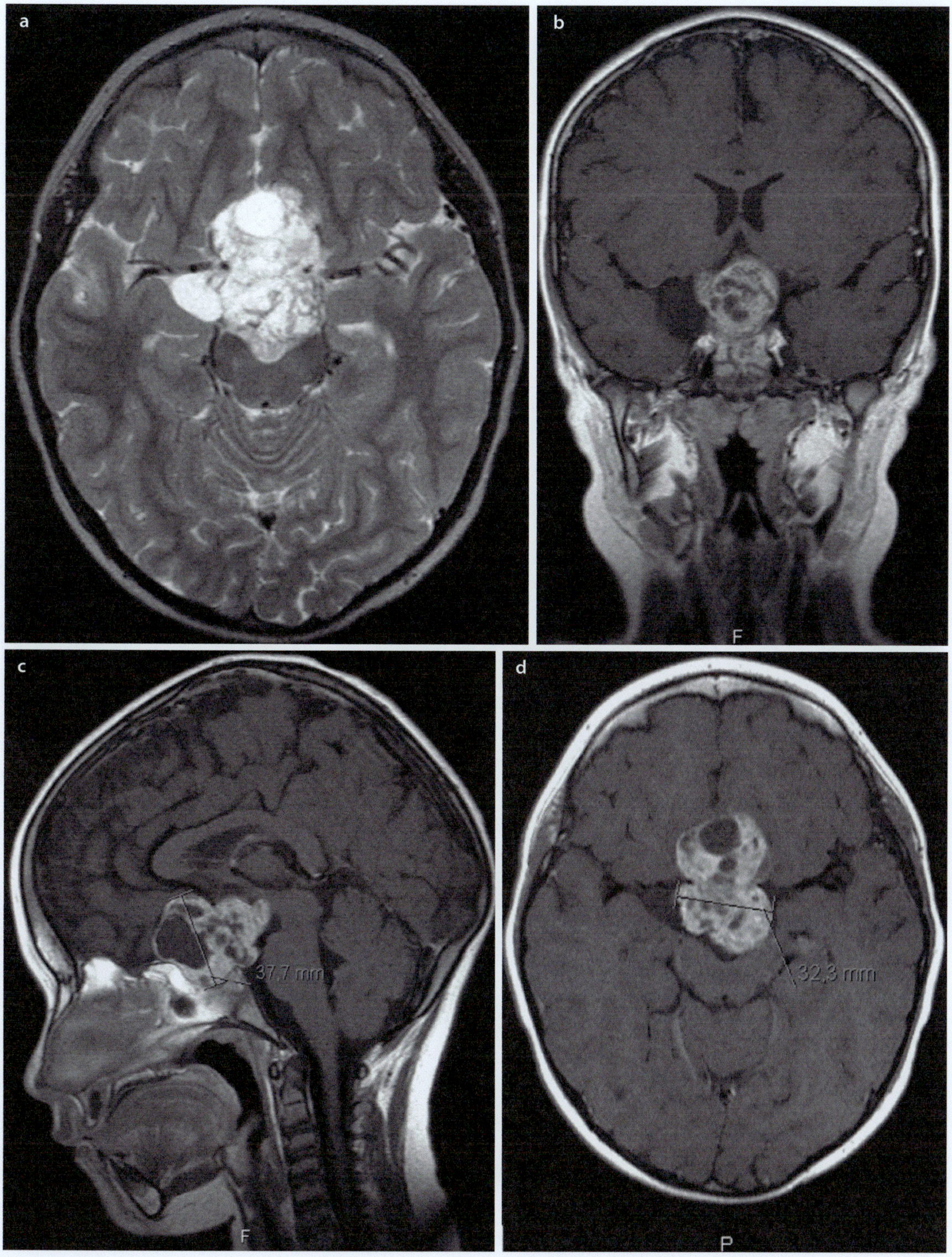

Fig. 5.64

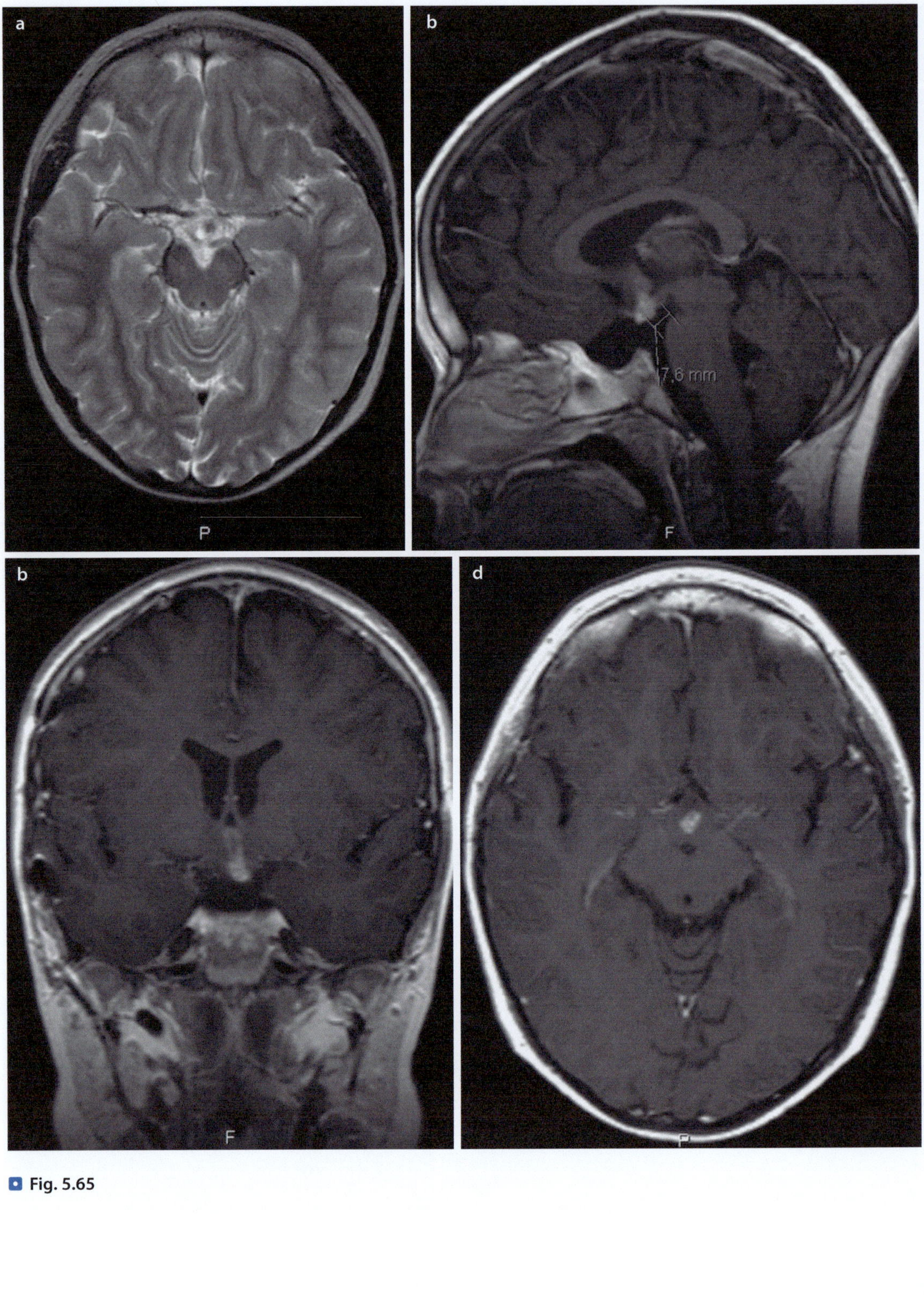

Fig. 5.65

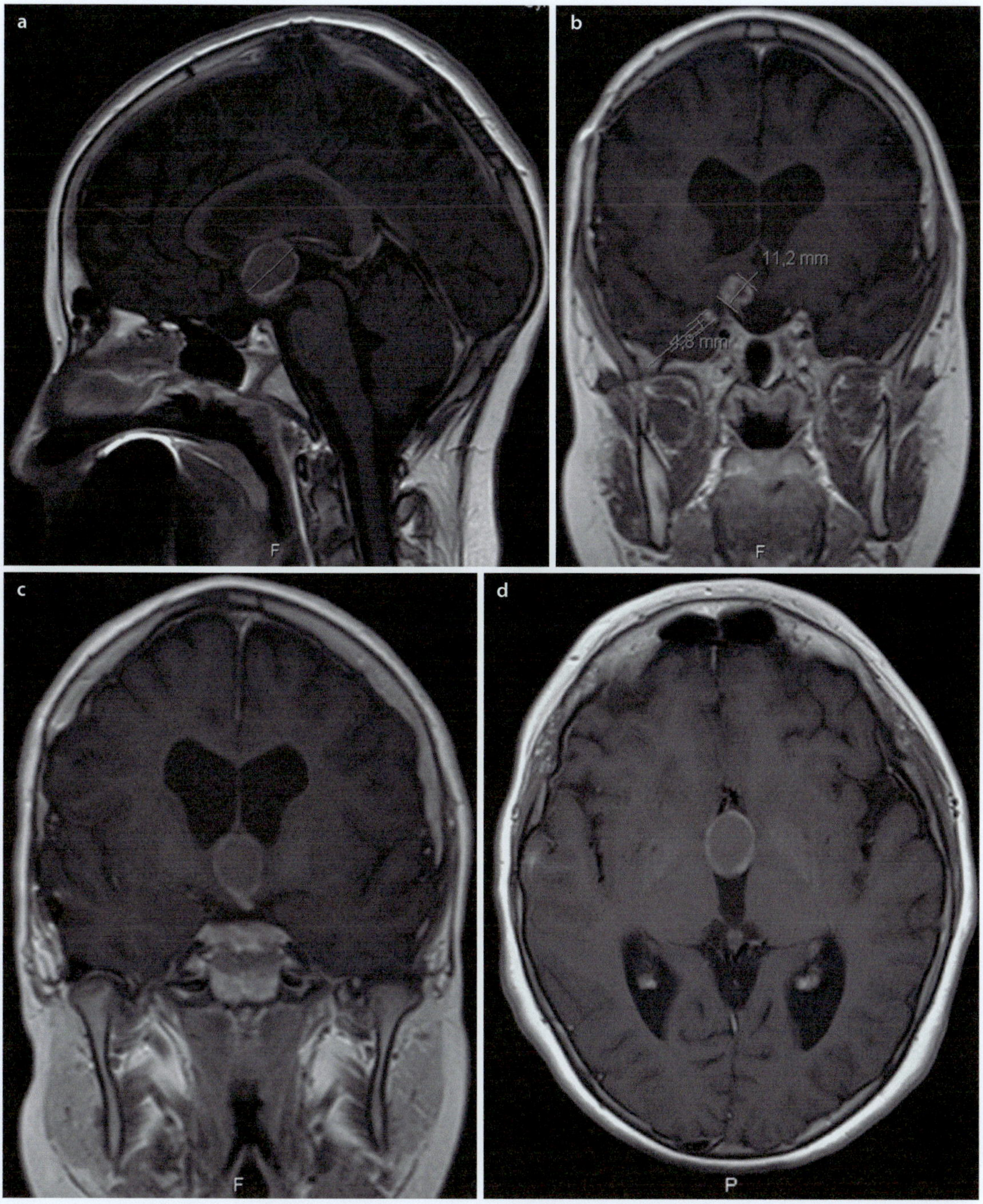

Fig. 5.66

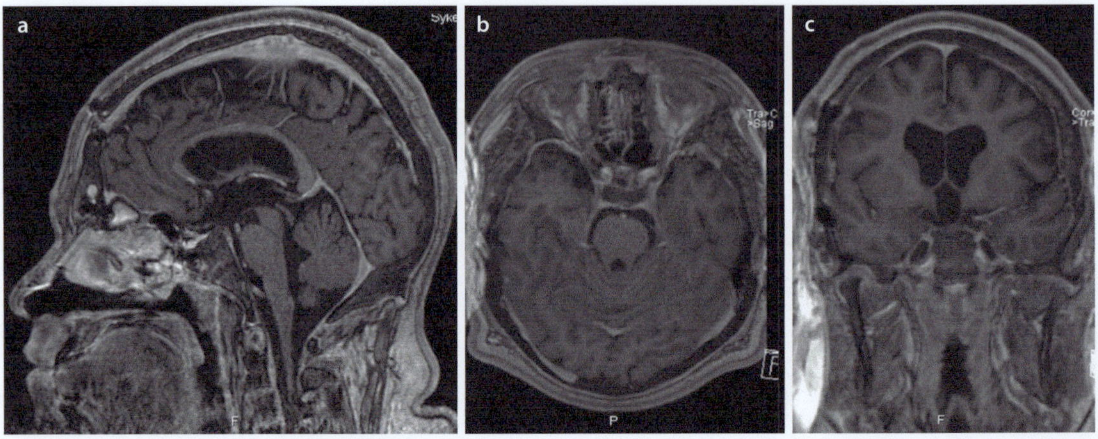

Fig. 5.67

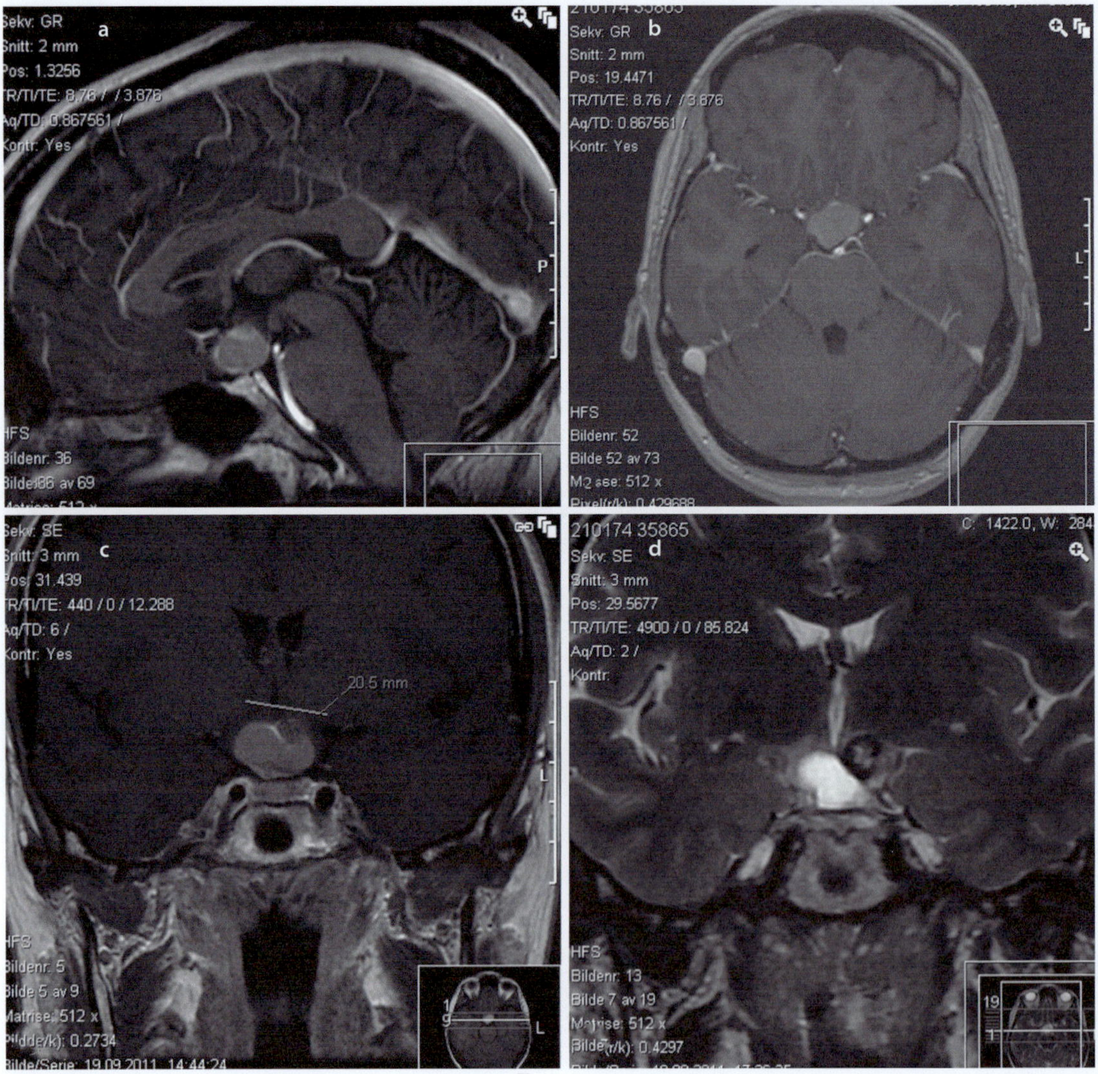

Fig. 5.68

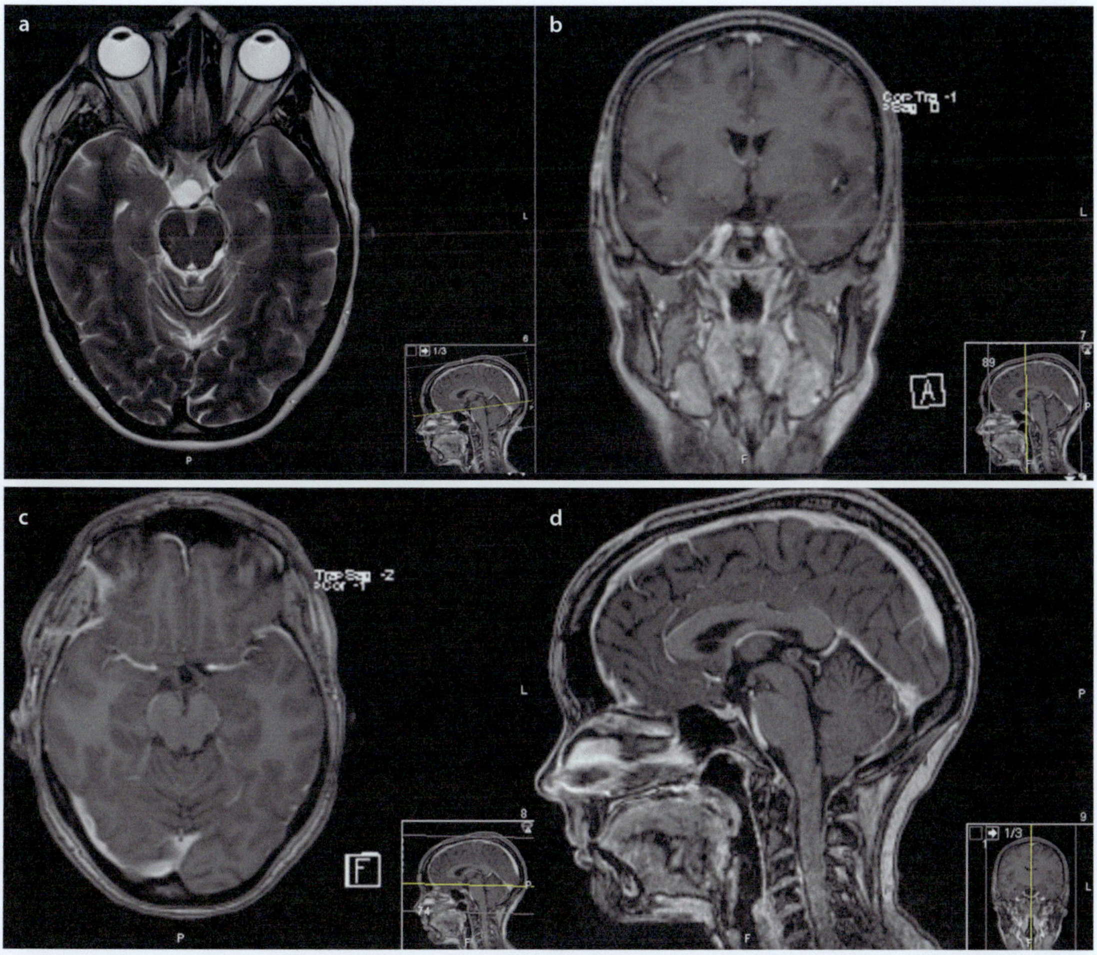

Fig. 5.69

left with a panhypopituitarism postoperatively. After 5 years of follow-up, there are no signs of recurrence.

Case 6: Mini-orbitofrontal (MOF) Craniotomy

Hx

A 42-year-old woman presented with headaches and personality changes, including memory disturbances. Her neuro-ophthalmological findings and endocrinological status were normal apart from an elevated serum prolactin.

Dx

MR showed a 32 mm large, partially cystic, and partially calcified craniopharyngioma extending sub- and retrochiasmatically from the pituitary stalk into the third ventricle, engaging the ACOM complex and causing an obstructive hydrocephalus, as well as posteriorly to engage the basilar apex complex (Fig. 5.70).

Sx

The patient underwent a right-sided mini-orbitofrontal craniotomy (MOF) for a transsylvian, translamina terminalis approach. The pituitary stalk, which was very firm and completely invaded by an adamantinomatous craniopharyngioma, was cut to obtain a complete excision of the tumor (Fig. 5.71).

F/O

She had an uneventful recovery and the hydrocephalus was completely resolved. As expected, she was left with a complete panhypopituitarism but has a normal quality of life on medication.

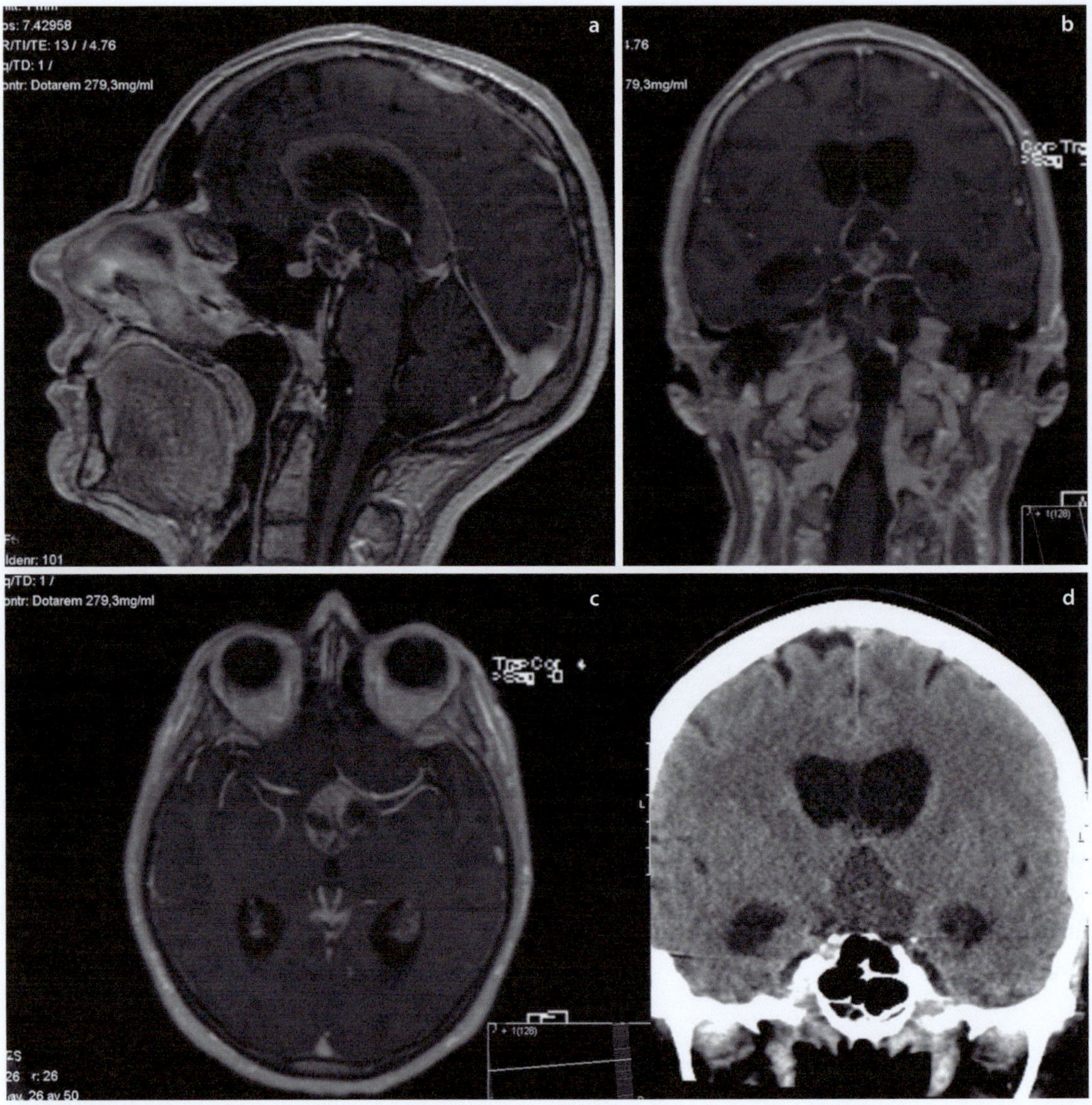

Fig. 5.70

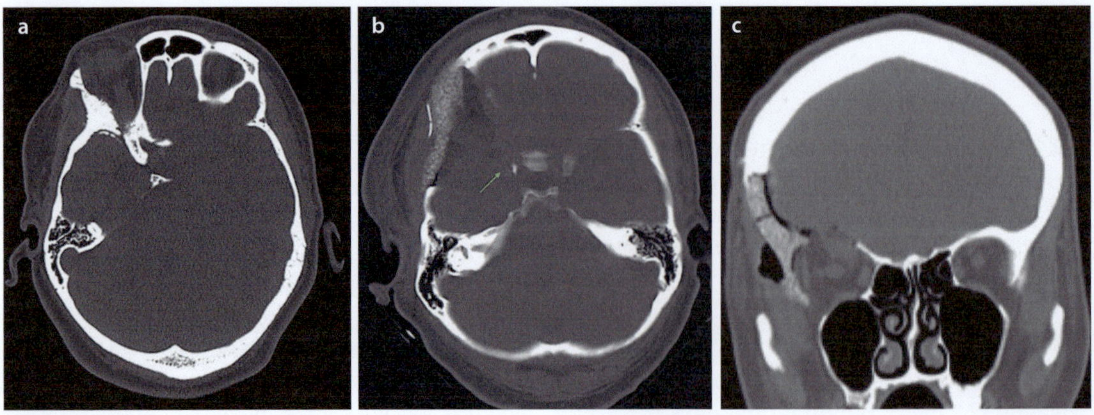

Fig. 5.71

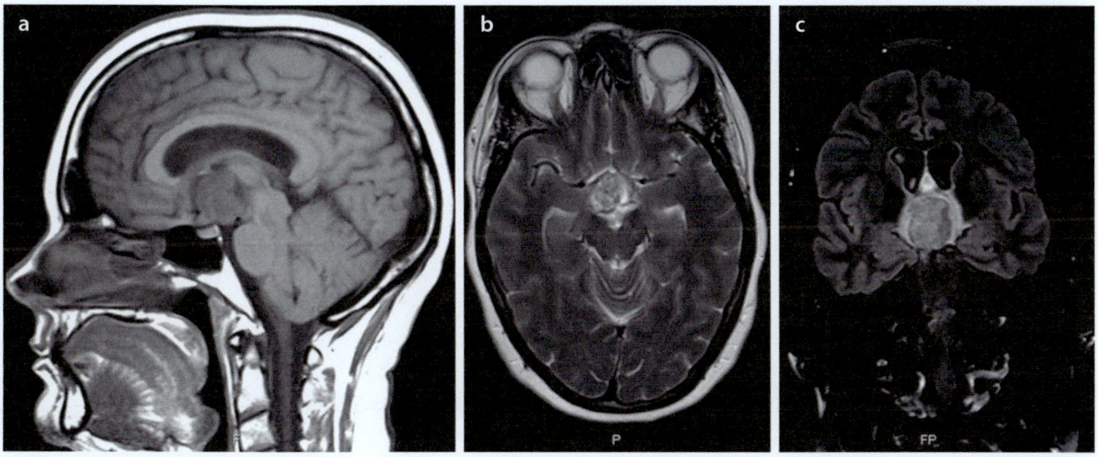

Fig. 5.72

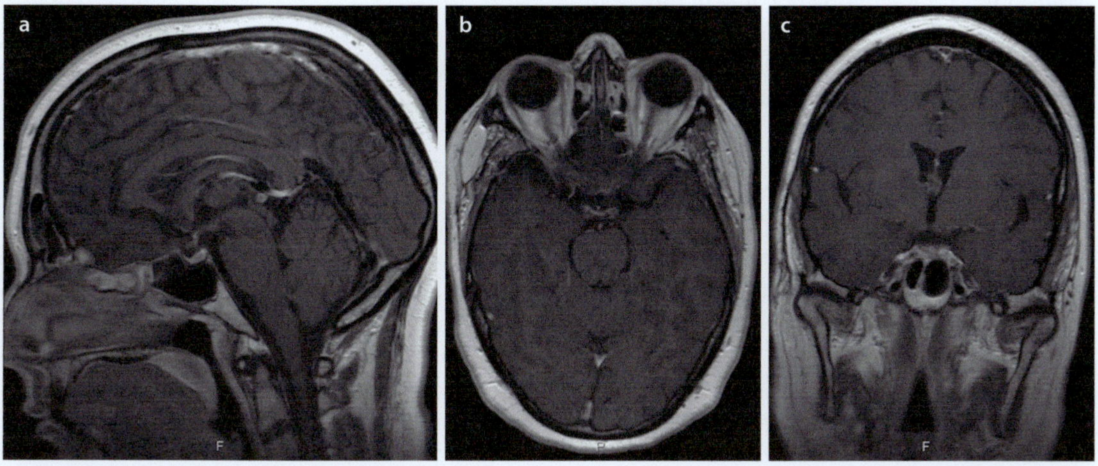

Fig. 5.73

After 3 years of follow-up, there are no signs of recurrence.

Case 7: Frontotemporal Orbitozygomatic (FTOZ) Craniotomy

Hx

A 46-year-old woman presented with headaches and bitemporal visual field deficits but normal endocrinological status.

Dx

MR showed a 29 mm large craniopharyngioma extending sub- and retrochiasmatically from the pituitary stalk into the third ventricle causing a moderate obstructive hydrocephalus, as well as engaging the ACOM complex and the basilar apex complex (Fig. 5.72).

Sx

The patient underwent a standard right-sided frontotemporal orbitozygomatic (FTOZ) craniotomy for a transsylvian and subfrontal translaminal approach for this adamantinomatous craniopharyngioma. The pituitary stalk was anatomically preserved, including its vessels. In the end, we were able to obtain a complete excision of the tumor (Fig. 5.73).

F/O

She had an uneventful recovery and her hydrocephalus was completely resolved. She had no new-onset optic pathway deficits. However, she was left with a partial hypopituitarism but has a normal quality of life on medication. After 4 years of follow-up, there are no signs of recurrence.

5.6 Epidermoid and Dermoid Tumors

G. Inoue and T. Fukushima

Surgery is the only effective treatment for intracranial epidermoids and dermoids at present. Even though they are encapsulated benign tumors, the size, the ability to spread out through cisterns, and the adherence to surrounding neurovascular structures make surgery challenging. With proper approach, instrumentation, and experienced hands, radical resection is possible in most cases. Radical total resection, including the capsule, should always be the goal for every case, to lower not only recurrence but complications as well.

5.6.1 General Information

Dermoid and epidermoid tumors are rare, usually benign, slow-growing tumors, categorized together due to their pathological background. They are both consequences of ectopic inclusion of ectoblasts, which are committed to cutaneous decent. Inclusion is believed to occur between weeks 3 and 5 of gestation when the medullary tube is forming from the neural groove McLendon et al [193]. The definitive histological difference between dermoid and epidermoid tumors is the existence of dermal elements within the capsule. Together, epidermoids and dermoids comprise 0.5–1.8% of all intracranial tumors. Epidermoids and dermoids tend to present from early to mid-ages of life and can occur anywhere within the cranium.

Epidermoid tumors can also occur after trauma [176]. Iatrogenic causes such as multiple lumbar punctures or an incidental formation of a skin pocket by suturing may also result in epidermoid tumor. The incidence of lumbosacral region epidermoids caused by a lumbar puncture has greatly decreased by insertion of a stilet to close the hollow barrel when inserting the puncture needle [199]. Since both of the tumors are composed of soft and malleable keratin, slowly accumulating within the docile capsule wall, it expands by insinuating into any available space, such as subarachnoid and cisternal spaces, often resulting in the tumor to grow to large sizes before intolerable symptoms develop and diagnosis occurs.

Dermoid Tumors

Dermoid tumors are rare, benign, congenital lesions considered to comprise approximately 0.04–0.6% of intracranial tumors. There is no consistency in the sex predominance. The dermoid tumor contains both dermal and epidermal elements such as keratin, hair, and hair follicles, as well as apocrine, sebaceous, or sweat glands. Less differentiation of epithelial cells may be observed in dermoid tumors compared to epidermoid tumors. Generally, they are well-defined, opaque, oval, or rounded masses in a variety of sizes. When there is persistence of the cutaneous tract with the overlying skin, a communicating dermal sinus may develop [196]. The lining of the capsule wall is simple squamous epithelium supported by collagen. The thickness of the wall varies with papillary projections. In the thicker parts, the lining is supplemented by the dermis containing hair follicles and sebaceous glands. Plaque of calcification may be found in the wall. The tumor often contains thick, foul smelling, yellow-brown liquid or mucoid (Fig. 5.74) as a result of the secretion of sebaceous glands and desquamated epithelium. Entangled hairs (Fig. 5.75) and less frequently teeth are found within. The bone, cartilage, and fat are occasionally found owing to the secondary induction of the primitive mesenchymal cells.

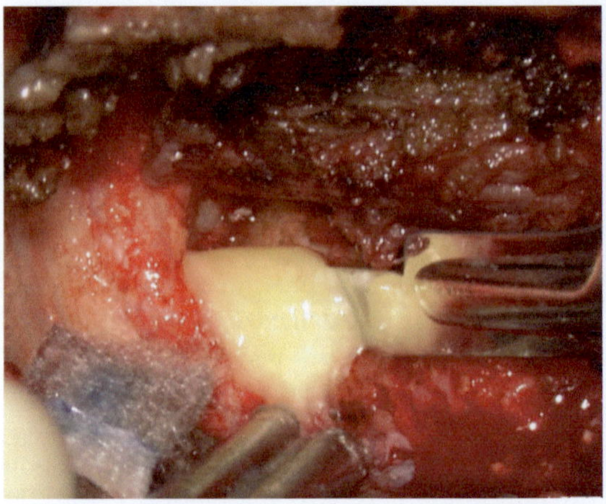

Fig. 5.74 Thick foul smelling *yellow-brown* liquid or mucoid bursting out after incising the dermoid capsule

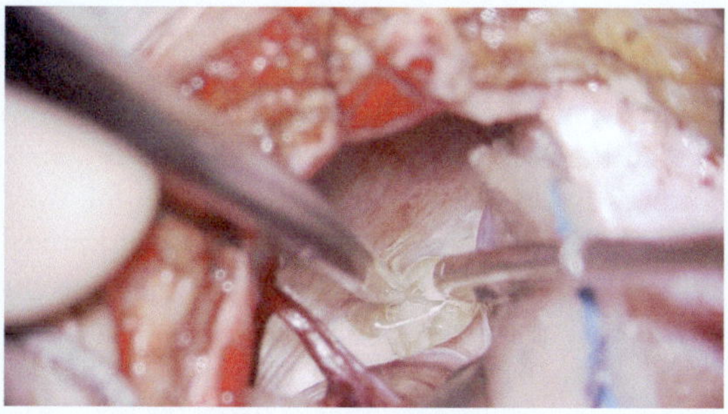

Fig. 5.75 Hair seen inside the dermoid tumor

Epidermoid Tumors

Epidermoid tumors are reported to constitute 0.5–1.5% of all intracranial tumors about three times more frequent than dermoids. Epidermoids are benign tumors, which grow slowly but most likely present in large sizes. Histopathologically, the capsule of the epidermoid tumors is circumscribed with a smooth simple stratified squamous epithelium supported by an outer layer of collagenous tissue. Calcification may be found in the capsule. Within the capsule, white shinny soft material is a result of a progressive desquamation and breakdown of keratin from the epithelial lining, which gained the name of «pearly tumor» by Cruveilhier [173] (Fig. 5.76). The contents could also present as viscid, brown, or gray, considered to be the result of a prior hemorrhage.

Epidermoids can occur anywhere in the cranium, but they prefer the cerebellopontine (CP) angle and suprasellar region. This lateral placement of epidermoids is explained by the displacements occurring during the closing of the otic and optic vesicles [177].

5.6.2 Clinical Signs and Symptoms

Dermoid Tumors

Dermoid tumors are congenital and could theoretically present at any age of life; however, they are most frequently diagnosed in the first and second decades of life [180]. Two possible explanations for this are as follows: first, dermoid tumors have thicker capsule walls, which grow more round or oval pushing away the normal structures, and, second, the oily components within the capsule cause irritation to the adjacent structures than keratin alone, as in the case of epidermoid tumor [164].

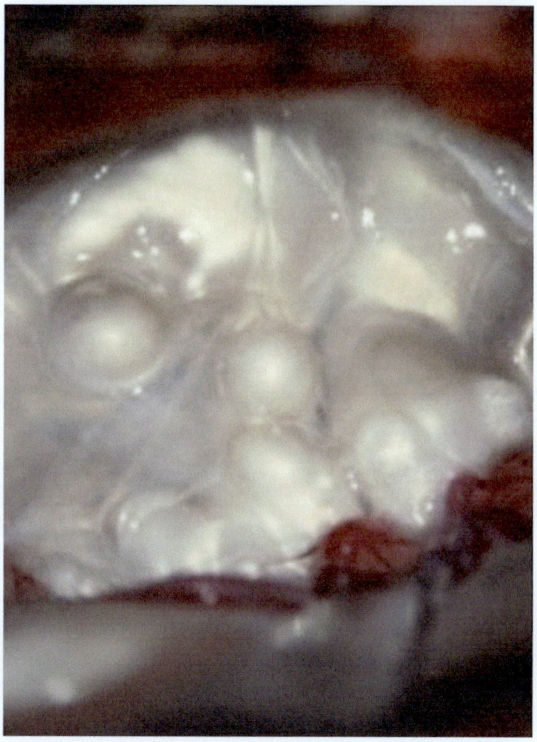

Fig. 5.76 Shiny epidermoid tumor

The average duration of symptoms for dermoids is reported to be 8.5 years [186], which is long compared to other intracranial tumors but slightly shorter than that of epidermoids. Symptoms vary with the location of the tumor and the surrounding neurovascular structures. It could present as local neural deficits or headache due to the mass effect or hydrocephalus, caused by obstruction of the cerebral spinal fluid pathways. Aseptic (chemical) meningitis is another distinctive feature, which leads to diagnosis of dermoid tumors. Spillage of the contents, especially cholesterol, into the cerebrospinal space causes excitement with a granulomatous form of meningitis most likely accompanied by a foreign body giant cell reaction.

The percentage of distribution is not declared, but midline in the posterior fossa is the favored site, involving the vermis and the adjacent meninges [178]. Other locations for intracranial dermoids are the orbit, cavernous sinus, CP angle [175], lateral ventricle [208], and anterior fontanel [183]. Suspected dermoids in the pineal region are rare, often part of germinomas or teratomas [184]. Intraparenchymal dermoids are rarely reported [168].

Nearly half of midline dermoids in infancy and childhood are associated with midline fusion defects such as Chiari malformation, Klippel–Feil syndrome [202], spina bifida, failure of vertebral segmentation, cleft palate, etc. Twenty-five percent of cases are connected by a congenital sinus or stalk to the intracranial structures or to the spinal canal.

Epidermoid Tumors

Epidermoids tend to be present and are diagnosed later than dermoids. The age of diagnosis ranges from birth up to 80s and even during autopsy but is most frequently seen in the 30s and 40s. There is no consistency in sex predominance, but the 334 case series of the senior author (TF) showed 1:2 female predominance with support of few other reports (◘ Fig. 5.77).

It is well known that epidermoids occur in the CP angle. The distribution of intracranial epidermoids was reported by Mahoney in 1936 [193]. It is reported to consist in 40–70% of all intracranial epidermoids and approximately 6% of all CP angle tumors. Other rather common locations are parasellar [204], middle fossa or intracavernous sinus, pineal region, intraosseous [172], and fourth ventricle [201]. Epidermoids are also seen more rarely in the dorsal vermis, interhemispheric fissure [163], frontal base, convexity, orbit, and third ventricle [185]. The distribution of epidermoid tumor within the cranium from the authors' experience is shown in ◘ Fig. 5.78. Tumors in the CP angle comprise 78%, followed by parasellar 5%, cavernous sinus 4%, and pineal region 4% (◘ Fig. 5.79). Other minor locations included intraosseous 3% (petrous and occipital bone), fourth ventricle 2% (◘ Fig. 5.80), dorsal vermis 1%, interhemispheric 0.6% (◘ Fig. 5.81), and frontal base 0.3%. In reports, the distribution of epidermoids, including large numbers of cases, varies; therefore, it is very difficult to derive a consistent result. This is possibly due to the infiltrating nature of the tumor which makes the decision of the location somewhat inconsistent. For example, the parasellar group often extends into the middle fossa; these tumors are usually embedded in the temporal lobe and often involve the temporal horn of the lateral ventricle. Also, paratrigeminal extradural epidermoids may be associated with the cavernous sinus or can cause erosion of the apex of the petrous bone [165] and may be related to those more obviously confined to that bone [194]. Or this is demonstrated in cases where the tumor spreads across the middle fossa and the posterior fossa via a narrow neck through Meckel's cave forming a dumbbell-shaped tumor.

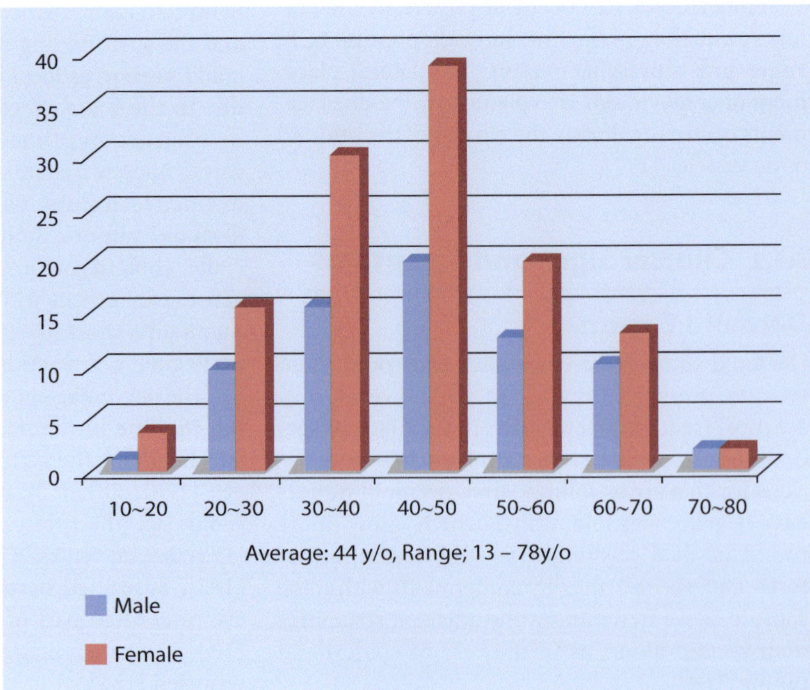

◘ **Fig. 5.77** Age and sex distribution of epidermoid tumor. Peek seen in the 30s and 40s. In all age distributions, female is dominant

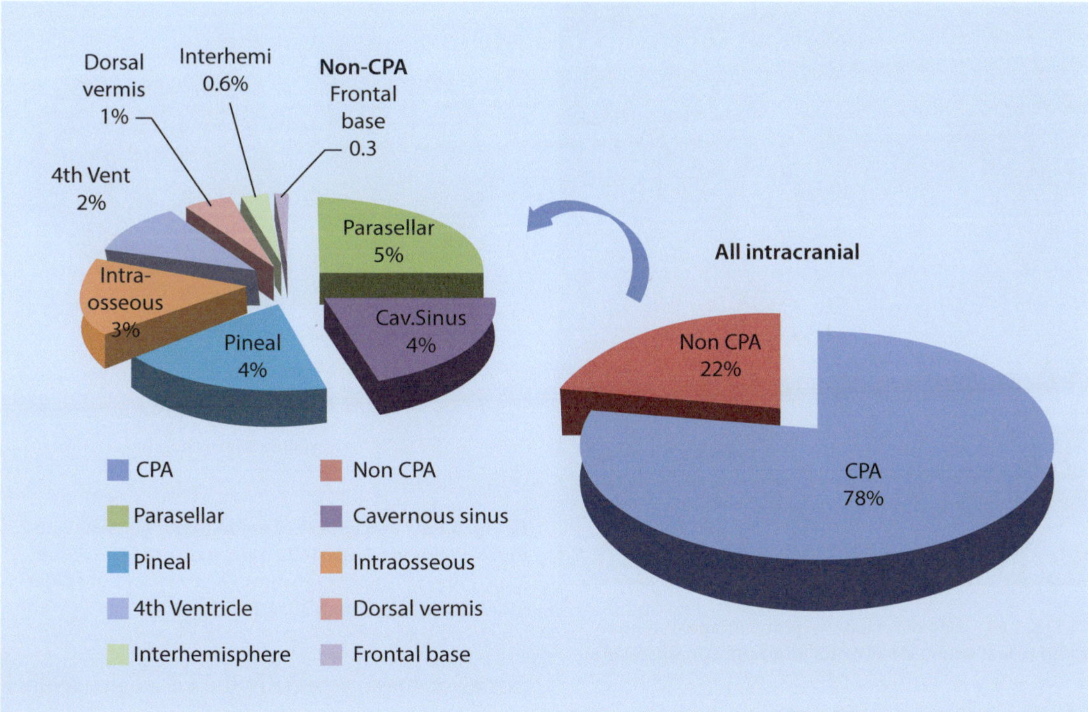

Fig. 5.78 Distribution of epidermoids

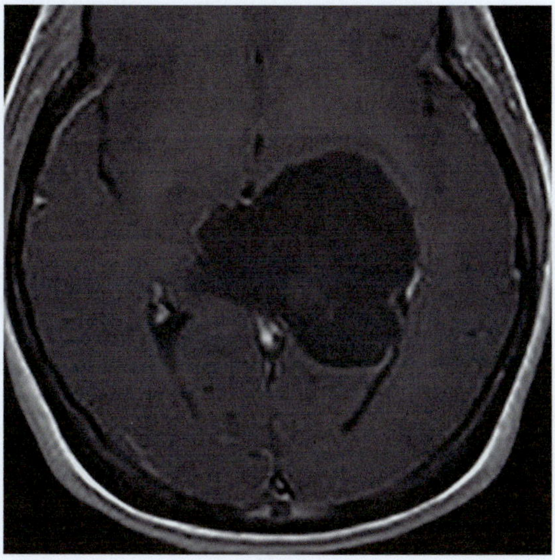

Fig. 5.79 MRI T1-weighted image after induction of contrast agent of giant epidermoid at pineal region. No enhancement seen

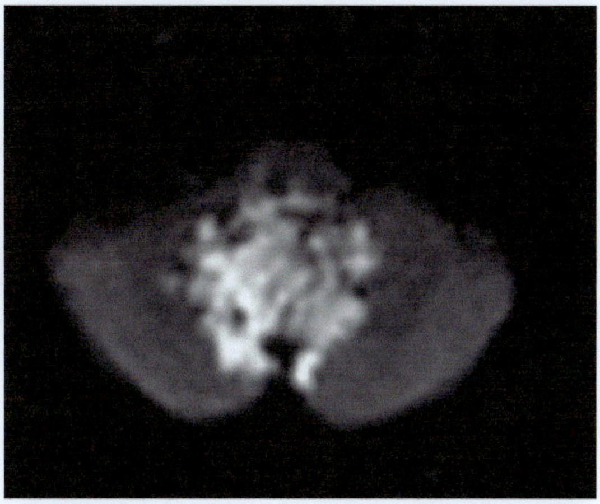

Fig. 5.80 MRI diffusion-weighted image of epidermoid tumor in fourth ventricle

Purely parenchymal epidermoids are considered very rare, with Chandler et al.'s [170] report of 5.8% being the highest. We have experienced one case of intraparenchymal epidermoid at the occipital lobe out of 334 cases (Fig. 5.82).

In terms of sizes, nearly 80% of the cases were over 30 mm in their largest diameter (Fig. 5.83). Seventy five percent of the epidermoids situated in the CP angle demonstrated involvement of more than one set of neurovascular structures. Also, 46% of CP angle tumors showed extension supratentorially or to the contralateral side. Tumors in the pineal region, forth ventricle, and dorsal vermis tended to be diagnosed over 40 mm. In

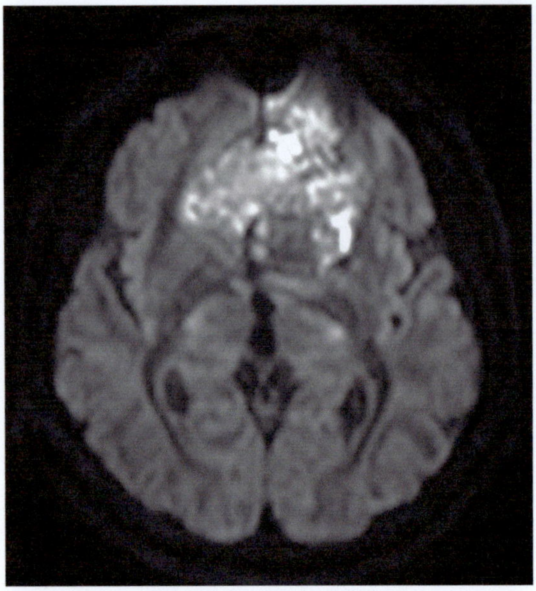

Fig. 5.81 MRI diffusion-weighted image of epidermoid tumor situated in frontal interhemispheric fissure

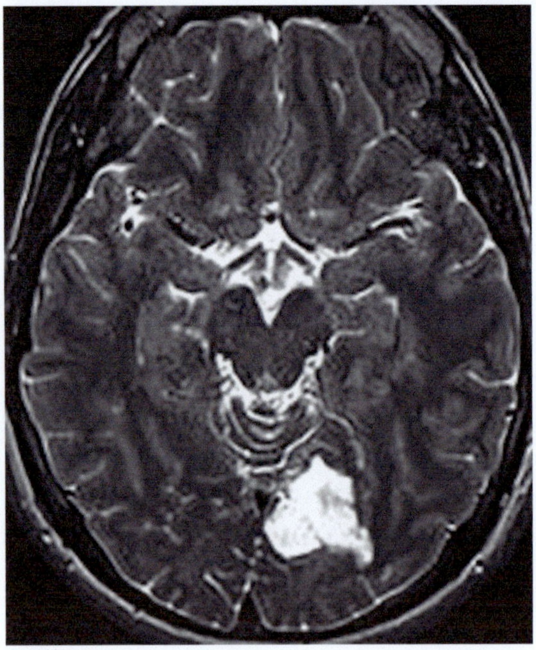

Fig. 5.82 T2-weighted MRI image of an intraparenchymal epidermoid tumor in left occipital lobe

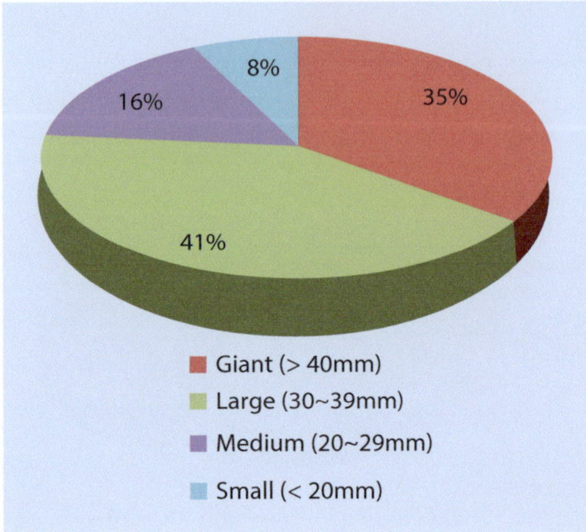

Fig. 5.83 Percentage of epidermoids classified into four size groups. Small (<20 mm), medium (20 ~ 29 mm), large (30 ~ 39), giant (>40 mm). Over 75% of the epidermoids were larger than 30 mm

contrast, cavernous sinus lesions tend to be found and treated at a smaller size.

Presenting symptoms for epidermoid tumors obviously rely on the location. Overall, percentages of symptoms seen in epidermoid tumors are shown in Fig. 5.84. Due to the preference to the posterior fossa, especially the CP angle, cerebellar symptoms such as unsteadiness and ataxia are the most common symptoms. For tumors in the CP angle, trigeminal neuralgia (42%) is the most common, followed by cerebellar symptoms (29%) and hearing loss (26%). Headache was only seen in 19% of patients with CPA epidermoid tumors despite the high percentage of large tumors. Symptoms of cranial nerve compression including diplopia (23%), dysphagia (8%), and facial nerve palsy (5%) are also observed preoperatively (Fig. 5.85). In the early stages of tumor growth, the tumor tends to enclose, rather than displace, the neural structures, due to its soft nature. This results in symptoms produced by irritation rather than dysfunction. Only 7% of patients present with seizures, presumably from supratentorial extension and irritation of the medial temporal lobe. Stroke as a presenting feature of CPA epidermoid is a rare phenomenon and appears related to stretching of the basilar artery [207]. The rate of repeated bouts of aseptic meningitis reported previously by other authors [162] seems to be decreasing over a period of time and is seen in only 1%. The mean duration of symptoms at the time of surgery is about 10 years with the longest duration being up to 40 years. Long duration symptoms are often mild and could wax, wane, and even remiss for a long time before any intervention to the tumor is performed. It is noteworthy that these slow-growing lesions tend

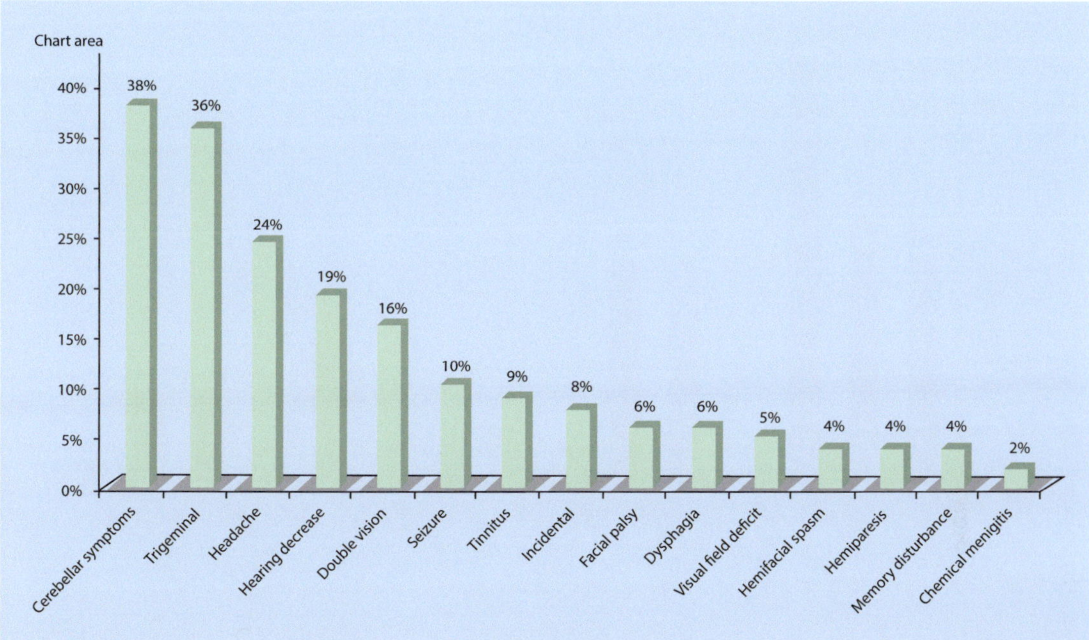

Fig. 5.84 Overall presenting symptoms for epidermoid tumors

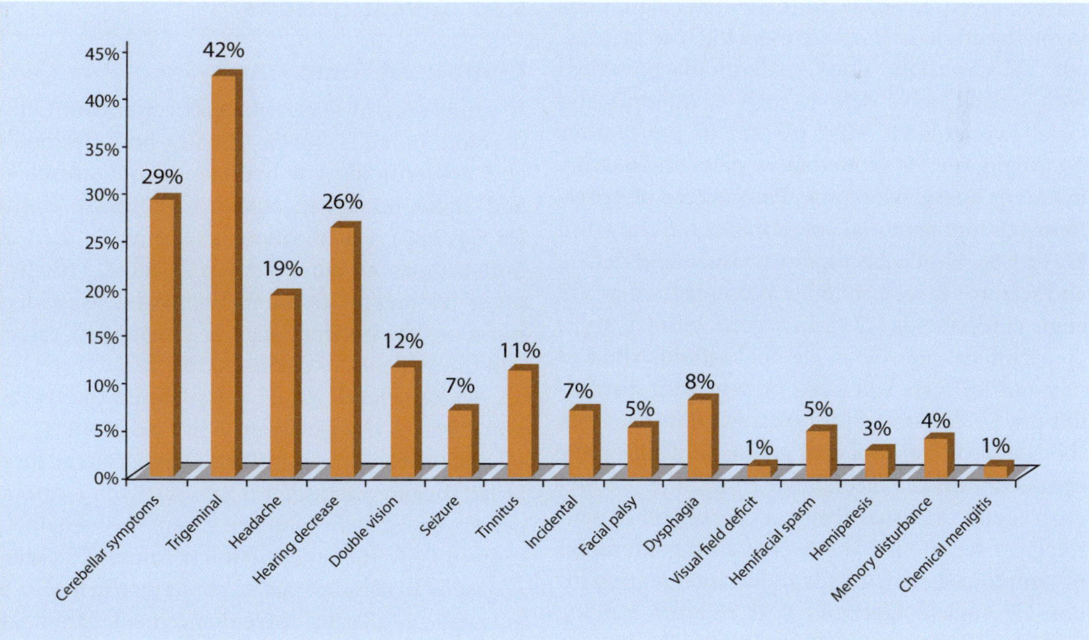

Fig. 5.85 Presenting symptoms of CP angle epidermoid tumors

to present with symptoms of nerve irritation such as trigeminal neuralgia and hemifacial spasm rather than facial numbness and weakness, suggesting that the pathology affects the nerve root in a manner similar to vascular compression.

On the other hand, the most common symptom for non-CP angle epidermoids is headache, which is seen in approximately 45% of cases; however, this is not the case when the tumor is located in more isolated spaces such as the cavernous sinus, dorsal

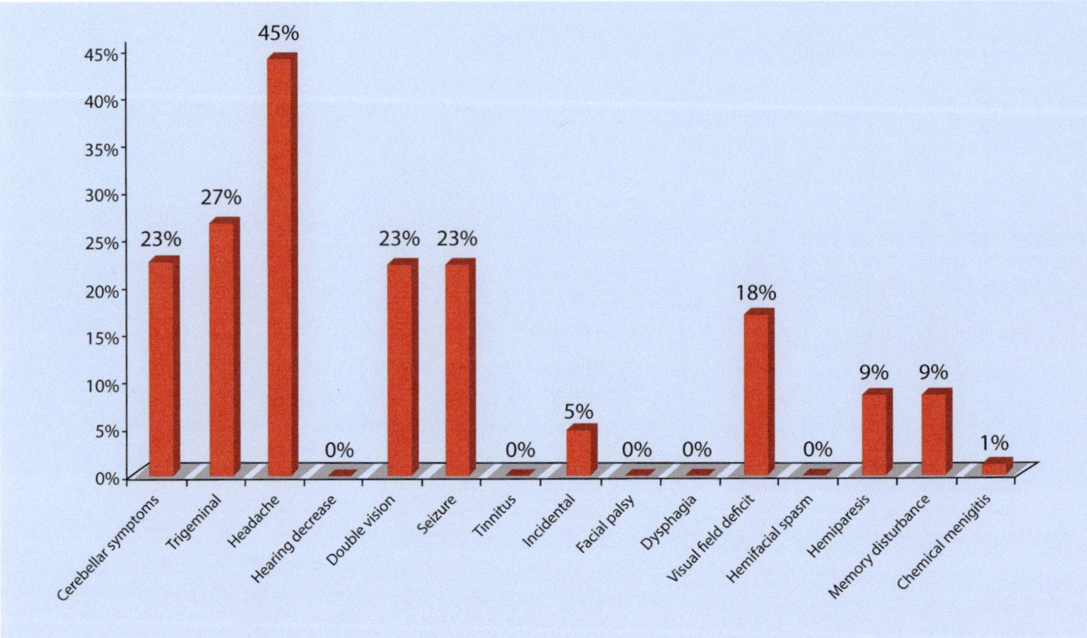

Fig. 5.86 Presenting symptoms of supratentorial epidermoid tumors

vermis, or intraosseous. In these areas, symptoms involving cranial nerves are more likely to be present. All cavernous sinus epidermoids presented with cranial nerve deficits such as diplopia and facial hypoesthesia. Fifty percent of the petrous bone epidermoids showed facial palsy and hearing loss as primary symptoms. Percentages of symptoms for supratentorial epidermoids are shown in Fig. 5.86. Headache, diplopia, visual field deficit, and seizure are seen at higher percentages than CP angle epidermoids [171]. In accord with CP angle epidermoids, non-CP angle epidermoids situated in posterior fossa will often present with disequilibrium [198]. Orbital tumors are said to rise from the lateral orbital roof and gradually displace the eye downward and medially, often without producing a change in visual acuity or causing other neurological symptoms. The overall average duration of symptoms before microsurgical intervention for non-CP angle epidermoid is 48 months, ranging from 1 to 240 months [192]. Among the various locations, only petrous bone lesions tend to have a short symptom duration of 3.3 months. This might be due to the limited space with no subarachnoid cistern to diffuse, causing sudden and intolerable symptoms, or the reason might be explained that extradural epidermoids tend to grow faster than intracranial epidermoids as stated by Gormley et al. [180].

5.6.3 Investigations

Computed Tomography

It is not easy to differentiate dermoid from epidermoid on a CT image. Usually, both dermoids and epidermoids are hypodense and avascular and show no enhancement to contrast agents (Fig. 5.87). Calcification is commonly seen in both tumors but more often in dermoids. The two other features of dermoid compared to epidermoid are the greater range of attenuation values and the evidence of dermal sinus tract.

An extradural cranial lesion shows the typical bony erosive changes seen with epidermoids. On CT scan, the epidermoid shows a similar attenuation as fat, thus hypodense. It is possible with a careful evaluation using the Hounsfield unit to differentiate trapped CSF. The other option is to use CT cisternography to demonstrate its contours when MRI is not applicable. Partial rim enhancement, peripheral calcification, and history of hemorrhage are rare but can appear as hyperdense areas [164].

Magnetic Resonance Imaging

Dermoid Tumors

A heterogeneous image is usually obtained in dermoids on both T1- and T2-weighted images of MRI (Fig. 5.87) [195]. The heterogeneity is

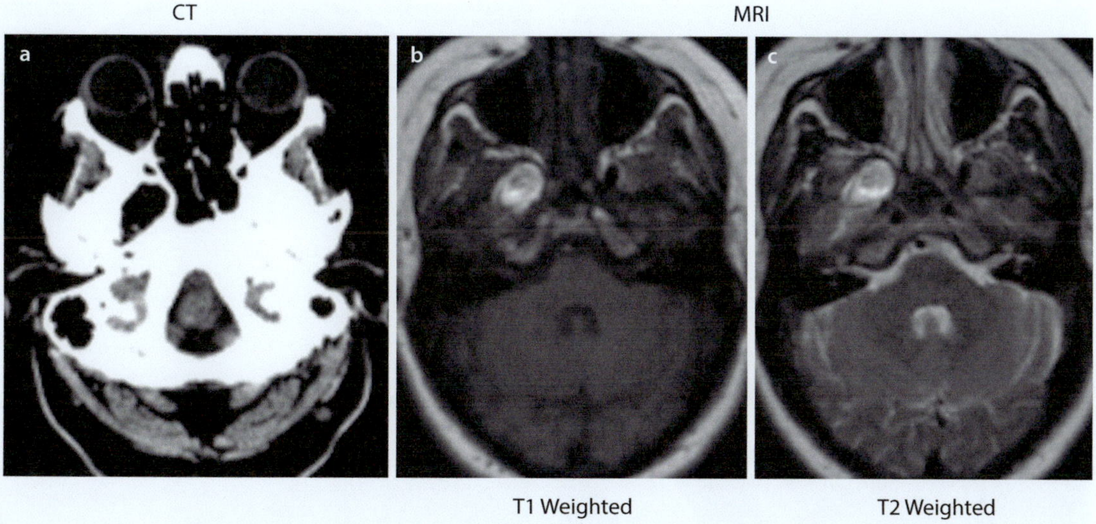

Fig. 5.87 CT and MRI images of a dermoid tumor in the right infratemporal fossa. **a** Hypodense appearance on CT, **b** heterogeneous intensity on MRI T1- and **c** T2-weighted images

originated by the various contents within the capsule such as the cholesterol, hair, calcification, and oily mixture containing lipids. Both T1- and T2- weighted images show some high signal. Consistent with CTs, contrast enhancement is scarcely seen accounting for the avascular feature of the tumor (Fig. 5.88), although reports on enhancing dermoids or mural nodules are found [167]. With thicker walls and more solid content than epidermoids, dermoids tend to demonstrate more local mass effect, rather than growing between the neurovascular structures. When the capsule of the dermoid ruptures, the MRI shows different patterns of distribution of the spilled contents [191]. Typically, the fatty droplets may be sprinkled throughout the ventricular and subarachnoid spaces, presenting as high signal areas on T1-weighted image.

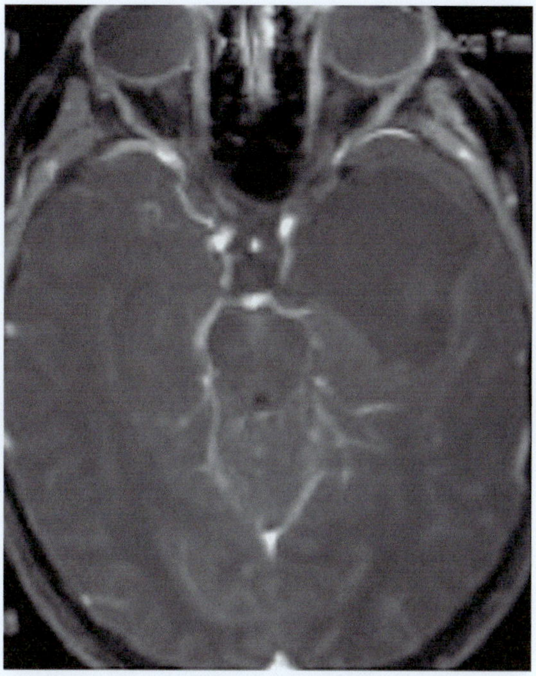

Fig. 5.88 T1-weighted MRI image (with contrast) of a left middle fossa dermoid tumor. No enhancement is observed

Epidermoid Tumors

An MRI image of an epidermoid tumor is usually hypointense to the parenchyma but hyperintense to isointense to CSF on T1-weighted images (Fig. 5.89). The tumor is often hyperintense on T2-weighted images with some heterogeneity (Fig. 5.90). Atypical MRI images are referred to as «white epidermoid,» which appears hyperintense on T1-weighted images and hypointense on T2-weighted images [181]. On FLAIR images, epidermoid will appear heterogeneous and partially hyperintense to CSF (Fig. 5.91). The tumor will restrict diffusion and appear hyperintense on a diffusion-weighted image (DWI). DWI is probably most suitable when diagnosing epidermoid and differentiating from other cystic pathologies such as arachnoid cysts. Enhancement is uncommon after an induction of contrast agent, but the capsule may show some enhancement. There are

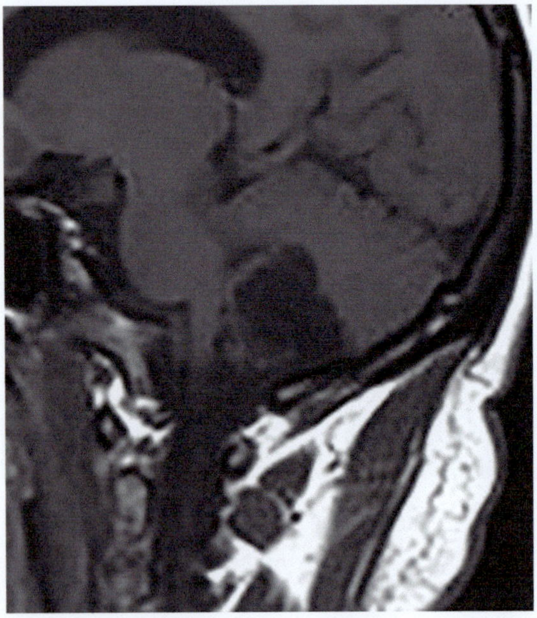

Fig. 5.89 T1-weighted MRI image of an epidermoid tumor located in the posterior vermis region

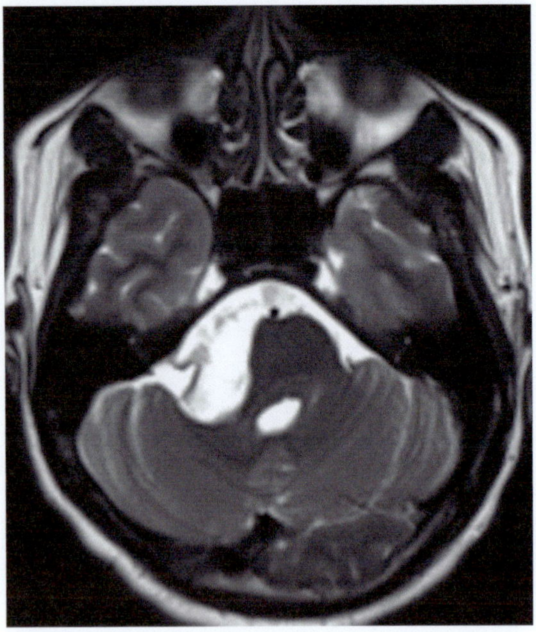

Fig. 5.90 T2-weighted MRI image of an epidermoid tumor in the CP angle. Mostly hyperintense, but partial hypointensity can be seen

two other features on imaging which could both be explained by a unique characteristic of epidermoid and dermoid tumors: The first is that it lacks parenchymal edema considering its size. The parenchymal edema of the surrounding neural

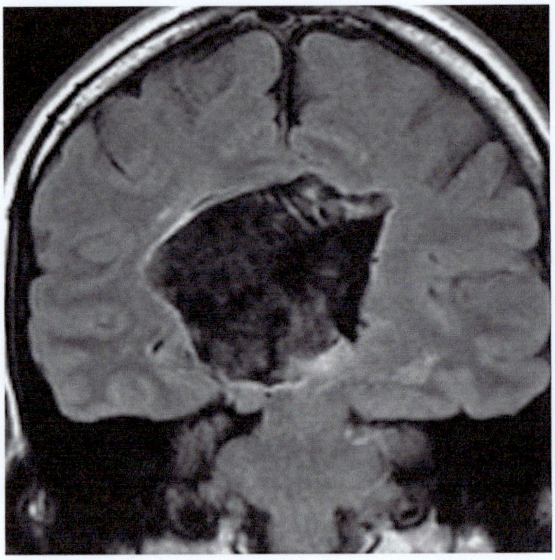

Fig. 5.91 T2 FLAIR MRI image of an epidermoid tumor in the pineal region. Mixed intensity of the tumor is present and notice very little brain edema is observed despite the size of the tumor

structures seen in epidermoids is very small compared to other solid tumors or inflammatory diseases. Second, the degree of hydrocephalus when the tumor obstructs the CSF pathways is very limited. These two features may both result from the slow growing and soft nature of the tumor, thereby allowing the CSF to percolate.

5.6.4 Surgical Technique, Instrumentation, and Management

Whether epidermoid or dermoid, the therapeutic goal of treatment is complete surgical excision of both the capsule lining and its contents, since this is the only effective treatment and there is no current role for radiotherapy or chemotherapy. Resection of the tumor starts by volume reduction of the internal content. Caution must be used to prevent spillage filling into the subarachnoid and ventricular spaces after opening the capsule, especially for dermoid tumors where oily mixture is encountered. To achieve this, the use of cottonoids is beneficial by placing them between the tumor wall and normal structures (Fig. 5.92). As some surgeons have reported, irrigation of the surgical field with a hydrocortisone added with Ringer's fluid will lower the inflammatory response

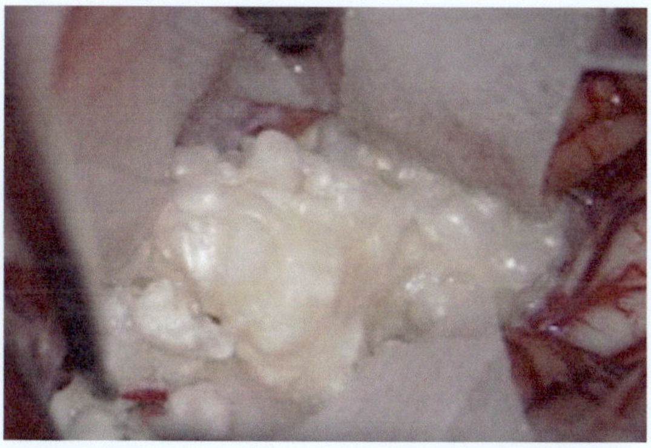

Fig. 5.92 Intraoperative image of cottonoids placed between the tumor and normal structures

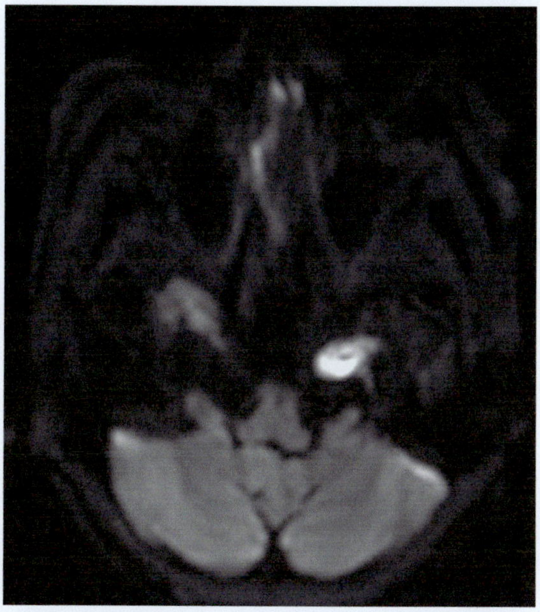

Fig. 5.93 MRI diffusion-weighted image of epidermoid tumor in petrous apex

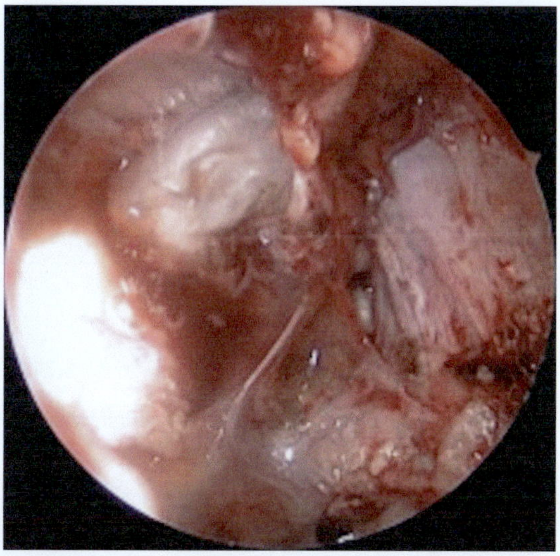

Fig. 5.94 Intraoperative endoscopic view demonstrating a hidden portion of the tumor, which was hard to see under direct view of a microscope

[169]. Once the debulking of the tumor content is achieved, surgery advances to the removal of the surrounding capsular wall. It is essential to identify the dissecting plane between the capsule and the arachnoid. Generally, it is feasible to find and follow the dissecting plane and attain radical total resection under high magnification. Adherence of the capsule to the surrounding neurovascular structures is occasionally encountered and becomes a major obstacle to radical resection. It is crucial that the capsule never be pulled or tugged from the cranial nerve surface as this trauma may result in permanent nerve injury. To prevent this, neuromonitoring such as auditory brain stem response recording (ABR), facial nerve EMG monitoring, SSEP, and MEP should be utilized. Through the authors' experience, the thick, shiny capsule is where the toughest adherence to the cranial nerves and the brain surface is found. This may be a chronic granulomatous reaction possibly formed over many years [203]. In such cases, a decision must be made to leave a thin piece of adherent capsule to avoid permanent damage to the neurovascular structures.

For intraosseous lesions (Fig. 5.93), scraping of the content and the capsule from the surrounding bone leads to successful removal of the tumor. If the periphery wall is irregular making it difficult to scrape, thereby forcing a residual piece of tumor to remain, then drilling into the normal bone will help extract the remaining tumor. On the other hand, intracranial tumors spread and infiltrate through multiple cisterns, separating neurovascular structures. This makes surgery more challenging. Recently, the adoption of neuronavigational equipment facilitates identifying the hidden portion of the tumor. Also, induction of an endoscope to help in visualizing elevates the resection rate, especially those with bilateral involvement around the ventral brain stem and those extending above and below the tentorium (Fig. 5.94). It is rare to encounter adherence between the tumor capsule and the lateral ventricle wall, therefore epidermoids are more easily removed. On the other hand, fourth ventricle

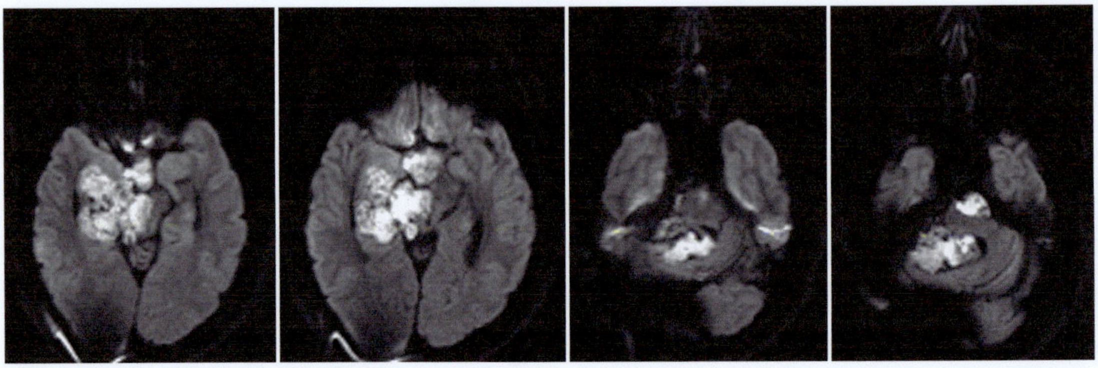

Fig. 5.95 Parasellar region epidermoid tumor, spreading down to the fourth ventricle, demanding two-staged operations

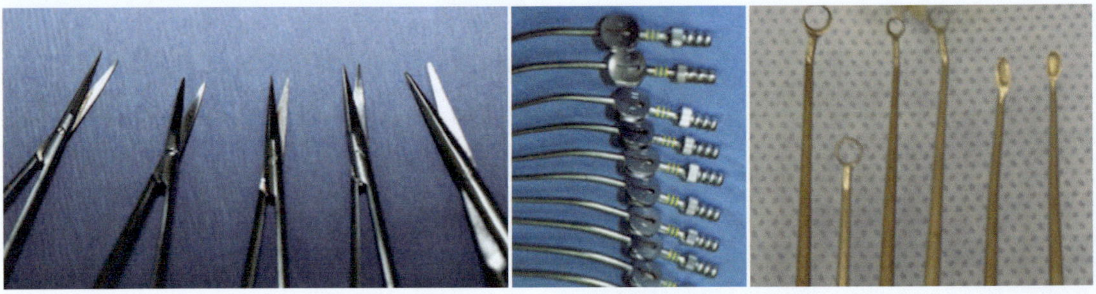

Fig. 5.96 Instruments necessary for meticulous dissection of the tumor. Microscissors: thick, medium, thin blade, curved and straight, long, medium, and short sizes are necessary. Suctions: various French pressure controllable suctions. Ring curettes: various size angle curettes are beneficial for volume reduction of the tumor. The rings should be flat and sharp in order to avoid unnecessary pull

epidermoids tend to have intense adhesion to the floor of the fourth ventricle producing a challenge for complete resection.

Historically, lesions of the CPA have been surgically challenging, and epidermoid tumors are of no exception. These slow-growing tumors advance throughout the basal cisterns and engulf and adhere to the surrounding neurovascular structures and brain stem making complete surgical resection very difficult. The authors' series showed that, except for the largest lesions, 90% of the cases (223 out of 249) could be resected through a small retromastoid retrosigmoid craniotomy. For more extensive tumors, the cranial opening was widened, and in some cases, the tentorium was incised from its inferior surface. When the tumor extends notably toward the supratentorial area, a combined supra- and infratentorial transpetrosal approach was used. In cases of complete hearing loss, a translabyrinthine approach was applied. For extensive lesions compressing the medulla at the level of the foramen magnum, an extreme lateral infrajugular transcondylar transtubercular exposure (ELITE) was utilized. In tumors which spread bilaterally, or spread from superior to inferior of the tentorium, two-staged operations were needed (Fig. 5.95). This is only applied in 3% of all the cases. In most cases, the tumor itself made the corridor and working space needed for resection of the tumor.

In the surgical resection of these lesions, a focus of calcification and dense adherence in the paratrigeminal region was occasionally observed, which may represent the origin of these lesions. With respect to the surgical treatment of these lesions, it is crucial that this focus of adherence be identified and completely dissected from the surrounding nerves, especially in patients presenting with symptoms of cranial nerve irritation in order to achieve a complete resection with symptomatic relief.

With precise microsurgical technique, most of the involved cranial nerves and vessels can be sharply dissected free of the tumor and preserved with proper instrumentation. Three to six French pressure controllable teardrop suctions are essential not only for suction but also to hold, pick up, and even dissect the tumor (Fig. 5.96). Various size and angled tip bipolars, ultra-fine microdissectors, and thin-blade microscissors are fundamental for meticulous removal. Sharp-edge ring curettes of various sizes and angles are very useful when debulking the flaky components and the capsule.

5.6.5 Operative Results and Complications

Operative Results

The total resection rate in the literature, including all locations in the cranium, has been reported to be 36–97% [171, 192, 206]. This diversity is most likely derived from the existence of surgeons whom their goal is not always gross total resection. Due to the adherent nature of the tumor capsule leading to possible damage to the eloquent structures and the slow-growing nature of the tumor, some authors have advocated conservative surgery with minimal or no removal of the adherent capsule [166]. Others recommend attempted complete removal except where the capsule is adherent to important structures [197]. As was originally expressed by Yasargil et al. [206], radical total excision including dissection of the tumor capsule should be the operative goal. Because the capsule is thought to represent the living, growing portion of the tumor, failure to remove the capsule will heighten the possibility of regrowth of the lesion. With the improvement of perioperative imaging, microneurosurgical technique, and instruments, the resection rate has improved remarkably during the course of this century.

The resection rate for epidermoid tumor was 75% overall in the authors' series. Even though there was no statistical significance, tumor location contributed to the different rate of resection as shown in ◘ Table 5.7. The lowest resection rate was observed in fourth ventricle epidermoids (44%), followed by parasellar region (60%). For CPA epidermoids, the GTR rate was 77%. As for fourth ventricle lesions, adhesion of the tumor capsule to the brain stem made radical resection difficult. In contrast, locations like dorsal vermis, interhemispheric fissure, and intraosseous where there was less neurovascular structure tended to result in higher resection rate. There was no significant relationship between recurrent epidermoid tumors and extent of resection. When the tumors were categorized into small or large by their maximum diameter, small-sized epidermoid tumors were 52% more likely to result in gross total resection compared to large tumors.

◘ **Table 5.7** Resection, complication, recurrence rate

Location	GTR (%)	Complication		Recurrence (%)
		Temporary (%)	Persistent[a] (%)	
Overall	75	23	10	11 (9[b])
CP angle	77	24	10	13
Non-CP angle	70	19	16	12
Parasellar	60	29	13	20
Cavernous sinus	80	13	25	8
Pineal region	73	17	22	0
Intraosseous	86	14	0	10
Fourth ventricle	44	28	12	11
Dorsal vermis	100	0		50
Interhemisphere	100	0		0
Frontal base	100	0		0

[a]New symptoms persisting after 1 year
[b]Percent of cases needed for reoperation

Operative Complications

The mortality after surgical treatment of epidermoids and dermoids has been reported to be as high as 20–57% in the past and decreasing since [197]. Yasargil et al. [206] reported no mortality after GTR in 22 patients in CPA epidermoids. Through the 334 case series, the mortality rate was 0.7% (2 cases), both with postoperative cardiopulmonary complications.

Postoperative complications occurred in 33% of the cases overall (◘ Table 5.7). In terms of tumor location, the highest rate of complication was for parasellar (42%), followed by fourth ventricle lesions (40%), cavernous sinus (38%), and CP angle (34%). The complications for parasellar region and cavernous sinus lesions were associated with cranial nerve deficits such as double vision and facial dysesthesia. Twenty-four percent of the complications which occurred after CP angle epidermoid were cranial nerve deficit resulting from manipulation of the nerves encased by the tumor. Most frequently encountered complications after CP angle epidermoid tumor resection were abducens nerve and facial nerve palsy (9%), followed by hearing decrease and cerebellar symptoms (4%). Ataxia, disequilibrium, dysphagia, and CSF leaks were more commonly seen after fourth ventricle epidermoids. Not only did fourth ventricle epidermoids have the lowest GTR rate, they also had higher chances of complications, making them one of the most challenging locations for epidermoid resection. Conversely, no complications were seen for interhemispheric and frontal base tumors. The important fact is that only 10% of those were permanent, and most of these complications resolved within a year as presented in the literature [200]. Diplopia and facial dysesthesia after parasellar and cavernous sinus lesions and disequilibrium after fourth ventricle lesions were the only persisting complications at 1 year follow-up. Postoperative chemical meningitis is used to be one of the most common complications after epidermoid/dermoid surgeries, encountered as high as 40% of the cases in the past. The incidence can now be reduced to 0.5% with gross total resection and with avoiding spillage of the tumor content. Guidetti and Gagliardi [182] stated that this complication occurs far more frequently when removal of the capsule was incomplete. Postoperative hydrocephalus is another uncommon complication following removal of epidermoids. It occurs more frequently in patients who develop postoperative aseptic meningitis, and it may be concurrent with an inflammatory condition in the postoperative period. Postoperative hematomas, subarachnoid hemorrhage caused by formation of pseudoaneurysm, and pseudomeningocele were experienced as rare complications, most likely caused by the damage to the outer membrane when dissecting the capsule from the vessel. Another interesting result found was that, for primary cases, complications occurred in only 28%, whereas in the recurrent group, this increased to 47%. This was statistically significant, in that prior surgery increased the chance of complications by 46%, suggesting epidermoids should be resected on the first attempt.

Recurrence

Recurrence of these tumors has been reported to be 0–24%. As described in the literature, there is no argument that subtotal resection leads to a higher recurrence rate [174, 182, 200, 205]. We experienced 11% of radiographic recurrence, and 9% needed reoperation due to recurrence of the tumor as shown in ◘ Table 5.7. The average intersurgical duration was 7 years, ranging from 1 to 11 years. There was a statistical significance in recurrence between the gross total group and the subtotal group. Gross total resection decreased the chance of recurrence by 51%. The recurrence rate for the gross total group was 6%, whereas the subtotal group showed a much higher recurrence rate of 25%. There was no significant relationship between the location of the tumor and size of the tumor with the incidence of recurrence .

Due to the linear slow-growing nature of the tumor, it may take a long time for these tumors to recur. The average interval for epidermoids and dermoids to recur and become symptomatic is approximately 9 years. There seems to be no significant intersurgical interval difference between the gross total group and subtotal group. For both groups, long-term follow-up with periodical neuroimaging is necessary.

Malignant Transformation

Malignant transformation of these tumors is considered rare. In dermoids, it primarily involves the squamous element and results in squamous cell carcinoma [188]. A rare transformation into atypical hidradenoma has been reported [187]. For epidermoid tumors, many have been illustrated in the literature on malignant progression to locally invasive squamous cell carcinoma with infiltration of the adjacent brain [190]. In some cases, transformation could also result in carcinomatosis of leptomeninges [189]. Malignant transformations can even occur over 30 years after the initial surgery [179]. We experienced 3 cases (0.8%) of malignant transformation through the authors' 334 case series.

5.6.6 Conclusion

Through the data of 334 cases, the series revealed that gross total resection significantly lowered the risk of recurrence and the chance of complications. Reoperations made the incidence of complication higher. These results led us to conclude that when treating dermoids and epidermoid tumors, total resection should always be the goal at the first surgery with the state-of-the-art meticulous and precise micro-techniques by experienced hands, utilizing indispensable micro-instruments.

5.7 Glomus Jugulare Tumors

Y. Nonaka and T. Fukushima

Glomus jugulare tumors (GJTs) involve neurootologic structures and lower cranial nerves (LCNs) and hence remain extremely difficult to achieve radical resection. They also often extend into the intradural and high cervical spaces. Therefore, GJTs continue to pose a significant challenge to skull base surgeons despite the development of the improved surgical approach. Management for GJTs includes preoperative feeder embolization, followed by surgical resection, and/or option of radiation.

5.7.1 General Information

GJTs are benign slow-growing neoplasm occupying the jugular foramen, hearing apparatus, and lower cranial nerves. Radical resection of GJTs may have risks of audio-facial and lower cranial nerve deficits because of their invasive character, hypervascularity, and involvement of critical structures. Surgical treatment has been associated with high rate of morbidity and mortality [218, 221]. GJTs mainly infiltrate into the base of the temporal bone; inner ear, supra- or infrajugular area, and larger tumors reach to the cavernous sinus, clivus, and infratemporal area. Neurological symptoms are related to the region affected by the tumor. The most common symptoms are headache, deafness, pulsatile tinnitus, vertigo, and multiple cranial nerve palsies. Advances in neuroimaging, microneurosurgery, and modern skull base surgery have facilitated radical resection of these tumors with lower rates of morbidity and mortality.

Two grading systems have been developed to classify GJTs on the basis of the location, size, and extent of disease. Fisch [212] introduced a classification of GJTs which guides surgical approach depending on tumor size and extension (■ Table 5.8). Jackson et al. [218] also reported a new classification which is focused upon intracranial extension (■ Table 5.9). We reported a simple tumor classification for jugular foramen schwannomas according to imaging results as follows: Type A, intradural tumor; Type B, dumbbell-shaped tumor; and Type C, dumbbell-shaped tumor with high cervical extension [211]. Our classification can also be applied to the glomus jugulare tumors. Type A tumors are purely intradural and can be approached via a retromastoid approach or ELITE. Type B tumors are intradural and involve the jugular bulb; these tumors are best approached via an intradural and transjugular approach. Type C tumors have an intradural component and involve both the jugular bulb and the IJV. In these tumors, an intradural and transjugular approach with possible ligation of the IJV may be necessary.

These classifications facilitate the operative planning for current skull base surgery techniques and provide a simplified method for better surgical outcomes.

5.7.2 Investigations

The size, extension, and stage of GJTs and the degree of ICA involvement are the most important factors to determine the surgical strategy. Computed tomography (CT) scan, magnetic resonance imaging (MRI), and angiograms are important radiologic diagnostics for GJTs. MRI with and without gadolinium enhancement is performed to delineate the tumor size, location,

Table 5.8 The Fisch classification of glomus tumors

Class	Description
A	Tumors confined to the tympanum and arising from the promontory, without evidence of bone erosion
B	Tumors involving the tympanum, with or without mastoid involvement but always arising from the hypotympanic region The cortical bone over the jugular bulb must be intact
C	Tumors eroding the bone over the jugular bulb; the tumor may extend into and destroy the bone of the infralabyrinthine and apical compartments of the temporal bone
C1	Tumors involving the foramen caroticum
C2	Tumors involving the vertical segment of the carotid canal
C3	Tumors involving the horizontal segment of the carotid canal
C4	Tumors extending to the ipsilateral foramen lacerum and cavernous sinus
D	Tumors with intracranial extension
De1	Tumors with intracranial extradural extension of up to 2 cm
De2	Tumors with intracranial extradural extension of more than 2 cm
Di1	Tumors with intracranial intradural extension of up to 2 cm
Di2	Tumors with intracranial intradural extension of more than 2 cm
D3	Tumors with inoperable intracranial extension

Fisch [212]

Table 5.9 The Glasscock–Jackson classification of glomus jugulare tumors

Grade	Description
1	Small tumor involving the jugular bulb, middle ear, and mastoid
2	Tumor extending under the internal auditory canal; may have intracranial extension
3	Tumor extending into petrous apex; may have intracranial extension
4	Tumor extending beyond petrous apex into clivus or infratemporal fossa; may have intracranial extension

Jackson (1982)

and extent. The relationship of the tumor to the jugular foramen (JF), cranial nerves, pars nervosa, brain stem, temporal bone, and neighboring vascular structures is examined carefully. Evidence of tumor involvement of ICA can be determined on these images. Thin slice CT scan of the skull base is useful to evaluate the anatomy and the extent of bony destruction by the tumor.

Angiographic studies are essential and critical to assess the feeding arteries and the venous drainage of the tumor. In patients who have tumor involvement of the ICA, a balloon occlusion test is performed to assess the risk involved with performing an ICA sacrifice and subsequent reconstruction of the ICA with a high-flow bypass. Preoperative feeder embolization is a key element of modality for reducing intraoperative blood loss [221]. Arterial feeders most commonly arise from the ascending pharyngeal artery and feeders from the external carotid artery.

5.7.3 Therapeutic Options

Surgical Approaches and Treatment

A microsurgical skull base approach is crucial to obtain a radical removal of GJTs. The most appropriate surgical approach and the extent of resection should be tailored to each case in order to preserve lower cranial nerves. The key anatomical issues for surgical management of GJTs are the fallopian segment of facial nerve, ICA, and LCNs [210, 214, 221, 223]. The conventional surgical technique is based on the temporal bone drilling, exposure of the JB and ICA with or without rerouting of the facial nerve, and high cervical exposure. Over the past three decades, these extensive postauricular approaches introduced by Fisch [212] have been the basis for GJT surgery. This technique has been recommended by many authors with some modifications and is advocated as a two-stage operation in some cases [219, 220, 224].

Over the past 20 years, we have attempted to modify the Fisch approach to make it a smaller less invasive exposure and minimize cranial nerve morbidity. Moreover, in recent years, we have developed a less invasive transjugular approach with fallopian bridge technique, which allows tumor resection while preserving hearing and protecting the facial nerve and the pars nervosa [222].

Transmastoid: High Cervical Approach for Extreme Large or Extensive GJTs (The Combined Transmastoid Retro- and Infralabyrinthine Transjugular Transcondylar Transtubercular High Cervical Approach)

For large or extensive GJTs, we perform one-stage transjugular posterior infratemporal fossa approaches that allow radical resection of tumors located around the JF, the lower clivus, and the high cervical region (■ Fig. 5.97). This approach is a combination of the transmastoid, retro- and

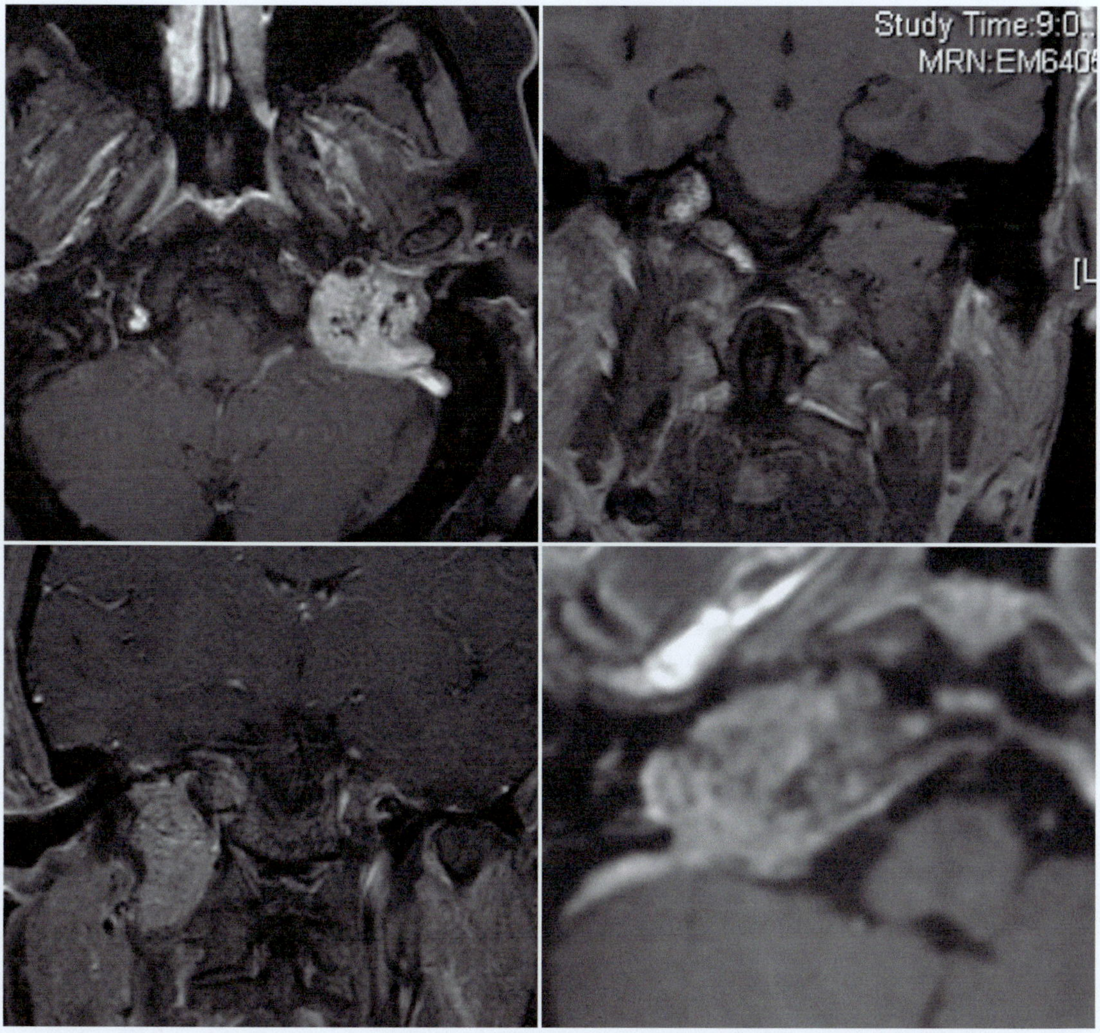

■ **Fig. 5.97** Representative four cases of large GJTs: each MRI reveals GJT expanding into the infratemporal fossa and high cervical area

infralabyrinthine, transjugular, extreme lateral infrajugular transcondylar transtubercular, and high cervical approaches [213, 220]. The bony labyrinth should be kept intact in case with serviceable hearing. Total exposure of the JF can be achieved, and multidirectional approaches can be performed from an anterolateral direction, including suprajugular, transjugular, and infrajugular exposures. Both intracranial and extracranial tumor can be removed in a one-stage procedure. Transection of the external ear canal and permanent rerouting of the facial nerve are not necessary; instead, slight anterior transposition of the facial nerve, on select cases, can provide adequate exposure of the infratemporal ICA (C7 segment), without anterior dislocation of the mandible.

This complex approach for total JF exposure can be simplified in a stepwise fashion: (1) retroauricular curvilinear skin incision; (2) high cervical exposure; (3) retrolabyrinthine mastoidectomy; (4) skeletonization and anterior translocation of the facial nerve; (5) lateral suboccipital craniotomy and transcondylar–transtubercular exposure; (6) ligation and removal of the internal jugular vein (IJV), jugular bulb (JB), and sigmoid sinus (SS); and (7) intradural exposure if necessary.

The patient is placed in a supine position with the head turned laterally away from the side of the lesion. A shoulder roll is used to elevate the ipsilateral side of the shoulder. For obese patients with short necks, a lateral position may be used. A retroauricular curvilinear sickle skin incision is started 2 cm posterior to the upper border of the ear. It continues posteroinferiorly into the neck over the anterior border of the sternocleidomastoid muscle and under the mandibular angle (Fig. 5.98).

The suboccipital muscles which include the sternocleidomastoid muscle, longissimus capitis, and splenius capitis muscles are reflected posteroinferiorly to expose the mastoid body, inferolateral part of occipital bone, suboccipital triangle, and transverse process of C1. The superior oblique muscle, which is composed of the upper part of the suboccipital triangle, is also elevated from the inferior nuchal line of the occipital bone then reflected inferiorly. The posterior belly of the digastric muscle is also detached from the digastric groove behind the mastoid tip and reflected anteriorly to protect the extracranial portion of the facial nerve. The transverse process of C1 is an important landmark to identify IJV, ICA, and the extracranial portion of the LCNs.

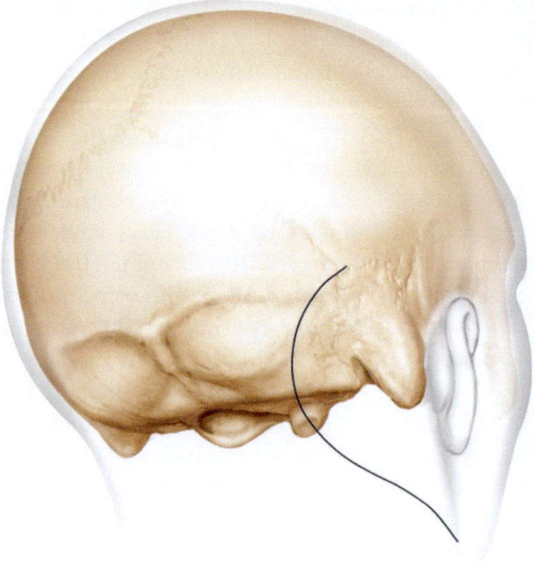

Fig. 5.98 A retroauricular curvilinear sickle skin incision

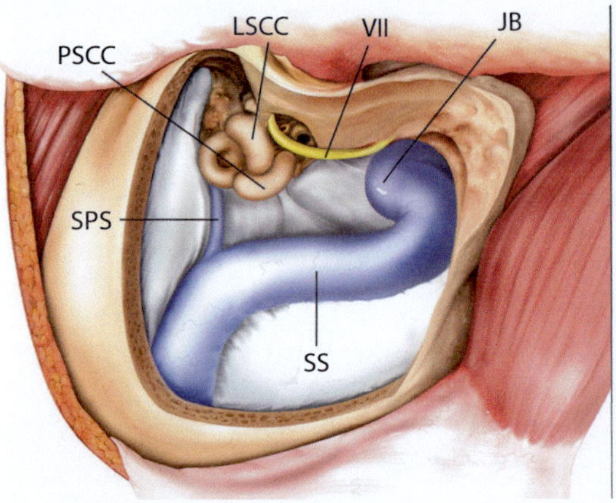

Fig. 5.99 The illustration demonstrates «transmastoid retrolabyrinthine exposure.» The infralabyrinthine–suprajugular area is exposed with the SS skeletonization all the way down to the JB

Transmastoid drilling is performed by using a diamond burr. The SS down to the JB are fully skeletonized, and the mastoid air cells are totally removed to expose the bony labyrinth, the presigmoid dura, the superior petrosal sinus, the sinodural angle, the temporal tegmen, and the retrosigmoid dura (Fig. 5.99). The facial nerve at the fallopian canal segment, which is located 12–15 mm deep from the cortical surface of the mastoid body, can be identified with an aid of a facial nerve stimulator. The fallopian canal is

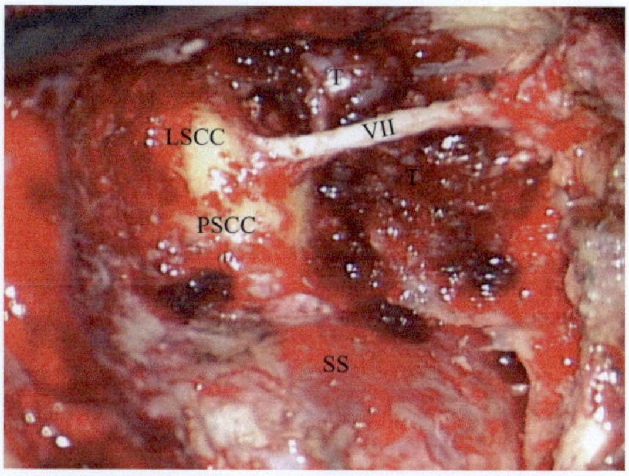

■ **Fig. 5.100** Intraoperative photo shows right side transmastoid retrolabyrinthine exposure. The fallopian segment of the facial nerve is skeletonized entirely, and facial recess is removed to visualize the tumor penetrating the upper wall of the JB

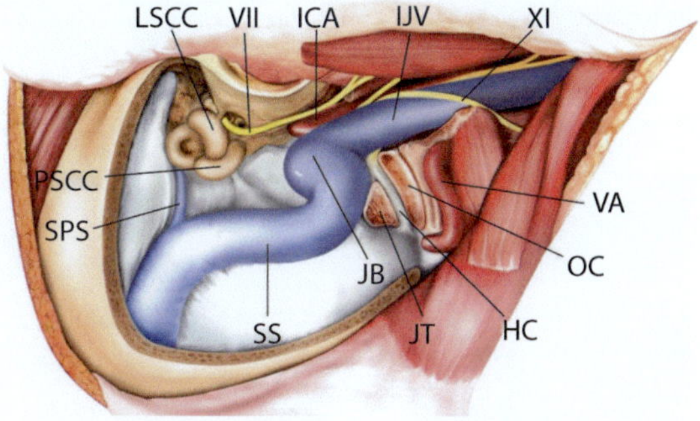

■ **Fig. 5.101** Transcondylar transtubercular drilling and high cervical dissection are performed to expose the HC, IJV, and extracranial portion of the LCNs

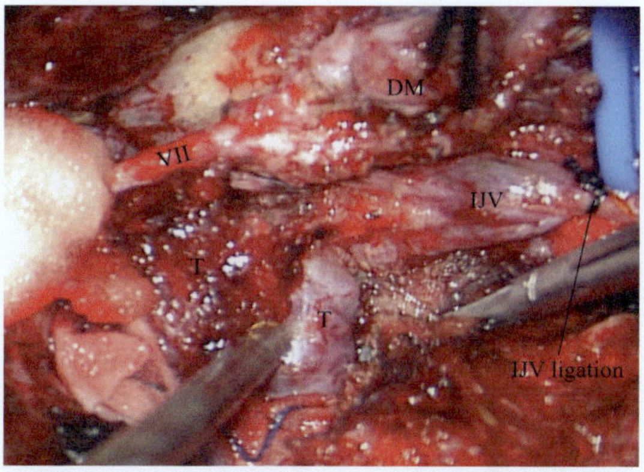

■ **Fig. 5.102** The facial nerve is slightly translocated anteriorly with the digastric muscle. The IJV is ligated with suture just below the intraluminal tumor. Complete exposure of the GJT located at SS and JB is done

carefully skeletonized from the genu to the stylomastoid foramen with a diamond burr under constant irrigation to avoid thermal injury of the facial nerve. In most of the cases, the tumor will be exposed during infralabyrinthine drilling around the JB (■ Fig. 5.100). The mastoid tip is removed carefully to decompress the facial nerve at the level of the stylomastoid foramen. If necessary, the fallopian segment of the facial nerve can be slightly translocated anteriorly to provide added exposure of the C7 vertical segment of the ICA. This maneuver is used selectively and produces less risk of facial nerve palsy in contrast with permanent facial nerve rerouting.

After transmastoid retrolabyrinthine drilling with the mastoid tip removal and anterior reflection of the digastric muscle, the rectus capitis lateralis, which overlies the IJV, is exposed. Removal of the rectus capitis lateralis finally allows full exposure from the SS to the IJV. A lateral suboccipital craniotomy is then performed to expose retrosigmoid posterior fossa dura. After the craniotomy, additional bone removal laterally inferior to the SS is mandatory. Further bone removal, which means extradural reduction of the occipital condyle (OC) and jugular tubercle (JT), is the key maneuver in this step. Removal of the posterior and medial one-third of the OC is adequate to increase the surgical corridor to the ventral side of brain stem. During this procedure, the posterior condyle emissary vein will be encountered as it travels from the JB and exits the condylar fossa via the condylar canal to join the extradural venous plexus. Bone removal of the posteromedial aspect of OC by using a drill should be done until the cortical layer of the bone that covers the hypoglossal canal is exposed (■ Fig. 5.101). The hypoglossal canal, which is situated superior to the OC and inferior to the JT, is an important landmark for condyle bone removal. Bone removal is next directed superiorly toward the JT. It is situated slightly medial and inferior to the JB, superior to the hypoglossal canal, and medial to the JF. The bone removal of the JT is the one of difficult procedures in this surgical approach because mechanical damage of the posterior fossa dura just superior to the JT may result in direct damage of LCNs.

After complete exposure of the SS, JB, and IJV, the tumor mass can be palpated within these venous structures through the venous wall. After all arterial feeders to the tumor are coagulated, the IJV is then ligated just inferior to the tumor (■ Fig. 5.102). The SS is occluded just above the

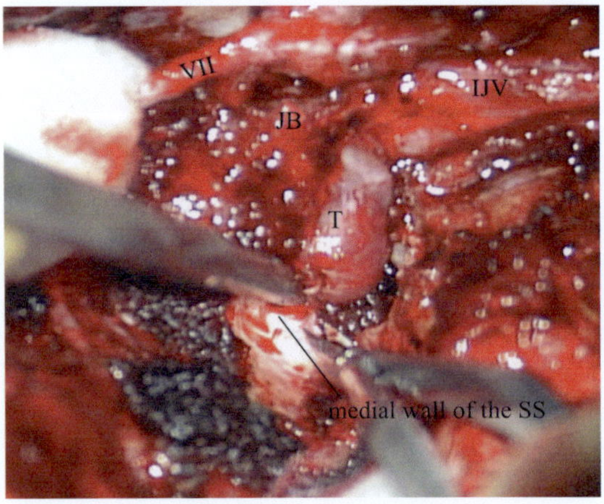

Fig. 5.103 The lateral wall of the SS is incised, and then the medial wall of the SS is visualized

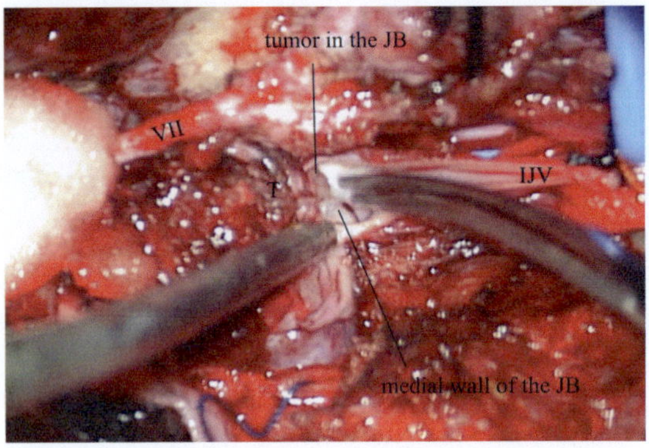

Fig. 5.104 The IJV is ligated and incised up to the JB to resect the intraluminal tumor

tumor with a suture ligature. Then, the lateral wall of the SS is incised and removed with the tumor down to the JB (Fig. 5.103). Inferior portion of the tumor also can be removed through an incision on the lateral wall of the IJV (Fig. 5.104). As the tumor is removed from the intraluminal space, bleeding will be encountered from remaining feeding vessels and venous channels around the JB, like the inferior petrosal sinus. It sometimes disturbs the surgeon to identify the correct dissection plane between the tumor and the medial wall of the JB overlying pars nervosa, which may lead to an unexpected LCN damage. These bleeding can be controlled with surgical packing and soft micro-paddies. However, «two-men, four-hand surgery» will be very helpful during tumor elevation of this portion. The dissection plane between the tumor and the medial wall of the JB is established proximally in the SS, in order to preserve the LCNs. The medial wall of the JB should be kept intact to decrease the risk of LCN damage (Fig. 5.105).

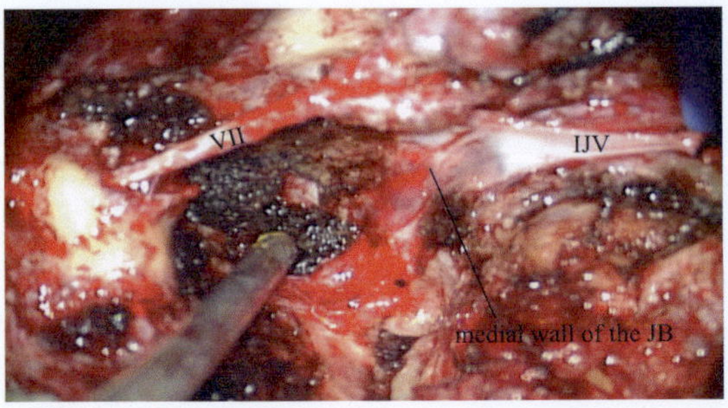

Fig. 5.105 Final picture of total tumor resection through the transmastoid retrolabyrinthine transjugular and high cervical approach. The medial wall of the JB and the IJV is left to protect the LCNs behind them. Complete hemostasis is done with Surgicel

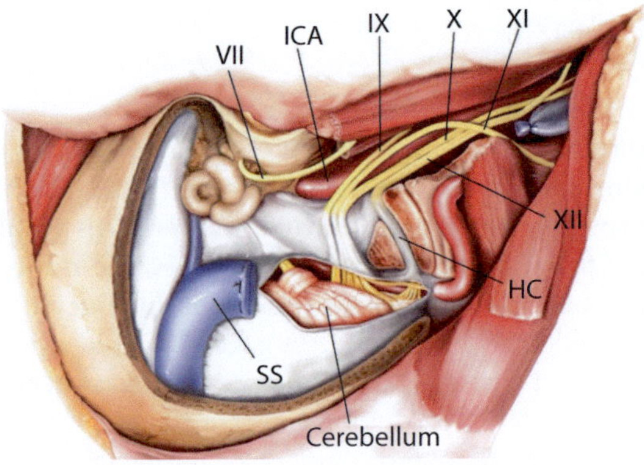

Fig. 5.106 A dural incision is made on the posterior fossa dura for resection of the intradural tumor

If there is tumor invasion into the intradural space, the retrosigmoid dura needs to be incised (Fig. 5.106). Adequate reduction of the OC and JT will provide a straight surgical trajectory to the ventral craniovertebral junction, parallel to the intracranial course of the vertebral artery. Structures of the inferior aspect of the cerebellopontine angle and the cerebellomedullary angle are visualized. The intradural aspect of the JF should be inspected for any tumor invasion. The tumor is carefully dissected from the LCNs and removed. Occasionally, the blood supply to the intradural tumor from posterior inferior cerebellar artery is seen. For these reasons, tumor removal of the intradural portion through the penetrated dura, which is not advisable, may result in unexpected bleeding or direct LCN damages.

We tailor the approach in terms of the retrojugular, transjugular, or infrajugular exposure with regard to the size and extension of the tumor. If the JB is already occluded and tumor has both intradural and JF components, we perform a combined intradural and extradural exposure. If the tumor involves the infrajugular component, infratemporal ICA, and JB, we do a combined transmastoid infralabyrinthine and combined transtemporal transjugular and infrajugular transcondylar and high cervical exposure. For extensive GJTs, we always expose the high cervical ICA for proximal control. Then the infratemporal ICA in front of the JB is exposed by drilling of the inferior bony tympanic ring to remove the tumor around the ICA.

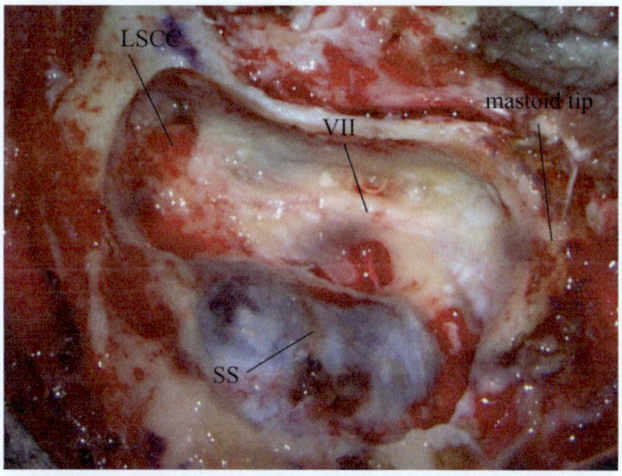

Fig. 5.107 Intraoperative transmastoid exposure of the sigmoid sinus (SS) and the facial nerve (VII) of the fallopian segment

Fallopian Bridge Technique for Small- to Large-Size GJTs (Less Invasive Transjugular Approach with Fallopian Bridge Technique)

Over the initial 10 years of our experience, we modified the Fisch technique. First, we moved away from performing a two-stage operation. Second, in patients with functional hearing, we did not close the external auditory canal (EAC). Then, we rarely perform extensive neck dissection in favor of a limited high cervical exposure. In our recent cases of small to large tumors with minimal extension to the high cervical region, we performed a transmastoid–transsigmoid–transjugular approach with slight anterior translocation of the fallopian segment of the facial nerve. We recognized that even with the less invasive transmastoid and high cervical approach, we experienced significant morbidity with facial weakness, hearing loss, and LCN dysfunction [220]. In order to decrease these complications, after extensive anatomic study, we have developed a much less invasive transmastoid, infralabyrinthine, transjugular approach with preservation of the fallopian canal so-called fallopian bridge technique [222]. The fallopian bridge technique was first used by Pensak and Jackler [225] for smaller tumors with no erosion of the EAC and no extension anterosuperior to the carotid genu. In the majority of their cases, satisfactory exposure of the region of the JF could be provided without facial nerve rerouting with favorable result.

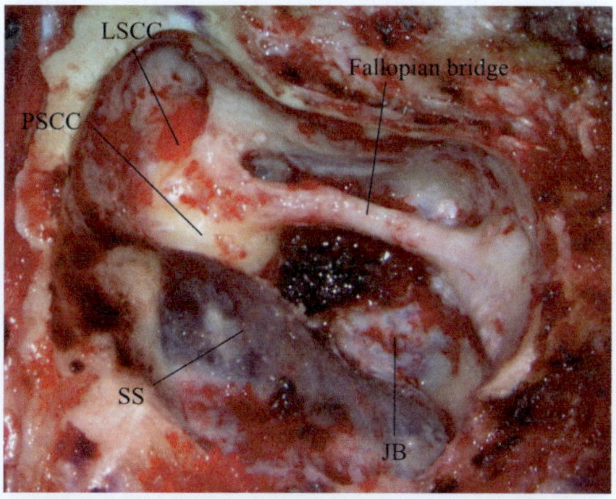

Fig. 5.108 Final exposure of the fallopian bridge technique through the transmastoid retrolabyrinthine drilling. The facial nerve (VII) is covered by thin cortical bone entirely

The patient is positioned in a supine position with head supported on an ENT pillow. A standard retroauricular C-shaped incision is made. An extended mastoidectomy is performed with total skeletonization of the sigmoid sinus, exposing both the retrosigmoid and presigmoid dura (Fig. 5.107). Maximum shaving of the labyrinth and fallopian canal, and full exposure of the jugular dome, is done next. A thin layer of the cortical bone like an eggshell is left to cover the entire fallopian segment of the facial nerve from the genu to the stylomastoid foramen, creating the «fallopian bridge» (Fig. 5.108). The mastoid tip is maximally skeletonized, the digastric groove is removed, and infrajugular drilling is carried down into the occipital condyle until the hypoglossal canal is exposed.

After creation of the fallopian bridge, further bone removal from the facial recess exposes the tumor in the inner ear and the hypotympanum area. This allows identification and preservation of the annulus of the tympanic membrane [214, 216]. While protecting the thin wall of the external auditory canal, the inferior bony tympanic ring is maximally drilled away. This removes the base of styloid process and exposes the vertical C7 segment of the ICA, which is located anterior to the JB. At this point, the viewing angle of the microscope can be manipulated allowing the surgeon full visualization of the jugular structures, the vertical ICA, and the hearing apparatus, looking from above or below the «fallopian bridge.» If the patient had already lost hearing function, or tumor has invaded the ventral side of the vertical ICA, the EAC can be closed followed by bony EAC drilling to obtain a wider operative field (◘ Figs. 5.109 and 5.110). The soft tissue of the EAC should be closed tightly by multiple-layer technique using the fascia to avoid postoperative infection [213, 217].

In a majority of GJTs, the retrofacial air cell space is filled with tumor. Resection of tumor from this suprajugular area must be done with extreme caution to prevent damage to the posterior semicircular canal and the basal turn of the cochlea. Additionally, care must be used while resecting tumor from around the ICA to prevent damage to cross the ninth nerve or the arterial adventitia. Transsigmoid and transjugular exposure facilitates resection of the major tumor mass. In cases of intradural extension, maximum effort is used to preserve anatomical continuity of the LCNs, unless the patient presents with LCN deficits. Tumor extension into the IJV through the JB can be removed with dissectors, ring curettes, and tumor forceps because this portion of the tumor usually does not adhere to the intimal surface of the IJV [217, 222] (◘ Figs. 5.111 and 5.112).

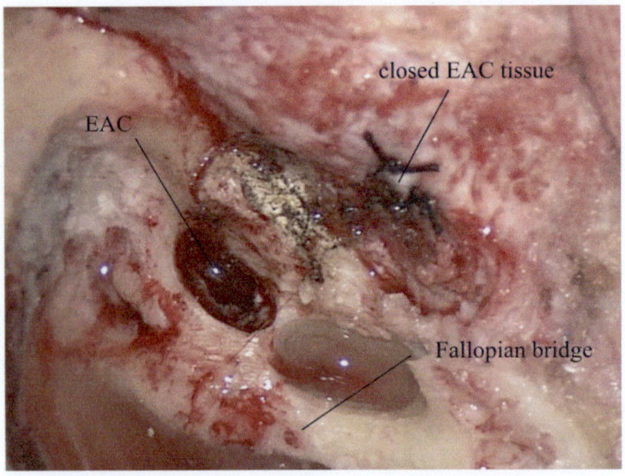

◘ **Fig. 5.109** The bony external acoustic canal (EAC) is exposed after EAC skin tissue elevation and closure

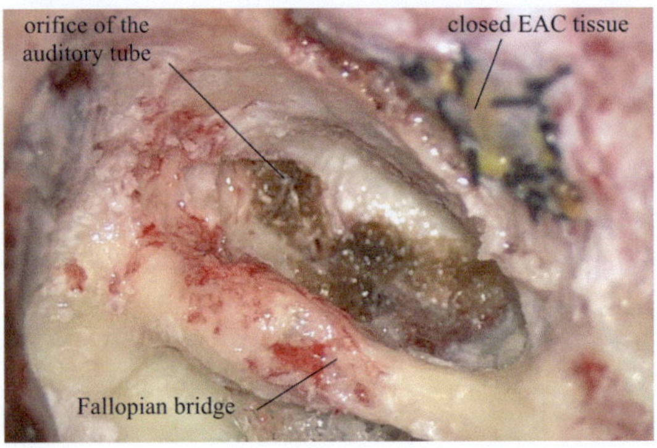

◘ **Fig. 5.110** Further drilling of the EAC, the facial recess, and the hypotympanum area creates a wider surgical field anteromedial to the fallopian bridge

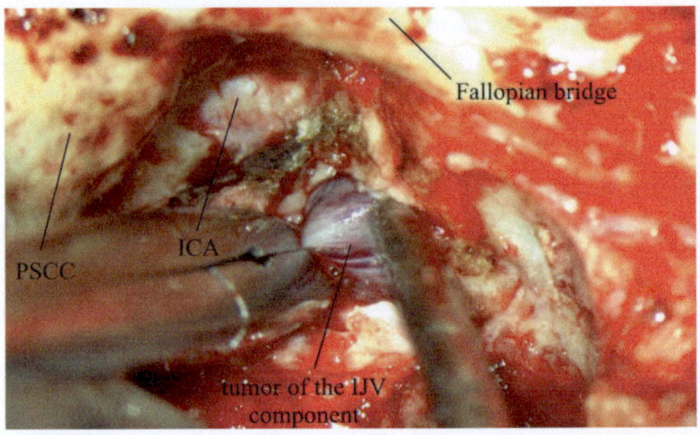

◘ **Fig. 5.111** After removal of the jugular bulb (JB) portion of the tumour, the internal jugular vein (IJV) portion of the tumor can be seen. A tumor forceps can grab the tip of the tumor

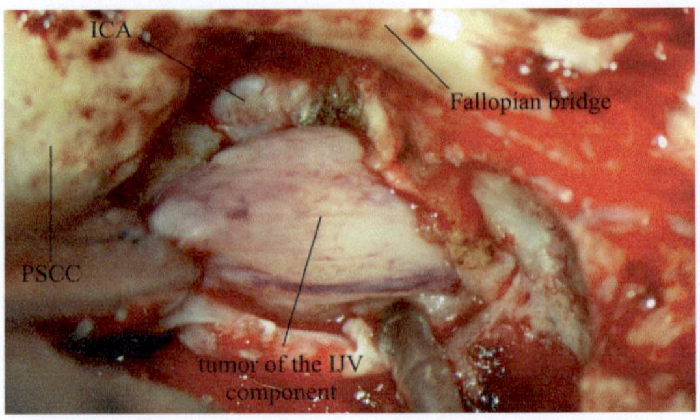

◘ **Fig. 5.112** The IJV component of the tumor is pulled out with the tumor forceps through the JB. No adhesion between the tumor and the endothelial surface of the IJV exists

Intraoperative Monitoring

Intraoperative monitoring that is indispensable for GJT surgery includes auditory brain stem response, somatosensory evoked potentials, motor evoked potentials, and facial nerve monitoring. The LCNs also can be monitored by using an electromyographic endotracheal tube.

Key Maneuvers for Complication Avoidance in GJT Surgery

GJTs are locally destructive, highly vascular lesions located in one of the most critical regions of the skull base. Tumor may be both intra- and extradural with engulfment of critical neurovascular structures. The key maneuvers to avoid surgical complications in the management of GJTs are how to treat the facial nerve at fallopian segment, C6 petrous and/or C7 vertical segments of ICA, and LCNs [210, 221, 223].

Facial Nerve Dislocation

Fallopian bridge technique has been advocated recently because it makes possible the removal of C1 and C2 GJTs without any need to dislocate the facial nerve and remove the external ear canal and middle ear. In case of small to large size of tumors, we specially choose not to reroute the facial nerve to avoid postoperative facial nerve palsy as much as possible. Even in the case with large aggressive tumor, if necessary, we used to translocate the descending fallopian and stylomastoid foramen segments of the facial nerve approximately 5 mm anteriorly to provide adequate exposure of the infratemporal ICA [220].

ICA Engulfment

One of the most important issues in the GJT surgery is the exposure and control of the ICA [210, 216]. GJTs frequently adhere or engulf the ICA (C7 vertical segment and/or C6 petrous segment) as well as LCNs. For extensive tumors, full exposure of the vertical portion of the ICA is mandatory. Complete dissection of the tumor from the C6 ICA is probably the most limiting factor for achieving radical resection of GJTs. And they often receive blood supply from the ICA. Therefore, controlled ICA dissection should be performed. A dissection plane can be developed between the adventitia and the tumor with the aid of the microscope. We do not recommend subadventitial dissection of the ICA because of the high risk of carotid rupture or occlusive complications.

The risk of permanent ICA occlusion is high, even in patients who passed a balloon occlusion test. In case of the extensive carotid involvement, the high-flow carotid bypass should be considered followed by permanent balloon occlusion of the ICA. However, it should be kept in mind that reconstruction of the ICA also has been associated with major risks as well as ICA sacrifice.

Preservation of LCNs

Cranial nerve preservation during the surgical resection of GJTs is the main factor in reducing the postoperative rate of morbidity. Especially, preservation of the LCN function is one of major management issues. The worsening or a new deficit of LCNs substantially diminishes patient's quality of life. There are four possible chances to damage the LCNs in the surgical procedure: (1) drilling of the JT, (2) tumor removal at the JB, (3) dissection of high cervical region, and (4) intradural tumor removal.

Extradural bone removal of the JT is a key maneuver in transcondylar–transtubercular exposure, because it reduces an obstructed view of the ventral side of the brain stem and clivus anterior to the LCNs while performing an intradural procedure. The JT should be drilled away as much as possible with extreme care, because the LCNs which cross over the posterior aspect of the JT into the JF are in very close proximity and may be at risk of damage by direct trauma, stretching of the dura, and heat generated by the drill.

After complete ligation of the SS, tumor within the JB can be removed with lateral wall of the JB. The tumor should be elevated sharply to leave the medial wall of the JB intact to preserve the LCNs at the pars nervosa. This procedure has been already introduced as «intrabulbar dissection technique» by Al-Mefty and Teixeira [209]. If there is obvious tumor invasion into the pars nervosa through the medial wall of the JB, it is controversial to leave or remove the tumor. Sanna et al. [226] advocated that it is not advisable to attempt to preserve the anatomic integrity of the LCNs when there is tumor involvement, which usually occurs when the lesion infiltrates the medial wall of the JB. In their experience, dissection of the involved nerves has always resulted in a complete palsy, with the additional risk of leaving some tumor remnants medial to the JF. They concluded that possible dural infiltrations managed conservatively might result in intradural recurrences after some years.

Sen et al. [227] studied the histopathological features of 11 glomus tumors involving the temporal bone, with respect to nerve invasion, associated fibrosis, and carotid artery adventitial invasion. Within the JF, the cranial nerves lie anteromedial to the JB and maintain a multifascicular histoarchitecture. GJTs of the temporal bone can invade the cranial nerve fascicles, and infiltration of these nerves can occur despite a normal function. In these situations, total resection may not be possible without sacrificing these nerves.

Even the patients who underwent gross total resection may have microscopic residual infiltration around the JB. Therefore, a long-time follow-up examination is necessary for such a slow-growing neoplasm to monitor if the residual infiltration may grow.

Radiosurgery

The treatment of GJTs with radiation therapy remains controversial. Conventional radiotherapy has no direct effect on the tumor cells, producing only fibrosis of the vessels supplying tumor. In addition, potentially life-threatening complications like osteoradionecrosis and induction of malignancy have been reported. Stereotactic radiotherapy (SRT) represented by Gamma Knife surgery (GKS) has been proposed as an alternative to surgery in the management of selected GJT patients, with high rate of tumor growth control, preserving or improving clinical status and with limited complications. It has the capability of delivering precise high-dose radiation to a small localized field increasing the changes of obliterating endarteritis while reducing complications by sparing adjacent normal structures. Hafez et al. [215] reported that the tumor progression-free survival in their patients was 95.5% at 5 and 7 years of the follow-up period post GKS.

SRT is suggested mainly for small GJTs confined to the JB. However, it does not seem indicated in large lesions with extensive bone infiltration, where its effects are questionable and the risks of osteoradionecrosis may be comparable to those of conventional radiotherapy. For these reasons, microsurgery remains the preferred treatment modality in most cases, at least in patients with a life expectancy of more than 20 years, even with the risk of recurrence.

SRT would seem to be an effective primary management for local tumor control with limited complications especially to those who do not have significant cranial or cervical extension, elderly, and surgically unfit patients; moreover, it is safe and highly effective as adjuvant therapy as well.

Management of Tumor Recurrences

Although the surgical indication and management of the GJTs are still controversial, a patient's age should be considered the main factor in reducing postoperative rates of morbidity and mortality related to pharyngolaryngeal paralysis. In our experience, young- and middle-aged patients (<60 years old) are candidates for radical tumor resection for the aim of surgical cure. Patients who had postoperative LCN deficits require a prolonged rehabilitation, often accompanied by surgical correction such as thyroplasty or Teflon paste injection of the paralyzed vocal cord. However, they are usually well tolerated. In elderly patients, we should be less aggressive in surgery because LCN palsies are poorly tolerated and should be avoided; if that happens, then consider postoperative radiotherapy.

«Wait and see» policy is also recommended currently only in selected cases, mainly those of elderly patients with intact LCN function. In elderly patients with advanced disease, radiotherapy must be preferred. Size of tumor, age, clinical symptoms, physical condition of the patient, social backgrounds, and cooperation should be considered as well as other skull base neoplasms.

Even patients in which gross total resection was performed may have some residual infiltration around the JB, ICA, or temporal bone in a minority of cases. We have been monitoring these residual tumors in follow-up examinations, and in many of these cases, the tumor shows no growth over a follow-up period of 5–10 years. If we see significant growth, the patient is referred for stereotactic radiotherapy or radiosurgery.

5.8 Pituitary Adenomas

K. Barkas, S. Barazi, and N. Thomas

Clinical manifestations of pituitary adenomas are mainly due to their space-occupying effect or due to endocrine hyper- or hypofunction. Besides ophthalmologic diagnostics, the endocrinological (pre-) therapeutic management plays a central role. Symptomatic pituitary adenomas are usually treated surgically whereupon the endoscopic technique gains more and more importance. Prolactinomas are an exception since they are treated medically in most cases. Radiotherapy is another treatment option after surgery when detecting persistent tumor growth or a recurrent tumor despite medical and surgical therapy. Stereotactic radiosurgery delivers high doses, a high efficacy, and a better comfort for the patient compared to conventional radiotherapy.

5.8.1 General Information

With the wider use of imaging, an increasing number of incidental pituitary adenomas are being identified, many of which require no treatment or intervention. The most common presenting symptoms relate to visual function followed by endocrine dysfunction. MRI can establish the diagnosis with a high degree of certainty.

A multidisciplinary team approach is essential in view of the potential complexity of the endocrinological diagnosis and management of the pituitary adenoma. Surgery should be performed by experienced and appropriately trained subspecialty neurosurgeons and rhinological surgeons.

Epidemiology

The incidence of pituitary tumors is probably the same worldwide, representing between 10% and 15% of all intracranial tumors. Pituitary adenomas are common with a prevalence of 78–94/100,000 and an incidence of 4/100,000 [228]. Depending on the studies of unselected adult autopsy material, their frequency as an incidental finding varies between 5% and 20% [229].

Pathophysiology

Clinical manifestations are mainly due to either mass effect or to endocrine hyper- or hypofunction. With a few exceptions, pituitary adenomas are not under the control of hypothalamic factors.

Multiple oncogene abnormalities may be involved in pituitary tumorigenesis, which is more heterogeneous than formerly thought. The vast majority of these tumors are benign, but certain factors involved in the genesis of the tumor may determine its rate of growth and aggression, with the presence of p53 correlating with more aggressive behavior.

Although the majority of pituitary adenomas are sporadic, approximately 5% of all cases occur in a familial setting, and over half of these are due to multiple endocrine neoplasia Type I (MEN-1) and Carney's complex (CNC) disorders (2). Important genetic causes of familial isolated pituitary adenoma (FIPA) are inactivating mutations or deletions in the aryl hydrocarbon receptor-interacting protein (AIP) gene [230].

Classification

Pathological Classification

The historical classification of adenomas being basophilic, eosinophilic, and chromophobic has been updated taking into consideration electromicroscopic and immunohistochemical analysis. These techniques have identified hormonal production in many chromophobe adenomas, and they have also demonstrated that many are plurihormonal. Functioning tumors are derived from cells of the anterior pituitary gland and can produce adrenocorticotrophic hormone (ACTH), growth hormone (GH), prolactin (PRL), gonadotrophins (FSH and LH), and thyroid-stimulating hormone (TSH). The differential diagnosis of a sellar lesion is wide and is summarized in ◘ Table 5.10.

Functioning Lactotroph Adenomas (PRL)

Functioning lactotroph adenomas are derived from the lactotroph cells of the adenohypophysis and secrete PRL and comprise approximately 50–60% of functioning tumors and around 30% of all adenomas [232, 233]. Most are microadenomas, but when they are macroadenomas, they tend to be more aggressive with possible invasion of the dura and the nasal sinuses [232, 233].

Functioning Somatotroph Adenomas (GH)

They are derived from somatotroph cells, which produce GH, and comprised of approximately 20% of pituitary adenomas [234–236]. They are usually macroadenomas with suprasellar and parasellar extension, but if they are microadenomas, then they are usually demarcated.

5

Table 5.10 Sellar region masses (4)

Tumors of pituitary origin	Metastatic/hematopoietic tumors
Tumors of adenohypophyseal origin	Carcinoma
Pituitary adenoma	Lymphoma
Intrasellar gangliocytoma	Plasmacytoma
Spindle cell oncocytoma	Leukemia
Pituitary carcinoma	Cysts/hamartomas/malformations/vascular
Tumor of neurohypophyseal origin	Rathke's cleft cyst
Pituicytoma (glioma)	Arachnoid cyst
Granular cell tumor	Epidermoid, dermoid, teratomatous cyst
Adenohypophyseal hyperplasia	Hamartomas
Primary nonpituitary tumors	Cavernous hemangioma
Craniopharyngioma	Arteriovenous malformation
Germ cell tumors	Inflammatory conditions
Meningioma	Lymphocytic hypophysitis
Chordoma	Langerhans cell histiocytosis
Gliomas	Sarcoidosis
Schwannoma	Other granulomatous conditions
Paraganglioma	Mucocele
Tumors of mesenchymal origin	Pyogenic/infectious abscess
Sarcomas (osteo-, chondro-, leiomyo-, etc.)	
Solitary fibrous tumors/hemangiopericytoma	
Lipoma	
Chondroma	
Giant cell tumor of the bone	

Functioning Gonadotroph Adenomas (FSH or LH)

Functioning gonadotroph adenomas account for approximately 20% of all adenomas [237]. They are derived from the gonadotroph cells, produce FSH or LH, and are usually large macroadenomas.

Functioning Corticotroph Adenomas (ACTH)

Functioning corticotroph adenomas are derived from corticotroph cells, and they produce ACTH. They comprise approximately 10–15% of pituitary adenomas, and the majority are microadenomas at presentation. There is a female predisposition (ratio 3:1), and they usually occur in the third and fourth decade of life [238, 239].

Functioning Thyrotroph Adenomas (TSH)

Functioning thyrotroph adenomas are derived from thyrotroph cells, and they produce TSH. They are the least common of the secreting tumors (0.5–3%), and they are usually macroadenomas. An inappropriately elevated TSH is identified in the setting of hyperthyroidism, although the patient may be euthyroid or even hypothyroid [240]. TSH-secreting cells are laterally placed in the pituitary, and tumors have a high propensity to become invasive with lateral extension of the tumor. They tend to adopt an aggressive pattern of growth, extend into the suprasellar space, and invade the cavernous sphenoid sinus, and they can be particularly fibrous.

Clinically Nonfunctioning Pituitary Adenomas

They account for approximately 7–14% of all adenomas but up to 30% of the surgically resected ones. The majority of them are identified as silent gonadotroph adenomas (14). Nonfunctioning corticotroph adenomas (ACTH positive) can also be observed and are thought to be more aggressive and are almost always macroadenomas with half of them exhibiting cavernous sinus or bony invasion [241]. Null cell adenomas (NCA) show no immunoreactivity for any pituitary hormone or weak immunoreactivity for beta FSH, beta LH, or alpha subunits and are negative for SF-1. It appears that they form a distinct subgroup within the NFPAs with possibly differing behavioral characteristics [242, 243].

Plurihormonal Pituitary Adenomas

The most common combination is GH and PRL or GH, PRL, and TSH. This is important in the medical management of the tumor as a combination of a somatostatin analogue, and a dopamine agonist may be used for medical control [244].

Atypical Adenoma

Atypical adenomas are characterized by an elevated Ki67 (>3%) and overexpression of p53 on immunohistochemistry [245], and they tend to have a more aggressive natural history requiring closer clinical observation.

Pituitary Carcinoma

Pituitary carcinoma is defined as a tumor that has metastasized, either by the cerebrospinal pathway or systemically. They are very rare, most commonly seen with secreting tumors (mainly prolactin and ACTH), and the Ki67 and expression of p53 are often elevated. Of note is that the invasiveness of a tumor in the adjacent structures is not considered a criterion of malignancy. Pituitary carcinomas carry a very poor prognosis [245, 246].

Pituicytoma

Pituicytomas arise from pituicytes, which are glial cells located in the neurohypophysis. The recently described spindle cell oncocytoma and the granular cell tumor of the pituitary appear to be variants of pituicytoma [247].

Surgical Classification

From a surgical point of view, pituitary tumors can be divided based on size into microadenomas (<1 cm diameter) and macroadenomas (>1 cm diameter).

5.8.2 Clinical Presentation and Syndromes

The clinical presentation of a pituitary adenoma can fall in one of three categories:

- Compression/invasion of adjacent neurovascular structures including apoplexy and CSF leak
- Hyper- or hyposecretion of hormones
- Incidental finding

Compression/Invasion of Adjacent Structures

The majority of the patients present with bitemporal hemianopia and/or visual acuity loss relating to chiasmatic compression. An early ophthalmological sign is impairment of color vision. At the same time, the majority of tumors are nonfunctioning and therefore do not exhibit secretion of any hormone. Ophthalmoplegia with diplopia and ptosis may occur when a tumor has undergone apoplexy. This does not necessarily denote invasion of the cavernous sinus. If cranial nerve palsies are a presenting feature and there is absence of apoplexy, one should be suspicious of cavernous sinus invasion with an atypical adenoma where the clinical picture may be more sinister. Compression of the dura, especially in the context of acute expansion, as in apoplexy, can cause headaches. Rarely the presentation can be that of a CSF rhinorrhea from extension into the sphenoid sinus. There are case reports with large macroadenomas presenting with symptoms of hydrocephalus with compression of the foramina of Monro or even proptosis [248].

Hyper- or Hyposecretion of Hormone

The term panhypopituitarism refers to the deficiency of several anterior pituitary hormones. If diabetes insipidus is a presenting feature, one should suspect a diagnosis other than an adenoma such as a craniopharyngioma or hypophysitis. Excessive secretion of prolactin can cause galactorrhoea even if it relates to stalk effect with a nonfunctioning adenoma. See ◘ Table 5.11 for a summary of the clinical manifestations.

Incidental Finding: The Incidentaloma

This is now a common phenomenon with the increasing availability of MR and CT imaging. Both micro- and macroadenomas may be found. A recent observational study of conservatively managed patients showed that those with macroadenomas were identified to have a cumulative probability of enlargement at 4 years' observation of 44%; the vast majority of the macroadenomas with an increase in size had chiasmatic involvement with or without visual field defects. In contrast patients with microadenoma have a small probability of tumor growth (19% at 4 years), which is not associated with visual compromise.

Table 5.11 Deficiency

Hormone	Oversecretion		Undersecretion	
GH	*Adults* Acromegaly: Changes in the size of the hand and feet Frontal bossing Prognathism Changes in voice Hirsutism Glucose intolerance (1/5 will progress to DM) Obstructive sleep apnea Cardiomyopathy Myopathy (→weakness) Carpal tunnel syndrome Lumbar canal stenosis Arthritis Colonic polyps	*Children* Gigantism	*Adults* Obesity Hypercholesterolemia Higher rate of cardiovascular disease Reduced muscle strength and exercise capacity	*Infants* Hypoglycemia *Children* Reduced growth rate Decreased height
Prolactin	*Men* Hypogonadism Decreased libido Impotence Galactorrhea (rare)	*Women* Hypogonadism Amenorrhea Galactorrhea Infertility		
TSH	Hyperthyroidism		Malaise Weight gain Lack of energy Cold intolerance Constipation	
FSH-LH	Not associated with a clinical syndrome		*Men:* Diminished libido and impotence; testes shrink in size (spermatogenesis generally preserved) *Women:* Diminished libido and dyspareunia, breast atrophy (if chronic deficiency) *Children:* Delayed puberty (or even absence)	
ACTH	Cushing's: Weight gain Centripetal obesity and moon face Violet striae in the skin, pigmentation Easy bruising Proximal myopathy Mood changes up to psychiatric Arterial hypertension Diabetes mellitus Cataracts Glaucoma Osteoporosis Libido disturbance		Weight loss Lack of energy Malaise Severe adrenal insufficiency	

Therefore, the authors conclude that the «watch and wait» policy seems reasonable for microadenomas but is probably not a safe approach for adenomas measuring ≥1 cm [249].

Pituitary Apoplexy

Pituitary apoplexy is a clinical syndrome, characterized by sudden onset of headache, vomiting, visual impairment, and decreased consciousness caused by hemorrhage and/or infarction of the pituitary gland. It usually occurs in patients with preexisting pituitary adenomas and evolves within hours or days. This is often associated with profound biochemical imbalance (particularly hyponatremia relating to hypocortisolemia) necessitating urgent administration of intravenous hydrocortisone. The major source of mortality associated with pituitary apoplexy is the acute secondary adrenal insufficiency, which can be present in up to two-thirds of the patients. The frequency of subclinical hemorrhagic infarction is around 25%, but this does not constitute a diagnosis of pituitary apoplexy.

The Society for Endocrinology has published the UK guidelines for the management of pituitary apoplexy, an effort that has contributed significantly in the treatment of this entity as well as in understanding that it is a medical emergency [250]. Pituitary apoplexy can be precipitated by multiple factors which are summarized in ► Box 5.1.

Box 5.1: Precipitating Factors of Pituitary apoplexy

Hypertension
Major surgery (especially coronary artery bypass)
Dynamic testing of the pituitary gland with GnRH, TRH, and CRH
Anticoagulation therapy
Coagulopathies
Initiation or withdrawal of dopamine receptor agonists
Estrogen therapy
Radiation therapy
Pregnancy
Head trauma

Patients with reduced visual acuity, persistent or deteriorating visual field defects, or deteriorating level of consciousness may require surgical intervention after being medically stabilized. Ophthalmoplegia due to involvement of cranial nerves III, IV, or VI, in the absence of visual field defects or visual acuity reduction, is not in itself an indication for immediate surgery. In our series, we have seen cases with rapid resolution of the ophthalmoplegia when operated promptly, and our advice is for expeditious surgery as soon as it is safe.

Visual acuity, visual field defects, and ophthalmoplegia have been reported to improve in the majority of the patients after surgical decompression but are less likely in patients presenting with monocular or binocular blindness. The latter is by no means a contraindication to urgent surgery as significant improvement has been observed in patients rendered blind by pituitary apoplexy if early surgical decompression is undertaken.

Nearly 80% of the patients will need some form of hormone replacement with GH being the most commonly deficient although not always requiring replacement. Long-term hormone replacement therapy following pituitary apoplexy includes corticosteroids in 60–80%, thyroid hormone in 50–60%, and desmopressin in 10–25% of patients and testosterone in 60–80% of men.

The proposed algorithm for the management of pituitary apoplexy is summarized in ◘ Fig. 5.113.

Conservatively managed patients need to be closely monitored. The pituitary apoplexy score is a tool for this monitoring and can help quantify the neuro-ophthalmological deficits and audit the outcome in surgically and conservatively managed patients (◘ Table 5.12).

5.8.3 Investigations and Preoperative Work-Up

Radiographic Evaluation

The primary imaging modality in the evaluation of the pituitary gland is MRI. Dedicated pituitary high-resolution MRI with and without contrast should be obtained so that primarily isointense lesions do not escape detection [251].

CT can be used when MRI is contraindicated or when identification of bony anatomy or calcification is required. We perform a thin slice CT scan in all of our reoperations and frequently use image guidance (◘ Fig. 5.114).

There is great variability in the dimensions of the pituitary gland. Elster's rule (24) can be used as a rule of thumb; as measured in the coronal

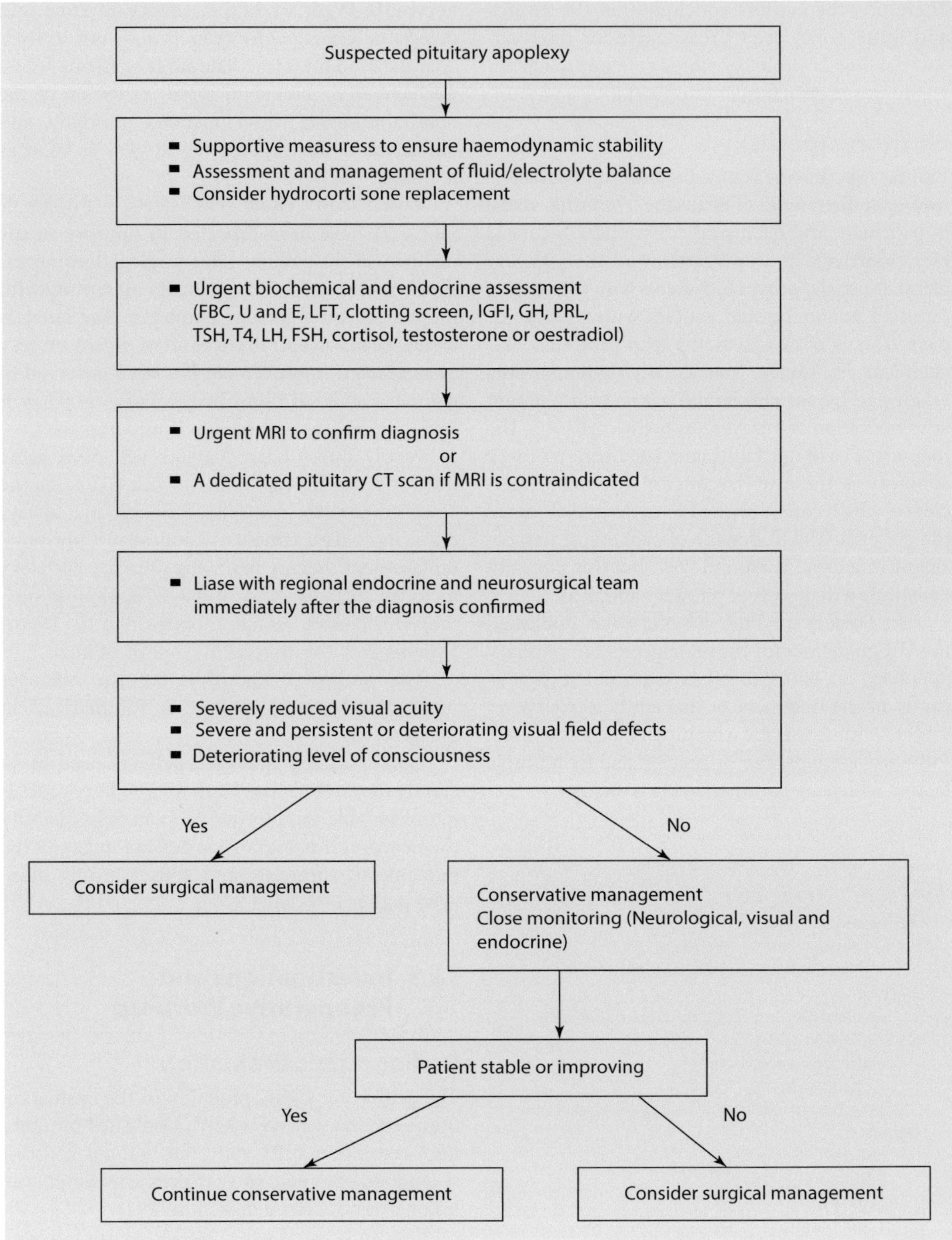

Fig. 5.113 Algorithm for the management of pituitary apoplexy (Rajasekaran et al. [250], © 2010 Blackwell Publishing Ltd)

Table 5.12 Pituitary apoplexy score

Pituitary apoplexy score	
Variable	*Points*
Level of consciousness	0
GCS 15	2
GCS 8–14	4
GCS <8	
Visual acuity	0
Normal [a] 6/6	1
Reduced–unilateral	2
Bilateral	
Visual field deficits	0
Normal	1
Unilateral defect	2
Bilateral defect	
Ocular paresis	0
Absent	1
Present–unilateral	2
Bilateral	

[a]No change from premorbid visual acuity

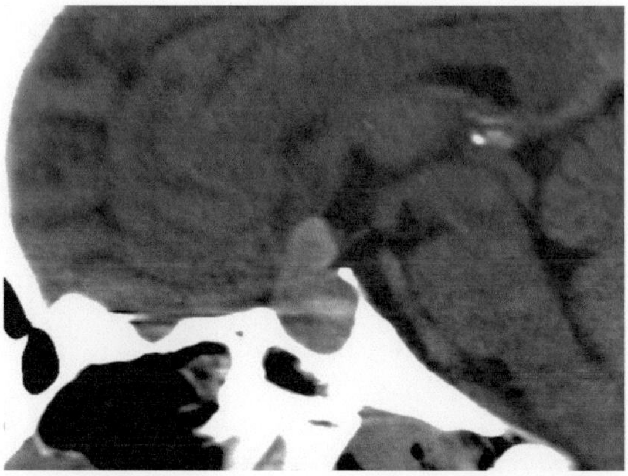

Fig. 5.114 Conchal type of sphenoid sinus. The use of CT and neuronavigation is of great importance for preoperative planning. Note the macroadenoma with suprasellar extension

plane, the height of the gland is 6 mm in infants and children, 8 mm in men and postmenopausal women, 10 mm in women in childbearing age, and 12 mm in pregnancy and postpartum. A normal stalk is less than 4 mm thick. The adenohypophysis is usually isointense and the neurohypophysis uniformly hyperintense on T1-weighted images. Stalk deviation has a high incidence in the normal population and therefore should not be used to support or refute the presence of a microadenoma.

Most microadenomas are hypointense on T1-weighted images. The minority that are isointense are usually evident in the gadolinium-enhanced studies. The majority of microadenomas are enhanced less compared to the normal gland post-Gd administration (Figs. 5.115, 5.116, 5.117, 5.118, and 5.119).

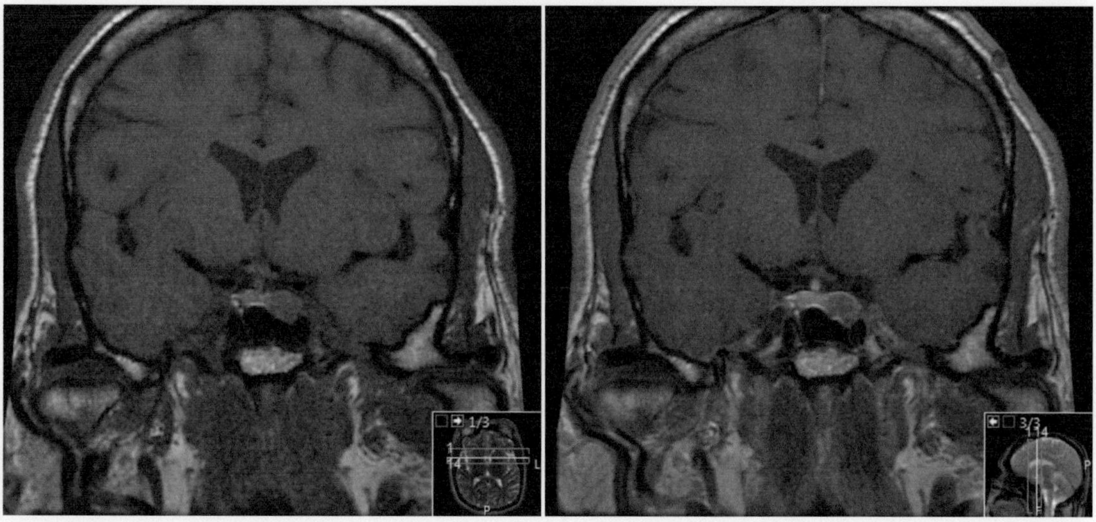

Fig. 5.115 Coronal T1-weighted pre- and post-Gd. Note the enhancement of the normal pituitary gland that makes the adenoma more obvious

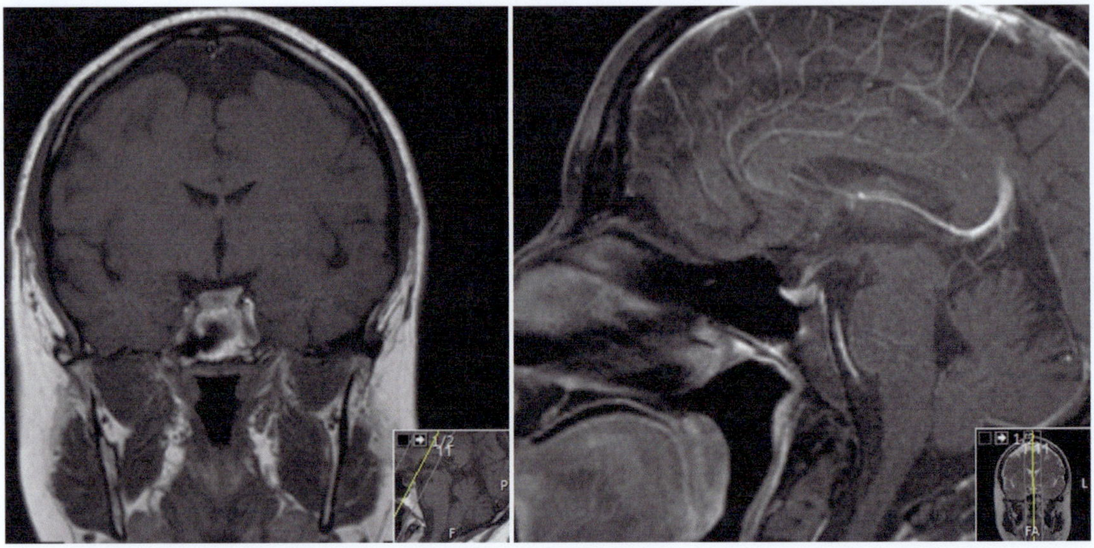

Fig. 5.116 Coronal and sagittal T1-weighted post-Gd. Small hypointensity in the posterior aspect of the pituitary gland, proven to be ACTH-secreting microadenoma

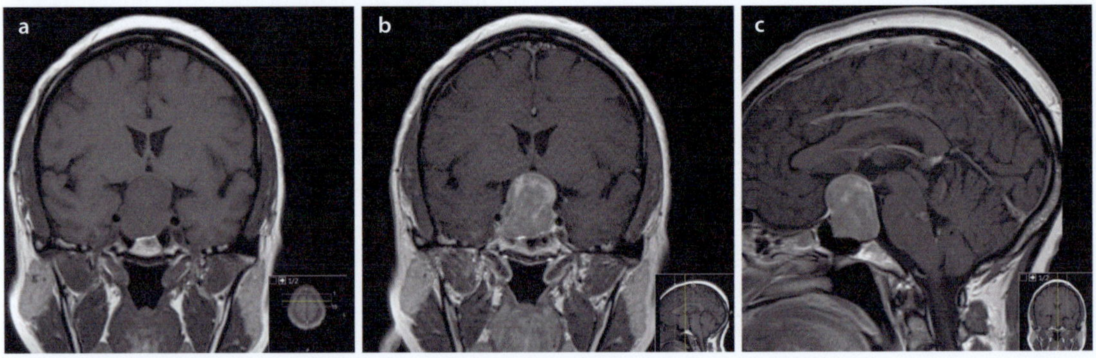

Fig. 5.117 Coronal T1-weighted and coronal and sagittal T1-wighted post-Gd: macroadenoma with suprasellar extension. Note the «snowman sign» from the constriction produced by the diaphragma sellae

The Hardy and Knosp classifications identify tumor extension beyond the confines of the sella and are particularly useful in assessing the likelihood of cure of invasive functioning adenomas (Fig. 5.120) [252, 253]. Despite the high frequency of cavernous sinus invasion, constriction of the ICA is very uncommon. This would be a finding favoring the diagnosis of a meningioma.

Anatomical variations such as a tortious carotid artery need to be identified preoperatively to avoid carotid injury (Fig. 5.121). The differential diagnosis of a sellar mass is extensive, and collaboration with a neuroradiologist is of outmost importance (Figs. 5.122 and 5.123).

Preoperative Endocrine Evaluation and Treatment

Close collaboration with endocrinologists is essential, and the preoperative evaluation is of great importance. In all macroadenomas, a PRL should be urgently obtained, even when there is significant visual compromise as a macroprolactinoma can rapidly diminish in size with improvement in visual fields on dopamine agonist therapy.

The adrenal and thyroid axes should be checked to ensure adequacy, because untreated adrenal insufficiency or hypothyroidism can be potentially life threatening in the perioperative period. Equally important is to ensure that

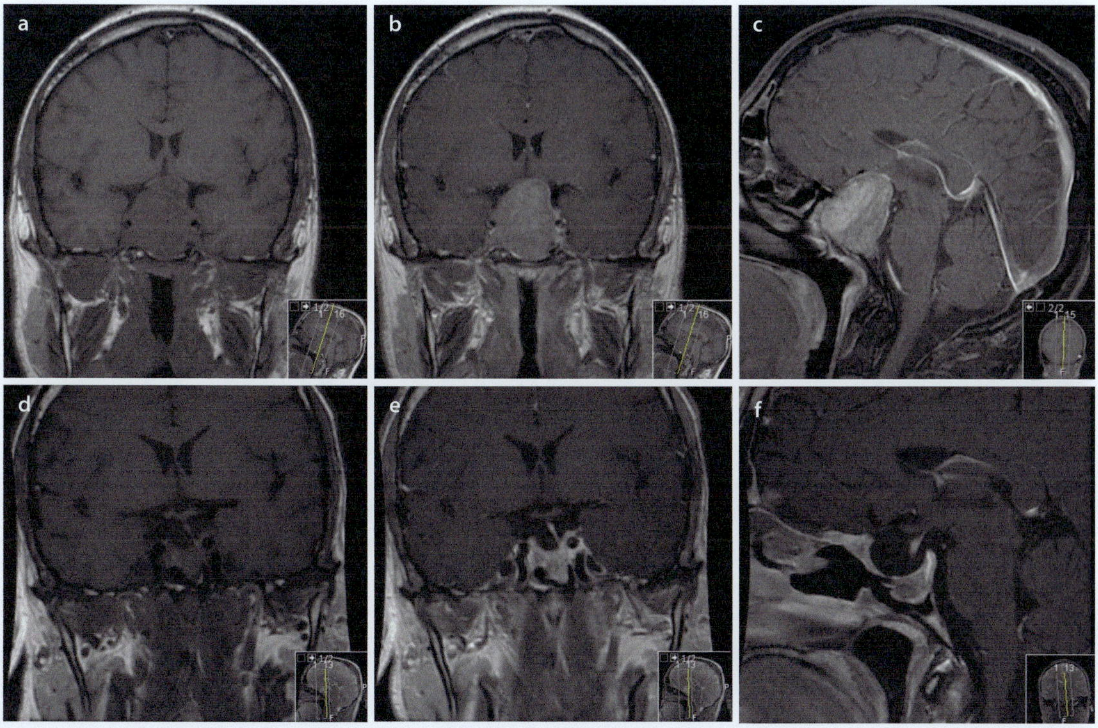

Fig. 5.118 Pre **a**, **b**, **c** and post-op **d**, **e**, **f** MRI images of a macroadenoma with cavernous sinus extension on the right

patients with uncontrolled hyperthyroidism due to a TSH-secreting tumor are treated prior to surgery, as they are at risk of a thyroid storm perioperatively, which is associated with increased mortality [231].

Cushing's Disease

The diagnosis of Cushing's disease can prove to be challenging. When assessing Cushing's disease, the endocrinologist aims to establish a clear diagnosis of a pituitary ACTH-dependent source. Inferior petrosal sinus sampling (IPSS) is often needed. This can be extremely helpful in diagnosing Cushing's disease where there is a greater than 2:1 central to peripheral gradient of measured ACTH after the administration of intravenous CRH. Care should be taken when interpreting lateralization of the lesion as the intercavernous sinuses allow for bilateral venous drainage of the pituitary gland. MRI of the pituitary may identify heterogeneity of the gland that may not represent an adenoma. When the MRI is positive, it is superior to IPSS in determining the intrapituitary location of an adenoma. When the MRI shows no clear adenoma, IPSS can be used to guide the initial gland exploration when there is a significant difference in the gradient on one side but cannot be used to guide hemihypophysectomy. In such case, the entire pituitary gland must be thoroughly explored since up to 31% of patients would harbor an untreated ACTH-secreting adenoma within the remaining gland if it were left unexplored [254].

Regarding the indication for pretreating Cushing's disease prior to operation, there is no consensus. In one series, results suggest that effective normalization of cortisol preoperatively is not associated with earlier normalization of hypocortisolism postoperatively but seems to be associated with a better long-term remission [255]. The pathophysiological hypothesis is that by regaining tissue eucortisolism preoperatively, there is reduction in intraoperative bleeding with improved intrasellar vision that may facilitate complete adenoma resection, thereby increasing the chance of both low postoperative cortisol and long-term remission.

In our department, we have started 3 months' pretreatment with blockade in those patients suffering from severe Cushing's disease where tissues are of poor quality. In our experience, operative conditions are more favorable with less bleeding,

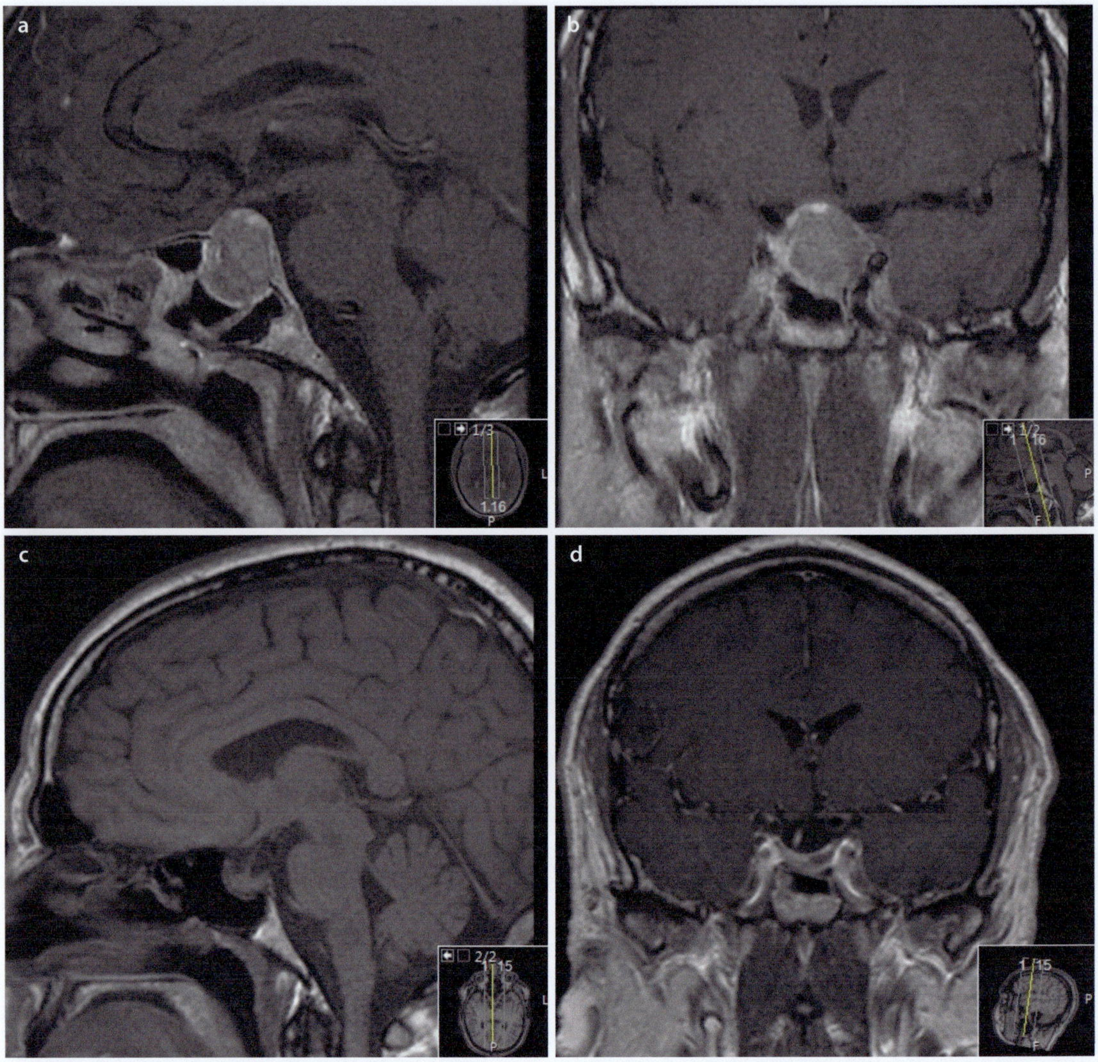

Fig. 5.119 Pre **a**, **b** and post-op **c**, **d** MRI images of a macroadenoma. There is expansion of the bony sella and a heterogeneously enhancing T1 intermediate intrasellar/suprasellar lesion. The pituitary infundibulum is displaced to the right, and there is impingement on the optic chiasm and prechiasmatic segment of the optic nerves. There is no obvious parasellar extension **a**, **b**. Resection of the sellar/suprasellar mass and the chiasm is no longer compressed. The stalk is deviated to the right side. There is a small amount of poorly enhancing non-specific tissue within the left side of the sella. This was a silent gonadotroph adenoma

and if a CSF leak is encountered, a repair has a far greater chance of being successful.

Postoperatively the patients usually require replacement therapy for 6–24 months, because it takes several months for the hypothalamic–pituitary–adrenal axis to recover.

Acromegaly

The incidence of acromegaly is approximately three per million, with no sex predilection. Patients with acromegaly are at significant risk of morbidity and mortality compared to age-matched population [236].

Pretreatment with a somatostatin analogue (SA) has been debated, but it is not supported by the current literature as a standard practice. However, «for an individual patient with advanced metabolic, cardiovascular and respiratory dysfunction SA pretreatment may help in reducing perioperative morbidity.» The pathophysiological mechanism is considered to be the improvement of the state of the soft tissues relating to the airways (reducing

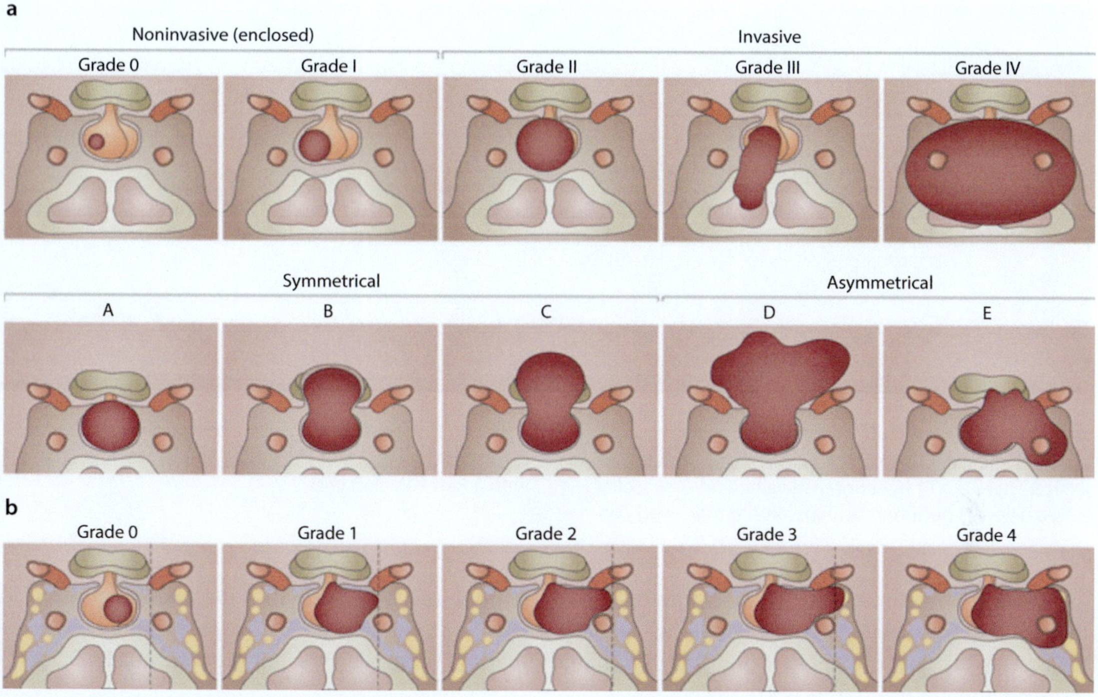

Fig. 5.120 **a** *Hardy classification system*. Sella turcica tumors can be noninvasive (grade 0, intact with normal contour; grade 1, intact with bulging floor; or grade 2, intact, enlarged fossa) or invasive (grade 3, localized sellar destruction; or grade 4, diffuse destruction). Suprasellar tumors can be symmetrical (grade A, suprasellar cistern only; grade B, recess of the third ventricle; or grade C, whole anterior third ventricle) or asymmetrical (grade D, intracranial extradural; or grade E, extracranial extradural [cavernous sinus]). **b** *Knosp classification system* used to quantify invasion of the cavernous sinus, in which only grades 3 and 4 define true invasion of the tumor into the cavernous sinus. Grade 0, no cavernous sinus involvement; grades 1 and 2, the tumor pushes into the medial wall of the cavernous sinus but does not go beyond a hypothetical line extending between the centers of the two segments of the internal carotid artery (grade 1), or it goes beyond such a line but without passing a line tangent to the lateral margins of the artery itself (grade 2); grade 3, the tumor extends laterally to the internal carotid artery within the cavernous sinus; grade 4, total encasement of the intracavernous carotid artery (26)

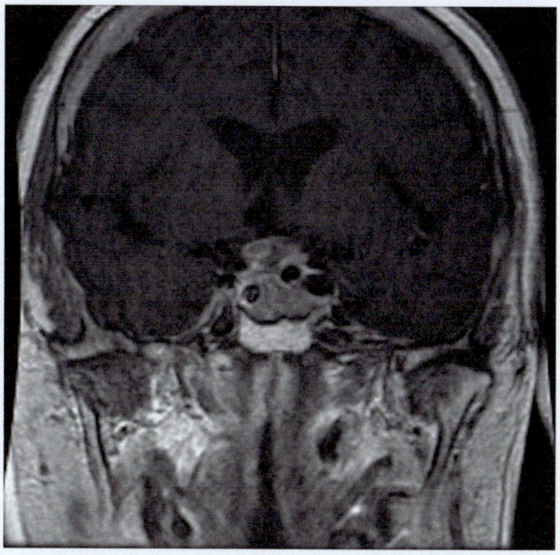

Fig. 5.121 Coronal T1-weighted post-Gd. Note the «kissing carotids.» Identification of this anatomical variation is of outmost importance in order to avoid carotid injury

postoperative respiratory complications), reduction of the blood pressure, and improvement of the cardiological physiology. If decided to do so, then patients should be pretreated for 3–6 months, with 3 months probably being sufficient when a high-dose SA loading regimen is employed from the outset [256]. In addition, prior knowledge that the tumor responds biochemically and anatomically to a somatostatin analogue is useful in case medical therapy is required postoperatively.

Prolactinomas

Despite an equal distribution between men and women, women are more likely to be symptomatic, and they can be challenging to treat during pregnancy. Only 1.4% of patients with microadenomas develop visual abnormalities during pregnancy, but this can be as high as 16% in patients with macroadenomas.

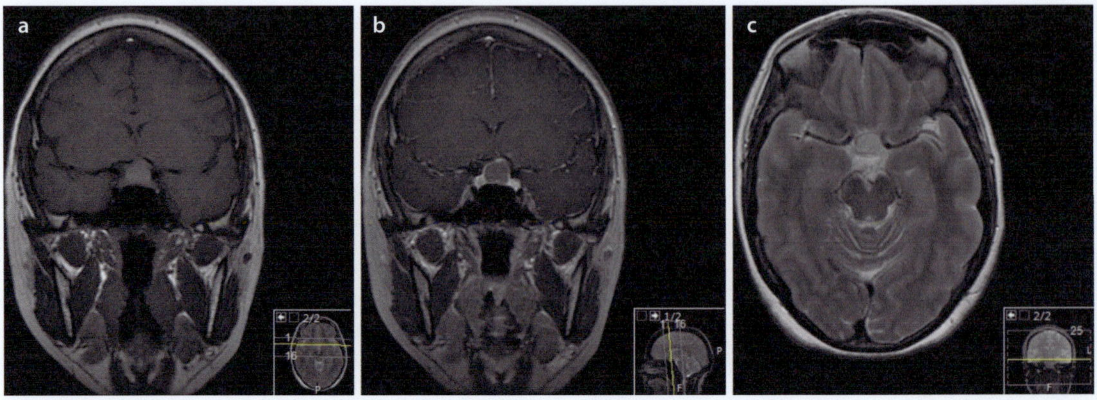

Fig. 5.122 Coronal T1-weighted pre **a** and post **b** contrast and axial T2-weighted **c**. The bony sella is normal in size. There is a T1 hyperintense sellar and suprasellar lesion. There is peripheral enhancement following contrast application. The suprasellar component abuts and displaces the optic chiasm. Appearances are in keeping with a Rathke's cleft cyst

Dopamine agonists are the first line of treatment for normalization of prolactin as well as tumor shrinkage. Indications for surgery have reduced and are limited to [257, 258]:

- Failed medical management
- Intolerable side effects
- Adjuvant therapy that provides cytoreduction to facilitate the effects of medical therapy
- Persistent chiasmal compression despite optimal medical therapy
- Medically unresponsive cystic prolactinoma
- In women seeking fertility, macroadenoma in close proximity to optic chiasm despite optimal medical therapy (prepregnancy debulking)
- Apoplexy
- Cerebrospinal fluid leak during administration of a dopamine agonist

Relative indications are:

- Female patients that want to get pregnant
- Patients with psychiatric background (dopamine agonist therapy may induce psychotic episodes)

FSH–LH Secreting

The diagnosis is usually made on assessment of the preoperative biochemistry, especially since the excessive secretion of FSH and LH is not associated with a clinical syndrome.

TSH Secreting

An inappropriately elevated TSH is identified in the setting of hyperthyroidism, although the patient may be euthyroid or even hypothyroid [240]. As mentioned before, thyroid axis abnormalities should be treated preoperatively.

Aims of Operation

Major goals are to protect vision, control hormonal hypersecretion, and symptom improvement. In hormone-secreting tumors, the aim is to achieve cure/long-term control, and sometimes sacrifice of the entire pituitary gland has to be considered. Preexisting hypopituitarism very rarely resolves.

Consenting the Patient

A detailed discussion with the patient should take place with a neurosurgeon and an endocrinologist and sometimes an oncologist being present (Table 5.13).

Moffett's Solution

Major Arthur James Moffett of the Royal Army Medical Corps published in 1941 the solution that has been synonymous with nasal preparation. There is variance in its preparation and use. In our daily practice, we use 1 ml of 10% cocaine (100 mg), 1 ml of 1:1000 adrenaline (1 mg), 2 ml of 8.4% w/v sodium bicarbonate, and 6 ml of 0.9% normal saline. Ten 4 cm patties soaked in the solution are applied in both nostrils for at least 20′. The pathophysiological mechanism behind its use has been summarized excellently by Benjamin et al. and is shown in the table [260].

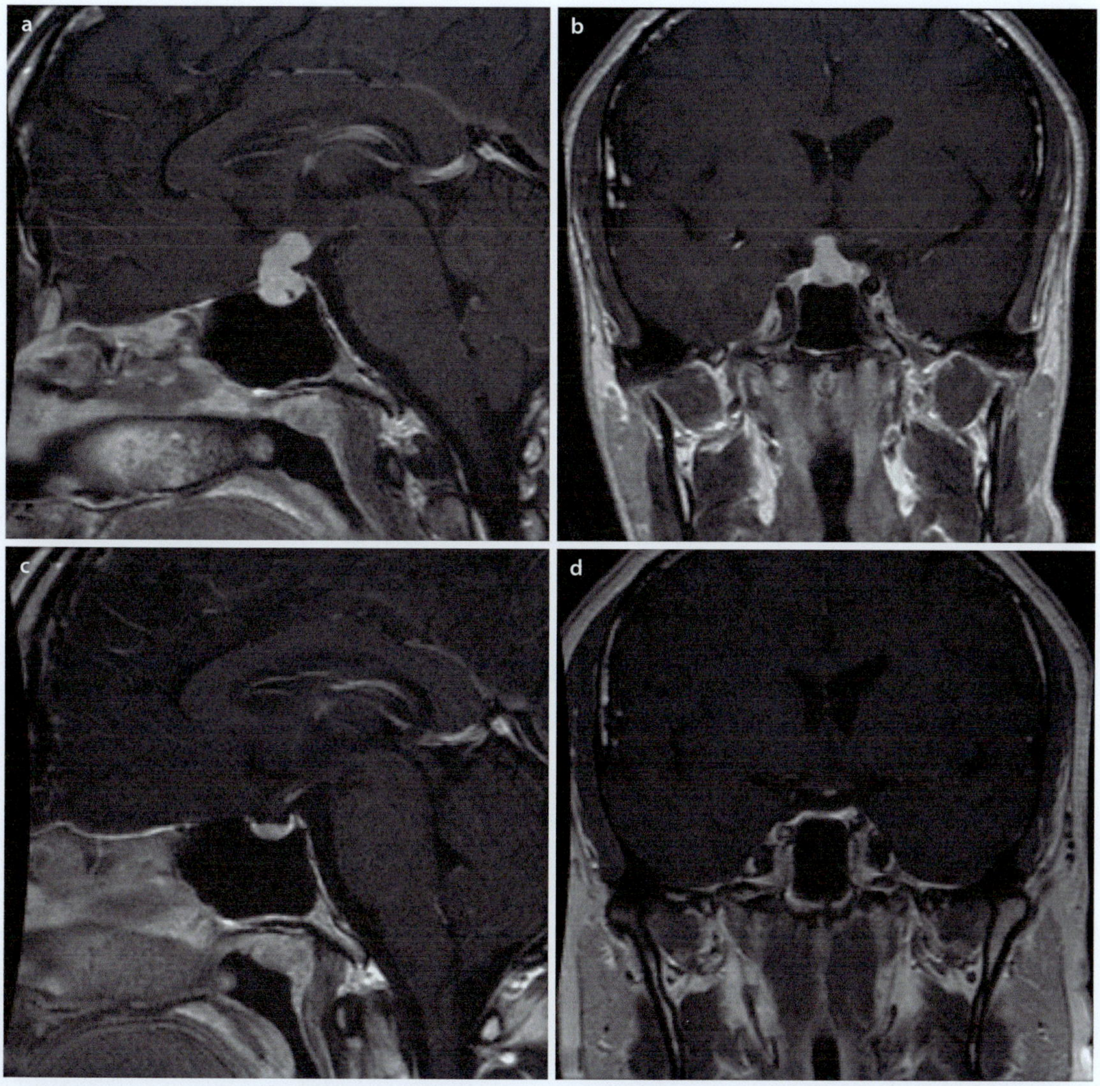

Fig. 5.123 **a, b** There is a homogenously enhancing intrasellar and suprasellar mass with expansion of the infundibulum. There is loss of the pituitary bright spot. The sella is not expanded. The mass has a broad point of contact with the optic chiasm, which is slightly elevated centrally. The imaging features are most in keeping with a hypophysitis. **c, d** Histology of peripheral lymph node confirmed sarcoid. Images 1 year posttreatment with steroids

Anesthetic Considerations

The preoperative assessment is crucial, especially in patients with acromegaly and Cushing's disease where obesity, cardiomyopathy, difficult airway, sleep apnea, and hypertension are common. If a patient suffers from preexisting sleep apnea, then we will opt for an overnight stay in the high dependency unit. It is of great importance that hyperthyroidism is controlled prior to surgery. All of our patients have a group and are screened, but we do not routinely crossmatch units of blood.

Standard oral endotracheal intubation is used. We routinely use a throat pack, in order to prevent efflux of blood and operative debris in the stomach. It is preferable to secure all the oral tubes to the left lower lip and cheek, as the surgeon will stand on the patient's right side. The eyes are carefully taped and closed and ten size 4 patties soaked in Moffett's solution are gently inserted in both nostrils. An arterial line is inserted, and intraoperatively we aim for a systolic blood pressure of <90 mmHg, for reduction in mucosal oozing, provided this is

5

Table 5.13 Complications to be discussed with patients preoperatively

Possible complications to be discussed with the patients preoperatively	
Type	**Manifestation**
Neurologic	CSF leak Meningitis Impaired visual acuity including blindness Ophthalmoparesis resulting in double vision Stroke Death
Endocrine	Diabetes insipidus Panhypopituitarism (necessitating lifelong replacement therapy)
Sino-nasal	Sinus congestion/sinusitis Reduced/altered smell Septal perforation Epistaxis
Failure to control hormonal overproduction	
Recurrence	

Adapted from Schwartz et al. [259]

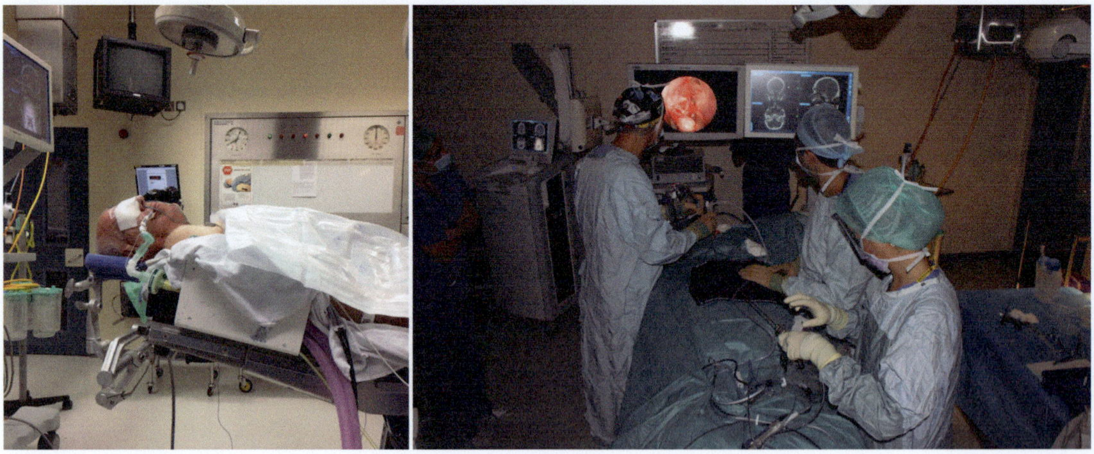

Fig. 5.124 Patient's head is elevated 30° to allow venous drainage. Surgeon and assistant are standing either side of the patient, anesthetic machine is at the patient's feet, and endoscopic stalk and neuronavigation screen are side by side

safe for the patient. Adequate intravenous access is important because of the rare occurrence of abrupt hemorrhage. A single dose of co-amoxiclav for antimicrobial cover is used, and we always administer 100 mg of hydrocortisone. We do not routinely insert a urinary catheter. Postoperative pain relief and regular use of antiemetics are extremely important for patient's comfort as well as for protection of the repair in cases of CSF leak.

Positioning

The patient is placed supine with the head resting on a horseshoe and up 30°, to facilitate venous drainage, with a degree of extension. Placing the head on a horseshoe and avoiding rigid fixation have the advantage of being able to move the head during the case in order to improve exposure. The patient is then rotated so that the anesthetic equipment is at the patient's feet (Fig. 5.124).

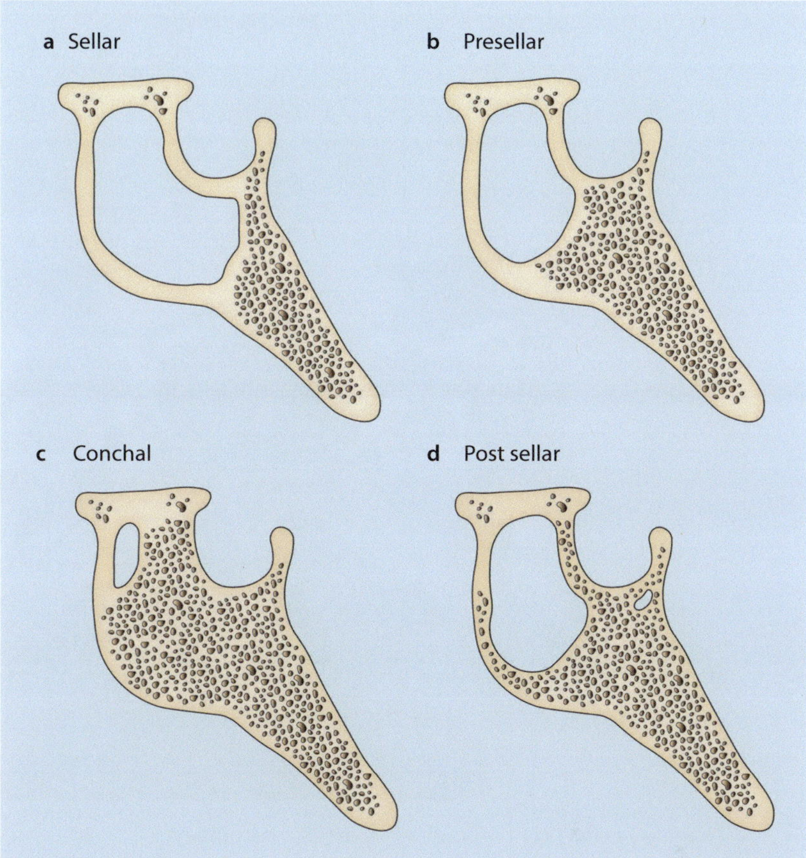

Fig. 5.125 Classification of the sphenoid sinus according to pneumatization. The sellar (A)represents 80% of the cases, the presellar 17%, and the conchal 3%. The postsellar type is not of great clinical significance. We advocate use of image guidance in the conchal type

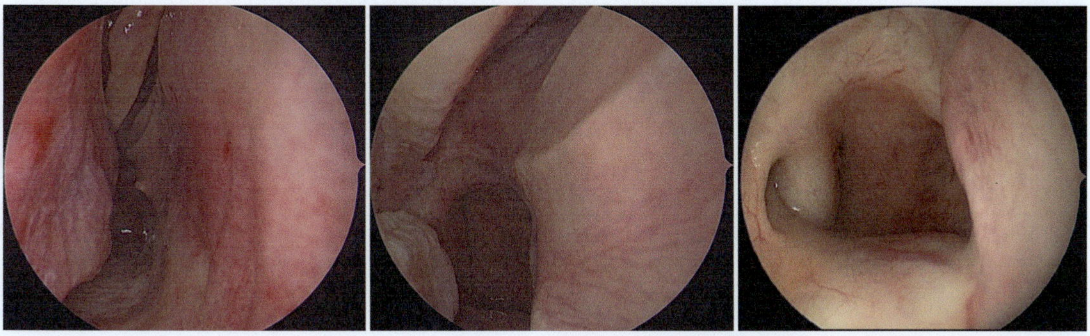

Fig. 5.126 Inferior and middle turbinates and choana identified. The sphenoid ostium is located in the anterosuperior aspect of the anterior sphenoid sinus wall and approximately 1.5 cm superior to the choana. The choana, the exit of the Eustachian tube, and the fossa of Rosenmuller should be inspected

Anatomy Pearls

Pneumatization of the sphenoid sinus is classified into sellar (80%), presellar (17%), and conchal (3%), and image guidance is strongly advised in the conchal type (Fig. 5.125).

The entrance in the sphenoid sinus will be achieved by identifying the sphenoid ostium. This is located in the anterosuperior aspect of the anterior sphenoid sinus wall and approximately 1.5 cm superior to the choanae. It is adjacent to the posterior tip of the middle turbinate and the inferior edge of the superior turbinate. The sphenopalatine artery runs in the inferolateral corner of the sphenoid sinus (Figs. 5.126, 5.127, 5.130,

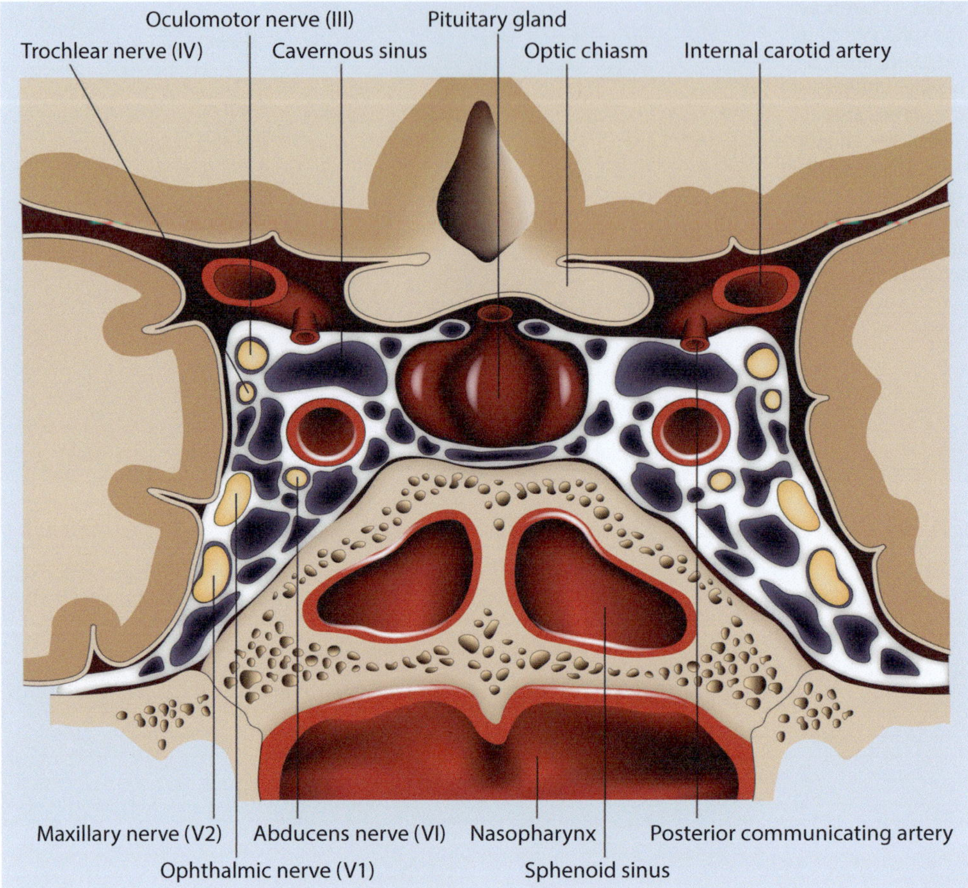

Fig. 5.127 Anatomy of the cavernous sinus. Note the intercavernous sinus, which can be a cause of significant bleeding. The intercavernous sinus should be coagulated and then divided in order to avoid bleeding. The abducens nerve, traveling within the cavernous sinus, is more often spared in the event of ophthalmoparesis from cavernous sinus involvement

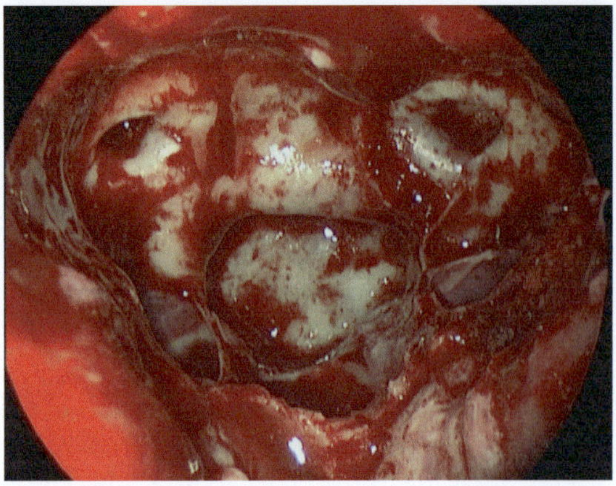

Fig. 5.128 Pituitary fossa, carotid pillars, and medial opticocarotid recess identified. The sphenoid septae are usually ending at the carotid pillars, and care should be taken not to fracture them as this can cause inadvertent carotid injury. Careful drilling is preferable

5.131, 5.132, 5.133, 5.134, 5.135, 5.136, 5.137 and 5.138).

An anatomical variation that is present in 7–25% of the patients is the so-called Onodi cell. This represents a pneumatization of a posterior ethmoid cell into the sphenoid sinus, and it may distort the identification of the true sphenoid sinus. The optic nerve passes in the lateral wall of the cell making it important to recognize preoperatively.

The carotid artery lies directly against the lateral wall of the sphenoid sinus forming the two carotid pillars (Figs. 5.126 and 5.129). The bone covering the carotid artery or the optic nerve is less than 0.5 mm in almost 90% and 80% of the patients, respectively. In up to 10% of patients, the bone separating the carotid artery from the sphenoid sinus may be missing, and the sphenoid mucosa rests directly on the internal

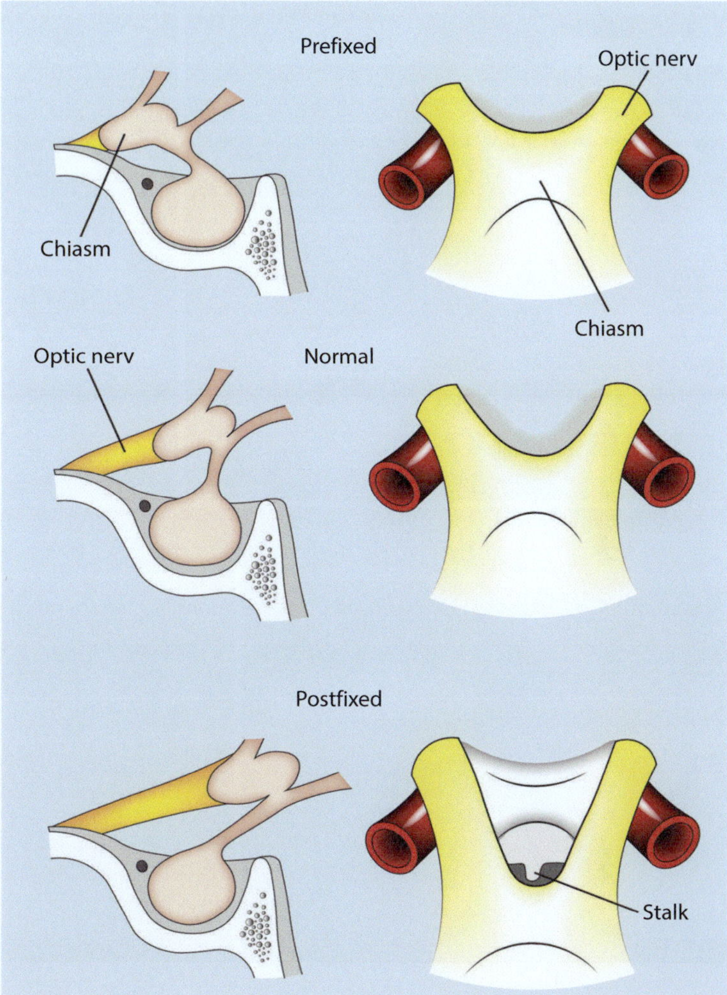

Fig. 5.129 Relationship of the optic chiasm in relation to the pituitary gland and infundibulum. This is defined as normal when it is above the diaphragm and pituitary gland (~70%), prefixed when it is above the tuberculum sellae (~15%) and postfixed chiasm when it is above the dorsum sella (~15%). This anatomical relationship is important in extended transsphenoidal procedures and even more so in the subfrontal approaches

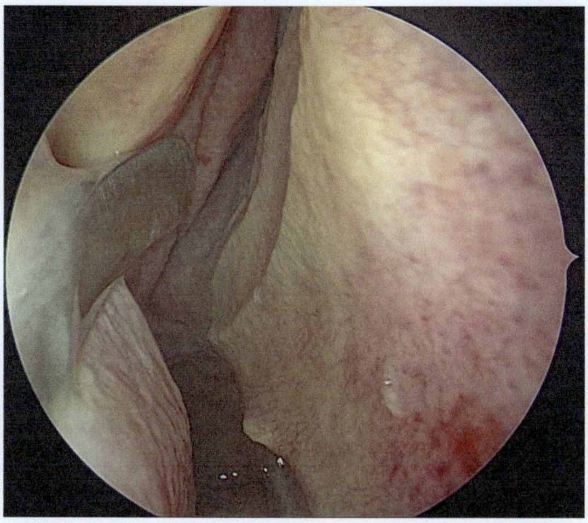

Fig. 5.130 Medial turbinate is outfractured using the Freer elevator along the entire length of the turbinate so that it is outfractured in one movement

carotid artery dehiscence. Optic nerve dehiscence can be found in up to 20% of patients.

The lateral opticocarotid recess corresponds to the optic strut and anterior clinoid process intracranially. It is bounded superomedially by the optic canal and inferomedially by the carotid protuberance; N. III is also found inferiorly within the confines of this recess.

The medial opticocarotid recess corresponds to the lateral aspect of the tuberculum sellae. It is bounded superolaterally by the optic canal and inferolaterally by the carotid protuberance. It corresponds with the medial clinoid intracranially and represents the space medial to the junction between the optic nerve and the carotid arteries.

The medial walls of the cavernous sinuses are usually separated from the pituitary gland by a single layer of dura. There are several venous

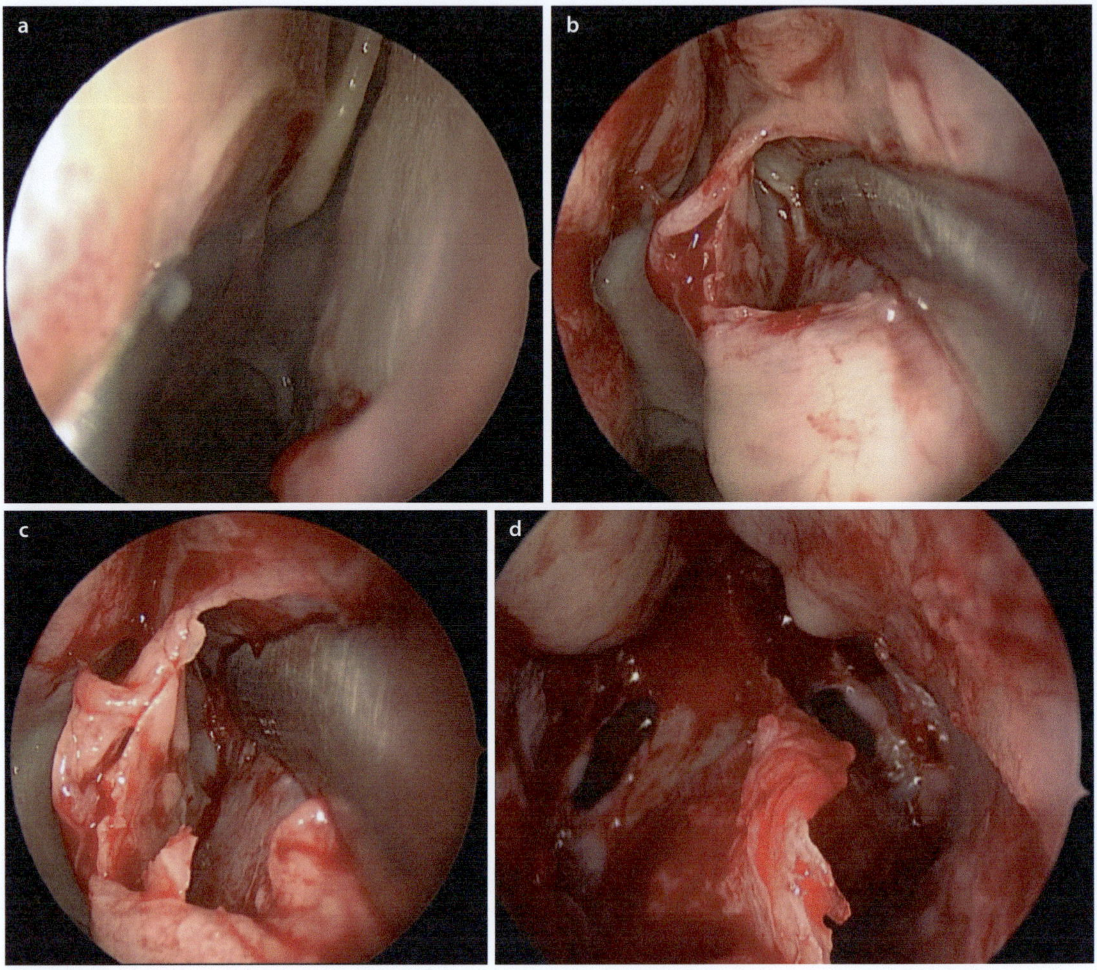

Fig. 5.131 The ostium is sometimes not easily identifiable, as it can be obstructed by a superior or supreme turbinate **a**. In such cases, we fracture the junction of the cartilaginous septum and the vomer **b**, and with a submucosal dissection, we find the contralateral ostium **c**. Identification of both ostia is important. The vomer will always be the landmark for midline **d**

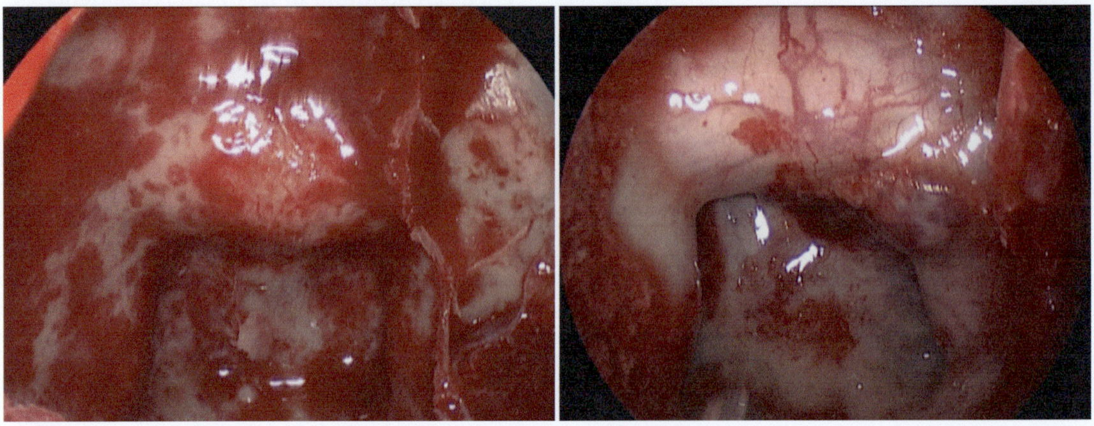

Fig. 5.132 Identifying the carotid pillars and the clival recess is extremely important. Tumor can sometimes erode the fossa

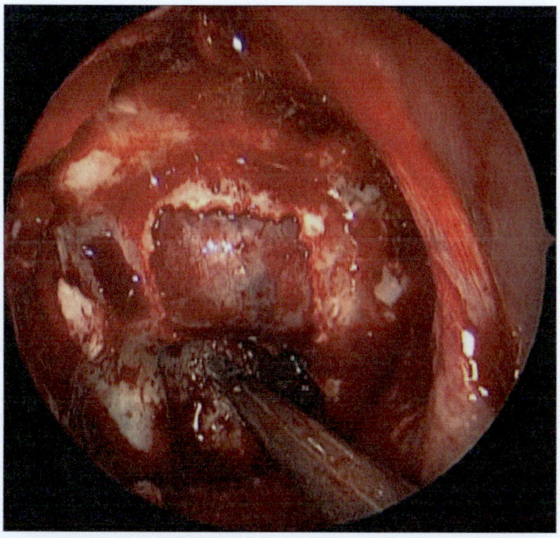

◘ **Fig. 5.133** The fossa should be opened from cavernous sinus to cavernous sinus, also exposing the superior and inferior intercavernous sinuses

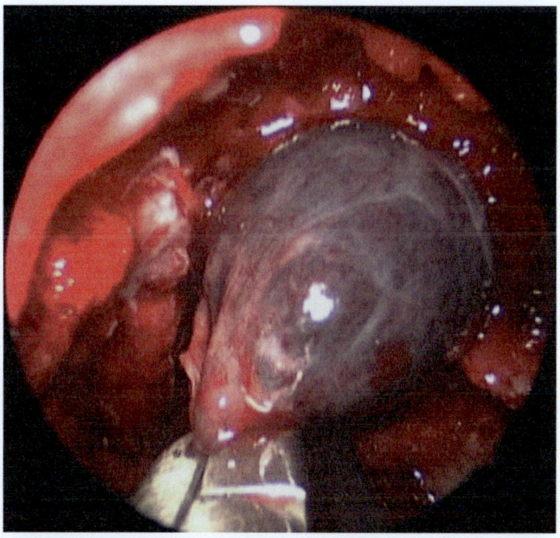

◘ **Fig. 5.134** Sometimes the capsule of the tumor is easily identifiable, and the lesion can be removed en bloc. This is not usually the case in very soft tumors

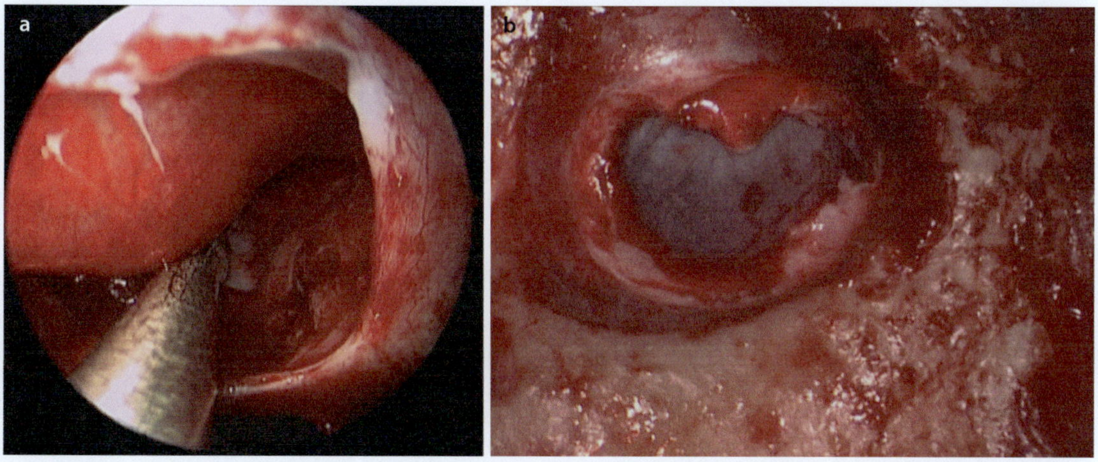

◘ **Fig. 5.135** The premature descent of the diaphragm can isolate and obscure vision of lateral and posterior components of the tumor. The diaphragm can be robust and amenable to maneuvers **a** or thin and susceptible to perforation and CSF leak **b**

sinuses connecting the cavernous sinuses, which are named based on their location to the pituitary gland and may occur anterior, inferior, or posterior to the gland. The anterior intercavernous sinus is usually larger than the posterior sinus and may sometimes cover the entire anterior part of the sella, a configuration which can cause significant bleeding (◘ Fig. 5.128).

An important relationship both for transsphenoidal and more importantly for transcranial routes is the relationship of the optic chiasm in relation to the pituitary gland and infundibulum. This is defined as normal (above the diaphragm and pituitary gland ~ 70%), prefixed (above the tuberculum sellae ~15%), and postfixed chiasm (above the dorsum sella ~15%) (◘ Fig. 5.129).

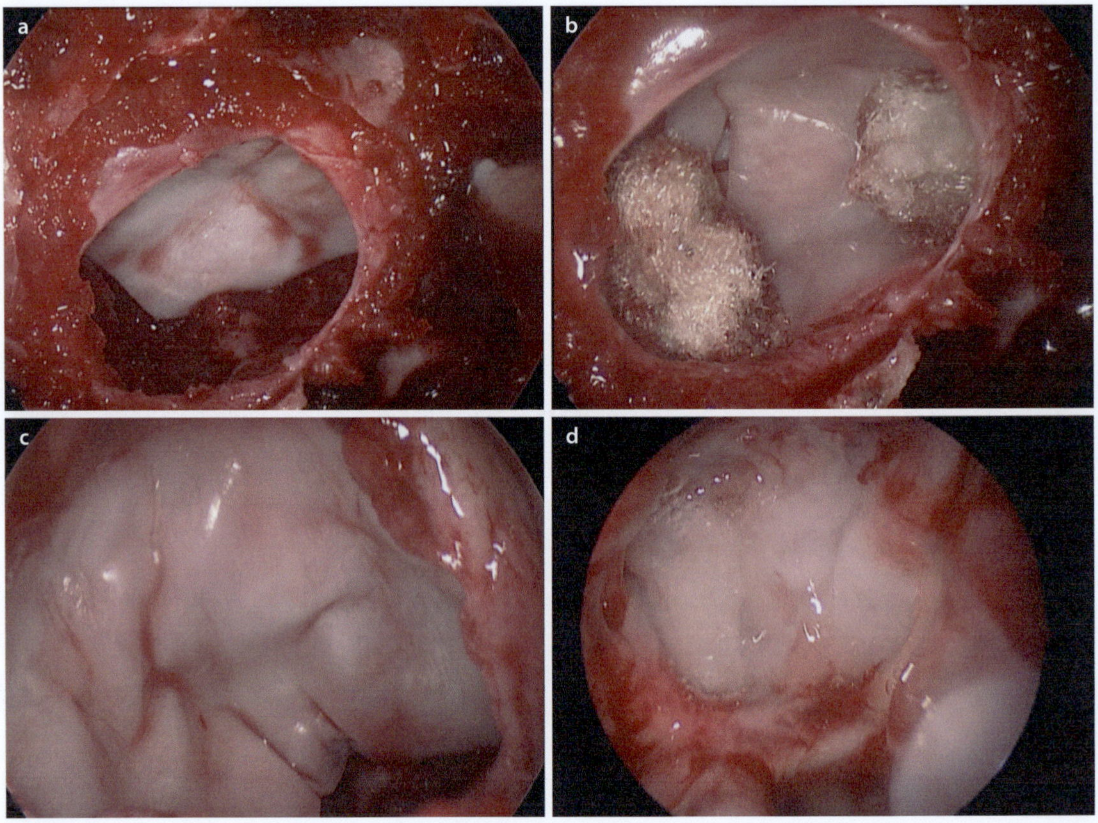

Fig. 5.136 Multilayer closure for sealing of intraoperative CSF leak. Inlay allograft (Lyoplant) **a**, followed by Fibrillar Surgicel **b**, second layer of allograft **c**, and at the end application of fibrin matrix (Tisseel) **d**

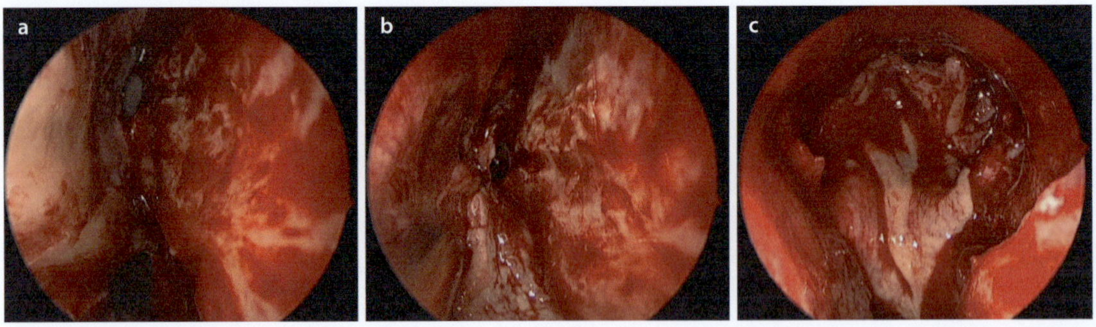

Fig. 5.137 Pedicled nasoseptal flap: **a** dissection from the septum **b** secured in the choana and **c** applied with the mucosal surface facing externally

5.8.4 Therapeutic Options

Surgical Treatment

Surgical Technique

Preoperative review of the images is important. Careful evaluation of the nasal septum and sphenoid sinus anatomy will help plan the surgery. A fine cut contiguous slice CT with neuronavigation is useful in the conchal type of sphenoid sinus and in revisional surgery, especially in the context of acromegaly (where there may be soft tissue and mucosal hypertrophy). Evaluation of the sphenoidal septae is helpful, as they can be used as landmarks both for identifying the carotids and aiding to locate microadenomas [268, 276].

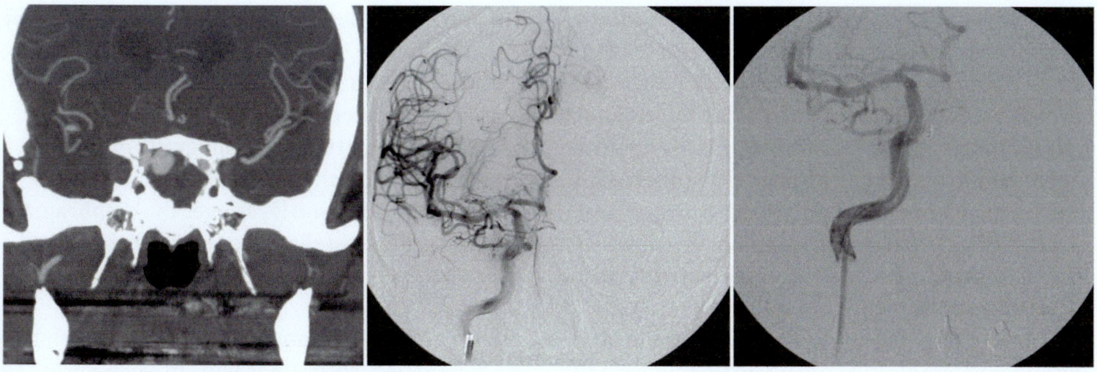

Fig. 5.138 CTA showing a pseudoaneurysm in the cavernous segment of the right ICA. DSA pre and post embolization. Patient had full fortunately recovery

The surgeon and the assistant stand on either side of the patient's shoulders.

We always use a binarial approach. The endoscope is introduced, and the inferior, middle, and superior turbinates are identified. The middle turbinate is outfractured, and the choana and the sphenoid ostium are identified. When outfracturing the middle turbinate using the Freer elevator, we are careful to place the elevator along the entire length of the turbinate so that it is outfractured in one movement, rather than working along the turbinate; this avoids hemorrhage from multiple mucosal injuries.

The ostium lies approximately 1.5 cm above the choana, medial to the inferior edge of the superior turbinate. Sometimes it is not easily identified as it can be obstructed by a superior or supreme turbinate or thickened mucosa. In such cases, we fracture the junction of the cartilaginous septum and the vomer, and with a submucosal dissection, we find the contralateral ostium (Fig. 5.131). If image guidance is not being used and there is uncertainty as to where the ostium is, it is invariably the case that the surgeon is too rostral and is entering the posterior ethmoidal air cells, and therefore dissection should proceed inferiorly. Injudicious probing with the Freer dissector may perforate the thin anterior fossa floor and cause a CSF leak. Correct identification of the ostium is sometimes confirmed with an air bubble appearing over the ostium (coming from the sphenoid sinus) in the presence of hemorrhage.

After identification of the ostium, a wide anterior sphenoidotomy is performed with the Kerrison rongeurs and the diamond drill. Care should be taken not to injure the sphenopalatine artery, which emerges inferolateral to the ostia. We then proceed to excise the posterior third of the cartilaginous septum. The vomer is identified, and it is the most important landmark since it will always represent the midline. The most common pitfall is disorientation from the midline, which can lead to suboptimal fossa opening or even inadvertent carotid injury. Whenever in doubt regarding the extent of the laterality of the approach, the endoscope should be removed, the vomer should be re-identified, and reorientation to the midline will have been re-achieved. The vomer should be adequately drilled in order to have sufficient maneuverability in the craniocaudal axis and to allow correct placement of a Hadad–Bassagasteguy flap along the floor of the sphenoid sinus if required. We use a diamond burr (usually 4 mm) and the drill in the right-to-left direction, i.e., opposite to the torque of the drill, to diminish the likelihood of the burr jumping. The sphenoid septae are drilled down until the sphenoid sinus is flat. This is always performed in preparation of a possible CSF leak, as one of the most important technical pearls of the repair is to apply one's flap of choice onto a flat surface. Both carotid pillars, optic nerves, and lateral opticocarotid recesses should be identified, but this is not always so easy as described in textbooks. Identifying the clival recess can be very helpful, especially in an expanded fossa. Correlation with up-to-date imaging is essential (Fig. 5.132).

In the case of an eroded fossa floor, the bone can usually be fractured with a dissector; otherwise, thinning with the drill is advocated. Kerrison rongeurs are then used to enlarge the opening. The fossa should be opened from cavernous sinus to cavernous sinus, also exposing the superior and inferior intercavernous sinuses. In cases where a residual was identified and a reoperation was performed, we have found that the opening was suboptimal in the majority of cases. Care should be taken while removing the bone at the tuberculum, since at that point, the upper aspect of the pituitary gland is directly related to arachnoid and pia and sometimes the subarachnoid space extends below the diaphragm (◘ Figs. 5.133, 5.134, and 5.135).

The dura is incised in a cruciate fashion starting superolaterally and cutting no further than the central part of the exposed dura to avoid entering the contralateral cavernous sinus. Ideally one would want to cut the dura without entering the pseudocapsule of the adenoma, which is sometimes evident. Using a dissector, care is taken to remove the adenoma en bloc, which can sometimes be achieved. Oldfield et al. have described in detail the advantage in using the pseudocapsule extraction surgical technique in Cushing's disease and have also pointed out that recurrent or persistent Cushing's disease consistently results from residual tumor. In many cases though this is not possible, particularly if the tumor is very soft or even liquefied. A wide variety of ring and «cup» curettes will help in this. The debulking should always start form the inferior portion of the tumor, followed by the lateral aspect. The superior part should be the last one to be addressed. With this strategy, the premature descent of the diaphragm is avoided, which can isolate and obscure vision of lateral and posterior components of the tumor.

Pituitary rongeurs should not be inserted into the sella itself, and care should be taken not to apply traction to the dural leaflets as this can cause significant cavernous sinus bleeding.

A Valsalva maneuver elevates the intracranial pressure and can cause inferior displacement of the mass and may facilitate tumor removal. Some surgeons advocate preoperative placement of a lumbar drain and slow instillation of saline to elevate the intracranial pressure. After removal of the tumor, a 45 degree scope is introduced to inspect the surgical cavity for residual tumor.

In case of a Rathke's cleft cyst, we aim for drainage of the cyst and subtotal cyst wall removal, as this is less likely to cause hypopituitarism [261].

After tumor removal, we always carefully pack the sella with Fibrillar Surgicel, and the closure depends on the presence or absence of CSF leak. If there is no CSF leak, then the abovementioned will suffice. If there is a small CSF leak, then we will close in one of two ways:

1. We will use a fascia lata graft and apply Tisseel (Baxter, Deerfield, IL) on top.
2. We will use a two-layer allograft (preferably Hemopatch, Baxter Healthcare Corp., Deerfield, IL), one layer over the diaphragm and one extra-sellar layer over the dura, and then apply fibrin matrix (Tisseel).

In cases of high-volume CSF leaks, we prefer to use a pedicled nasoseptal flap. In such cases, an overnight intranasal pack of Merocel (Medtronic Inc., Minneapolis, MN, USA) is used, and nasal douches are encouraged from day 5 post-op. Lumbar drainage is not routinely used.

In case of a CSF leak, it is important to remember to remove the mucosa from the sphenoid sinus and prepare the bone surface with drilling down to the septae. An uneven surface will cause accumulation of the CSF behind the flap and inevitable failure.

Nasopore (Polyganics, Groningen, the Netherlands) is used to lightly pack the sphenoid sinus. The medial turbinate is medialized, and blood and debris are sucked from the choana and laterally to the middle turbinate.

Postoperative visual deterioration necessitates urgent CT scan to look for hematoma or overpacking of the fossa, both of which will require urgent surgical evacuation.

CSF Leak Repair

Despite the best efforts to repair an intraoperative CSF leak, a significant percentage (around 5% in our series) will need reoperation. In these cases, one has to tailor the approach depending on the initial findings. In cases where a small leak is encountered and a nasoseptal flap was not utilized, then this will most likely suffice. In cases where a larger leak is identified or a nasoseptal flap has failed, a decision will be taken intraoperatively as to whether repositioning of the flap will suffice or whether a contralateral nasoseptal flap will need to be raised because of constriction of the first. An adjunct fascia lata may be employed with a 3-day lumbar drainage in addition. In cases where a CSF leak has been proven but cannot be identified intraoperatively, then fluorescein is used with high sensitivity [262].

The mucosa of the middle turbinate can also be used for a repair of a small CSF leak. This can be vascularized, which is technically more demanding, or nonvascularized. This also carries a low risk of causing a neurogenic anosmia.

Nasoseptal Flap (Hadad–Bassagasteguy Vascularized Nasoseptal Pedicled Flap)

Angled needle-tip monopolar cautery is very helpful in harvesting the nasoseptal flap. The first incision should start from the superolateral part of the choana on the sphenoidal ethmoidal recess passing medially onto the vomer and then inferiorly to the nasal floor. The second incision is the continuation of the first through the nasal floor up to the squamociliary junction. The third starts from the ostium and curves sharply toward the septum anterosuperiorly, with the superior border correlating with the superior level of the middle turbinate. The fourth interconnects the second and third at the level of the squamociliary junction. The flap is elevated in the submucoperichondrial and submucoperiosteal planes. Dissection should be slow and careful to avoid penetrating the flap. When applying the flap, the mucosal side should be facing externally, the flap should not be folded, and the pedicle should not be kinked.

Control of Bleeding

Preparation with Moffett's solution or an alternative vasoconstrictive solution and systolic BP of <90 mmHg play a significant role. Adrenaline-soaked patties will help in diffuse mucosal oozing. Bipolars are routinely used, but we have found that they are not always reliable. If bleeding from the sphenopalatine artery is encountered, then meticulous coagulation of the vessel is important. Once avulsed, it can be difficult to coagulate since it tends to retract to the maxilla. This may result in delayed epistaxis which may be life threatening. Intercavernous sinus or cavernous sinus bleeding is easily controlled with Fibrillar Surgicel or Surgiflo (Johnson & Johnson Wound Management, Somerville, NJ) and patience. Head elevation will facilitate venous drainage. Sometimes the use of Tisseel (Baxter Healthcare Corp., Deerfield, IL) can be of help with difficult to control cavernous sinus bleeding with injection of the material in the sinus.

Carotid artery injury will result in torrential bleeding. The first step is for the surgeon to remain calm and to avoid removing the endoscope. Appropriate suction should be used and a pattie applied to control bleeding and avoid excessive blood loss. Hemostasis can be achieved with a combination of Surgiflo (halve the quantity of diluent to make product more viscous) and muslin. Compression of the ipsilateral carotid at the cervical level may be of benefit to reduce the bleeding. The anesthesiologist should resuscitate the patient, and a postoperative angiography should follow to rule out pseudoaneurysm [279]. In situations where immediate control cannot be achieved, then a Fogarty catheter can be inserted and inflated in the sphenoid sinus until the endovascular intervention.

Complication Avoidance

Adequate exposure prior to undertaking operations independently is of outmost importance. Anatomical and endocrinological theoretical background and cadaveric courses are important, but an accredited fellowship in pituitary surgery is becoming essential [263].

Stereotaxis and Intraoperative MRI

In the majority of our reoperations, we use the electromagnetic-based neuronavigation (AxiEM, Medtronic, and Zimmer, Warsaw, IN, USA). Inserting the AxiEM probe into the suction provides continuous navigation and is useful in small recurrent or residual tumors (◘ Figs. 5.139 and 5.140).

The use of intraoperative MRI is debatable. Zaidi et al. found that iMRI can be useful in detecting unexpected residual tumor, and they reported improved rate of gross total removal of

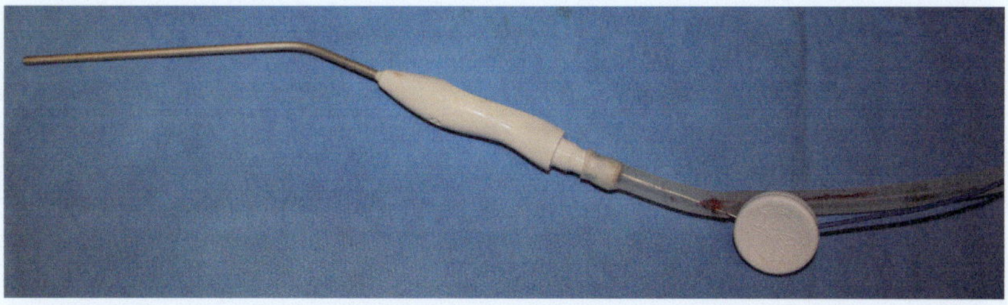

◘ **Fig. 5.139** Inserting the AxiEM probe into the suction provides continuous navigation

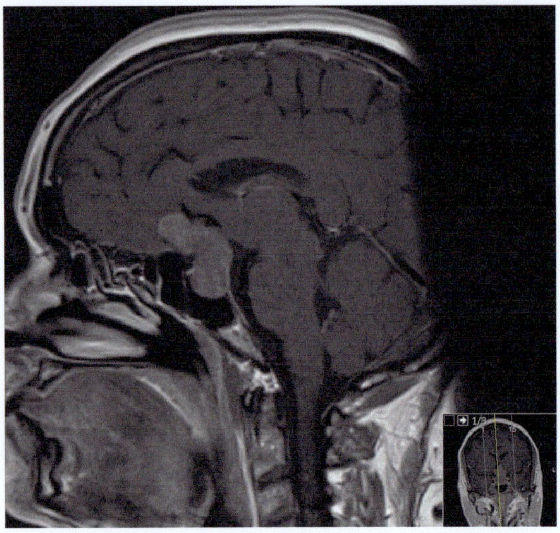

Fig. 5.140 One of the indications for a craniotomy is the anterior extension of the tumor. This macroadenoma was treated with planned two-stage operations. First was the endoscopic transsphenoidal and the second stage was a supraorbital craniotomy

the tumor. The cost-effectiveness of this tool is yet to be determined [264].

Transcranial Surgery

The indications for transcranial surgery have declined significantly. It is used for a second stage operation, after the primary procedure has been performed, via the endoscopic transsphenoidal route. Depending on the characteristics of the residuum, a second stage transcranial approach is planned, and it is most likely a pterional craniotomy or a subfrontal approach via a supraorbital craniotomy.

Comparison of Endoscopic Versus Microscopic

Endoscopic transnasal transsphenoidal surgery for pituitary adenomas is becoming the favored approach to more and more neurosurgical departments. Nevertheless, it has not yet been proven to be superior to microscopic approach for pituitary surgery. Zaidi et al. compared the results of a less experienced surgeon using a full endoscopic technique to those of a very experienced surgeon using a microscopic technique in a cohort of patients with nonfunctioning tumors smaller than 60 cm^3. With the fully endoscopic technique, the surgeon was able to achieve similar outcomes. In a recent study, the endoscopic approach was found to be the most cost-effective intervention compared to the microscopic approach for patients requiring resection of their pituitary adenoma [265]. A meta-analysis found that the only difference was that endoscopic surgery was associated with higher risk of vascular injury ($p < 0.0001$) [266], and at the moment, microsurgical techniques may still be the gold standard method of treating pituitary adenomas. Clearly there are advantages of the endoscope when considering extended approaches [267].

Postoperative Management

The patients are hospitalized in a neurosurgical ward, and they are monitored for DI using our local protocol (Table 5.14 and Fig. 5.141). Strict fluid monitoring is essential, and daily bloods with Na will help in the diagnosis of DI or SIADH.

There are no restrictions to mobilization, LMWH is administered from the first postoperative day, and the patients are advised to avoid blowing their nose, strenuous activities, and heavy lifting for a period of 3 weeks. Stool softeners are prescribed for the same period of time. In case of a nasoseptal flap, we advocate nasal douche with normal saline from day 5 post-op.

In cases that a CSF leak is suspected, then a CT scan is performed to look for air within the pituitary fossa, and if there is doubt, then a sample is sent for β2-transferrin.

Follow-Up

We have found that early postoperative MRI is of no benefit, and we therefore obtain a baseline MRI 3 months postoperatively. Patients with gross total removal confirmed in MRI and endocrinological cure run a lifelong risk of recurrence which is up to 16% in 10 years. Therefore, lifelong endocrinological and imaging surveillance is required [238].

In cases of Cushing's disease that no cure has occurred, we usually opt for a re-exploration within the same admission. In cases of persistent hormonal hypersecretion, there is sometimes difficulty in localizing the lesion, especially in microadenomas and recurrent tumors. In these cases with equivocal MRI results, there have been promising results with the use of (11) C-methionine PET–CT, which can aid in the

Table 5.14 Pathophysiological mechanism of action of Moffett's solution

Moffett's solution	
Cocaine	Crosses the axon lipid membrane in its uncharged form → becomes ionized intracellularly → binds and blocks the sodium channel → prevents sodium influx → blocks the propagation of the action potential of the nerve → anesthetic properties In addition to its anesthetic effect, cocaine is the only local anesthetic to have vasoconstrictive properties. Cocaine acts by preventing the binding and reuptake of free catecholamines to their receptors at adrenergic terminals
Adrenaline	When cocaine is used with adrenaline, there is some evidence that the additional direct vasoconstrictive action of adrenaline reduces the systemic absorption of cocaine
Bicarbonate	Alkalinization of aqueous solutions of cocaine speeds the onset of action and the duration of its effect. This is because of the increased proportion of the lipidophilic, uncharged amine, which passes easily through the axon membranes to reach the sodium channels

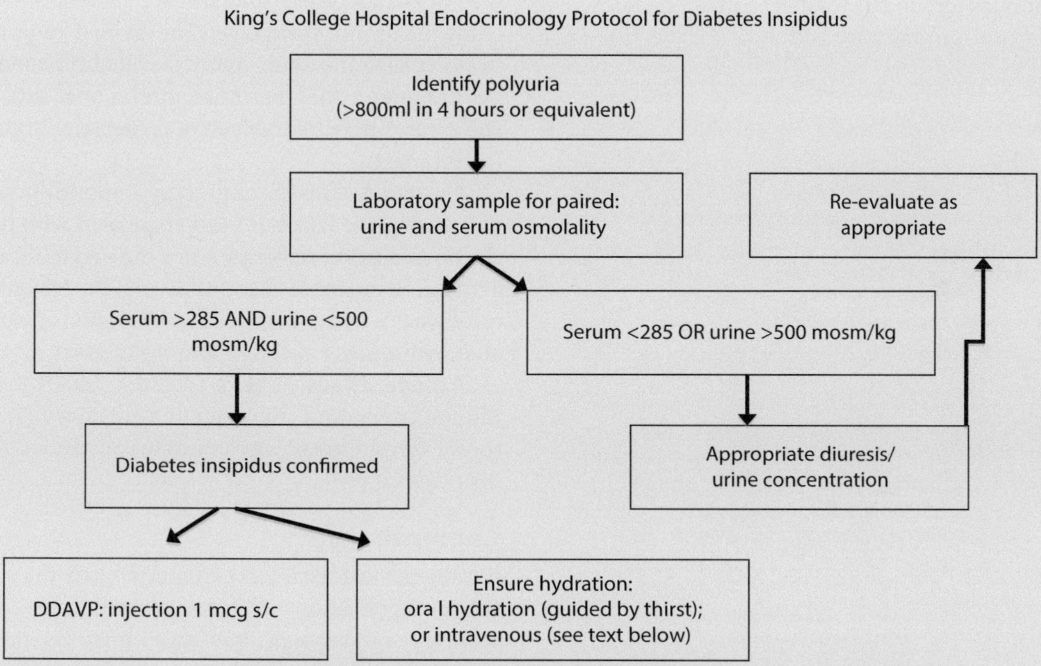

- Patients with known or suspected DI are at risk of severe dehydration and hypernatremia if they are kept nil by mouth or if they have reduced level of consciousness for any reason
- In these circum stances the maintenance of a fluid balance chart is essential to identify if a patient is developing a significant negative fluid balance
- Patients who are nil by mouth should have intravenous fluids prescribed
- The rate of infusion should be adjusted to mai ntain a neutral fluid balance
- One method is to administer each hour the amount of fluid lost in urine the previous hour

Fig. 5.141 KCH protocol for DI

detection of secreting tumors (especially ACTH-secreting and GH-secreting tumors) and facilitate targeted therapy [269, 270].

Prognostication and Further Management

A new clinicopathological classification has been proposed, taking into account tumor invasion and proliferation (▶ Box 5.2). This classification of pituitary tumors into grades displayed a highly significant prognostic value for predicting post-operative disease-free outcome or recurrence-/progression-free status, across all tumor types and for each type of tumor. Raverot et al. showed that «at 8-year follow-up, the probability of a patient showing evidence of disease or showing tumour progression was 25- and 12-fold higher, respectively, if he had an invasive and proliferative tumours (grade 2b) than if he had a non-invasive and non-proliferative tumours (Grade 1a)» [271, 272]. Of note is that MRI is needed to evaluate the invasion because the histological proof of invasion is rare.

Box 5.2: Clinicopathological Classification of Pituitary Endocrine Tumors

The classification is based on the three following characteristics:

1. Tumor diameter by MRI:
   - Micro (<10 mm)
   - Macro (≥10 mm)
   - Giant >40 mm
   - Tumor type into GH, PRL, ACTH, FSH/LH, and TSH by immunocytochemistry
2. Tumor grade based on the following criteria:
   - Invasion defined as histological and/or radiological (MRI) signs of cavernous or sphenoid sinus invasion
   - Proliferation considered on the presence of at least two of the three criteria:
     - Ki-67: >1% (Bouin–Hollande fixative) or ≥3 (formalin fixative)
     - Mitoses: n > 2/10 HPF
     - P53: Positive (>10 strongly positive nuclei/10 HPF)

The five grades are the following:

- Grade 1a: Noninvasive tumor
- Grade 1b: Noninvasive and proliferative tumor
- Grade 2a: Invasive tumor
- Grade 2b: Invasive and proliferative tumor
- Grade 3: Metastatic tumor (cerebrospinal or systemic metastases)

HPF High power filed (0.30 mm 2, 400× magnification)

Radiotherapy

Radiation therapy is a further treatment option after surgery if there is persistent tumor growth or recurrence despite medical and/or surgical therapy. Stereotactic radiosurgery (SRS) delivers high-dose radiation and offers good efficacy and enhanced patient convenience. Fractionated radiotherapy over 4–6 weeks can be employed if the tumor targets approximate radiation-sensitive normal tissues that cannot be spared from the radiation.

The RTx response rates are hard to assess as technique, doses administered, and definitions of biochemical response employed vary significantly between studies. Radiotherapy exhibits a tumoristatic effect and in rare instances may result in tumor shrinkage. The period required to normalize the abnormally elevated biochemical parameter may be more than a year and in some cases may be ineffective (especially in prolactinomas).

Cessation of medical therapy 1 month before and during the RTx has been correlated with better biochemical responses, since the metabolically active cells are more susceptible to RTx. A smaller tumor has a better response to RTx and is associated with a lower risk of hypopituitarism.

Complications of RTx include risk of brain radionecrosis and subsequent secondary brain tumor development, hypopituitarism, and visual disturbance [273].

Chemotherapy

Recent clinical trials have demonstrated the successful application of temozolomide, to treat pituitary carcinomas, but care must be taken since some tumors develop secondary resistance during follow-up [273]. Despite these encouraging results with temozolomide treatment showing long-term control for some patients, it should be emphasized that it is not effective for all pituitary carcinomas or aggressive adenomas.

TMZ has been recently used as a salvage therapy in the treatment for malignant and highly aggressive prolactinomas. There are two potential factors that might predict a response to TMZ in pituitary tumors:

1. The histological type (i.e., prolactinoma)
2. The low or negative MGMT staining

Current clinical practice supports the use of temozolomide as a salvage therapy for malignant and highly aggressive prolactinomas, which have failed to respond to dopamine agonist therapy, multiple surgical interventions, and radiotherapy [274].

5.8.5 The Future of Pituitary Surgery

Recent developments in image guidance, endoscopy, and instrument design have underpinned many of the major technical advances in the surgical management of pituitary adenomas. In the near future, synergistic technologies such as augmented reality, three-dimensional high-definition endoscopy, and robotic articulated instruments may allow for even more delicate and precise surgery. Such technologies may be particularly helpful for less experienced surgeons or when performing challenging cases [275, 277].

5.8.6 Conclusion

Pituitary adenomas necessitate a multidisciplinary collaborative approach. Surgery should be undertaken in high-volume specialized centers from highly skilled subspecialized neurosurgeons and ENT surgeons [277, 278]. These centers should be able to provide comprehensive care to patients and specialized training ideally with fellowship training and contribute to research in pituitary disorders.

5.9 Metastatic and Invasive Tumors of the Skull Base

A. König, S. Ranguis, and U. Spetzger

Metastatic neoplasia is a systemic disease of the body, and therefore, treatment planning should be determined via a multidisciplinary approach. Usually medical oncologists, radiation oncologists, and specialists treating the primary tumor, along with the allied health professionals, are involved in the treatment discussions. A fundamental question is whether or not to primarily treat the cranial metastasis. Furthermore, the treatment modality (surgery, radiotherapy, chemotherapy, or a combination thereof) needs to be determined. In general, it is accepted that readily accessible solitary metastases without infiltration of critical neurovascular structures can be treated by surgical excision (e.g., in the region of the anterior skull base). In select anterior skull base cases, an endoscopic endonasal approach by an ENT surgeon may be indicated. Carcinomas of the paranasal sinuses with direct invasion of the skull base should be considered for surgical resection and postoperative radiotherapy.

5.9.1 General Information

Metastatic tumors can appear in every region of the skull base. Usually, their origin is in the bony skull base and with further progression infiltrate adjacent neural and vascular structures. Tumors with a propensity to metastasize to the skull base include prostate, renal, thyroid, and breast carcinoma [284–287]. Less commonly metastases from gastrointestinal tumors may be observed [280, 283].

In most cases of metastatic skull base tumors, radiotherapy is considered as the first option. Surgery is considered in cases of solitary tumors and/or in younger patients with neurological deficits significantly affecting their quality of life. In many cases, the extent of the underlying disease demands a palliative approach. The treatment modality should be considered by the multidisciplinary team and taking into account the tumor stage and the patient's age and general condition. This requires collaboration between primary specialists (medical oncologists, urologists, gynecologists, ENT surgeons, etc.) and neurosurgeons and radiation oncologists.

Infiltrative tumors of the skull base usually originate from the paranasal sinuses with a predilection for the anterior skull base. Histologically the tumor is often a squamous cell carcinoma with mucosal or cutaneous origin [281].

Therapy involves radical surgical resection followed by postoperative radiotherapy. With this modality, 5-year survival rates of 65% can be achieved [281]. Typically, surgery is a collaboration between the ENT surgeon (transnasal endoscopic approach) and the neurosurgeon (transcranial microsurgical approach). Optimal surgical outcomes are achieved in cases without neurovascular involvement as this allows complete resection of the tumor. In cases with diffuse neurovascular involvement, primary radiation therapy is the treatment of choice.

5.9.2 Clinical Signs and Symptoms

Clinical symptoms depend on the location of the tumor in the anterior, middle, or posterior fossa. Furthermore, there are general symptoms that can appear independent of tumor position:

- Headache
- Nausea
- Partial or generalized seizures

Metastases of the anterior skull base cause specific symptoms:

- Mood changes
- Apathy
- Organic depressive disorders
- Disinhibition
- Loss of judgment
- Exophthalmus (in cases of infiltration of the orbit)
- Diplopia and strabismus (with involvement of the oculomotor, trochlear, and/or abducens nerve within the superior orbital fissure)
- Loss of vision (due to involvement of the optic nerve within the optic canal or inside the orbit)
- Rhinorrhea (due to a CSF leak)

Metastases in the middle fossa including the sella turcica, cavernous sinus, and petrous apex can cause the following location-related symptoms [280, 283–286]:

- Memory loss
- Temporal lobe epilepsy
- Diplopia (with involvement of the oculomotor, trochlear, and/or abducens nerve within the cavernous sinus)
- Endocrine disorders (mainly hypopituitarism, due to tumors in the sella turcica)
- Paresthesia, anesthesia, or pain in the distribution of the trigeminal nerve divisions
- Balance problems, vertigo, and hearing loss (due to involvement of vestibulocochlear nerve in the petrous bone)
- Facial palsy (due to involvement of the facial nerve in the petrous bone)

In the posterior fossa, metastases can cause:

- Ataxic gait
- Generalized ataxia
- Vertigo
- Nystagmus
- Dysphagia
- Atlanto-occipital instability

5.9.3 Investigations

A CT scan to investigate the patient with headaches, first-time seizures, or focal neurological deficits may demonstrate only indirect signs of skull base metastases, especially if acquired without contrast agent. This may show the following:

- Edema and mass effect of the adjacent cerebral parenchyma
- Osteolysis of the bony skull base

Nowadays, an MRI scan is performed in most cases (Figs. 5.142, and 5.143) and will demonstrate the suspected lesion and associated features such as other cerebral metastases or meningeal carcinomatosis. Such findings have important consequences for the planning of further treatment:

- Surgical treatment versus radiation therapy
- Curative versus palliative aims

If the cranial metastasis is the index presentation of the tumor, staging investigations are further required to detect the primary site and to allow planning for further treatment. In the patient with the known primary with a new cerebral metastasis, re-staging may be necessary.

The first step in the detection of a primary neoplasm is usually a CT scan of the thorax and abdomen since most primary tumors are located here. If this does not yield a diagnosis, a CT scan of the neck should be added to detect a tumor of the upper aerodigestive tract or a thyroid cancer. PET–CT or PET–MRI are further alternatives to a conventional staging CT.

If the CT scan is suspicious for a primary tumor in the breast or urogenital region, then the use of further imaging modalities (mammography, ultrasonography, MRI of the pelvis) may be required to obtain information about the TNM staging and to set up therapy. Primary tumors of the bone or bone marrow or tumors with osseous metastases require scintigraphy as part of the staging to assess the spread of disease.

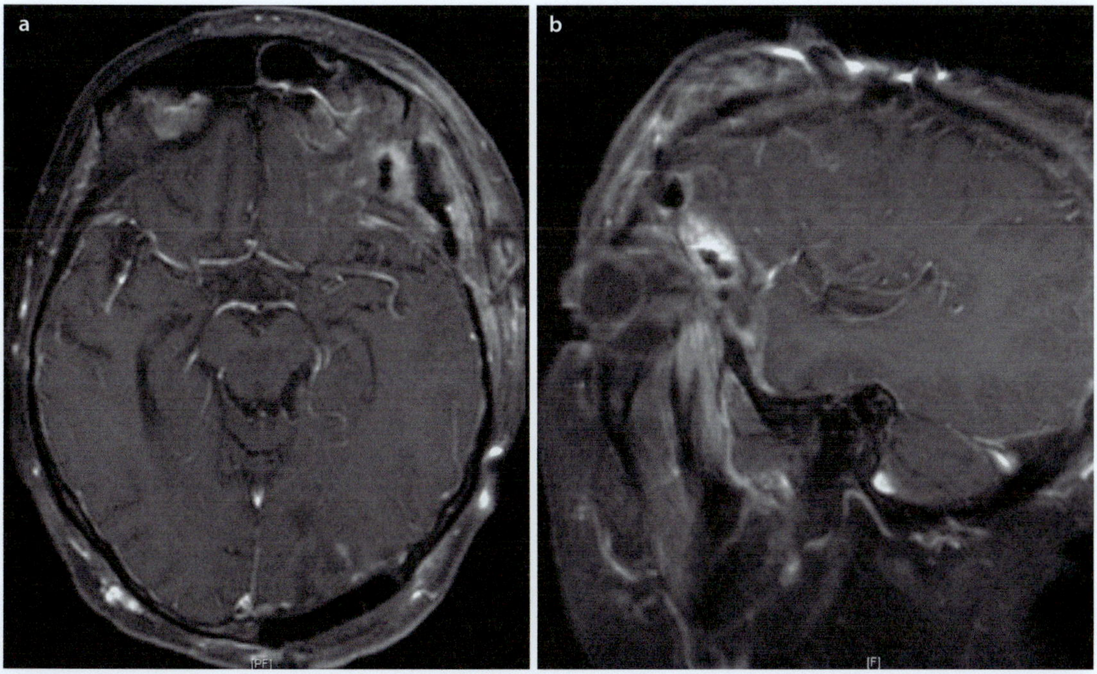

Fig. 5.142 Left-sided frontobasal metastatic prostate cancer presenting with ophthalmoplegia. T1-weighted MRI scan with contrast enhancement, axial **a** and sagittal **b** images

5.9.4 Therapeutic Options

Metastatic neoplasia is a systemic disease of the body, and therefore, treatment planning should be determined via a multidisciplinary approach. Usually medical oncologists, radiation oncologists, and specialists treating the primary tumor, along with the allied health professionals, are involved in the treatment discussions. A fundamental question is whether or not to primarily treat the cranial metastasis. Furthermore, the treatment modality (surgery, radiotherapy, chemotherapy, or a combination thereof) needs to be determined. In general, it is accepted that readily accessible solitary metastases without infiltration of critical neurovascular structures (e.g., the cavernous sinus) can be treated by surgical excision (e.g., in the region of the anterior skull base). Stereotactic radiosurgery needs to be discussed as an alternative to microsurgery. In select anterior skull base cases, an endoscopic endonasal approach by an ENT surgeon may be indicated [287].

If the tumor resection of the anterior skull base results in a large bony and/or dural defect, the surgeon needs to consider a complex reconstruction of the skull base [282].

Carcinomas from the paranasal sinuses that invade into the skull base (Figs. 5.144, 5.145, 5.146, 5.147, and 5.148) should be surgically resected first and then offered with postoperative radiation therapy. If the tumor presents with extensive infiltration of critical neurovascular structures, then radiation therapy is indicated as the primary treatment modality.

5.9.5 Surgical Technique

Since most skull base metastases and infiltrating sinonasal tumors affect the anterior skull base, we describe the surgical technique for this region below.

Tumors of the medial sphenoid wing and the cavernous sinus can be approached via a classical pterional or a supraorbital craniotomy. In these cases, an extended biopsy is all that may be indicated as tumors in these regions usually infiltrate critical neurovascular structures. Metastases in the sellar region (Fig. 5.143) can be reached by a transnasal transsphenoidal microsurgical approach or an endoscopic approach via the same route.

5

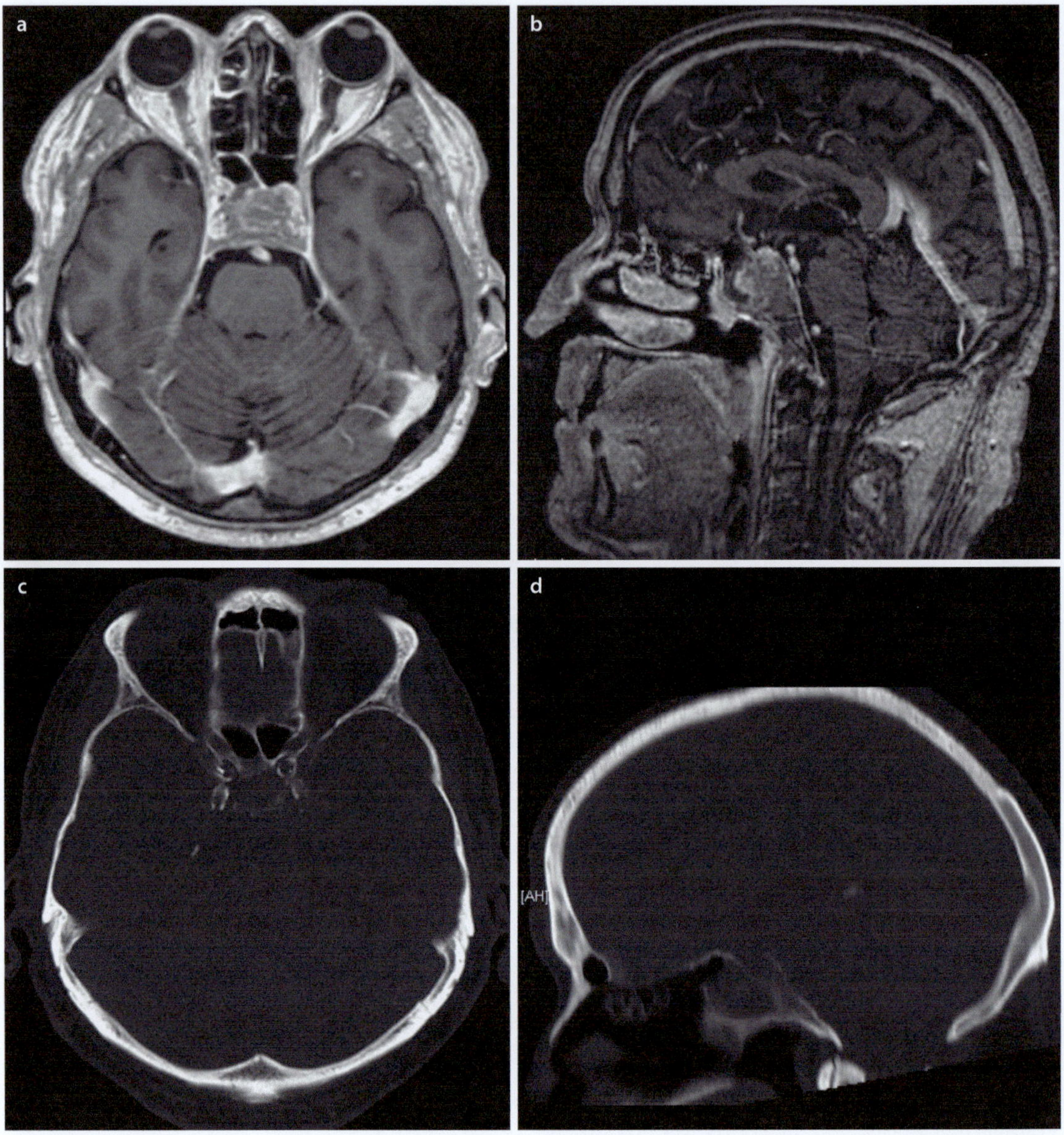

Fig. 5.143 Renal cancer metastasis of the sellar region and upper clivus presenting with ophthalmoplegia. T1-weighted MRI scan with contrast enhancement showing a lesion infiltrating the skull base, axial **a** and sagittal **b** images. CT scan (bone window) with moderate widening of the sella turcica and radiodensity of the sphenoid sinus, axial **c** and sagittal **d** slices

Since aggressive tumor growth and radical surgical resection may result in a significant bony defect, the surgical strategy has to account for a skull base reconstruction (Figs. 5.149, 5.150, and 5.151). Midline tumors of the anterior skull base can be easily approached via a bifrontal craniotomy (Fig. 5.151a). This approach facilitates surgical reconstruction after the tumor resection (Fig. 5.151b).

If the tumor shows a significant sinonasal portion, then surgery is performed in a multidisciplinary fashion. The endonasal portion is resected by an ENT surgeon, and the intracranial portion is accessed microsurgically via the bifrontal cra-

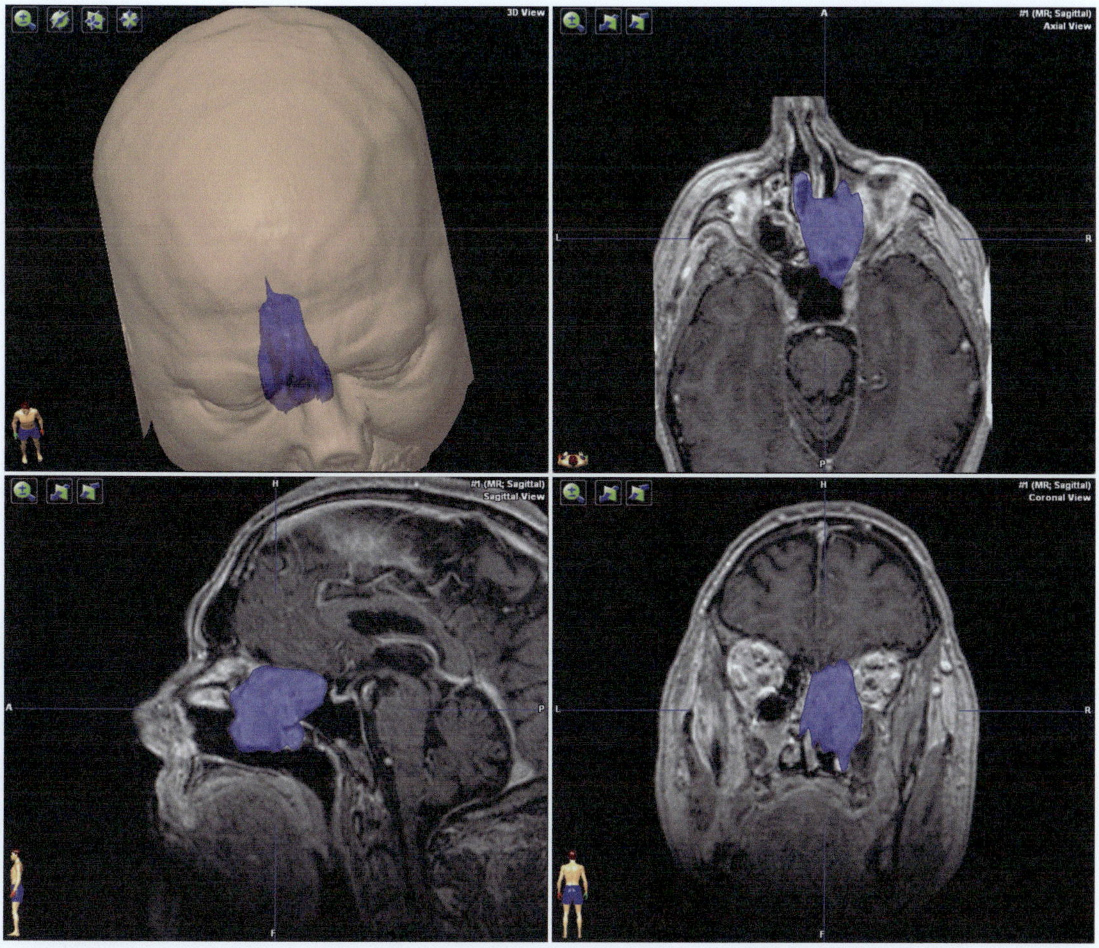

Fig. 5.144 Squamous cell carcinoma originating from the paranasal sinuses with infiltration of the right medial anterior skull base. 3D volume rendering and MRI imaging in three planes for surgical planning

niotomy. Reconstruction using a pericranial flap covers the bony defect and is fixed into place using a tailored piece of titanium mesh. The surgical technique of anterior skull base reconstruction is described in detail in ► Sect. 4.1.5 and illustrated in Figs. 4.13, 4.14, 4.15, 4.16, 4.17, 4.18, 4.19, 4.20, 4.21, 4.22, 4.23, 4.24, 4.25, 4.26, 4.27, 4.28, 4.29, and 4.30.

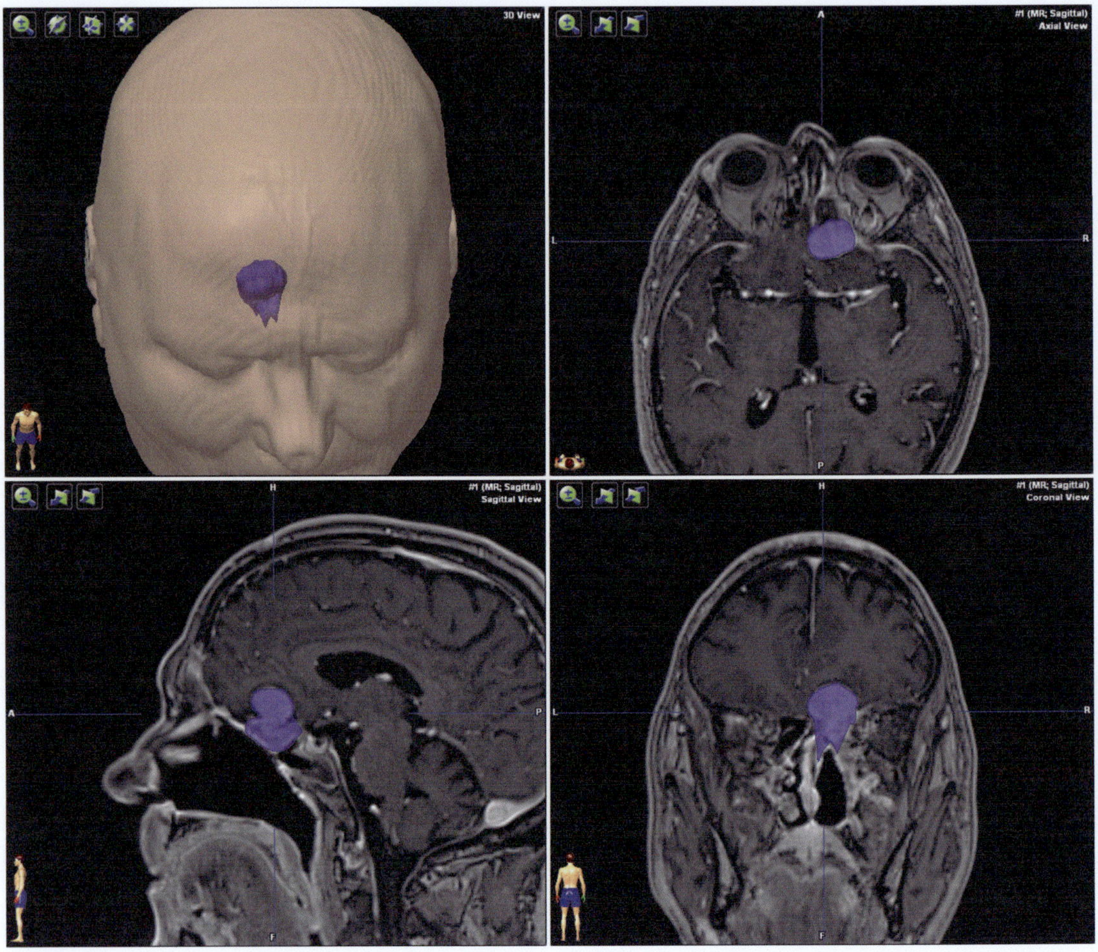

Fig. 5.145 Recurrent small intracranial tumor 1 year after resection of the squamous cell carcinoma from the previous figure. Planning of secondary resection using a navigation data set including 3D volume rendering and MRI in three planes

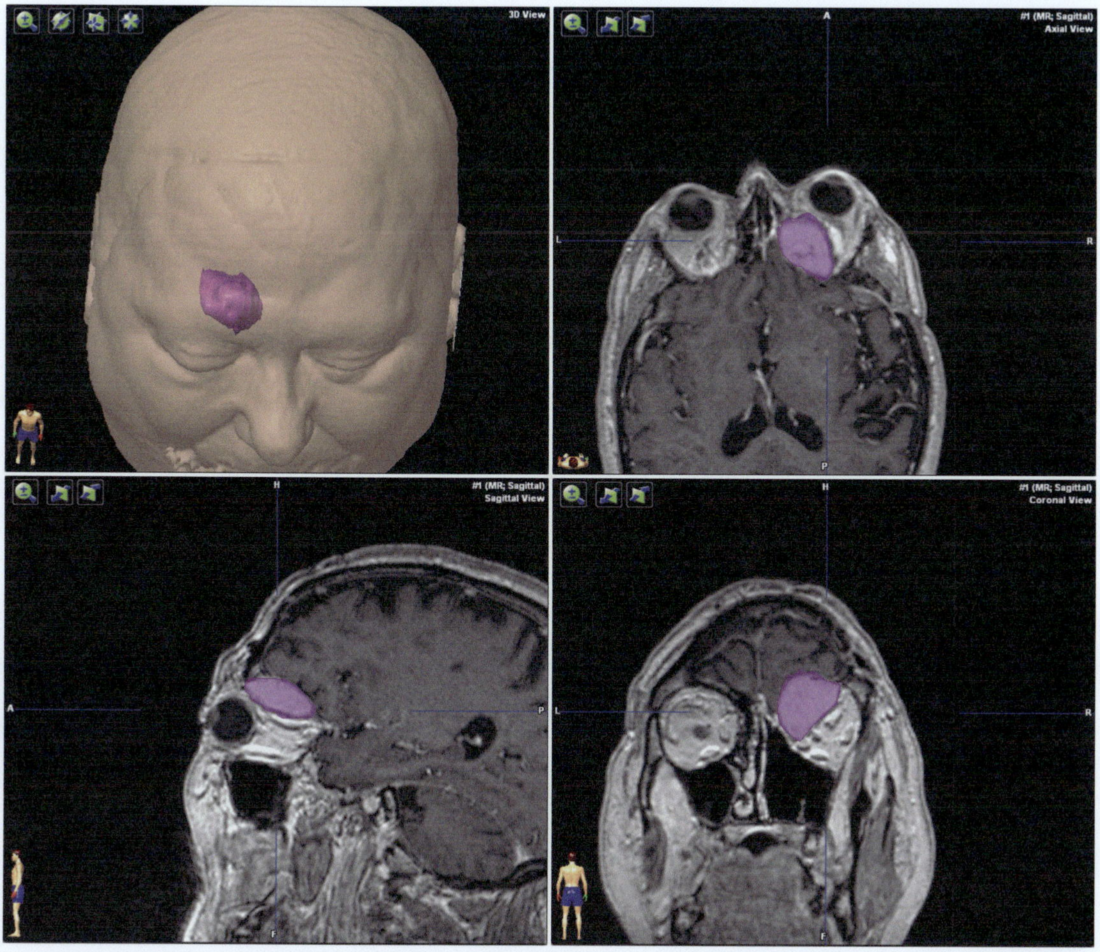

Fig. 5.146 Further recurrence 3 years after resection of the recurrent tumor from the previous figure. Note the infiltration of the right orbit. Indication for further surgical excision

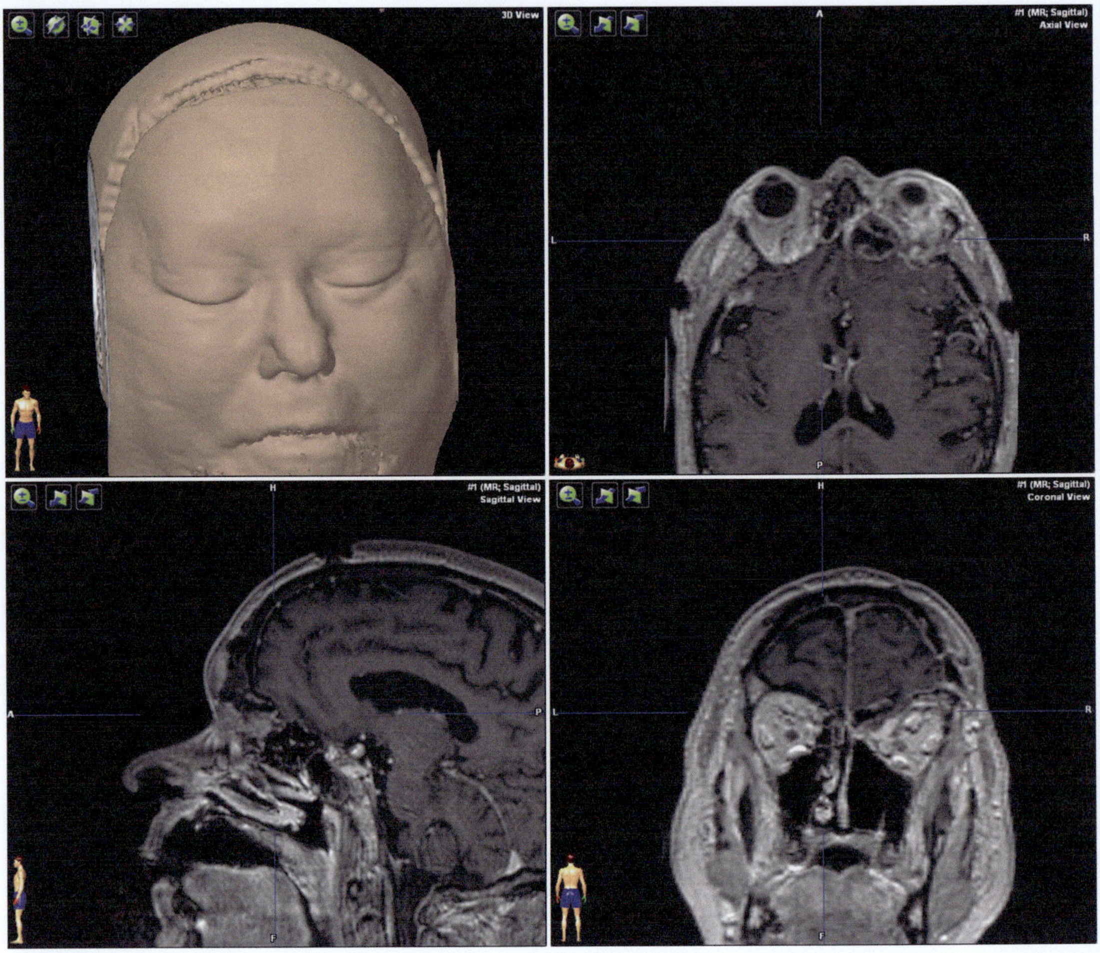

Fig. 5.147 Postoperative MRI scan in three planes and 3D volume rendering for controlling resection of the tumor from Fig. 5.146

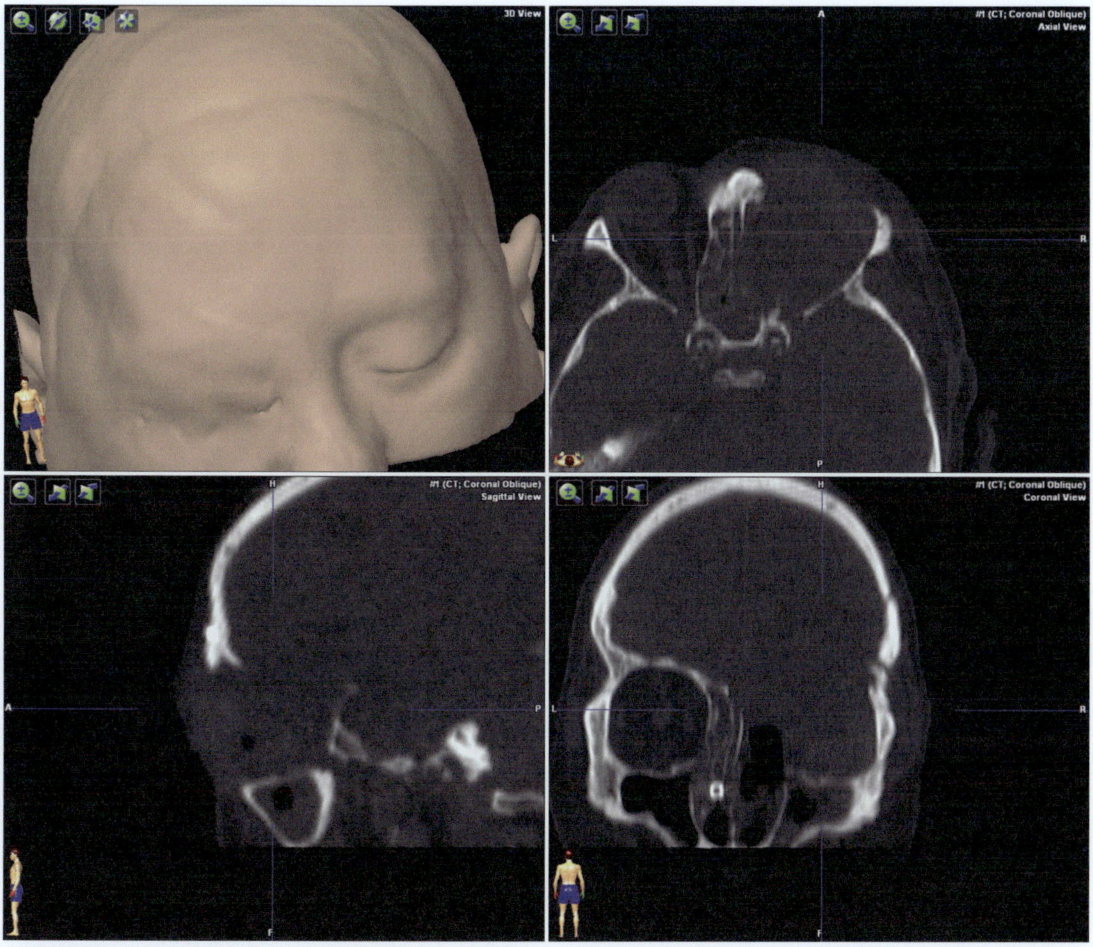

Fig. 5.148 Following recurrence of the tumor shown in Figs. 5.144, 5.145, 5.146, and 5.147, an exenteration of the orbit was required. The defect was filled with temporalis muscle. Postoperative CT in three planes and 3D volume rendering

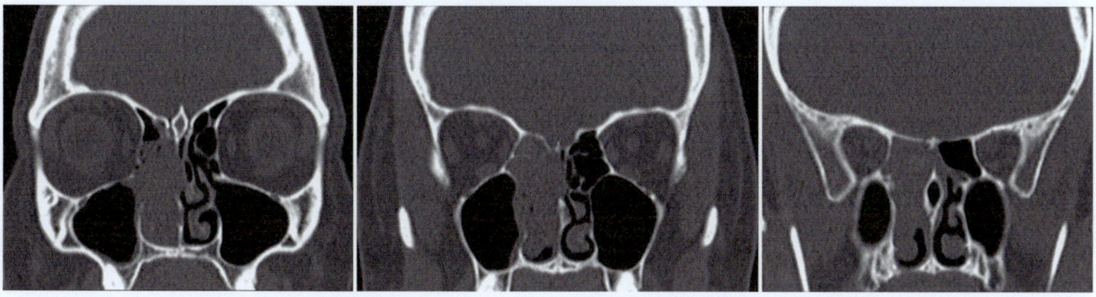

Fig. 5.149 Right paranasal sinus carcinoma. Preoperative coronal CT imaging (bone window) before endoscopic resection by ENT surgeons. The histopathology confirmed a squamous cell carcinoma. Thus, the ENT surgeons performed a secondary, radical resection with transcranial reconstruction of the anterior skull base (see figures below)

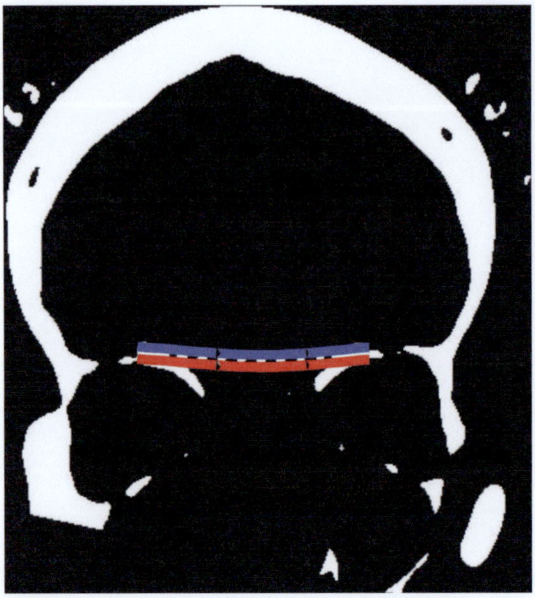

Fig. 5.150 Schema of the surgical reconstruction of the anterior skull base. After placement of the pericranial flap (*red line*), the latter is pressed against and fixed at the bony skull base by a custom-fitted piece of titanium mesh (*blue line*)

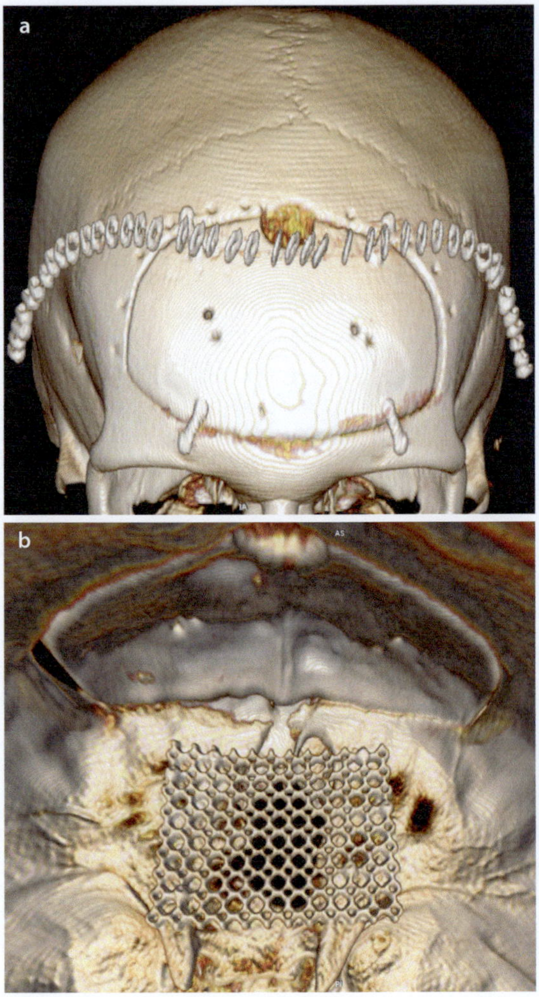

Fig. 5.151 Postoperative result of the case from Figs. 5.149 and 5.150. Bifrontal osteoplastic craniotomy **a**. Intracranial view of the reconstruction of the anterior skull base by titanium mesh **b**

References

Meningiomas of the Skull Base

1. Schick U, Dott U, Hassler W. Surgical management of meningiomas involving the optic nerve sheath. J Neurosurg. 2004;101(6):951–9.
2. Schick U, Jung C, Hassler WE. Primary optic nerve sheath meningiomas: a follow-up study. Cent Eur Neurosurg. 2010;71(3):126–33. https://doi.org/10.1055/s-0029-1246136. Epub 2010 Feb 1.
3. Zweckberger K, Unterberg AW, Schick U. Pre-chiasmatic transection of the optic nerve can save contralateral vision in patients with optic nerve sheath meningioms. Clin Neurol Neurosurg. 2013;115(12):2426–31. https://doi.org/10.1016/j.clineuro.2013.08.027. Epub 2013 Sep 17.
4. Mortazavi MM, Brito da Silva H, Ferreira M Jr, Barber JK, Pridgeon JS, Sekhar LN. Planum sphenoidale and tuberculum sellae meningiomas: operative nuances of a modern surgical technique with outcome and proposal of a new classification system. World Neurosurg. 2015;86:270–86. https://doi.org/10.1016/j.wneu.2015.09.043. Epub 2015 Sep 25.PMID: 26409085.
5. Schick U, Hassler W. Surgical management of tuberculum sellae meningiomas: involvement of the optic canal and visual outcome. J Neurol Neurosurg Psychiatry. 2005;76(7):977–83.
6. Lehmberg J, Krieg SM, Meyer B. Anterior clinoidectomy. Acta Neurochir. 2014;156(2):415–9; discussion 419. https://doi.org/10.1007/s00701-013-1960-1. Epub 2013 Dec 10.
7. Hashemi M, Schick U, Hassler W, Hefti M. Tentorial meningiomas with special aspect to the tentorial fold: management, surgical technique, and outcome. Acta Neurochir. 2010;152(5):827–34. https://doi.org/10.1007/s00701-009-0591-z. Epub 2010 Feb 11.
8. Schick U, Bleyen J, Bani A, Hassler W. Management of meningiomas en plaque of the sphenoid wing. J Neurosurg. 2006;104(2):208–14.
9. Borghei-Razavi H, Tomio R, Fereshtehnejad SM, Shibao S, Schick U, Toda M, et al. Pathological location of cranial nerves in petroclival lesions: how to avoid their injury during anterior petrosal approach. J Neurol Surg Part B: Skull Base. 2015;77(1):6–13. http://doi.org/10.1055/s-0035-1555137 (E First).
10. Ichimura S, Kawase T, Onozuka S, Yoshida K, Ohira T. Four subtypes of petroclivalmeningiomas: differences in symptoms and operative findings using the anterior transpetrosal approach. Acta Neurochir. 2008;150:637–45.
11. Chang SW, Wu A, Gore P, Beres E, Porter RW, Preul MC, Spetzler RF, Bambakidis NC. Quantitative comparison of Kawase's approach versus the retrosigmoid approach: implications for tumors involving both middle and posterior fossae. Neurosurgery. 2009;64(3 Suppl):ons44–51; discussion ons 51–2. https://doi.org/10.1227/01.NEU.0000334410.24984.
12. Borghei-RazaviH, SchickU. Multi-size, multi-angle micro-bipolar forceps for skull base surgery: technical note. J Neurol Surg Rep. 2016;76(1):e146–50. https://doi.org/10.1055/s-0035-1549313. Epub 2015 Jun 1.
13. Watanabe T, Igarashi T, Fukushima T, Yoshino A, Katayama Y. Anatomical variation of superior petrosal vein and its management during surgery for cerebellopontine angle meningiomas. Acta Neurochir. 2013;155:1871–8.
14. Borghei-Razavi H, Tomio R, Fereshtehnejad SM, Shibao S, Schick U, Toda M, Kawase T, Yoshida K. Anterior petrosal approach: the safety of Kawase triangle as an anatomical landmark for anterior petrosectomy in petroclival meningiomas. Clin Neurol Neurosurg. 2015;139:282–7. https://doi.org/10.1016/j.clineuro.2015.10.032. Epub 2015 Oct 28.
15. Lanzino G, Paolini S, Spetzler RF. Far-lateral approach to the craniocervical junction. Neurosurgery. 2005;57 (4 Suppl):367–71.

Optic Pathway and Hypothalamus Gliomas

16. Dalla Via P, Opocher E, Pinello ML, et al. Visual outcome of a cohort of children with neurofibromatosis type 1 and optic pathway glioma followed by a pediatric neuro-oncology program. Neuro-Oncology. 2007;9(4):430–7.
17. Nicolin G, Parkin P, Mabbott D, et al. Natural history and outcome of optic pathway gliomas in children. Pediatr Blood Cancer. 2009;53(7):1231–7.
18. Ben S, Shlomi C, Felix B, Zvi R, Liat B-S, Sigal F, Gilad V, Anat K. Optic pathway gliomas in adults. Neurosurgery. 2014;74:273–80.
19. Chikai K, Ohnishi A, Kato T, et al. Clinico-pathological features of pilomyxoid astrocytoma of the optic pathway. Acta Neuropathol. 2004;108:109–14. 15168135.
20. Shofty B, Ben-Sira L, Freedman S, et al. Visual outcome following chemotherapy for progressive optic pathway gliomas. Pediatr Blood Cancer. 2011;57(3): 481–5.
21. Shofty B, Ben-Sira L, Kesler A, Constantini S. Optic pathway gliomas. Adv Tech Stand Neurosurg. 2015;42:123–46. https://doi.org/10.1007/978-3-319-09066 -5_7.
22. Binning MJ, Liu JK, Kestle JR, Brockmeyer DL, Walker ML. Optic pathway gliomas: a review. Neurosurg Focus. 2007;23(5):E2.
23. Schick U, Hassler W. Pediatric tumors of the orbit and optic pathway. Pediatr Neurosurg. 2003;38(3):113–21.

Acoustic Neuromas

24. Andrews RJ, Bringas JR. A review of brain retraction and recommendations for minimizing intraoperative brain injury. Neurosurgery. 1993;33(6):1052–63.
25. Atlas MD, Lowinger DS. A new technique for hypoglossal-facial nerve repair. Laryngoscope. 1997;107(7):984–91.
26. Baricich A, Cabrio C, Paggio R, Cisari C, Aluffi P. Peripheral facial nerve palsy: how effective is rehabilitation? Otol Neurotol. 2012;33(7):1118–26.
27. Bashir A, Poulsgaard L, Broholm H, Fugleholm K. Late malignant transformation of vestibular schwannoma in the absence of irradiation: case report. Ahead of print. J Neurosurg. 2015;125(2):372–7.
28. Biglioli F, Frigerio A, Colombo V, Colletti G, Rabbiosi D, Mortini P, Dalla TE, Lozza A, Brusati R. Masseteric-facial nerve anastomosis for early facial reanimation. J Craniomaxillofac Surg. 2012;40(2):149–55.
29. Biglioli F. Facial reanimations: part II–long-standing paralyses. Br J Oral Maxillofac Surg. 2015;53(10):907–12.

30. Biglioli F, Colombo V, Rabbiosi D, Tarabbia F, Giovanditto F, Lozza A, Cupello S, Mortini P. Masseteric-facial nerve neurorrhaphy: results of a case series. J Neurosurg. 2016;126(1):312–8.
31. Brooks DN, Weber RV, Chao JD, Rinker BD, Zoldos J, Robichaux MR, Ruggeri SB, Anderson KA, Bonatz EE, Wisotsky SM, Cho MS, Wilson C, Cooper EO, Ingari JV, Safa B, Parrett BM, Buncke GM. Processed nerve allografts for peripheral nerve reconstruction: a multicenter study of utilization and outcomes in sensory, mixed, and motor nerve reconstructions. Microsurgery. 2012;32(1):1–14.
32. Carlson ML, Tveiten OV, Driscoll CL, Goplen FK, Neff BA, Pollock BE, Tombers NM, Lund-Johansen M, Link MJ. What drives quality of life in patients with sporadic vestibular schwannoma? Laryngoscope. 2015;125(7):1697–702.
33. Carlson ML, Habermann EB, Wagie AE, Driscoll CL, Van Gompel JJ, Jacob JT, Link MJ. The changing landscape of vestibular schwannoma management in the United States–a Shift toward conservatism. Otolaryngol Head Neck Surg. 2015a;153(3):440–6.
34. Carlson ML, Jacob JT, Habermann EB, Glasgow AE, Raghunathan A, Link MJ. Malignant peripheral nerve sheath tumors of the eighth cranial nerve arising without prior irradiation. Ahead of print. J Neurosurg. 2016;125(5):1120–9.
35. Charabi S, Tos M, Thomsen J, Borgesen SE. Suboccipital acoustic neuroma surgery: results of decentralized neurosurgical tumor removal in Denmark. Acta Otolaryngol. 1992;112(5):810–5.
36. Chen Z, Prasad SC, Di LF, Medina M, Piccirillo E, Taibah A, Russo A, Yin S, Sanna M. The behavior of residual tumors and facial nerve outcomes after incomplete excision of vestibular schwannomas. J Neurosurg. 2014;120(6):1278–87.
37. Crowson MG, Cunningham CD III, Moses H, Zomorodi AR, Kaylie DM. Preoperative lumbar drain use during acoustic neuroma surgery and effect on CSF leak incidence. Ann Otol Rhinol Laryngol. 2016;125(1):63–8.
38. Delgado TE, Bucheit WA, Rosenholtz HR, Chrissian S. Intraoperative monitoring of facila muscle evoked responses obtained by intracranial stimulation of the facila nerve: a more accurate technique for facila nerve dissection. Neurosurgery. 1979;4(5):418–21.
39. Evans DG, Baser ME, O'Reilly B, Rowe J, Gleeson M, Saeed S, King A, Huson SM, Kerr R, Thomas N, Irving R, MacFarlane R, Ferner R, McLeod R, Moffat D, Ramsden R. Management of the patient and family with neurofibromatosis 2: a consensus conference statement. Br J Neurosurg. 2005;19(1):5–12.
40. Evans DG, Ramsden RT, Gokhale C, Bowers N, Huson SM, Wallace A. Should NF2 mutation screening be undertaken in patients with an apparently isolated vestibular schwannoma? Clin Genet. 2007;71(4):354–8.
41. Gerganov VM, Pirayesh A, Nouri M, Hore N, Luedemann WO, Oi S, Samii A, Samii M. Hydrocephalus associated with vestibular schwannomas: management options and factors predicting the outcome. J Neurosurg. 2011;114(5):1209–15.
42. Gleeson MJ, Cox TC, Strong AJ. Aneurysm of the anterior inferior cerebellar artery mimicking an intracanalicular acoustic neuroma. J Laryngol Otol. 1989;103(1):107–10.
43. Hahn CH, Stangerup SE, Caye-Thomasen P. Residual tumour after vestibular schwannoma surgery. J Laryngol Otol. 2013;127(6):568–73.
44. House WF, Hitselberger WE. Acoustic tumors: diagnosis and management. Minn Med. 1967;50(6):873–7.
45. Iacoangeli M, Salvinelli F, Di RA, Gladi M, Alvaro L, Greco F, Carassiti M, Scerrati M. Microsurgical endoscopy-assisted presigmoid retrolabyrinthine approach as a minimally invasive surgical option for the treatment of medium to large vestibular schwannomas. Acta Neurochir. 2013;155(4):663–70.
46. Kanzaki J, Tos M, Sanna M, Moffat DA, Monsell EM, Berliner KI. New and modified reporting systems from the consensus meeting on systems for reporting results in vestibular schwannoma. Otol Neurotol. 2003;24(4):642–8.
47. Koerbel A, Gharabaghi A, Safavi-Abbasi S, Samii A, Ebner FH, Samii M, Tatagiba M. Venous complications following petrosal vein sectioning in surgery of petrous apex meningiomas. Eur J Surg Oncol. 2009;35(7):773–9.
48. Koos WT, Perneczky A. Suboccipital approach to acoustic neurinomas with emphasis on preservation of facial nerve and cochlear nerve function. In: Rand W, editor. Microneurosurgery. 3rd ed. St Louis: CV Mosby; 1985. p. 335–65.
49. Liu JK, Jyung RW. Retractorless translabyrinthine approach for resection of a large acoustic neuroma: operative video and technical nuances. Neurosurg Focus. 2014;36(1 Suppl):1.
50. Lloyd SK, Glynn FJ, Rutherford SA, King AT, Mawman DJ, O'Driscoll MP, Evans DG, Ramsden RT, Freeman SR. Ipsilateral cochlear implantation after cochlear nerve preserving vestibular schwannoma surgery in patients with neurofibromatosis type 2. Otol Neurotol. 2014;35(1):43–51.
51. Matthies C, Raslan F, Schweitzer T, Hagen R, Roosen K, Reiners K. Facial motor evoked potentials in cerebellopontine angle surgery: technique, pitfalls and predictive value. Clin Neurol Neurosurg. 2011;113(10):872–9.
52. Matthies C, Brill S, Kaga K, Morita A, Kumakawa K, Skarzynski H, Claassen A, Hui Y, Chiong C, Muller J, Behr R. Auditory brainstem implantation improves speech recognition in neurofibromatosis type II patients. ORL J Otorhinolaryngol Relat Spec. 2013;75(5):282–95.
53. May M, Sobol SM, Mester SJ. Hypoglossal-facial nerve interpositional-jump graft for facial reanimation without tongue atrophy. Otolaryngol Head Neck Surg. 1991;104(6):818–25.
54. Monfared A, Corrales E, Theodosopoulos P, Blevins NH, Oghalai JS, Selesnick SH, Lee H, Gurgel RK, Hansen MR, Nelson RF, Gantz B, Kutz W, Isaacson B, Roland P, Amdur R, Jackler R. Facial nerve outcome and tumor control rate as a function of degree of resection in treatment of large acoustic neuromas: preliminary report of the acoustic neuroma subtotal resection study. Neurosurgery. 2015;79(2):194–203.
55. Nakatomi H, Miyazaki H, Tanaka M, Kin T, Yoshino M, Oyama H, Usui M, Moriyama H, Kojima H, Kaga K, Saito N. Improved preservation of function during

acoustic neuroma surgery. J Neurosurg. 2015;122(1): 24–33.
56. Nejo T, Kohno M, Nagata O, Sora S, Sato H. Dorsal displacement of the facial nerve in acoustic neuroma surgery: clinical features and surgical outcomes of 21 consecutive dorsal pattern cases. Neurosurg Rev. 2015;39(2):277–88; discussion 288.
57. Oghalai JS, Driscoll CLW. Atlas of neurotologic and lateral skull base surgery. Berlin: Springer; 2016.
58. Päsler D, Baldauf J, Runge U, Schroeder HW. Intrameatal thrombosed anterior inferior cerebellar artery aneurysm mimicking a vestibular schwannoma. J Neurosurg. 2011;114(4):1057–60.
59. Plotkin SR, Merker VL, Halpin C, Jennings D, McKenna MJ, Harris GJ, Barker FG. Bevacizumab for progressive vestibular schwannoma in neurofibromatosis type 2: a retrospective review of 31 patients. Otol Neurotol. 2012;33(6):1046–52.
60. Pothula VB, Lesser T, Mallucci C, May P, Foy P. Vestibular schwannomas in children. Otol Neurotol. 2001;22(6):903–7.
61. Roche PH, Moriyama T, Thomassin JM, Pellet W. High jugular bulb in the translabyrinthine approach to the cerebellopontine angle: anatomical considerations and surgical management. Acta Neurochir. 2006;148(4):415–20.
62. Rowe J, Radatz M, Kemeny A. Radiosurgery for type II neurofibromatosis. Prog Neurol Surg. 2008:21176–82.
63. Sameshima T, Morita A, Tanikawa R, Fukushima T, Friedman AH, Zenga F, Ducati A, Mastronardi L. Evaluation of variation in the course of the facial nerve, nerve adhesion to tumors, and postoperative facial palsy in acoustic neuroma. J Neurol Surg B Skull Base. 2013;74(1):39–43.
64. Sampath P, Rini D, Long DM. Microanatomical variations in the cerebellopontine angle associated with vestibular schwannomas (acoustic neuromas): a retrospective study of 1006 consecutive cases. J Neurosurg. 2000;92(1):70–8.
65. Setty P, D'Andrea KP, Stucken EZ, Babu S, LaRouere MJ, Pieper DR. Endoscopic resection of vestibular schwannomas. J Neurol Surg B Skull Base. 2015;76(3):230–8.
66. Shahinian HK, Eby JB, Ocon M. Fully endoscopic excision of vestibular schwannomas. Minim Invasive Neurosurg. 2004;47(6):329–32.
67. Shahinian HK, Ra Y. 527 fully endoscopic resections of vestibular schwannomas. Minim Invasive Neurosurg. 2011;54(2):61–7.
68. Spielmann PM, Sillars H. Assessing the threshold for vestibular schwannoma resection and the behavior of residual tumor. Otol Neurotol. 2013;34(5):935–8.
69. Spiriev T, Poulsgaard L, Fugleholm K. Techniques for preservation of the frontotemporal branch of facial nerve during orbitozygomatic approaches. J Neurol Surg B Skull Base. 2015;76(3):189–94.
70. Springborg JB, Fugleholm K, Poulsgaard L, Caye-Thomasen P, Thomsen J, Stangerup SE. Outcome after translabyrinthine surgery for vestibular schwannomas: report on 1244 patients. J Neurol Surg B Skull Base. 2012;73(3):168–74.
71. Stepanidis K, Kessel M, Caye-Thomasen P, Stangerup SE. Socio-demographic distribution of vestibular schwannomas in Denmark. Acta Otolaryngol. 2014;134(6):551–6.
72. Storrs LA. Acoustic neurinomas presenting as middle ear tumors. Laryngoscope. 1974;84(7):1175–80.
73. Strauss C. The facial nerve in medial acoustic neuromas. J Neurosurg. 2002;97(5):1083–90.
74. Taoka T, Hirabayashi H, Nakagawa H, Sakamoto M, Myochin K, Hirohashi S, Iwasaki S, Sakaki T, Kichikawa K. Displacement of the facial nerve course by vestibular schwannoma: preoperative visualization using diffusion tensor tractography. J Magn Reson Imaging. 2006;24(5):1005–10.
75. Temple RH, Axon PR, Ramsden RT, Keles N, Deger K, Yucel E. Auditory rehabilitation in neurofibromatosis type 2: a case for cochlear implantation. J Laryngol Otol. 1999;113(2):161–3.
76. Tomita Y, Tosaka M, Aihara M, Horiguchi K, Yoshimoto Y. Growth of primary and remnant vestibular schwannomas: a three-year follow-up study. World Neurosurg. 2015;83(6):937–44.
77. Tos M, Drozdziewicz D, Thomsen J. Medial acoustic neuromas. A new clinical entity. Arch Otolaryngol Head Neck Surg. 1992;118(2):127–33.
78. Wanibuchi M, Friedman AH, Fukushima T. Photo atlas of skull base dissection; techniques and operative approaches. New York: Thieme; 2009.

Chordomas

79. Amichetti M, Cianchetti M, Amelio D, Enrici RM, Minniti G. Proton therapy in chordoma of the base of the skull: a systematic review. Neurosurgery. 2009;32:403–16.
80. Barry JJ, Jian BJ, Sughrue ME, Kane AJ, Mills SA, Tihan T, Parsa AT. The next step: innovative molecular targeted therapies for treatment of intracranial chordoma patients. Neurosurgery. 2011;68:231–41.
81. Bohman LE, Koch M, Bailey RL, Alonso-Basanta M, Lee JY. Skull base chordoma and chondrosarcoma: influence of clinical and demographic factors on prognosis; a SEER analysis. World Neurosurg. 2014;82(5): 806–14.
82. Boeuf S, Bovée JVM, Lehner B, Hogendoorn PCW, Richter W. Correlation of hypoxic signalling to histological grade and outcome in cartilage tumours. Histopathology. 2010;56:641–51.
83. Chambers KJ, Lin DT, Meier J, Remenschneider A, Herr M, Gray ST. Incidence and survival patterns of cranial chordoma in the united states. Laryngoscope. 2014;124(5):1097–102.
84. Chibbaro S, Cornelius JF, Froelich S, Tigan L, Kehrli P, Debry C, Romano A, Herman P, George B, Bresson D. Endoscopic endonasal approach in the management of skull base chordomas–clinical experience on a large series, technique, outcome, and pitfalls. Neurosurg Rev. 2014;37(2):217–24;discussion 224–5.
85. Colli BO, Al-Mefty O. Chordomas of the craniocervical junction: follow-up review and prognostic factors. J Neurosurg. 2001;95:933–43.
86. Di Maio S, Rostomily R, Sekhar LN. Current surgical outcomes for cranial base chordomas: cohort study of 95 patients. Neurosurgery. 2012;70(6):1355–60; discussion 1360.

87. Frank G, Sciarretta V, Calbucci F, Farneti G, Mazzatenta D, Pasquini E. The endoscopic transnasal transsphenoidal approach for the treatment of cranial base chordomas and chondrosarcomas. Neurosurgery. 2006;59(1 Suppl 1):ONS50–7; discussion ONS50–7.
88. Gay E, Sekhar LN, Rubinstein E, Wright DC, Sen C, Janecka IP, Snyderman CH. Chordomas and chondrosarcomas of the cranial base: results and follow-up of 60 patients. Neurosurgery. 1995;36(5):887–96; discussion 896–7.
89. George B. Chordomas – Report. Neurochirurgie. 2014;60(3):63–140.
90. Kano H, Iqbal FO, Sheehan J, Mathieu D, Seymour ZA, Niranjan A, Flickinger JC, Kondziolka D, Pollock BE, Rosseau G, Sneed PK, McDermott MW, Lunsford LD. Stereotactic radiosurgery for chordoma: a report from the North American gamma knife consortium. Neurosurgery. 2011;68(2):379–89.
91. Komotar RJ, Starke RM, Raper DM, Anand VK, Schwartz TH. The endoscope-assisted ventral approach compared with open microscope-assisted surgery for clival chordomas. World Neurosurg. 2011;76(3–4):318–27; discussion 259–62.
92. Krishnan S, Foote RL, Brown PD, Pollock BE, Link MJ, Garces YI. Radiosurgery for cranial base chordomas and chondrosarcomas. Neurosurgery. 2005;56(4):777–84; discussion 777–84.
93. Koutourousiou M, Gardner PA, Tormenti MJ, Henry SL, Stefko ST, Kassam AB, Fernandez-Miranda JC, Snyderman CH. Endoscopic endonasal approach for resection of cranial base chordomas: outcomes and learning curve. Neurosurgery. 2012;71(3):614–24; discussion 624–5.
94. Noël G, Habrand JL, Mammar H, Pontvert D, Haie-Méder C, Hasboun D, Moisson P, Ferrand R, Beaudré A, Boisserie G, Gaboriaud G, Mazal A, Kérody K, Schlienger M, Mazeron JJ. Combination of photon and proton radiation therapy for chordomas and chondrosarcomas of the skull base: the Centre de Protonthérapie D'Orsay experience. Int J Radiat Oncol Biol Phys. 2001;51(2):392–8.
95. Pamir MN, Ozduman K. Tumor-biology and current treatment of skull-base chordomas. Adv Tech Stand Neurosurg. 2008;33:35–129.
96. Sahgal A, Chan MW, Atenafu EG, Masson-Cote L, Bahl G, Yu E, Millar BA, Chung C, Catton C, O'Sullivan B, Irish JC, Gilbert R, Zadeh G, Cusimano M, Gentili F, Laperriere NJ. Image-guided, intensity-modulated radiation therapy (IG-IMRT) for skull base chordoma and chondrosarcoma: preliminary outcomes. Neuro-Oncology. 2015;17(6):889–94.
97. Samii A, Gerganov VM, Herold C, Hayashi N, Naka T, Mirzayan MJ, Ostertag H, Samii M. Chordomas of the skull base: surgical management and outcome. J Neurosurg. 2007;107:319–24.
98. Sekhar L, Schramm VL, Jones NF. Subtemporal-preauricular infratemporal fossa approach to large lateral and posterior cranial base neoplasms. J Neurosurg. 1987;67(4):488–99.
99. Sen C, Triana AL, Berglind N, Godbold J, Shrivastava RK. Clival chordomas: clinical management, results & complications in 71 patients. J Neurosurg. 2010;113(5):1059–71.
100. Stippler M, Gardner PA, Snyderman CH, Carrau RL, Prevedello DM, Kassam AB. Endoscopic endonasal approach for clival chordomas. Neurosurgery. 2009;64:268–78.
101. Takahashi S, Kawase T, Yoshida K, Hasegawa A, Mizoe J. Skull base chordomas: efficacy of surgery followed by carbon ion radiotherapy. Acta Neurochir. 2009;151:759–69.
102. Uhl M, Mattke M, Welzel T, Roeder F, Oelmann J, Habl G, Jensen A, Ellerbrock M, Jäkel O, Haberer T, Herfarth K, Debus J. Highly effective treatment of skull base chordoma with carbon ion irradiation using a raster scan technique in 155 patients: first long-term results. Cancer. 2014;120(21):3410–7.
103. Wu Z, Zhang J, Zhang L, Jia G, Tang J, Wang L, Wang Z. Prognostic factors for long-term outcome of patients with surgical resection of skull base chordomas-106 cases review in one institution. Neurosurg Rev. 2010;33(4):451–6.
104. Yasuda M, Bresson D, Chibbaro S, Cornelius JF, Polivka M, Feuvret L, Takayasu M, George B. Chordomas of the skull base and cervical spine: clinical outcomes associated with a multimodal surgical resection combined with proton-beam radiation in 40 patients. Neurosurg Rev. 2012;35(2):171–82; discussion 182–3.

Craniopharyngiomas

105. Abrams LS, Repka MX. Visual outcome of craniopharyngioma in children. J Pediatr Ophthalmol Strabismus. 1997;34:223–8.
106. Ansari SF, Moore RJ, Boaz JC, Fulkerson DH. Efficacy of phosphorus-32 brachytherapy without external-beam radiation for long-term tumor control in patients with craniopharyngioma. J Neurosurg Pediatr. 2015;17(4):439–45.
107. Barlas O, Bayindir C, Can M. Interstitial irradiation for craniopharyngioma. Acta Neurochir. 2000;142:389–95.
108. Bunin GR, Surawicz TS, Witman PA, Preston-Martin S, Davis F, Bruner JM. The descriptive epidemiology of craniopharyngioma. J Neurosurg. 1998;89:547–51.
109. Cavalheiro S, Di Rocco C, Valenzuela S, Dastoli PA, Tamburrini G, Massimi L, Nicacio JM, Faquini IV, Ierardi DF, Silva NS, Pettorini BL, Toledo SR. Craniopharyngiomas: intratumoral chemotherapy with interferon-alpha: a multicenter preliminary study with 60 cases. Neurosurg Focus. 2010;28:E12.
110. Cavalheiro S, Sparapani FV, Franco JO, da Silva MC, Braga FM. Use of bleomycin in intratumoral chemotherapy for cystic craniopharyngioma. Case report. J Neurosurg. 1996;84:124–6.
111. Cavallo LM, Frank G, Cappabianca P, Solari D, Mazzatenta D, Villa A, Zoli M, D'Enza AI, Esposito F, Pasquini E. The endoscopic endonasal approach for the management of craniopharyngiomas: a series of 103 patients. J Neurosurg. 2014;121:100–13.
112. Clark AJ, Cage TA, Aranda D, Parsa AT, Auguste KI, Gupta N. Treatment-related morbidity and the management of pediatric craniopharyngioma: a systematic review. J Neurosurg Pediatr. 2012;10:293–301.
113. Clark AJ, Cage TA, Aranda D, Parsa AT, Sun PP, Auguste KI, Gupta N. A systematic review of the results of surgery and radiotherapy on tumor control for pedi-

atric craniopharyngioma. Childs Nerv Syst. 2013;29:231–8.
114. Conroy R, Gomes L, Owen C, Buchsbaum J, Ahern V. Clinical equipoise: protons and the child with craniopharyngioma. J Med Imaging Radiat Oncol. 2015;59:379–85.
115. Dastoli PA, Nicacio JM, Silva NS, Capellano AM, Toledo SR, Ierardi D, Cavalheiro S. Cystic craniopharyngioma: Intratumoral chemotherapy with alpha interferon. Arq Neuropsiquiatr. 2011;69:50–5.
116. Eldevik OP, Blaivas M, Gabrielsen TO, Hald JK, Chandler WF. Craniopharyngioma: radiologic and histologic findings and recurrence. AJNR Am J Neuroradiol. 1996;17:1427–39.
117. Fernandez-Miranda JC, Gardner PA, Snyderman CH, Devaney KO, Strojan P, Suarez C, Genden EM, Rinaldo A, Ferlito A. Craniopharyngioma: a pathologic, clinical, and surgical review. Head Neck. 2012;34:1036–44.
118. Gutin PH, Klemme WM, Lagger RL, MacKay AR, Pitts LH, Hosobuchi Y. Management of the unresectable cystic craniopharyngioma by aspiration through an ommaya reservoir drainage system. J Neurosurg. 1980;52:36–40.
119. Ha EJ, Gwak HS, Rhee CH, Youn SM, Choi CW, Cheon GJ. Intracavitary radiation therapy for recurrent cystic brain tumors with holmium-166-chico: a pilot study. J Korean Neurosurg Soc. 2013;54:175–82.
120. Hargrave DR. Does chemotherapy have a role in the management of craniopharyngioma? J Pediatr Endocrinol Metab. 2006;19(Suppl 1):407–12.
121. Hasegawa T, Kobayashi T, Kida Y. Tolerance of the optic apparatus in single-fraction irradiation using stereotactic radiosurgery: evaluation in 100 patients with craniopharyngioma. Neurosurgery. 2010;66:688–94; discussion 694–685.
122. Hasegawa T, Kondziolka D, Hadjipanayis CG, Lunsford LD. Management of cystic craniopharyngiomas with phosphorus-32 intracavitary irradiation. Neurosurgery. 2004;54:813–20; discussion 820–812.
123. Hashizume C, Mori Y, Kobayashi T, Shibamoto Y, Nagai A, Hayashi N. Stereotactic radiotherapy using novalis for craniopharyngioma adjacent to optic pathways. J Neuro-Oncol. 2010;98:239–47.
124. Hoffman HJ. Surgical management of craniopharyngioma. Pediatr Neurosurg. 1994;21(Suppl 1):44–9.
125. Hoffmann A, Boekhoff S, Gebhardt U, Sterkenburg AS, Daubenbuchel AM, Eveslage M, Muller HL. History before diagnosis in childhood craniopharyngioma: associations with initial presentation and long-term prognosis. Eur J Endocrinol. 2015a;173:853–62.
126. Hoffmann A, Postma FP, Sterkenburg AS, Gebhardt U, Muller HL. Eating behavior, weight problems and eating disorders in 101 long-term survivors of childhood-onset craniopharyngioma. J Pediatr Endocrinol Metab. 2015b;28:35–43.
127. Hoffmann A, Warmth-Metz M, Gebhardt U, Pietsch T, Pohl F, Kortmann RD, Calaminus G, Muller HL. Childhood craniopharyngioma – changes of treatment strategies in the trials kraniopharyngeom 2000/2007. Klin Padiatr. 2014;226:161–8.
128. Honegger J, Barocka A, Sadri B, Fahlbusch R. Neuropsychological results of craniopharyngioma surgery in adults: a prospective study. Surg Neurol. 1998;50:19–28; discussion 28–19.
129. Iwata H, Tatewaki K, Inoue M, Yokota N, Baba Y, Nomura R, Shibamoto Y, Sato K. Single and hypofractionated stereotactic radiotherapy with cyberknife for craniopharyngioma. J Neuro-Oncol. 2012;106:571–7.
130. Jeswani S, Nuno M, Wu A, Bonert V, Carmichael JD, Black KL, Chu R, King W, Mamelak AN. Comparative analysis of outcomes following craniotomy and expanded endoscopic endonasal transsphenoidal resection of craniopharyngioma and related tumors: a single-institution study. J Neurosurg. 2016;124:627–38.
131. Karavitaki N, Brufani C, Warner JT, Adams CB, Richards P, Ansorge O, Shine B, Turner HE, Wass JA. Craniopharyngiomas in children and adults: systematic analysis of 121 cases with long-term follow-up. Clin Endocrinol. 2005;62:397–409.
132. Kickingereder P, Maarouf M, El Majdoub F, Fuetsch M, Lehrke R, Wirths J, Luyken K, Schomaecker K, Treuer H, Voges J, Sturm V. Intracavitary brachytherapy using stereotactically applied phosphorus-32 colloid for treatment of cystic craniopharyngiomas in 53 patients. J Neuro-Oncol. 2012;109:365–74.
133. Kim SD, Park JY, Park J, Lee JB, Kim SH, Lim DJ. Radiological findings following postsurgical intratumoral bleomycin injection for cystic craniopharyngioma. Clin Neurol Neurosurg. 2007;109:236–41.
134. Kobayashi T. Long-term results of gamma knife radiosurgery for 100 consecutive cases of craniopharyngioma and a treatment strategy. Prog Neurol Surg. 2009;22:63–76.
135. Koutourousiou M, Gardner PA, Fernandez-Miranda JC, Tyler-Kabara EC, Wang EW, Snyderman CH. Endoscopic endonasal surgery for craniopharyngiomas: surgical outcome in 64 patients. J Neurosurg. 2013;119:1194–207.
136. Laprie A, Hu Y, Alapetite C, Carrie C, Habrand JL, Bolle S, Bondiau PY, Ducassou A, Huchet A, Bertozzi AI, Perel Y, Moyal E, Balosso J, radiotherapy committee of S, and France H. Paediatric brain tumours: a review of radiotherapy, state of the art and challenges for the future regarding protontherapy and carbontherapy. Cancer Radiother. 2015;19:775–89.
137. Lovstad M, Funderud I, Endestad T, Due-Tonnessen P, Meling TR, Lindgren M, Knight RT, Solbakk AK. Executive functions after orbital or lateral prefrontal lesions: neuropsychological profiles and self-reported executive functions in everyday living. Brain Inj. 2012;26:1586–98.
138. Luo S, Pan J, Qi ST, Fang LX, Fan J, Liu BG. Analysis of the factors contributing to diabetes insipidus after surgeries for craniopharyngiomas. Nan Fang Yi Ke Da Xue Xue Bao. 2009;29:544–7.
139. Merchant TE, Kiehna EN, Kun LE, Mulhern RK, Li C, Xiong X, Boop FA, Sanford RA. Phase ii trial of conformal radiation therapy for pediatric patients with craniopharyngioma and correlation of surgical factors and radiation dosimetry with change in cognitive function. J Neurosurg. 2006;104:94–102.
140. Mortini P, Gagliardi F, Bailo M, Spina A, Parlangeli A, Falini A, Losa M. Magnetic resonance imaging as

predictor of functional outcome in craniopharyngiomas. Endocrine. 2016;51:148–62.
141. Mortini P, Losa M, Pozzobon G, Barzaghi R, Riva M, Acerno S, Angius D, Weber G, Chiumello G, Giovanelli M. Neurosurgical treatment of craniopharyngioma in adults and children: early and long-term results in a large case series. J Neurosurg. 2011;114:1350–9.
142. Mottolese C, Szathmari A, Berlier P, Hermier M. Craniopharyngiomas: our experience in lyon. Childs Nerv Syst. 2005;21:790–8.
143. Muller HL, Gebhardt U, Etavard-Gorris N, Korenke E, Warmuth-Metz M, Kolb R, Sorensen N, Calaminus G. Prognosis and sequela in patients with childhood craniopharyngioma – results of hit-endo and update on kraniopharyngeom 2000. Klin Padiatr. 2004;216:343–8.
144. Olsson DS, Andersson E, Bryngelsson IL, Nilsson AG, Johannsson G. Excess mortality and morbidity in patients with craniopharyngioma, especially in patients with childhood onset: a population-based study in sweden. J Clin Endocrinol Metab. 2015;100:467–74.
145. Ozyurt J, Muller HL, Thiel CM. A systematic review of cognitive performance in patients with childhood craniopharyngioma. J Neuro-Oncol. 2015;125:9–21.
146. Pascual JM, Prieto R, Castro-Dufourny I, Carrasco R, Strauss S, Barrios L. Development of intracranial approaches for craniopharyngiomas: an analysis of the first 160 historical procedures. Neurosurg Focus. 2014;36:E13.
147. Prieto R, Pascual JM, Barrios L. Optic chiasm distortions caused by craniopharyngiomas: clinical and magnetic resonance imaging correlation and influence on visual outcome. World Neurosurg. 2015;83:500–29.
148. Pulsifer MB, Sethi RV, Kuhlthau KA, MacDonald SM, Tarbell NJ, Yock TI. Early cognitive outcomes following proton radiation in pediatric patients with brain and central nervous system tumors. Int J Radiat Oncol Biol Phys. 2015;93:400–7.
149. Rahmathulla G, Barnett GH. Minimally invasive management of adult craniopharyngiomas: an analysis of our series and review of literature. Surg Neurol Int. 2013;4:S411–21.
150. Rushing EJ, Giangaspero F, Paulus W, Burger PC. Craniopharyngioma. In: Louis DN, Ohgaki H, Wiestler OD, Canevee WK, editors. Who classification of tumours of the central nervous system. 4th ed. Lyon: International Agency for Research on Cancer; 2007. p. 238–40.
151. Sanford RA. Craniopharyngioma: results of survey of the american society of pediatric neurosurgery. Pediatr Neurosurg. 1994;21(Suppl 1):39–43.
152. Shi XE, Wu B, Fan T, Zhou ZQ, Zhang YL. Craniopharyngioma: surgical experience of 309 cases in china. Clin Neurol Neurosurg. 2008;110:151–9.
153. Sklar CA. Craniopharyngioma: endocrine abnormalities at presentation. Pediatr Neurosurg. 1994;21(Suppl 1):18–20.
154. Steno J, Bizik I, Steno A, Matejcik V. Craniopharyngiomas in children: how radical should the surgeon be? Childs Nerv Syst. 2011;27:41–54.
155. Sughrue ME, Yang I, Kane AJ, Fang S, Clark AJ, Aranda D, Barani IJ, Parsa AT. Endocrinologic, neurologic, and visual morbidity after treatment for craniopharyngioma. J Neuro-Oncol. 2011;101:463–76.
156. Voges J, Sturm V, Lehrke R, Treuer H, Gauss C, Berthold F. Cystic craniopharyngioma: long-term results after intracavitary irradiation with stereotactically applied colloidal beta-emitting radioactive sources. Neurosurgery. 1997;40:263–9; discussion 269–270.
157. Wang KC, Hong SH, Kim SK, Cho BK. Origin of craniopharyngiomas: implication on the growth pattern. Childs Nerv Syst. 2005;21:628–34.
158. Yang I, Sughrue ME, Rutkowski MJ, Kaur R, Ivan ME, Aranda D, Barani IJ, Parsa AT. Craniopharyngioma: a comparison of tumor control with various treatment strategies. Neurosurg Focus. 2010;28:E5.
159. Yasargil MG, Curcic M, Kis M, Siegenthaler G, Teddy PJ, Roth P. Total removal of craniopharyngiomas. Approaches and long-term results in 144 patients. J Neurosurg. 1990;73:3–11.
160. Yeung JT, Pollack IF, Panigrahy A, Jakacki RI. Pegylated interferon-alpha-2b for children with recurrent craniopharyngioma. J Neurosurg Pediatr. 2012;10:498–503.
161. Zhang YQ, Ma ZY, Wu ZB, Luo SQ, Wang ZC. Radical resection of 202 pediatric craniopharyngiomas with special reference to the surgical approaches and hypothalamic protection. Pediatr Neurosurg. 2008;44:435–43.

Epidermoid and Dermoid Tumours

162. Achard JM, Lallement PY, Veyssier P. Recurrent aseptic meningitis secondary to intracranial epidermoid cyst and Mollaret's meningitis: two distinct entities or a single disease? A case report and a nosologic discussion. Am J Med. 1990;89(6):807–10.
163. Agarwal V, Vijayan A, Velho V, Mally R. Pearl in interhemispheric fissure: a rare phenomenon. Asian J Neurosurg. 2012;7(4):229–32. https://doi.org/10.4103/1793-5482.106663.
164. Bailey IC. Dermoid tumors of the spinal cord. J Neurosurg. 1970;33(6):676–81. https://doi.org/10.3171/jns.1970.33.6.0676.
165. Baumann CH, Bucy PC. Paratrigeminal epidermoid tumors. J Neurosurg. 1956;13(5):455–68. https://doi.org/10.3171/jns.1956.13.5.0455.
166. Berger MS, Wilson CB. Epidermoid cysts of the posterior fossa. J Neurosurg. 1985;62(2):214–9. https://doi.org/10.3171/jns.1985.62.2.0214.
167. Brown JY, Morokoff AP, Mitchell PJ, Gonzales MF. Unusual imaging appearance of an intracranial dermoid cyst. AJNR Am J Neuroradiol. 2001;22(10):1970–2.
168. Caldarelli M, Colosimo C, Di Rocco C. Intra-axial dermoid/epidermoid tumors of the brainstem in children. Surg Neurol. 2001;56(2):97–105.
169. Cantu RC, Ojemann RG. Glucosteroid treatment of keratin meningitis following removal of a fourth ventricle epidermoid tumour. J Neurol Neurosurg Psychiatry. 1968;31(1):73–5.
170. Chandler WF, Farhat SM, Pauli FJ. Intrathalamic epidermoid tumor. Case report. J Neurosurg. 1975;43(5):614–7. https://doi.org/10.3171/jns.1975.43.5.0614.

171. Chowdhury FH, Haque MR, Sarker MH. Intracranial epidermoid tumor; microneurosurgical management: an experience of 23 cases. Asian J Neurosurg. 2013;8(1):21–8. doi:10.4103/1793-5482.110276.
172. Ciappetta P, Artico M, Salvati M, Raco A, Gagliardi FM. Intradiploic epidermoid cysts of the skull: report of 10 cases and review of the literature. Acta Neurochir. 1990;102(1–2):33–7.
173. Cruveilhier J. Anatomie pathologique du corps humain; ou, Descriptions, avec figures lithographiées et coloriées, des diverses altérations morbides dont le corps humain est susceptible. Paris etc.: Chez J.B. Baillière; 1829.
174. deSouza CE, deSouza R, da Costa S, Sperling N, Yoon TH, Abdelhamid MM, et al. Cerebellopontine angle epidermoid cysts: a report on 30 cases. J Neurol Neurosurg Psychiatry. 1989;52(8):986–90.
175. Di Rienzo L, Artuso A, Lauriello M, Coen Tirelli G. Pauci-symptomatic large epidermoid cyst of cerebellopontine angle: case report. Acta Otorhinolaryngol Ital. 2004;24(2):92–6.
176. Enchev Y, Kamenov B, William A, Karakostov V. Posttraumatic giant extradural intradiploic epidermoid cysts of posterior cranial fossa : case report and review of the literature. J Korean Neurosurg Soc. 2011;49(1):53–7. https://doi.org/10.3340/jkns.2011.49.1.53.
177. Fleming JF, Botterell EH. Cranial dermoid and epidermoid tumors. Surg Gynecol Obstet. 1959;109:403–11.
178. Goh GJ, Page RD, Nixon TE. An unusual CT and MR appearance of a posterior fossa dermoid. Eur J Radiol. 1995;20(1):46–7.
179. Goldman SA, Gandy SE. Squamous cell carcinoma as a late complication of intracerebroventricular epidermoid cyst. Case report. J Neurosurg. 1987;66(4):618–20. https://doi.org/10.3171/jns.1987.66.4.0618.
180. Gormley WB, Tomecek FJ, Qureshi N, Malik GM. Craniocerebral epidermoid and dermoid tumours: a review of 32 cases. Acta Neurochir. 1994;128(1–4):115–21.
181. Gualdi GF, Di Biasi C, Trasimeni G, Pingi A, Vignati A, Maira G. Unusual MR and CT appearance of an epidermoid tumor. AJNR Am J Neuroradiol. 1991;12(4):771–2.
182. Guidetti B, Gagliardi FM. Epidermoid and dermoid cysts. Clinical evaluation and late surgical results. J Neurosurg. 1977;47(1):12–8. https://doi.org/10.3171/jns.1977.47.1.0012.
183. Hashiguchi K, Morioka T, Yokoyama N, Mihara F, Sasaki T. Subgaleal dermoid tumors at the anterior fontanelle. Pediatr Neurosurg. 2005;41(1):54–7. https://doi.org/10.1159/000084868.
184. Hudgins RJ, Rhyner PA, Edwards MS. Magnetic resonance imaging and management of a pineal region dermoid. Surg Neurol. 1987;27(6):558–62.
185. Iaconetta G, Carvalho GA, Vorkapic P, Samii M. Intracerebral epidermoid tumor: a case report and review of the literature. Surg Neurol. 2001;55(4):218–22.
186. Grafton Love J, Kernohan JW. Dermoid and epidermoid tumors (Cholesteatomas) of central nervous system. JAMA. 1936;107(23):1876–83. https://doi.org/10.1001/jama.1936.02770490030009.
187. Keogh AJ, Timperley WR. Atypical hidradenoma arising in a dermoid cyst of the spinal canal. J Pathol. 1975;117(4):207–9. https://doi.org/10.1002/path.1711170403.
188. Kobayashi T, Kuchiwaki H, Inao S, Nakashima N. A squamous cell carcinoma originated from intracranial dermoid cyst. Neurochirurgia (Stuttg). 1993;36(1):26–9. https://doi.org/10.1055/s-2008-1053791.
189. Landers JW, Danielski JJ. Malignant intracranial epidermoid cyst. Report of a case with leptomeningeal spread. Arch Pathol. 1960;70:419–23.
190. Link MJ, Cohen PL, Breneman JC, Tew JM Jr. Malignant squamous degeneration of a cerebellopontine angle epidermoid tumor. Case report. J Neurosurg. 2002;97(5):1237–43. https://doi.org/10.3171/jns.2002.97.5.1237.
191. Liu JK, Gottfried ON, Salzman KL, Schmidt RH, Couldwell WT. Ruptured intracranial dermoid cysts: clinical, radiographic, and surgical features. Neurosurgery. 2008;62(2):377–384; discussion 384. https://doi.org/10.1227/01.neu.0000316004.88517.29.
192. Lynch JC, Aversa A, Pereira C, Nogueira J, Goncalves M, Lopes H. Surgical strategy for intracranial dermoid and epidermoid tumors: an experience with 33 patients. Surg Neurol Int. 2014;5:163. https://doi.org/10.4103/2152-7806.145764.
193. McLendon RE, Rosenblum MK, Bigner DD, Russell DS, Rubinstein LJ. Russell and Rubinstein's pathology of tumors of the nervous system. 7th ed. London: Hodder Arnold; 2006.
194. Nadkarni T, Dindorkar K, Muzumdar D, Goel A. Epidermoid tumor within Meckel's cave– case report. Neurol Med Chir (Tokyo). 2000;40(1):74–6.
195. Osborn AG, Preece MT. Intracranial cysts: radiologic-pathologic correlation and imaging approach. Radiology. 2006;239(3):650–64. https://doi.org/10.1148/radiol.2393050823.
196. Sachs E Jr, Horrax G. A cervical and a lumbar pilonidal sinus communicating with intraspinal dermoids; report of two cases and review of the literature. J Neurosurg. 1949;6(2):97–112. https://doi.org/10.3171/jns.1949.6.2.0097.
197. Samii M, Tatagiba M, Piquer J, Carvalho GA. Surgical treatment of epidermoid cysts of the cerebellopontine angle. J Neurosurg. 1996;84(1):14–9. https://doi.org/10.3171/jns.1996.84.1.0014.
198. Schiefer TK, Link MJ. Epidermoids of the cerebellopontine angle: a 20-year experience. Surg Neurol. 2008;70(6):584–590; discussion 590. https://doi.org/10.1016/j.surneu.2007.12.021.
199. Shaywitz BA. Epidermoid spinal cord tumors and previous lumbar punctures. J Pediatr. 1972;80(4):638–40.
200. Talacchi A, Sala F, Alessandrini F, Turazzi S, Bricolo A. Assessment and surgical management of posterior fossa epidermoid tumors: report of 28 cases. Neurosurgery. 1998;42(2):242–51; discussion 251–242.
201. Tancredi A, Fiume D, Gazzeri G. Epidermoid cysts of the fourth ventricle: very long follow up in 9 cases and review of the literature. Acta Neurochir. 2003;145(10):905–910; discussion 910–901. https://doi.org/10.1007/s00701-003-0008-3.
202. Turgut M. Klippel-Feil syndrome in association with posterior fossa dermoid tumour. Acta Neurochir. 2009;151(3):269–76. https://doi.org/10.1007/s00701-009-0203-y.
203. Ulrich J. Intracranial epidermoids. A study on their distribution and spread. J Neurosurg. 1964;21:1051–8. https://doi.org/10.3171/jns.1964.21.12.1051.

204. Wong SW, Ducker TB, Powers JM. Fulminating parapontine epidermoid carcinoma in a four-year-old boy. Cancer. 1976;37(3):1525–31.
205. Yamakawa K, Shitara N, Genka S, Manaka S, Takakura K. Clinical course and surgical prognosis of 33 cases of intracranial epidermoid tumors. Neurosurgery. 1989;24(4):568–73.
206. Yasargil MG, Abernathey CD, Sarioglu AC. Microneurosurgical treatment of intracranial dermoid and epidermoid tumors. Neurosurgery. 1989;24(4):561–7.
207. Yilmazlar S, Kocaeli H, Cordan T. Brain stem stroke associated with epidermoid tumours: report of two cases. J Neurol Neurosurg Psychiatry. 2004;75(9):1340–2. https://doi.org/10.1136/jnnp.2003.029520.
208. Yoshimoto K, Nishio S, Suzuki S, Fukui M, Hasuo K. Movable oil in the brain: intracranial ruptured dermoid tumors. Case illustration. J Neurosurg. 1997;86(4):734. https://doi.org/10.3171/jns.1997.86.4.0734.

5

Glomus Jugulare Tumours

209. Al-Mefty O, Teixeria A. Complex tumors of the glomus jugulare tumors: criteria, treatment, and outcome. J Neurosurg. 2002;97:1356–66.
210. Borba LA, Araujo JC, de Oliveria JG, et al. Surgical management of glomus jugulare tumors: a proposal of approach selection based on tumor relationships with the facial nerve. J Neurosurg. 2010;112:88–98.
211. Bulsara KR, Sameshima T, Friedman AH, Fukushima T. Microsurgical management of 53 jugular foramen schwannomas: lessons learned incorporated into a modified grading system. J Neurosurg. 2008;109:794–803.
212. Fisch U. Infratemporal fossa approach for glomus tumors of the temporal bone. Ann Otol Rhinol Laryngol. 1982;91:474–9.
213. Fukushima T, Nonaka Y. Fukushima ELITE approach. In: Fukushima T, editor. Fukushima manual of skull base dissection. 3rd ed. Raleigh: AF-Neuro Video Inc; 2010.
214. Gjuric M, Bilic M. Transmastoid-infralabyrinthine tailored surgery of jugular paragangliomas. Skull Base. 2009;19:75–82.
215. Hafez RF, Morgan MS, Fahmy OM. An intermediate term benefits and complications of gamma knife surgery in management of glomus jugulare tumor. World J Surg Oncol. 2016;14:36. https://doi.org/10.1186/s12957-016-0779-7.
216. Inserra MM, Pfister M, Jackler RK. Anatomy involved in the jugular foramen approach for jugulotympanic paraganglioma resection. Neurosurg Focus. 2004;17:E6.
217. Jackler RK. Jugular Foramen. In: Jackler RK, editor. Atlas of neurotology and skull base surgery. Mosby-Year Book, Inc: St. Louis; 1996. p. 131–56.
218. Jackson CG, Glasscock ME III, Nissen AJ, et al. Glomus tumor surgery: the approach, results, and problems. Otolaryngol Clin N Am. 1982;15:897–916.
219. Kaylie DM, Wittkopf JE, Coppit G, Warren FM 3rd, Netterville JL, Jackson CG. Revision lateral skull base surgery. Otol Neurotol. 2006;27:225–33.
220. Liu JK, Sameshima T, Gottfried ON, Couldwell WT, Fukushima T. The combined transmastoid retro- and infralabyrinthine transjugular transcondylar transtubercular highcervical approach for resection of glomus jugulare tumors. Neurosurgery. 2006;59:ONS115–25.
221. Michael LM II, Robertson JH. Glomus jugulare tumors: historical overview of the management of this disease. Neurosurg Focus. 2004;17:E1.
222. Nonaka Y, Fukushima T, Watanabe K, Zomorodi AR, Friedman AH, McElveen JT, Cunningham CD III. Less-invasive transjugular approach for glomus jugulare tumors: fallopian-bridge technique with hearing preservation. Neurosurg Rev. 2013;36:579–86.
223. Pareschi R, Righini S, Destito D, Raucci AF, Colombo S. Surgery of glomus jugulare tumors. Skull Base. 2003;13:149–57.
224. Patel SJ, Sekhar LN, Cass SP, Hirsch BE. Combined approaches for resection of extensive glomus jugulare tumors. A review of 12 cases. J Neurosurg. 1994;80:1026–38.
225. Pensak ML, Jackler RK. Removal of jugular foramen tumors: the fallopian bridge technique. Otolaryngol Head Neck Surg. 1997;117:586–91.
226. Sanna M, Khrais T, Menozi R, Piazza P. Surgical removal of jugular paragangliomas after stenting of the infratemporal internal carotid artery: a preliminary report. Laryngoscope. 2006;116:742–6.
227. Sen C, Hague K, Kacchara R, Jenkins A, Das S, Catalano P. Jugular foramen: microscopic anatomic features and implications for neural preservation with reference to glomus tumors imvolving the temporal bone. Neurosurgery. 2001;48:838–48.

Pituitary Adenomas

228. Karavitaki N. Prevalence and incidence of pituitary adenomas. Ann Endocrinol (Paris). 2012;73(2):79–80.
229. Daly AF, Tichomirowa MA, Beckers A. The epidemiology and genetics of pituitary adenomas. Best Pract Res Clin Endocrinol Metab. 2009;23(5):543–54.
230. Daly AF, Beckers A. Familial isolated pituitary adenomas (FIPA) and mutations in the aryl hydrocarbon receptor interacting protein (AIP) gene. Endocrinol Metab Clin N Am. 2015;44(1):19–25.
231. Scognamiglio T, Lavi E. Histology of pituitary tumours. In: Shwartz T, Anand VK, editors. Endocopic pituitary surgery, endocrine, Neuro-ophthalmologic and surgical management. New York: Thieme; 2012.
232. Asa SL, Ezzat S. The pathogenesis of pituitary tumors. Annu Rev Pathol. 2009;4:97–126.
233. Thorner MO (2002) Hyperprolactinemia in Besser GM, Thorner MO. Comprehensive clinical endocrinology. UK Mosby, Edinburgh.
234. Kreutzer J, Vance ML, Lopes MB, et al. Surgical management of GH-secreting pituitary adenomas: an outcome study using modern remission criteria. J Clin Endocrinol Metab. 2001;86(9):4072–7.
235. Yamada S, Aiba T, Sano T, et al. Growth hormone-producing pituitary adenomas: correlations between clinical characteristics and morphology. Neurosurgery. 1993;33(1):20–7.
236. Katznelson L, Laws ER Jr, Melmed S, et al. Acromegaly: an endocrine society clinical practice guideline. J Clin Endocrinol Metab. 2014;99(11):3933–51.
237. Asa SL, Ezzat S, Watson RE Jr, et al. Gonadotropin producing adenoma. In: RA DL, Lloyd RV, Heitz PU,

Eng C, editors. World Health Organization classification of tumours. Pathology and genetics of tumours of endocrine organs. Lyon: IARC Press; 2004.
238. Nieman LK, Biller BM, Findling JW, et al. Treatment of Cushing's syndrome: an endocrine society clinical practice guideline. J Clin Endocrinol Metab. 2015;100(8):2807–31.
239. Newell-Price J, Bertagna X, Grossman AB, Nieman LK. Cushing's syndrome. Lancet. 2006;367(9522):1605–17.
240. Osamura RY, Sano T, Ezzat S, et al. TSH producing adenoma. In: RA DL, Lloyd RV, Heitz PU, Eng C, editors. World Health Organization classification of tumours. Pathology and genetics of tumours of endocrine organs. Lyon: IARC Press; 2004.
241. Webb KM, Laurent JJ, Okonkwo DO, et al. Clinical characteristics of silent corticotrophic adenomas and creation of an internet-accessible database to facilitate their multi-institutional study. Neurosurgery. 2003;53(5):1076–85.
242. Sano T, Yamada S, Watson RE Jr, et al. Null cell adenoma. In: RA DL, Lloyd RV, Heitz PU, Eng C, editors. World Health Organization classification of tumours. Pathology and genetics of tumours of endocrine organs. Lyon: IARC Press; 2004.
243. Balogun JA, Monsalves E, Juraschka K, et al. Null cell adenomas of the pituitary gland: an institutional review of their clinical imaging and behavioral characteristics. Endocr Pathol. 2015;26(1):63–70.
244. Horvath E, Lloyd RV, Kovacs K, et al. Plurihormonal adenoma. In: RA DL, Lloyd RV, Heitz PU, Eng C, editors. World Health Organization classification of tumours. Pathology and genetics of tumours of endocrine organs. Lyon: IARC Press; 2004.
245. Salehi F, Agur A, Scheithauer BW, et al. Ki-67 in pituitary neoplasms: a review–part I. Neurosurgery Sep. 2009;65(3):429–37.
246. Scheithauer BW, Kovacs K, Horvath E, et al. Pituitary carcinoma. In: RA DL, Lloyd RV, Heitz PU, Eng C, editors. World Health Organization classification of tumours. Pathology and genetics of tumours of endocrine organs. Lyon: IARC Press; 2004.
247. Mete O, Lopes MB, Asa SL. Spindle cell oncocytomas and granular cell tumors of the pituitary are variants of pituicytoma. Am J Surg Pathol. 2013;37(11):1694–924.
248. Cackett P, Eunson G, Bath L, et al. Proptosis as the presenting sign of giant prolactinoma in a prepubertal boy: successful resolution of hydrocephalus by use of medical therapy. Future Oncol. 2012;8(12):1621–6.
249. Karavitaki N, Collison K, Halliday J, et al. What is the natural history of nonoperated nonfunctioning pituitary adenomas? Clin Endocrinol. 2007;67(6):938–43.
250. Rajasekaran S, Vanderpump M, Baldeweg S, et al. UK guidelines for the management of pituitary apoplexy. Clin Endocrinol. 2011;74(1):9–20.
251. Elster AD. Imaging of the sella: anatomy and pathology. Semin Ultrasound CT MR. 1993;14(3):182–94.
252. Knosp E, Steiner E, Kitz K, et al. Pituitary adenomas with invasion of the cavernous sinus space: a magnetic resonance imaging classification compared with surgical findings. Neurosurgery. 1993;33(4):610–8.
253. Di Ieva A, Rotondo F, Syro LV, et al. Aggressive pituitary adenomas–diagnosis and emerging treatments. Nat Rev Endocrinol. 2014;10(7):423–35.
254. Wind JJ, Lonser RR, Nieman LK, et al. The lateralization accuracy of inferior petrosal sinus sampling in 501 patients with Cushing's disease. J Clin Endocrinol Metab. 2013;98(6):2285–93.
255. van den Bosch OF, Stades AM, Zelissen PM. Increased long-term remission after adequate medical cortisol suppression therapy as presurgical treatment in Cushing's disease. Clin Endocrinol. 2014;80(2):184–90.
256. Jacob JJ, Bevan JS. Should all patients with acromegaly receive somatostatin analogue therapy before surgery and, if so, for how long? Clin Endocrinol. 2014;81(6):812–7.
257. Klibanski A. Clinical practice. Prolactinomas. N Engl J Med. 2010;362(13):1219–26.
258. Ali S, Miller KK, Freudenreich O. Management of psychosis associated with a prolactinoma: case report and review of the literature. Psychosomatics. 2010;51(5):370–6.
259. Schwartz M, Swearingen B, Black P. Transsphenoidal surgery for pituitary tumors. In: Black P, Kaye A, editors. Operative neurosurgery. New York: Churchill Livingstone; 2000.
260. Benjamin E, Wong DK, Choa D. Moffett's' solution: a review of the evidence and scientific basis for the topical preparation of the nose. Clin Otolaryngol Allied Sci. 2004;29(6):582–7.
261. Aho CJ, Liu C, Zelman V, et al. Surgical outcomes in 118 patients with Rathke cleft cysts. J Neurosurg. 2005;102(2):189–93.
262. Raza SM, Banu MA, Donaldson A, et al. Sensitivity and specificity of intrathecal fluorescein and white light excitation for detecting intraoperative cerebrospinal fluid leak in endoscopic skull base surgery: a prospective study. J Neurosurg. 2016;124(3):621–6.
263. Royal College of Surgeons. 2017. https://www.rcseng.ac.uk/surgeons/training/accreditation/fellowships/national-fellowship-register/neurosurgery.
264. Zaidi HA, De Los RK, Barkhoudarian G, et al. The utility of high-resolution intraoperative MRI in endoscopic transsphenoidal surgery for pituitary macroadenomas: early experience in the advanced multimodality image guided operating suite. Neurosurg Focus. 2016;40(3):E18.
265. Zaidi HA, Awad AW, Bohl MA, et al. Comparison of outcomes between a less experienced surgeon using a fully endoscopic technique and a very experienced surgeon using a microscopic transsphenoidal technique for pituitary adenoma. J Neurosurg. 2015;16:1–9.
266. Rudmik L, Starreveld YP, Vandergrift WA, et al. Cost-effectiveness of the endoscopic versus microscopic approach for pituitary adenoma resection. Laryngoscope. 2015;125(1):16–24.
267. Ammirati M, Wei L, Ciric I. Short-term outcome of endoscopic versus microscopic pituitary adenoma surgery: a systematic review and meta-analysis. J Neurol Neurosurg Psychiatry. 2013;84(8):843–9.
268. Mortini P. Cons: endoscopic endonasal transsphenoidal pituitary surgery is not superior to microscopic

transsphenoidal surgery for pituitary adenomas. Endocrine. 2014;47(2):415–20.
269. Koulouri O, Steuwe A, Gillett D, et al. A role for 11C-methionine PET imaging in ACTH-dependent Cushing's syndrome. Eur J Endocrinol. 2015;173(4):M107–20.
270. Feng Z, He D, Mao Z, et al. Utility of 11C-methionine and 18F-FDG PET/CT in patients with functioning pituitary adenomas. Clin Nucl Med. 2016;41(3): e130–4.
271. Trouillas J, Roy P, Sturm N, et al. A new prognostic clinicopathological classification of pituitary adenomas: a multicentric case-control study of 410 patients with 8 years post-operative follow-up. Acta Neuropathol. 2013;126(1):123–35.
272. Raverot G, Jouanneau E, Trouillas J. Management of endocrine disease: clinicopathological classification and molecular markers of pituitary tumours for personalized therapeutic strategies. Eur J Endocrinol. 2014;170(4):R121–32.
273. Heaney AJ. Management of aggressive pituitary adenomas and pituitary carcinomas. Neurooncol. 2014;117(3):459–68.
274. Whitelaw BC, Dworakowska D, Thomas NW, et al. Temozolomide in the management of dopamine agonist-resistant prolactinomas. Clin Endocrinol. 2012;76(6):877–86.
275. Marcus HJ, Hughes-Hallett A, Kwasnicki RM, et al. Technological innovation in neurosurgery: a quantitative study. J Neurosurg. 2015;123:174–81.
276. Marcus HJ, Cundy TP, Hughes-Hallett A, et al. Endoscopic and keyhole endoscope-assisted neurosurgical approaches: a qualitative survey on technical challenges and technological solutions. Br J Neurosurg. 2014;28:606–10.
277. McLaughlin N, Laws ER, Oyesiku NM, et al. Pituitary centers of excellence. Neurosurgery. 2012;71(5): 916–26.
278. Faustini-Fustini M, Pasquini E, Zoli M, et al. Comment in: pituitary centers of excellence. Neurosurgery. 2013;73(3):E557.
279. Tantongtip D, Fratianni A, Jenkner J, Arnold S, Spetzger U. Surgical treatment of inadvertent internal carotid artery lesion by Extraintracranial high-flow bypass. A case report and review of the literature. J Neurol Surg Rep. 2015;76(1):e100–4.

Metastatic and Invasive Tumours of the Skull Base

280. Carey RA, Nathaniel SD, Das S, Sudhakar S. Cavernous sinus syndrome due to skull base metastasis: a rare presentation of hepatocellular carcinoma. Neurol India. 2015;63:437–9.
281. Kim YS, Moon KS, Kim GW, Lim SC, Lee KH, Jang WY, Jung TY, Kim IY, Jung S. Role of craniofacial resection for malignant tumors involving the anterior skull base: surgical experience in a single institution. Brain Tumor Res Treat. 2015;3:81–8.
282. König SA, Ranguis S, Gramlich V, Spetzger U. Reconstruction of the anterior skull base after major trauma or extensive tumour resection. Acta Neurochir. 2015;157:139–44.
283. Lee A, Chang KH, Hong H, Kim H. Sixth cranial nerve palsy caused by gastric adenocarcinoma metastasis to the clivus. J Korean Neurosurg Soc. 2015;57:208–10.
284. Minniti G, Esposito V, Clarke E, Scaringi C, Bozzao A, Falco T, De Sanctis V, Enrici MM, Valeriani M, Osti MF, Enrici RM. Fractionated stereotactic radiosurgery for patients with skull base metastases from systemic cancer involving the anterior visual pathway. Radiat Oncol. 2014;9:110.
285. Tunio MA, Al Asiri M, Al-Qahtani KH, Aldandan S, Riaz K, Bayoumi Y. Skull base metastasis from papillary thyroid carcinoma: a report of three cases. Int Med Case Rep J. 2015;8:127–31.
286. Tunio MA, AlAsiri M, Riaz K, Abdulmoniem R. Optic nerve metastasis from squamous cell carcinoma of the uterine cervix. J Coll Physicians Surg Pak. 2015;25:694–5.
287. Zacharia BE, Romero FR, Rapoport SK, Raza SM, Anand VK, Schwartz TH. Endoscopic endonasal management of metastatic lesions of the anterior skull base: case series and literature review. World Neurosurg. 2015;84:1267–77.

Check for updates

Vascular Lesions of the Skull Base

The original version of this chapter was revised. An erratum to this chapter can be found at https://doi.org/10.1007/978-3-319-64018-1_9

Electronic Supplementary Material The online version of this chapter (https://doi.org/10.1007/978-3-319-64018-1_6) contains supplementary material, which is available to authorized users.

A. König, U. Spetzger (eds.), *Surgery of the Skull Base*,
https://doi.org/10.1007/978-3-319-64018-1_6

6

Editor's Comment

Cerebrovascular diseases of the skull base represent a separate entity. Especially aneurysms located close to the skull base as well as dural arteriovenous fistulas require highly specialized neuroradiological diagnostics and an individualized treatment strategy being exactly tailored to the lesion. For different reasons there has been a shift to endovascular treatment of these vascular lesions of the skull base over the years. Modern supraselective microcatheters and further development and improvement of the different embolization materials nowadays allow a very selective occlusion of arteriovenous malformations. Furthermore, the ongoing development of endovascular coil technology and especially the modern methods of vessel wall reconstruction by stents have pushed back the complex surgical procedures for the microsurgical clipping of skull base aneurysms. But nevertheless, endovascular procedures will not completely replace microsurgical therapy in the foreseeable future. A problem for the younger generation and especially for the practical training of young skull base surgeons is the decreasing number of neurovascular cases due to the increasing number of endovascular cases. Furthermore, often very complex cases that are very difficult to operate on remain for microsurgical therapy.

According to the philosophy of this book which aims to mainly demonstrate neurosurgical treatment strategies, we abstain from a detailed description of the endovascular technique but focus on microsurgical therapy. Due to his unique expertise which is unlikely to be reached by the younger generation due to the increasing number of endovascular therapeutic options, Takanori Fukushima will illustrate the whole spectrum of microsurgical clip occlusion and reconstructive vascular microsurgery, especially his highly differentiated bypass surgery, in the chapter about the surgery of complex and difficult skull base aneurysms. Thus, the focus here is on very complex aneurysms and revascularizing microneurosurgery.

6.1 Surgery of Complex and Difficult Aneurysms with Skull Base Approaches and Microsurgical Flow Diversion

T. Fukushima, G. Inoue, and A. Zomorodi

Complex and difficult aneurysms are defined as giant-sized aneurysms (larger than 2 cm), fusiform or mega-sized serpentine, and intracavernous-pericavernous aneurysms. Management of these aneurysms remains difficult and challenging. Most of them can be repaired with combination clipping technique with or without small vessel microanastomosis backup bypass. However, some of the very large serpentine or mega-giant aneurysms may require microsurgical skull base high-flow bypass designated as «microsurgical flow diversion.» This chapter summarizes the author's personal operative series of 402 cases of complex and difficult aneurysms. Various updated skull base surgical approaches and microanatomy are described in details as well as the importance of refined skull base micro-instruments and special equipment.

6.1.1 General Information

The treatment of cerebral aneurysms is a major subject in neurosurgery. In general, aneurysm treatment is recommended to prevent rupture or progressing growth to large or giant size (larger than 2 cm) [18, 19, 35, 36, 44]. Complex and difficult aneurysms are those which have already reached a giant size, are large and fusiform or serpiginous, or are paracavernous in location. These aneurysms share a very aggressive natural history and frequently cause morbidity or mortality through rupture, mass effect on vital neural structures, or ischemic sequelae [2, 5, 16, 17, 22, 33, 36]. Another feature common to these aneurysms is a high rate of morbidity and mortality associated with microsurgical treatment and related morbidity. Multiple series in the literature underscore the fact that surgery must be performed by expert cerebrovascular neurosurgeons who have superb neurovascular operative skills and extensive experience, working in high-volume centers [11, 16, 25, 28, 29, 35]. To lessen the morbidity of treatment and increase treatment options, in recent years, endovascular treatment has been advocated and popularized. However, coiling and/or stenting of giant aneurysms has resulted in mostly incomplete obliteration of aneurysms and carries its own significant procedure-related risks [1, 6–9, 12, 15, 20, 24, 26, 27, 30, 31, 40–43]. Therefore, the surgical management of these lesions remains a necessary option, and every effort must be made to refine the techniques and improve the outcomes from microsurgery.

The high-flow skull base saphenous vein bypass, designated as «microsurgical flow diversion» by the senior author, has provided excellent results for the total obliteration and cure of complex and difficult aneurysms. Even extracranial skull base aneurysms can be treated safely with a high success rate with this saphenous vein microsurgical flow diversion surgery. The senior author developed the world's first successful skull base cavernous sinus carotid bypass procedure in 1986. Since then, five variations of skull base high-flow bypass operations named «Fukushima Bypass» have been developed and performed in a total of 136 cases [32, 39] (◘ Table 6.2, ◘ Fig. 6.34). This article presents the author's personal series of 402 consecutive cases of complex and difficult aneurysms. All cases were treated with direct clipping obliteration with or without the help of microvascular backup bypass or with the saphenous vein microsurgical flow diversion. Additionally, this article will present operative technical details, indications of direct clipping methods, various backup bypass methods, and the high-flow saphenous microsurgical diversion technique with detailed operative nuances, pearls, and complication avoidance.

6.1.2 Clinical Materials and Methods

Since the author became chief of service in 1980, his cerebrovascular database shows that a total of 2429 cases with cerebral aneurysms were treated surgically till the end of 2016. The author's cerebrovascular database, available clinical records, imaging studies, and detailed operative notes and illustrations from 3 hospitals in Raleigh-Durham and 13 hospitals in Japan were reviewed and analyzed. The patient demographics, operative approaches, surgical results, and complications are studied.

Of these 2429 cases, there were 253 cases of intracavernous or pericavernous aneurysms, 230 cases of giant aneurysms (≥20 mm), and 40 fusiform aneurysms of various etiologies (◘ Fig. 6.1 and ◘ Table 6.1). ◘ Figure 6.1 represents the author's classification of the various intracavernous and pericavernous aneurysms, including carotid fibrous ring aneurysms, paraclinoid aneurysms, and ophthalmic aneurysms (total of 253 cases). ◘ Table 6.1 demonstrates the number of giant aneurysms (≥20 mm) in various locations: anterior circulation giants, 173 cases (Acom 12, MCA 24, P-com 7, A2–3 4, A1 1, IC distal bifurcation 4, cavernous sinus 121), and posterior circulation giants, 57 cases (BA-SCA 5, BA-trunk 8, VA 25, PICA 4, PCA 3).

Clinical cases in this article involve 253 cases of intracavernous and pericavernous aneurysms (including 121 cases of cavernous giant aneurysms), 52 cases of anterior circulation giant aneurysms, and 57 cases of posterior circulation aneurysms. Of these 362 cases (230 cases of giant aneurysms and 132 cases of non-giant cavernous sinus aneurysms), there were 224 female patients and 138 male patients. Age ranged from 4 to 86 years old with the mean age of 56 years old. There are 130 cases of complex aneurysms located on the right and 230 cases on the left, and 2 patients had bilateral intracavernous giant aneurysms.

6.1.3 Classification of Cerebral Aneurysms and Nomenclature of Internal Carotid Artery Segments

A number of papers were published in the past in regard to the size and classification of cerebral aneurysms [21, 34, 35]. Kassell (1983) designated the standard aneurysm as less than 12 mm and giant aneurysms larger than 25 mm [21]. Wiebers (2003) classified small aneurysms as less than 7 mm, medium-size aneurysms as 7–12 mm, large aneurysms as 13–24 mm, and giant aneurysms as larger than 25 mm in size [44]. The author has been using his own classification of aneurysms as category I average A-class (standard small) aneurysms less than 10 mm, category II B-class aneurysms between 11 and 19 mm, and category III complex and difficult (C/D class) aneurysms including fusiform, cavernous sinus location, and giant aneurysms larger than 20 mm. Based upon the principle of the author's «Rule of Three», namely, class A aneurysms are the average standard small, and class B aneurysms are bulbous, bit bigger, or moderately large aneurysms (11–19 mm). Class C/D aneurysms are very large and giant, fusiform, or in cavernous sinus location (≥20 mm). The author believes this simple three-class classification of category I, II, and III or class A, B, and C/D is the best for designating

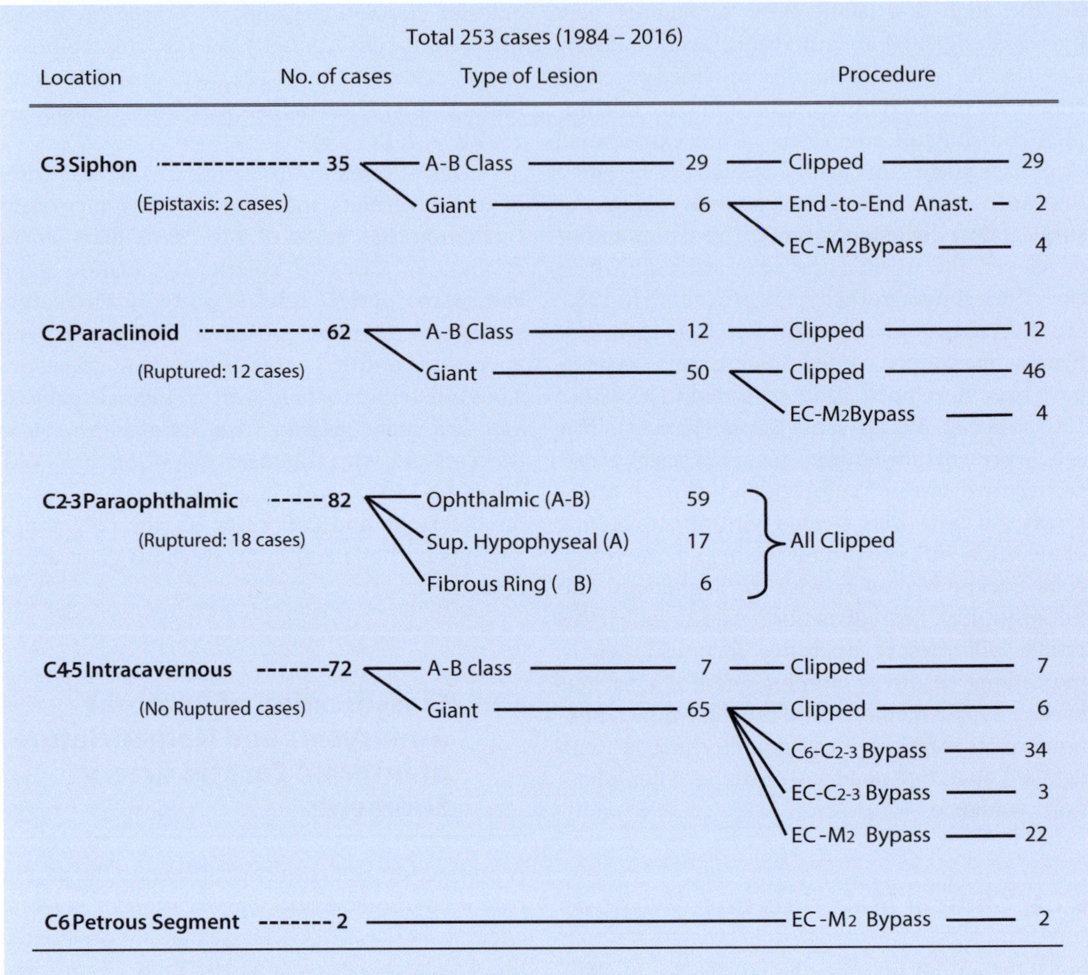

Fig. 6.1 Microsurgical repair of intracavernous and pericavernous aneurysms

surgical approaches and clipping methods and for determining the requirements of any bypass procedures. In the author's series, the majority of class A and class B aneurysms were obliterated with the direct clipping method, either by single clip or with a combination of several clips. Category C/D aneurysms are the subject of this chapter. The author believes that for any aneurysm, once it bleeds, the prognosis of subarachnoid hemorrhage is very grave. Aneurysm rupture carries a 30-day mortality rate of 40% with approximately half of survivors sustaining irreversible brain damage [36]. The best management of any aneurysm is the microsurgical one-time curative clipping treatment with or without bypass technique before it bleeds.

Nomenclature of Internal Carotid Artery Segments

The essential purpose of a surgical nomenclature system is to capture relevant details of surgical anatomy and to facilitate communication among surgeons by providing a common frame of reference. Fischer in 1938 reported the world's first nomenclature of segments of cerebral vascular tree with precise analysis of cerebral angiography [13] (Fig. 6.2a). Internal carotid segments are described as C1, C2, and C3; anterior cerebral artery segments as A1, A2, and A3; and middle cerebral artery segments as M1, M2, and M3, starting from the distal carotid bifurcation. This was a short neuroradiological report; however, using the internal carotid bifurcation as the starting point for

Table 6.1 Microsurgical repair of giant aneurysms (≥2 cm) (1981–2016), 35-year summary, 230 cases

Location of the aneurysms	No. of cases	Procedure	No. of cases
Anterior circulation	*52*	*(Ruptured: 27)*	
Acom giants	12	Clip	8
		Bonnet bypass	2
		A3-A3 anastomosis	2
MCA giants	24	Clip with STA-MCA back up bypass	10
		Clip only	8
		EC-M2 bypass	6
P-com	7	All clip	
A2-A3	4	End-to-End bypass	1
		A3-A3 bypass	1
		Clip	2
A1	1	Clip	
IC-bifurcation	4	Clip	2
		EC-M2 bypass	2
Posterior circulation	*57*	*(Ruptured: 12)*	
BA-tip giants	12	Clip	8
		EC-P2 bypass	4
BA-SCA giants	5	All clip	
BA-trunk	8	All EC-P2 bypass and clip	
VA giants	25	Clip, aneurysmorrhaphy, OA-PICA, PICA repositioning	
VA-PICA	4	All clip	
PCA(P2-P3)	3	STA-PCA transventricular End-to-end bypass	
Cavernous sinus giants	*121*	*(Ruptured: 12)*	
Paraclinoid giants	50	Clip	46
		EC-M2 bypass	4
C3 siphon	6	End-to-end anastomosis	2
		EC-M2	4
Intracavernous	65	Clip	6
(C4-C5)		C6-C2–3	34
		EC-M2	22
		EC- C2–3	3

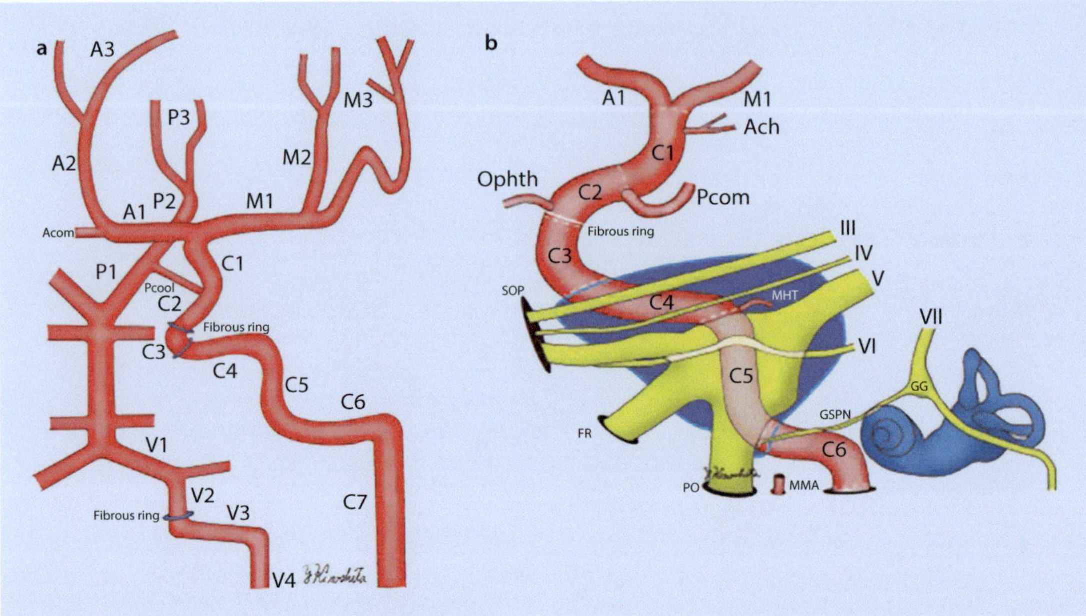

Fig. 6.2 **a** Nomenclature traditional German and Japanese nomenclature of the carotid artery segments and vertebrobasilar artery segments. **b** The nomenclature of the cavernous carotid segments in relation to the cavernous sinus cranial nerves, geniculate ganglion, and the cochlear

this system makes perfect sense for the neurosurgeon who operates standing at the patient's head. Thus, Fischer's nomenclature was adopted by the German and Japanese Neurosurgical Societies. In Japan, since the 1940s, Fischer's nomenclature has been extended to include cavernous carotid segments and the infratemporal carotid artery (Fig. 6.2b). Likewise, the posterior cerebral artery was named as P1, P2, and P3 and the vertebral artery from the vertebrobasilar junction as intradural segments V1 and V2, extracranial horizontal segment V3, and vertical segment V4. Again, given the intuitive and surgically oriented nature of this nomenclature, all members of the Japan Neurosurgical Society adopted this traditional nomenclature. In the early 1990s, Dr. Jeffrey Keller, Department of Neurosurgery, University of Cincinnati, published his own carotid nomenclature as a new classification system by reversing the order of segments to start from the cervical ICA as C1, petrous carotid segment as C2, clinoidal segment as C5, and intradural segments as C6 to C7 [3]. We believe this system runs counter to the surgical anatomy and introduces some confusion into the discussion of cerebral aneurysms. We continue to use and encourage the use of the traditional and more surgically relevant vascular nomenclature.

6.1.4 Skull Base Approaches and Operative Techniques

Instrumentation

In order to achieve appropriate skull base exposure, secure handling of high-speed power motor drills; maintaining a clean, dry, operative field with precise and meticulous hemostasis; and understanding of all relevant microanatomy of the cranial base are the key elements for success. Skull base drill shaving must be done as eggshelling style, leaving a thin shell of cortical bone to be elevated with sharp-rigid dissectors or curettes. The surgeon will need updated refined skull base micro-instruments such as tapered suckers with teardrop side ports (French sizes #3–12 and shaft length from short, medium, long, to extra-long) (Fig. 6.3a). Using teardrop suckers with continuously graded pressure adjustment with three fingertips is the #1 important maneuver in skull base surgery (Fig. 6.3b). A suction irrigator is extremely useful during skull base drilling (Fig. 6.3c), to cool down the shaving area and to clear up bone dust. The second important instrument is nonstick slim shape micro-bipolar forceps, such as Tokyo micro-bipolar, nonstick SilverGlide bipolar, and recent development of high-frequency

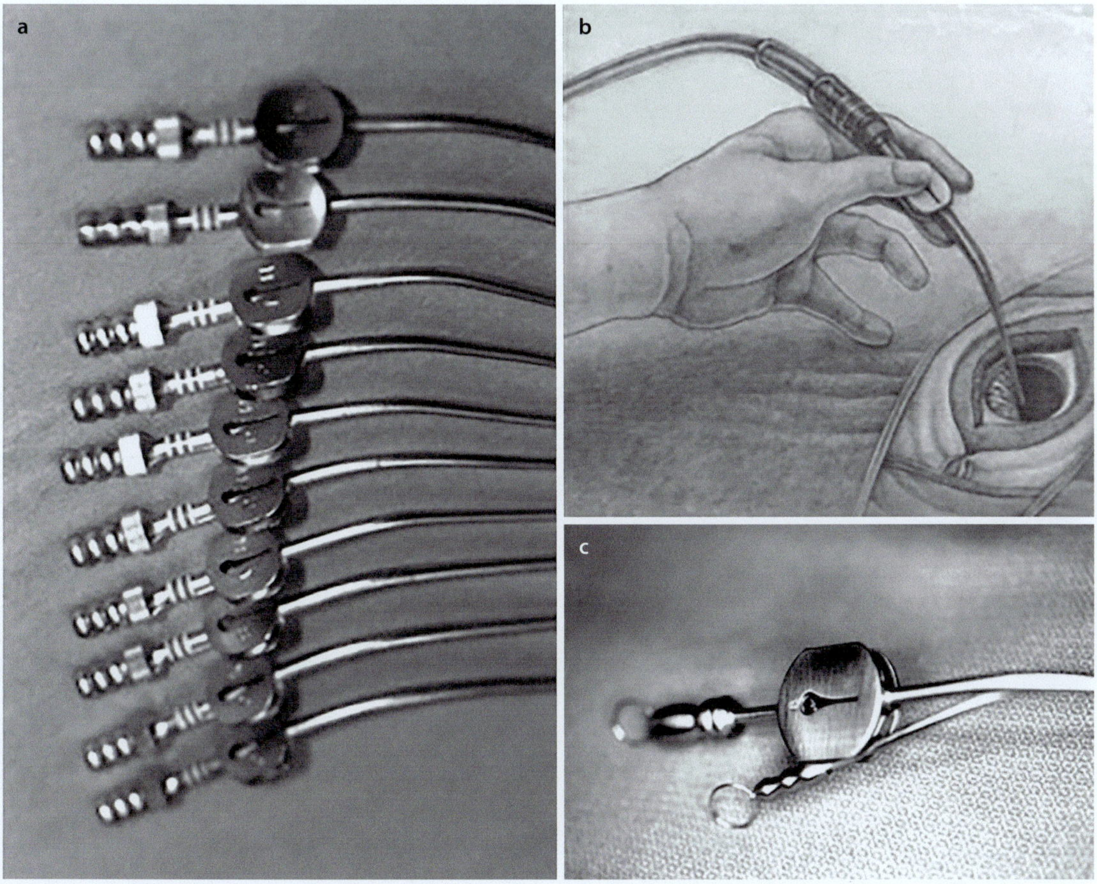

Fig. 6.3 **a** Teardrop side port-tapered suckers from French #3 to #12 with various lengths of short, medium, long, and extra-long. **b** Three-fingertip holding, adjusting suction pressure freely during the operation. **c** Suction irrigator for skull base drilling procedure

silver slim bipolar forceps (Fig. 6.4). The third important micro-instruments are hybrid super-microscissors with thin blade, medium blade, and thick rigid blades (Fig. 6.5). The medium blade and rigid blade are used for incising tumor capsules, dural membrane, and for other fibrous tissues. Thin blade microscissors are the key instrument for bloodless, sharp dissection of the arachnoid membrane. The fourth important instruments are various sized and shapes of rigid semi-sharp skull base dissectors, microprobe with smooth tapered bullet-type tips, micro-cup curettes, 90° bullet-tip neuro-dissectors, sharp hook knife, and flat thin blade sharp-edge micro-ring curettes (Fig. 6.6). These rigid dissectors, microprobes, and ring curettes super micro-dissectors are extremely important to perform precise and efficient skull base dissection and exposure. For obliterating aneurysms properly, the use of high-grade titanium clips (140 various sizes and shapes) and very thin-slim size, keyhole clip appliers (16 different holding appliers) is mandatory (Fig. 6.7) [38]. Figure 6.8 demonstrates preparation of micro-cottonoid from very thin 2 mm and 4 mm size to 10–15 mm, various sizes and length of delicate micro-cottonoid. Preparation of various sizes of square or rectangular shape of small Surgicel pieces is extremely helpful to accomplish precise hemostasis (variable sizes from 1 to 30 mm with 0.5 or 1 mm increments). Figure 6.9 demonstrates the universal holding system, which provides a wide dynamic range of circular holding of the soft tissue and multiple flexible snake holders. The universal holding system consists of two table clamps, four vertical posts, and six curved bars designed as surgeon bars, front bars, and sidebars. Blunt skin hooks, soft tissue hooks, flexible silicon rubber bands, multiple flexible snake holders, tapered 2 mm brain spatula (regular width and slim type), continuous irrigation, and patty holder

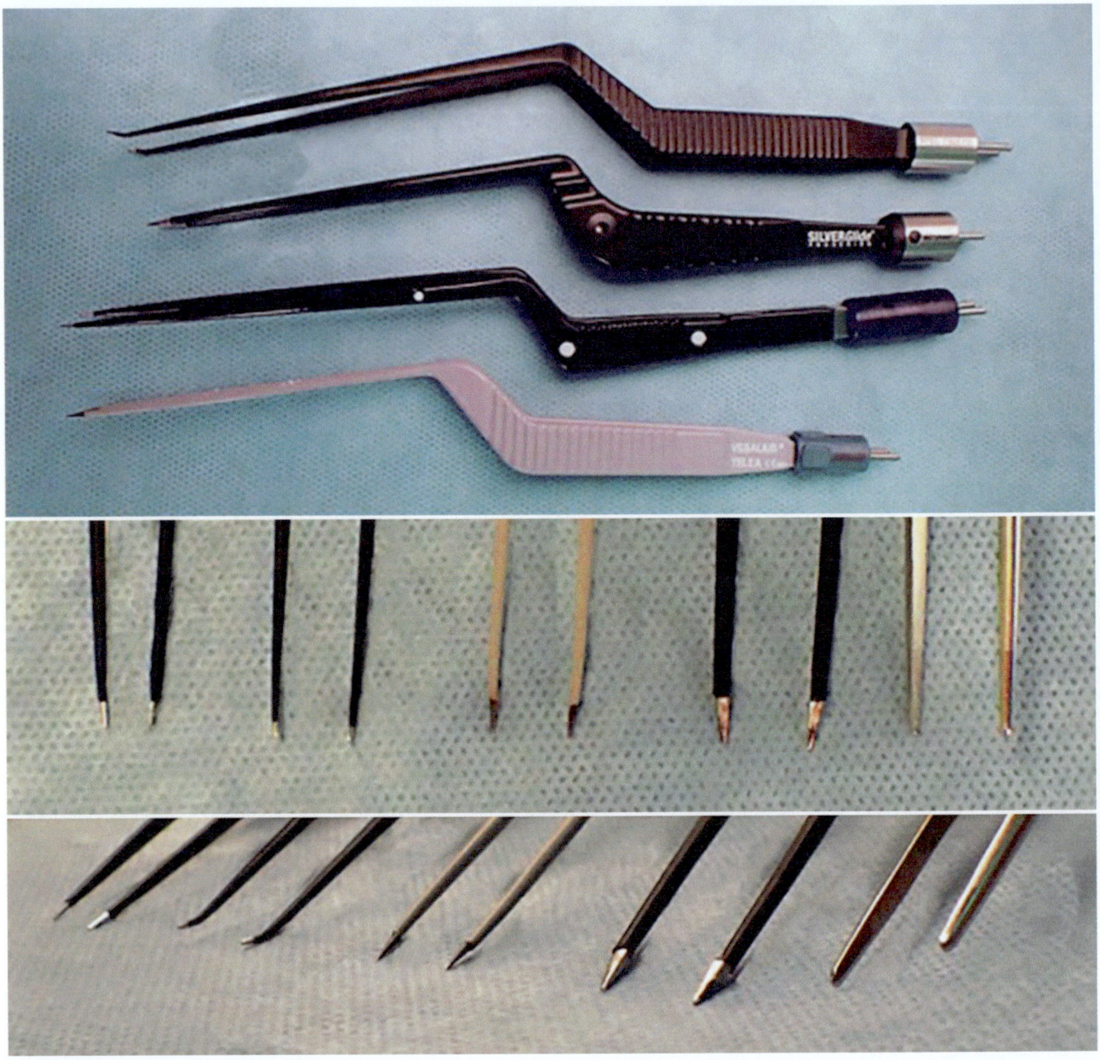

Fig. 6.4 Various keyhole micro-bipolar forceps designed by Fukushima

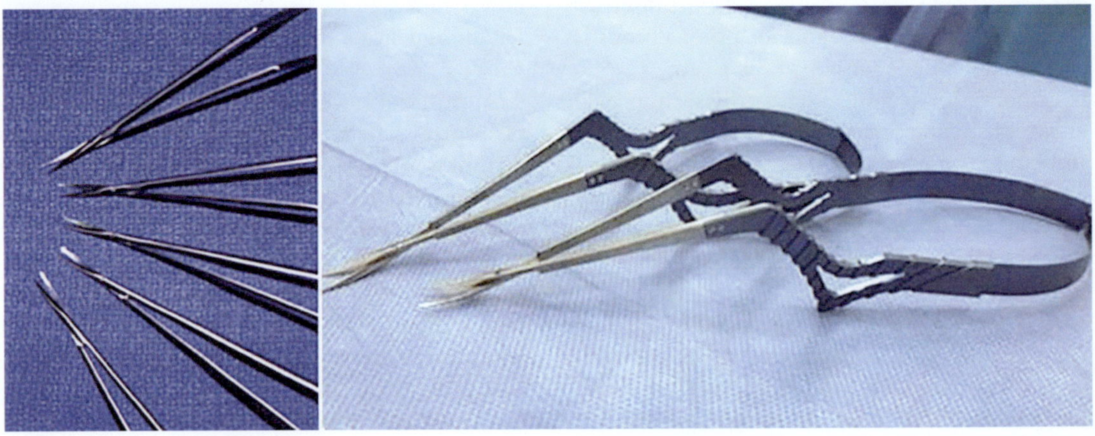

Fig. 6.5 Thin-blade hybrid super-microscissors designed by Fukushima

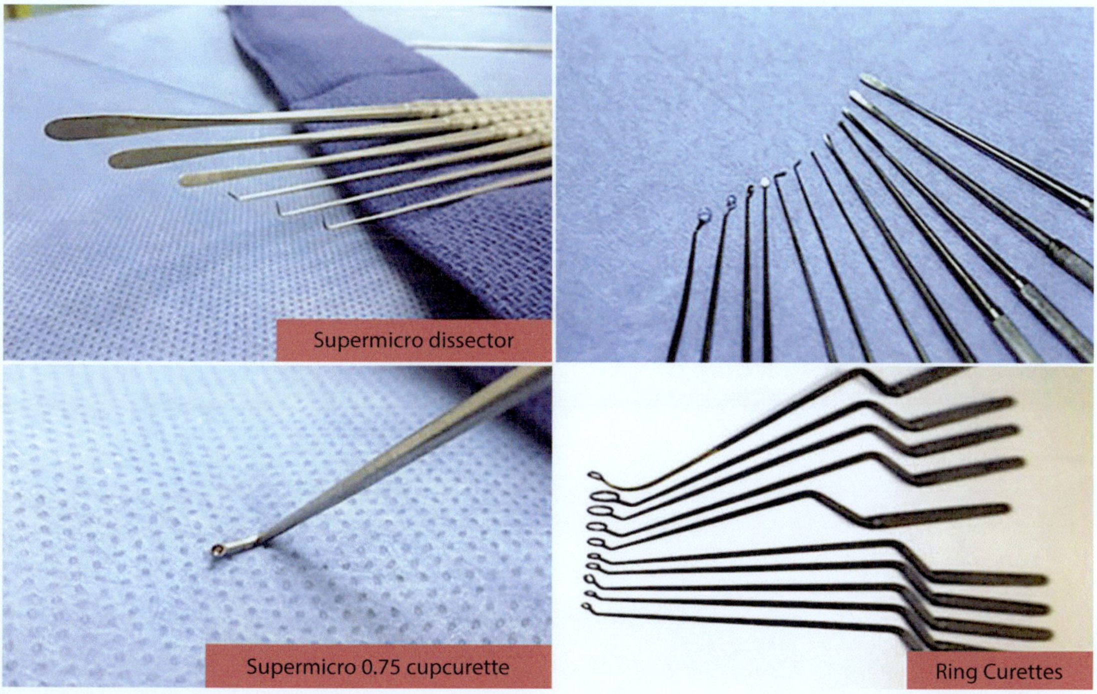

Fig. 6.6 Various skull base rigid semi-sharp skull base dissectors, super micro-dissectors, such as micro-sickle knife, bullet-tip 90° and 45° neuro-dissector, 90° and 45° sharp hook knives, 0.75 mm and 1 mm 90° micro-cup dissectors, and from 1.5, 2 mm, 2.5mm to 3 mm, 4 mm, 5 mm, and 6 mm and sharp-edge ring curettes. These micro-dissectors and ring curettes are extremely useful for total resection of skull base tumors, such as meningioma, acoustic neuromas, and epidermoid tumors

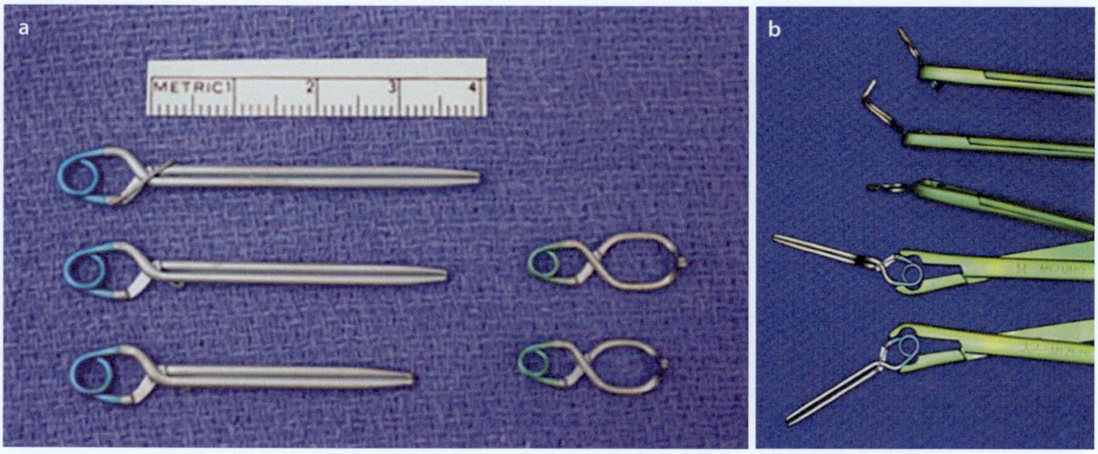

Fig. 6.7 **a** High-grade titanium clips to yield high-tension closure, manufactured using contemporary advanced metallurgical technology Giant long clips, 3 cm and 4 cm, and long window-locking clips designed by Fukushima. There are 140 different shapes and sizes of clips. **b** Fukushima keyhole aneurysm clips, slim appliers (16 variations)

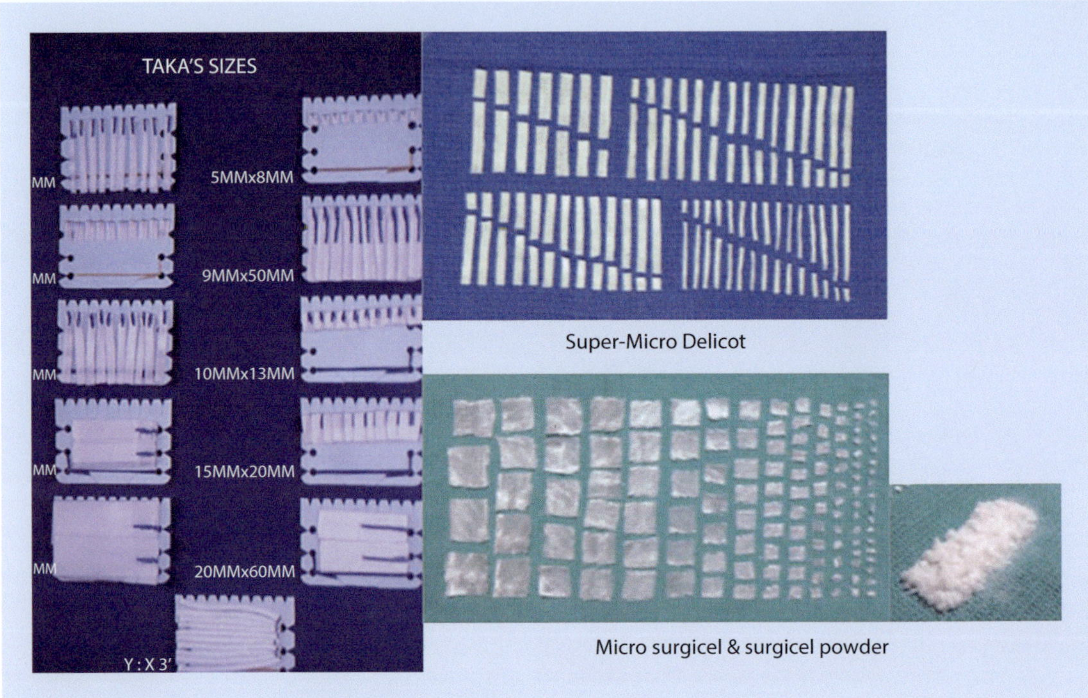

Fig. 6.8 Super micro-cottonoids and 80 Surgicel pieces of different millimeter sizes

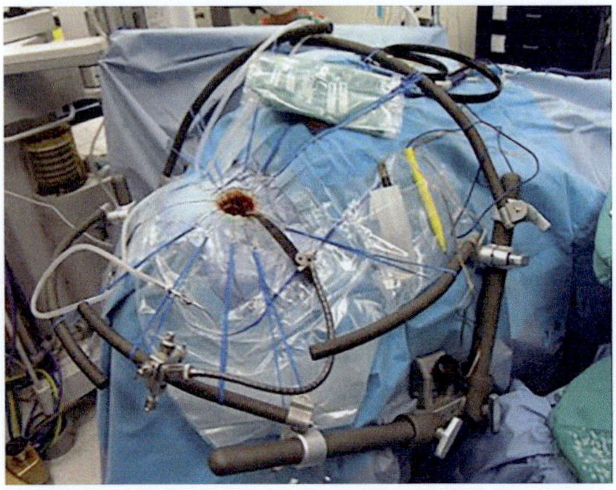

Fig. 6.9 Wide dynamic range universal holding system consisting of 2 table clamps, 4 vertical posts, and 6 bars (2 surgeon bars, 2 front bars and 2 side bars). Multiple blunt scalp hooks (small, medium, large, giant), silicone rubber bands, flexible snake holders, 2 mm tapered spatula, continuous drip irrigating needle, and patty-Surgicel holder. These all facilitate the surgeon's operative work while providing a wide open operative field

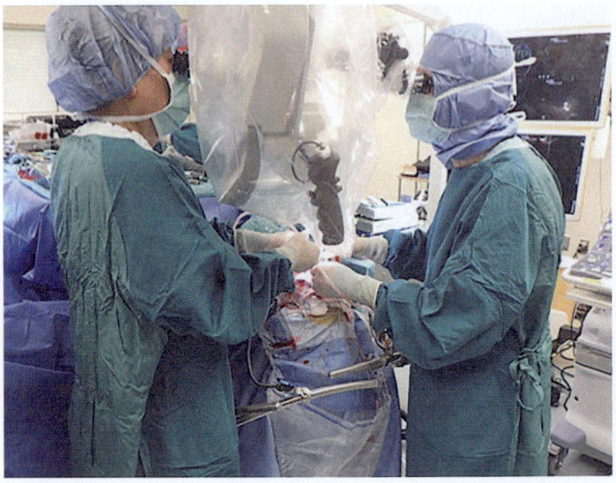

Fig. 6.10 Face-to-face (3D arrangement of microscope oculars. Two surgeon-4 hand microsurgeries facilitate efficient and rapid skull base surgery and bypass procedures. Double-suction performance and double bipolar actions by two surgeons simultaneously

will facilitate surgeons' micro-work in skull base surgery. This holding system provides wide and free operative areas to surgeon. Figure 6.10 demonstrates the arrangement of the face-to-face (3D) operating microscope and two surgeons, four hands» efficient microsurgery plus four additional robotic snake holder arms [45]. This style will provide very fast and efficient dissection, clipping, and bypass microanastomosis and is extremely valuable for practical operative education of younger neurosurgeons by guidance and assistance of senior faculty.

Skull Base Approaches

According to the location and complexity of the aneurysms, various skull base approaches have been utilized including transzygomatic, orbitocranial, orbitozygomatic, combined petrosal approach, extended middle fossa approach, and retrosigmoid or transsigmoid approaches. Extreme lateral infrajugular transcondylar approach (ELITE approach) is particularly useful for obliteration of aneurysms of the vertebral artery and PICA and vertebral basilar junction aneurysms. The optimal skull base operative approach given the location of the aneurysm is listed in ◘ Table 6.1. Sophisticated intraoperative monitoring methods were used such as EEG monitoring, MEP motor-evoked potential recording, intraoperative micro-Doppler monitoring and intraoperative ICG or fluorescence angiography monitoring. Lumbar spinal catheter placement for CSF drainage was used whenever indicated. During the bypass procedure with temporary clipping, mild-to-moderate hypothermia and pharmacological brain protection with the barbiturate or propofol, steroids, mannitol, phenytoin, or other pharmacological agents were used.

Frontotemporal Orbitocranial Approach

The frontotemporal pterional craniotomy is the most frequently used and popular approach in neurosurgery. The majority of anterior circulation aneurysms can be repaired using this standard craniotomy. However, some of the complex-difficult aneurysms require skull base dissection through the orbitocranial or orbitozygomatic or transzygomatic cranial base approach. Several modifications of orbitozygomatic craniotomy have been described. Over the past three decades, the authors have been performing and teaching younger neurosurgeons «less invasive» craniotomy with minimal bone loss technique. ◘ Figure 6.11 illustrates variations of orbitozygomatic and transzygomatic approaches. In principle, the authors advocate a minimally invasive smaller bone flap. Pterion (sphenoid ridge) and anterior temporal groove drilling are performed before turning the frontotemporal bone flap. Conventional large burr holes will not be performed. In the conventional craniotomy, four or five big burr holes are made to turn the bone flap; then surgeons bite and remove the skull base bones using rongeurs and Kerrison punch, resulting in a large amount of bone loss. With the author's less invasive method, cranial base

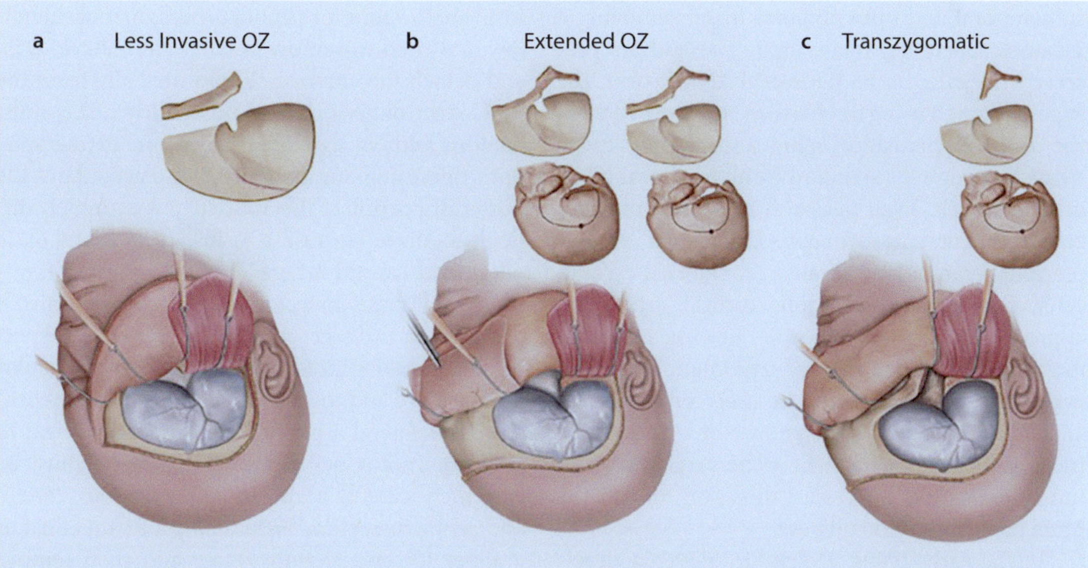

◘ **Fig. 6.11** Variations of orbitozygomatic, transzygomatic, and orbitocranial skull base approaches. **a** Less invasive orbitozygomatic approach with removal of only 3 cm length supraorbital bar between the supraorbital foramen and frontal zygomatic suture. **b** Extended orbitozygomatic craniotomy, one-piece method, or two-piece method. **c** Transzygomatic approach with osteotomy and removal of T-bone zygomatic arch using periosteal and fascial envelope method bone is shaved first before turning the bone flap; no large perforators are used. Surgeons use only 2 mm cone-shaped cutting burr or 4 mm extra-course diamond burr to shave the subtemporal skull base areas before craniotomy. After the triangular pterional drilling is finished, orbitotemporal detachment is performed at the far anterior temporal pole under an operating microscope. The anterior basal subtemporal groove is made for 15 mm length. Making one or two small bone openings (5 mm small space) posteriorly, where the pediatric or mini craniotome footplate can pass, minimal bone loss cosmetic craniotomy can be performed. In most cases, continuous lumbar spinal drainage may be placed to facilitate extradural frontotemporal basal dura elevation. Orbital roof, sphenoid ridge, and the lateral orbital wall are shaved flat like an eggshell. ◘ Figure 6.11a illustrates a less invasive orbitocranial approach without cutting the zygomatic arch. Temporal muscle is reflected inferiorly and posteriorly using multiple blunt scalp hooks and silicon rubber bands. About 3 cm length of supraorbital bar is removed using a sagittal saw, lateral to the supraorbital foramen and medial to the frontozygomatic suture. ◘ Figure 6.11b illustrates extended orbitozygomatic craniotomy in two-piece way or in one-piece fashion. ◘ Figure 6.11c illustrates a transzygomatic cranial base approach to the subtemporal and infratemporal fossa, removing a T-bone-shaped zygomatic arch. The authors preserve the galeofascial-periosteal tissue over the zygomatic arch using the envelope method. Most of the anterior circulation giant aneurysms can be treated through the standard frontotemporal pterional approach. Even pericavernous and intracavernous aneurysms are approached via regular pterional craniotomy, because the internal carotid, A1, M1, and the cavernous carotid artery are approached with microscope viewing angle at looking down direction. Transzygomatic or orbitozygomatic approach would be used for the excessive mega-giant aneurysms or serpentine mega-sized aneurysms, where the surgeon's viewing angle is looking upward direction toward the brain base from the skull base.

In the early 1980s, Dolenc in Slovenia developed a revolutionary extradural transcavernous operative method, for direct transcavernous exposure, which propagated all over the world to open the new horizon of the direct surgical access to the cavernous sinus for the management of intracavernous vascular and neoplastic lesions [10, 11]. ◘ Figures 6.12, 6.13a, b, and 6.14 illustrate details of operative method of Dolenc transcavernous techniques. The key elements of Dolenc operation are shaving of the orbital roof, removal of the sphenoid ridge and the lateral orbital wall to expose the superior orbital fissure, optic canal unroofing, and removal of the anterior clinoid process. Optic canal unroofing must be started from the distal part and from the lateral aspect. Medially, the ethmoid band should be preserved to maintain the posterior ethmoidal artery circulation. Medial to the orbit and optic canal, the ethmoid sinus and the sphenoid sinus cavities exist; therefore, optic canal unroofing must be done only through superior wall unroofing around 180° range. Shaving and removal of the anterior clinoid process and optic canal unroofing must be performed with running irrigating water to cool down the diamond drill burr and to clean up the bone dust. Removal of the anterior clinoid process, namely, anterior clinoidectomy, is the most important operative work for this approach. Using various sizes of diamond burrs (4, 3, 2 extra-course or course diamond), the first step, as illustrated in ◘ Fig. 6.12, is to shave the inside of the anterior clinoid process to make it hollow and then to remove medial half. Shave, drill, and detach the anterior clinoid medially from the optic strut (anteriorly and posteriorly). This must be done without damaging any of the extracranial optic nerve and dural membranes. Particularly, the posterior portion of the optic strut is extremely difficult to shave because it is just next to the optic nerve and carotid artery. Then, using rigid semisharp skull base dissectors (such as A dissector, B dissector, or D dissector), separate the lateral aspect of the anterior clinoid process off from the oculomotor nerve and toward the tip of the clinoid process. This lateral aspect of the dura is just next to the oculomotor nerve, and the surgeon must be extremely careful to perform meticulous careful and gentle dissection. Next, using a 2 mm alligator grabber forceps, slightly rotate and then remove the remaining anterior clinoid process from the C3 siphon angle (anteromedial cavernous sinus). The

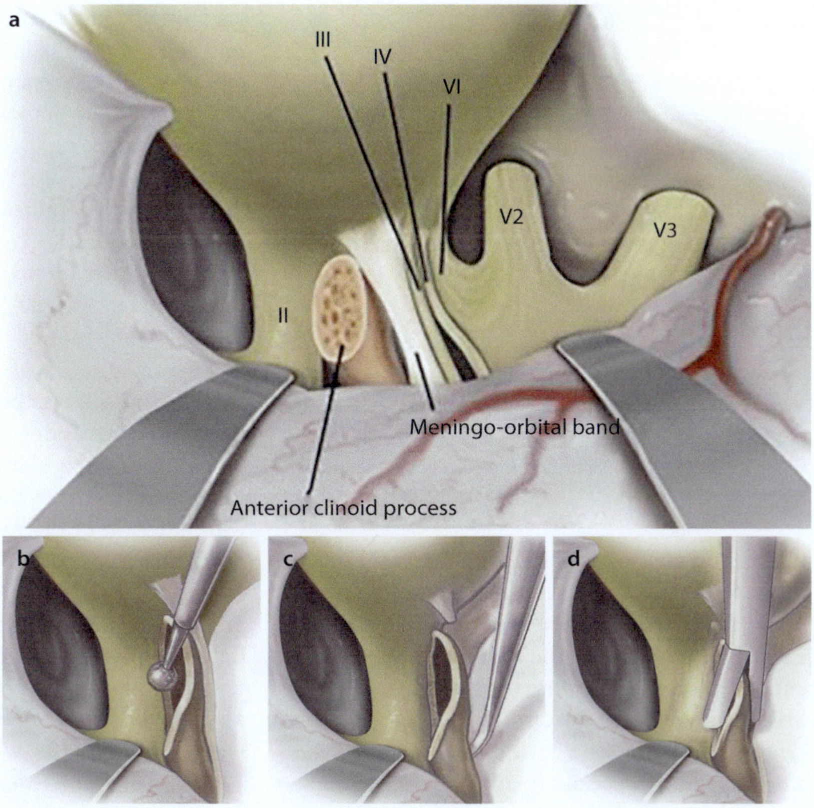

■ **Fig. 6.12** Extradural orbitobasal dissection, exposing the meningo-orbital band, extradural optic canal, anterior clinoid process, superior orbital fissure, and V2-V3 trigeminal peripheral nerves. The meningo-orbital band can be incised 7–8 mm lengths safely. **b** Precise and meticulous shaving using 2-3-4 diamond burrs with continuous irrigation cooling showing the initial step of making the anterior clinoid process halo. **c** Removal of the medial half of the clinoid process and detachment from the optic strut. **d** Careful removal of the lateral half of the anterior clinoid process without damaging the oculomotor nerve

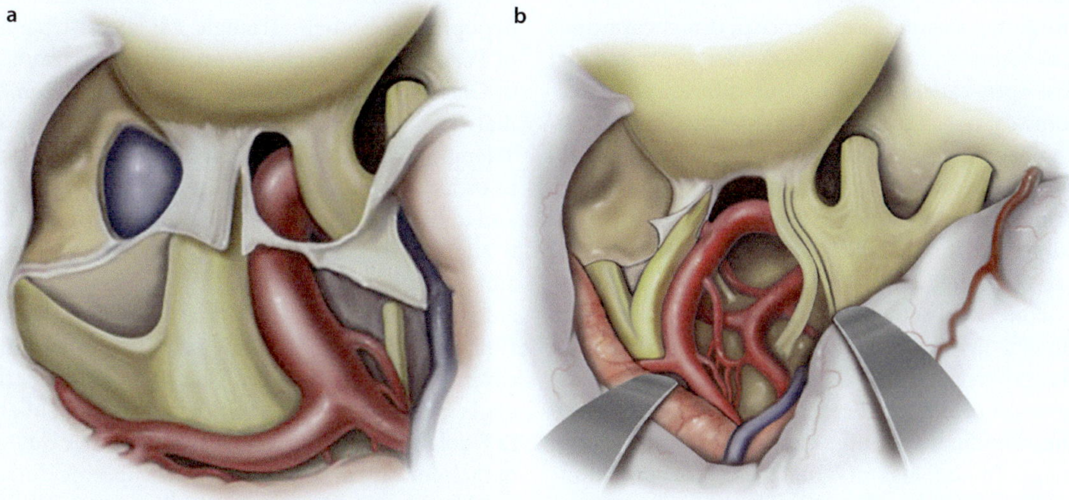

■ **Fig. 6.13** Combined extradural and intradural exposure following the optic canal unroofing and removal of the anterior clinoid process. Optic nerve dura can be incised **a** along the lateral border about 8 mm while preserving the ophthalmic artery and then the distal carotid fibrous ring can be excised to make Figure **b** style exposure. That this anteromedial transcavernous exposure toward the upper basilar artery

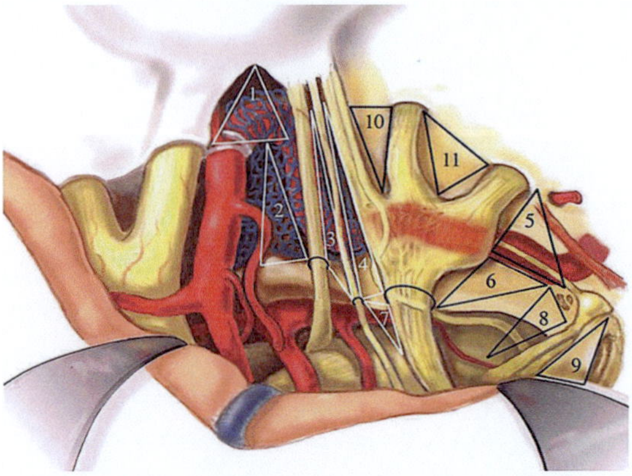

Fig. 6.14 Fukushima scheme of cavernous sinus entry triangles (1986–1990) including the concept of Hakuba and Dolenc

tip of the anterior clinoid process has a significant fibrous adhesion with the true cavernous membrane; therefore, this maneuver must be performed extremely gently. After the removal of the anterior clinoid process, the surgeon always encounters brisk venous bleeding from the anteromedial cavernous sinus (Dolenc triangle). This cavernous sinus bleeding can be easily controlled by filling the venous lake with 2 mm, 3 mm, or 4 or 5 mm adequate pieces of Surgicel and secure with Delicot cottonoids. Any cavernous sinus bleeding can be controlled in a few minutes using this method. In the author's clinical experience of direct cavernous sinus surgery over three decades demonstrated that just optic canal unroofing and anterior clinoidectomy carry 1–2% risks of postoperative visual deficit. If surgeons do not follow this extremely careful stepwise removing method (Figs. 6.12 and 6.13), visual deficit may increase to 10–30% risks. The surgeon at first needs a lot of skull base drilling exercise attending a cadaveric head hands-on microanatomy course (at least 10 times, possibly 20 times), then, learn clinical skull base practice from the expert surgeons. Figure 6.13a illustrates the location of the distal carotid fibrous ring between the intradural C2 and extradural C3 carotid segment. In the majority of cases, the ophthalmic artery is medial and intradural to this fibrous ring. However, in about 20% of the cases, the ophthalmic artery may be within the fibrous ring or at the extradural location. While controlling the cavernous sinus venous bleed with small pieces of Surgicel, if one performs very carefully, the excision of this fibrous ring, aneurysms of C3 clinoidal segment, superior hypophyseal aneurysms, dorsal or ventral paraclinoid giant aneurysms or any of the ophthalmic and paraophthalmic aneurysms become simple carotid aneurysms, such as P-com ones. Figure 6.13b demonstrates the anteromedial transcavernous exposure and access to the upper basilar trunk and basilar tip aneurysms. Figure 6.14 demonstrates the summary of the triangular operative corridors around the cavernous sinus. After learning the epidural transcavernous approach in June 1986 from Prof. Dolenc, in the following month, the author established the first systematic triangular transcavernous surgical corridors which was published in a Japanese journal (The 6th Mount Fuji Workshop, [14]). The scheme has been elaborated over the ensuing 5 years using cadaver dissection research. In 1991, with addition of the middle fossa rhomboids and premeatal and postmeatal triangles, the author established the 11 cavernous sinus triangles [14]. The author named each cavernous triangle after the pioneers who worked in this area.

Transcavernous Surgical Entry Corridors (Fig. 6.14)

Triangle #1: anteromedial triangle of Dolenc. Triangle #2: medial triangle of Hakuba and Dolenc. Triangle #3: superior triangle between the 3 and 4 of Fukushima triangle to make access to the C4 horizontal segment and to the meningohypophyseal branch. Triangle #4: lateral triangle of Parkinson. Triangle #5: posterolateral triangle of Glascock and Paulus. Triangle #6: posteromedial triangle of Kanzaki, Shiobara, and Kawase. Triangle #7: posteroinferior triangle of Fukushima in order to make access to the Gruber's ligament and to the abducens nerve. Triangle #8: premeatal triangle of Day- Fukushima. Triangle #9: postmeatal triangle of Day- Fukushima. Triangle #10: anterolateral triangle of Mullan where the superior and inferior ophthalmic vein merges into the cavernous sinus. Triangle #11: lateral Vidian triangle of Dolenc, Fukushima, and Froehlich. Figure 6.15 demonstrates two typical cases of paraclinoid giant aneurysm with superior dorsal projection. Case A shows a smaller neck and case B demonstrates a wider neck. Figure 6.16 demonstrates two cases of ventral-type paraclinoid giant aneurysms. For the majority of ventral paraclinoid giant aneurysms, the surgeon needs the proximal control either at C3 segment or C6 segment or simply at the submandibular neck internal carotid artery. In general, for any cerebral

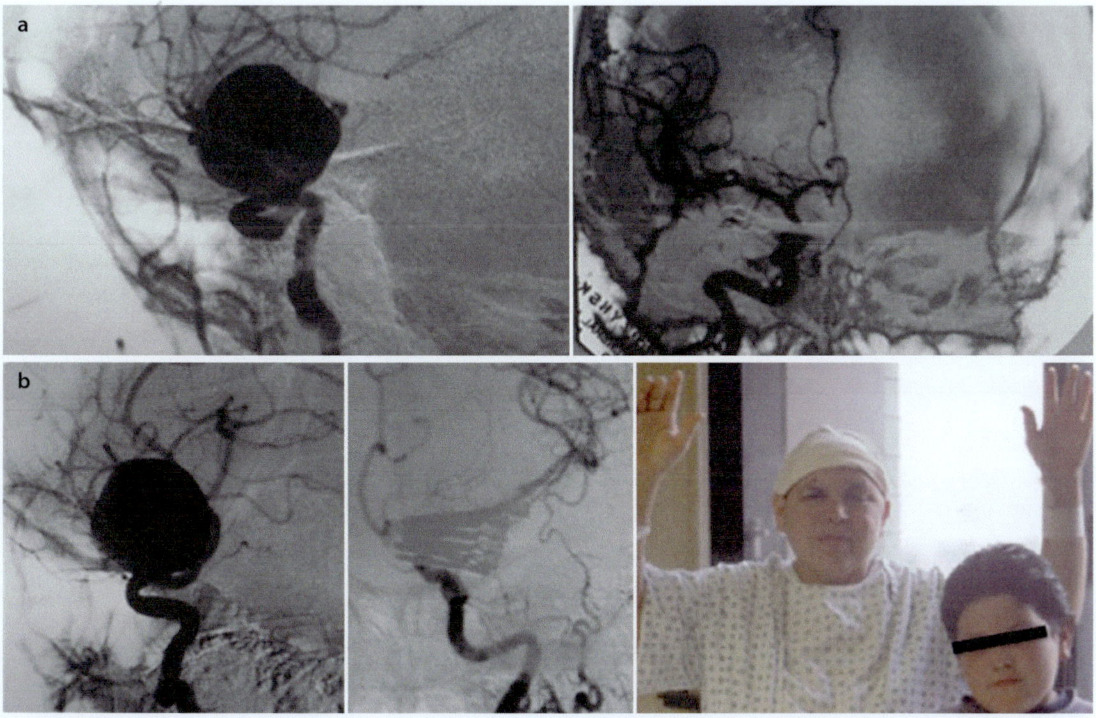

Fig. 6.15 Two examples of paraclinoid giant aneurysms. **a** Giant aneurysms of superior and dorsal projection with smaller neck obliterated with only two clips (56 y/o, female, right side). **b** A giant aneurysm with wider neck, which occluded totally using the required six large clips to totally obliterate the aneurysm (60 y/o, female, left side)

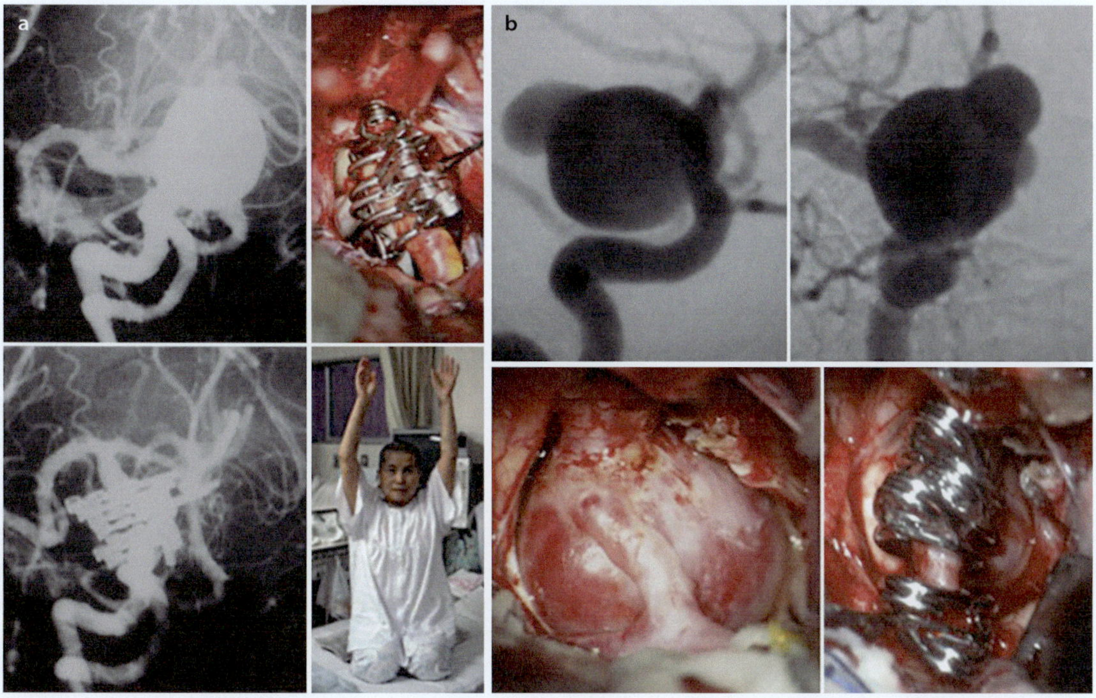

Fig. 6.16 Two cases of ventral projection paraclinoid giant aneurysm, optic canal unroofing, and anterior clinoidectomy make application of fenestrated clips much easier. **a** 65 y/o female, *right side*. **b** 36 y/o female, *right side*

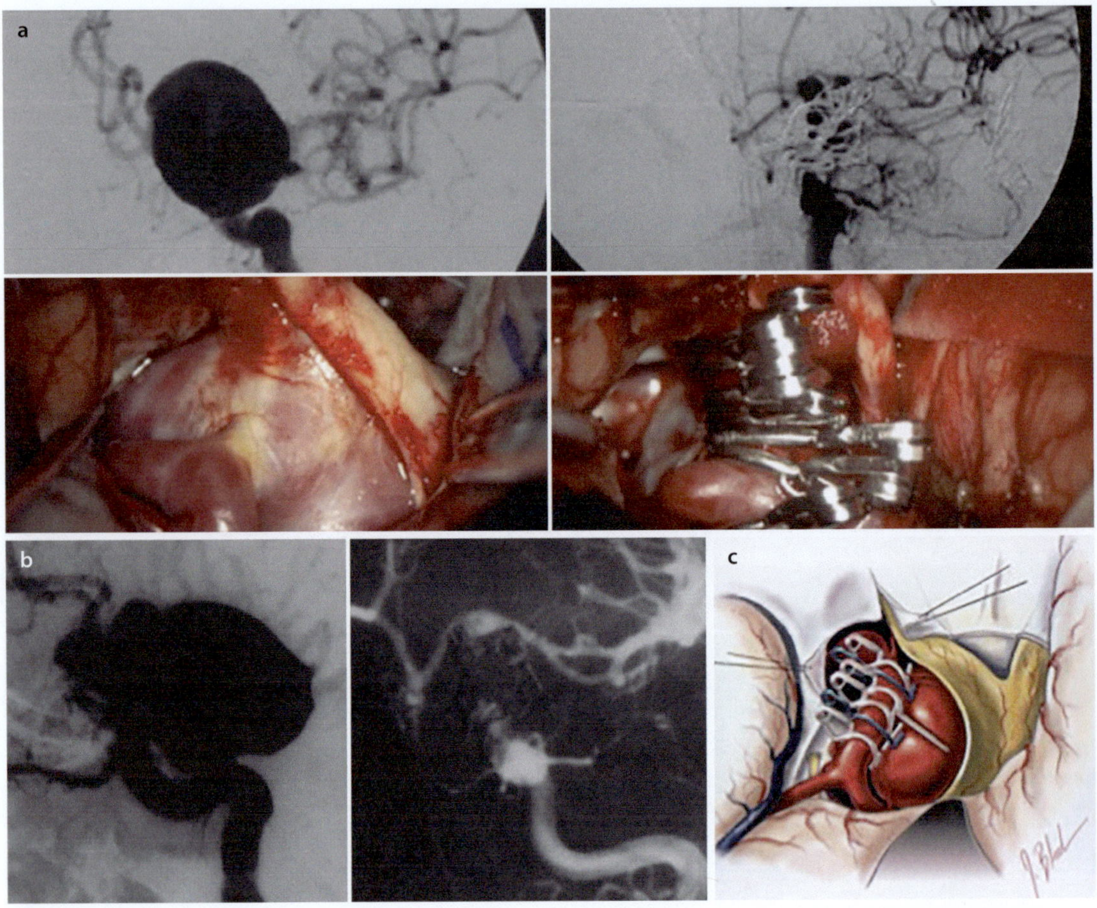

Fig. 6.17 Two cases of very difficult paraclinoid giant aneurysms. **a** This case shows the involvement of the P-com and anterior choroidal arteries, and special arrangement of the seven fenestrated clips was successful to totally obliterate the aneurysm, sparing fetal type of PCA and the anterior choroidal artery (38 y/o, female, *left side*). **b** A 50-year-old very exceptional patient who presented with four severe subarachnoid hemorrhages prior to Fukushima operation. Six fenestrated clips just obliterated the mega-giant aneurysm in Belfast, Ireland. This patient had a previous right carotid occlusion for the ophthalmic aneurysm, and this was one carotid patient. This patient was followed for 20 years without any neurological deficit (50 y/o, female, *left side*). **c** The typical fenestrated clip arrangement for the paraclinoid giant aneurysms with middle dome bisecting long blade straight fenestrated clips, series of various lengths of 90°-angled fenestrated clips and application of the long window-locking clips

aneurysms, the surgeon must be aware of the cardinal importance of the proximal control of the aneurysms to prepare for inadvertent intraoperative rupture of the aneurysm. For the majority of these paraclinoid or infraclinoid giant aneurysms, the surgeon needs careful application of various fenestrated clips: starting with a middle dome bisecting straight fenestrated clip and then applying various lengths (3, 4, 5, 6, 7 mm) of 90°-angled fenestrated clips. Figure 6.17 demonstrates two more clinical cases of extremely difficult infraclinoid giant aneurysms. Case A is a young patient, a 38-year-old female, left side. This patient's aneurysm involved the P-com and anterior choroidal arteries; therefore, clipping was extremely difficult to preserve these vital carotid branches. Intraoperative motor-evoked potential (MEP) monitoring and intraoperative ICG control is extremely useful. Case B was a mega-giant infraclinoid aneurysm, whom the author operated in Belfast, Ireland. This patient had previous right internal carotid ligation and remaining left one carotid developed mega-size aneurysm that bled severely four times to coma. Amazingly, this patient recovered to the normal condition, and I was invited to Belfast to obliterate this complex aneurysm. Using a primitive microscope, I used all seven fenestrated clips I brought, and the

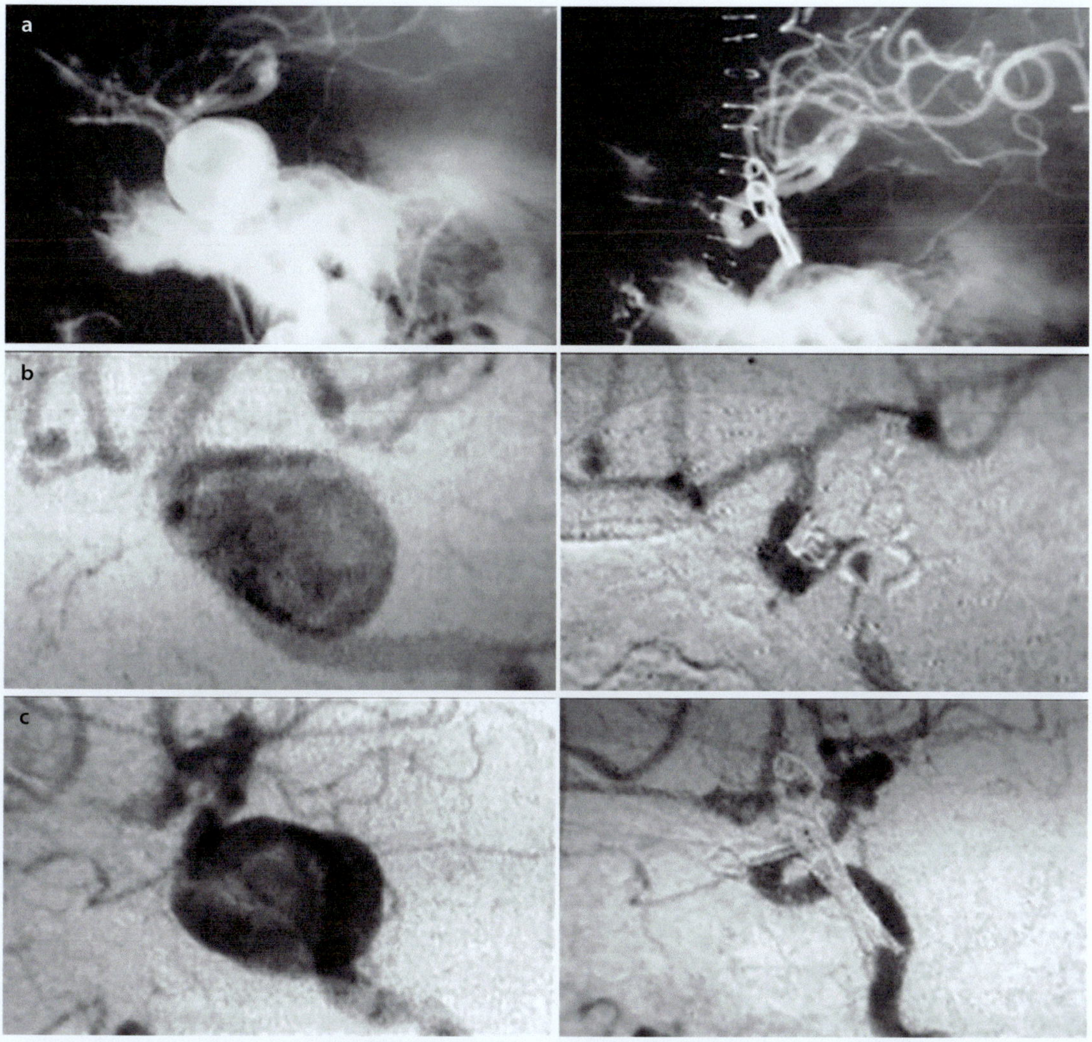

Fig. 6.18 **a-c** Three representative cases of direct transcavernous clipping of intracavernous giant aneurysms

surgery was successful. The author has followed this patient postoperatively for over 20 years, and the patient had no deficit from this aneurysm surgery. Figure 6.17c illustrates the typical clip arrangement for obliteration of this type of aneurysms preserving the ophthalmic artery, superior hypophyseal artery, P-com, and the anterior choroidal branches. Arrangement of the first clip being a long fenestrated dome bisecting clip and long window-locking clips (blue) to prevent slippage of the clips. Figure 6.18a–c demonstrates three cases of direct transcavernous clipping and repair of the intracavernous giant aneurysms. Using the Dolenc technique, this can be performed. However, in the initial series of the author's direct transcavernous surgery from 1986 to 1990, this direct clipping method was performed in six patients, and I could not clip in two cases which resulted in performing interpositional saphenous vein bypass. In addition, these six cases demonstrated some degree of postoperative sequelae of persistent diplopia or facial numbness. Therefore, I abandoned direct transcavernous clipping and switched my management to the various types of microsurgical flow diversion method using skull base high-flow saphenous vein bypass.

Middle Fossa Subtemporal Approach

The majority of subtemporal approaches can be done with the patient in the supine position and with the head rotated in a head lateral position.

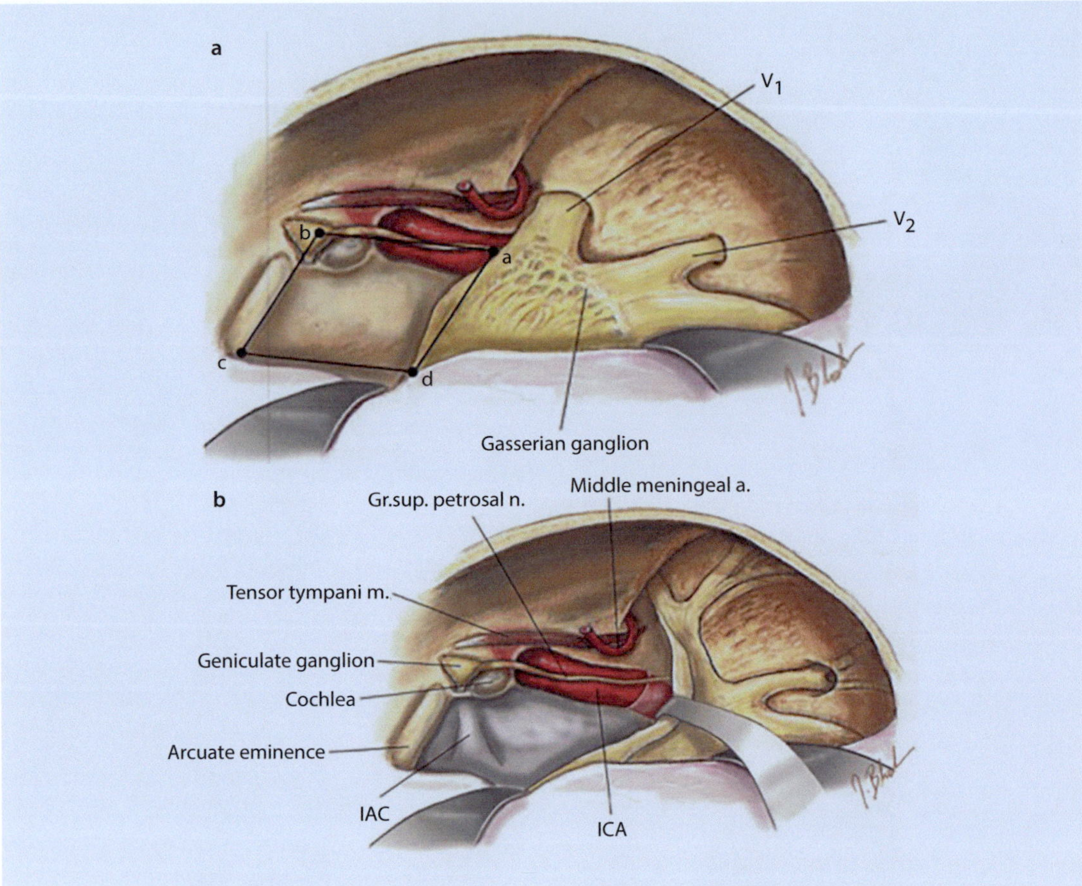

Fig. 6.19 Extradural exposure of the subtemporal middle fossa (superior petrosa). **a** Superior orbital fissure, foramen rotundum, foramen ovale, and middle meningeal artery. Posterior cavernous rhomboid construct is from the junction of the trigeminal third branch, GSPN, petrous carotid artery to the geniculate ganglion, superior semicircular canal, medial petrosal ridge, and the trigeminal fibrous ring, which forms the middle fossa rhomboid construct. **b** After drilling and shaving of the rhomboid area and anterior petrosectomy, exposure of the premeatal and postmeatal triangles and the internal auditory canal dura in the middle fossa and the posterior fossa dura toward the abducens nerve toward the inferior petrosal sinus and the abducens nerve. Gentle anterior translocation of the Gasserian ganglion using 2 mm tapered rigid spatula demonstrates posterolateral fibrous ring of the C6 and C5 junction

Mostly, a continuous lumbar spinal drainage tube is placed for relaxation of the temporal lobe and to avoid postoperative temporal lobe edema contusion or blood clot. In all cases, the temporal muscle is retracted anteriorly using multiple blunt scalp hooks in a one-layer fashion. In case of preauricular mid-subtemporal approach, temporal muscle is split in the middle and widened with a Gelpi retractor. The surgeon should know the anatomical landmarks around the anterior, middle, and posterior portion of the subtemporal cranial base, such as the foramen rotundum, Vidian loop, Ovale, MMA, and the root of zygoma. Before opening the dura, the base of the temporal lobe dura is held using a pair of 2 mm extradural rigid spatula (Fig. 6.19). In recent years, an increasing number of reports appeared in the international neurosurgical meeting that some neurosurgeons advocate no use of the brain spatula. These surgeons utilize suckers and instruments to retract and jiggle the brain tissue, which will result in more damage to the brain surface. In the author's 40 years of neurosurgical micro-operative experience, the best method of brain protection is to place on the brain surface mozaic Surgicel pieces or small collagen sheet and to cover with micro-cottonoid. Then, the brain is held gently with 2 mm tapered brain spatula preventing sagging of the brain and to provide the surgeon adequate operative space to work with his two hands freely. To perform clipping of aneurysms or to resect brain tumors, this gentle brain-holding method using one or two 2 mm tapered spatula is the best brain protection technique proven through the author's 40 years of experience of neurosurgery. It is not recommended to perform clumsy microsurgical dissection without using this brain-holding method.

In order to make access to the deep subtemporal base, the surgeon will have a lot of advantages by using a pair of 2 mm rigid dural holders. The surgeon encounters significant amount of bleeding from the subtemporal bone and venous connection, which is controlled by diamond drill shaving, by monopolar cautery, or by using bone wax and Surgicel application. After sufficient shaving and flattening of the subtemporal base and confirmation of the foramen rotundum, ovale, and middle meningeal artery, the dura can be opened at the far deep in the subtemporal base in order to make an easier intradural subtemporal approach and to protect the temporal brain with the dural coverage. In the majority of cases, the edge of the tentorium should be retracted laterally with two sutures to the temporal basal dura that makes transtentorial exposure much wider. Occasionally, fourth nerve and oculomotor dural sleeves are opened to make much wider access for the transtentorial approach to the basilar tip and upper basilar segment aneurysms.

In some cases of difficult large aneurysms, posterior transcavernous dissection can be made. The dura propria of the temporal base is elevated from the trigeminal second and third branches using a 15-blade knife and sharp A rigid dissector, exposing the trigeminal Gasserian ganglion. Then, using a 2 mm rigid spatula, anterior translocation of the third branch and Gasserian ganglion can be made to expose the anterior petrous bone. Anterior petrosectomy exposes the posterior fossa dura through the middle fossa rhomboid construct medial to the greater superficial petrosal nerve (GSPN) and anterior to the arcuate eminence (superior semicircular canal) and geniculate ganglion (◘ Fig. 6.19). When the trigeminal dural fibrous ring is excised and the superior petrosal sinus is divided, much wider transtentorial approach can be made just through this extended middle fossa approach. ◘ Figure 6.19a demonstrates the extended middle fossa epidural exposure of the triangle complex, C6 petrous carotid, GSPN, geniculate ganglion, and the superior semicircular canal. The rhomboid (◘ Fig. 6.19a a-b-c-d) space drilling is the anterior petrosectomy (◘ Fig. 6.20b).

Combined Petrosal Approach

Complex aneurysms of the basilar trunk, basilar tip, and the posterior cerebral artery are the most difficult to operate in neurosurgery. The deep location, complex anatomy, and the involvement of multiple cranial nerves, vessels, and the brain stem present neurosurgeons with the real challenge to achieve adequate cranial base approaches with negligible morbidity. The basilar tip and the basilar trunk can be accessed through the subtemporal transtentorial approach, through the extended middle fossa anterior petrosectomy approach, or through the retrosigmoid or transsigmoid posterior fossa approach. For the management of giant aneurysms of the basilar artery or to perform the P2 high-flow Fukushima Bypass (Type 5), the combined supra- and infratentorial transpetrosal approach is the best. In order to perform the proper combined petrosal approach with prevention of cosmetic deformity, postoperative CSF leakage or infection, very precise harvest of the STA-enhanced vascularized galeofascial pericranial flap is mandatory. ◘ Figure 6.20 demonstrates the so-called Fukushima lateral position. The important element of this Fukushima lateral positioning is bringing the patient's shoulder and the back exactly on the edge of the surgeon's side of the operating table. The upper shoulder and the arm need to be held 45° caudal and anterior. The upper shoulder rotates anteriorly to three-fourth lateral prone position. The patient's hip must be in the middle of the operating table with the lower leg bent 90°. Placing a couple of large, soft pillows, the upper leg will be crossing over the lower extremity. Most of the time, in order to harvest abdominal fat, the upper hip will be rotated posteriorly to make access to the lower abdomen. The head is fixated with the Mayfield three-pin head clamp and kept horizontal, slightly vertex down (◘ Fig. 6.20a). The entire head is elevated to make sufficient space between the lower neck and the lower arm (◘ Fig. 6.20b). The face is slightly rotated toward the floor to make the external auditory canal and the mastoid bone at the highest point, and the head and neck are moderately flexed. The upper shoulder must be positioned anteriorly and caudally to make easier access to the entire retroauricular retromastoid region and the entire

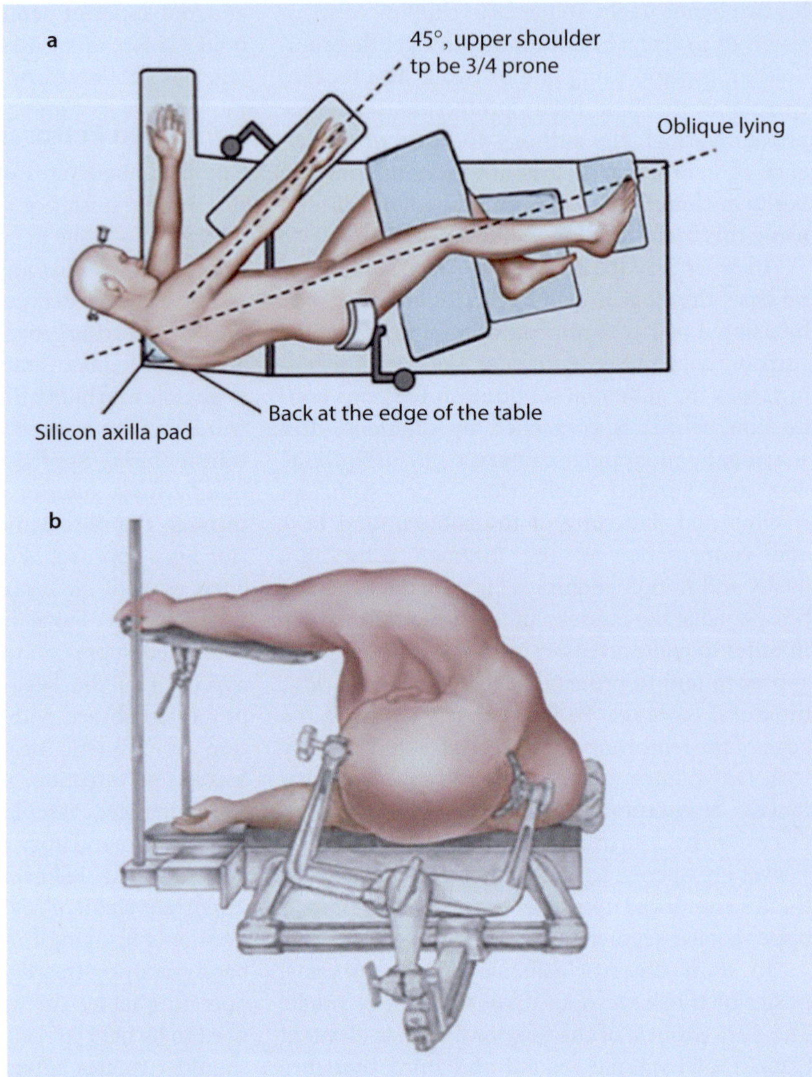

Fig. 6.20 Fukushima lateral position. This position is used uniformly for any transmastoid retrosigmoid approach, subtemporal approach, or combined petrosal approach. **a** The patient is positioned obliquely on the operating table with the hip in the middle rotated posteriorly for preparation of abdominal fat harvest. The upper shoulder is rotated anteriorly to make three-fourth lateral prone position with the arm placed 45° caudally and anteriorly. **b** The head is fixated with a three-pin head clamp. The forehead is elevated to make space between the neck and the lower shoulder and lower arm, vertex down and the nose slightly rotated toward the floor to make the mastoid and retrosigmoid line in the highest position

temporo-occipital region. The skin incision is either a postauricular large C incision or, in order to harvest an STA, enhanced highly vascularized flap; a preauricular incision is necessary in a so-called «*chef hat*» skin incision. Figure 6.21a illustrates the so-called chef hat scalp incision for dissection of the superficial temporal artery. Figure 6.21b illustrates the landmarks of the outer mastoid triangle, inner mastoid triangle, and the Macewen's triangle. At first, surgeons dissect the superficial temporal artery from the preauricular inferior zygomatic point all the way along the parietal branch of the STA and also dissect the frontalis branch of the STA. Therefore, the first layer of the skin and subcutaneous tissue is retracted in the anterior inferior direction using multiple small, medium, and large blunt hooks and silicon rubber bands. When the STA branches are dissected, we can make a large galeofascial pericranial flap, the second layer with wide pedicle from STA to EAC. It is extremely important to make a very thick and wide STA-enhanced highly vascularized galeofascial and pericranial flap (second layer) which is reflected inferior posteriorly with many blunt hooks. After this second vascularized flap is elevated, then the temporal muscle will be cleanly separated from the temporal bone and reflected anteriorly. Then, the suboccipital muscles are elevated from the mastoid and retracted posteriorly and inferiorly. The surgeon should know the outer landmarks of the root of the zygoma, that is, the glenoid cap 15° to the temporal

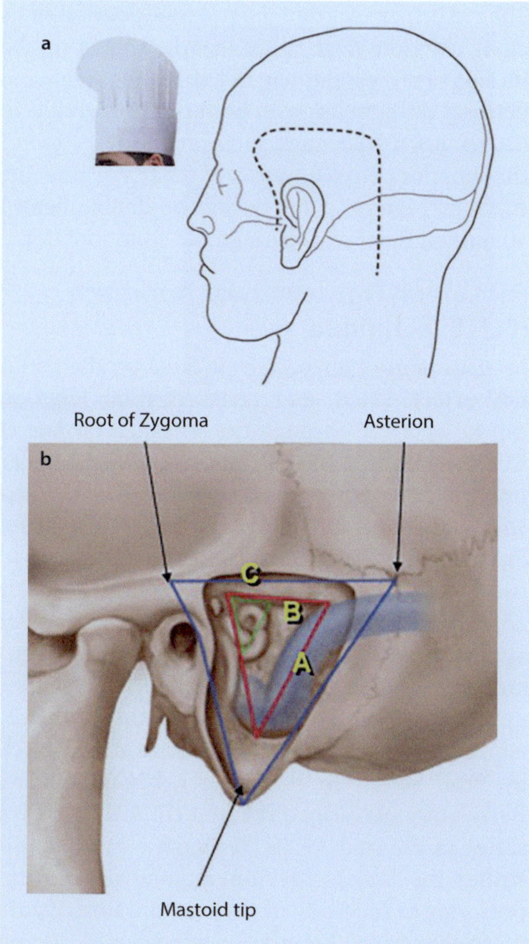

Fig. 6.21 **a** The so-called chef hat incision for the dissection and the harvest of the STA-enhanced highly vascularized galeofascial-pericranial flap. **b** The outer (C: *Blue line*) and inner mastoid triangles showing landmarks of transmastoid drilling. The inner triangle is similar to transitional Troutman's triangle (A: *Red line*). Small triangles demonstrate the anterior surface triangle of Macewen, which indicates the direction toward the mastoid antrum. Spine of Henle indicates the genu of the facial nerve junction of the tympanic segment and descending fallopian canal (B: *Green line*)

baseline. The length is about 22 mm. All bony landmarks such as the anterior temporal, pterion, superior squamosal point, middle temporal, posterior temporal, supramastoid ridge, and the occipital and suboccipital region must be secured before making a long L-shaped petrosal craniotomy. Asterion is the junction of the parietomastoid, lambdoid, and occipitomastoid sutures (Fig. 6.21b). The asterion is evident in all patients and serves to identify the transverse sinus and the mastoid outer triangle. From the asterion, it passes the middle of the supramastoid crest to the posterior point of the root of the zygoma and then passes inferiorly to the spine of Henle to the mastoid tip that confirms Fukushima's outer mastoid triangle. Figure 6.21b illustrates the outer mastoid triangle where the surgeon evenly drills the mastoid to expose the posterior temporal tegmen and transverse and sigmoid sinus and exposes the mastoid antrum, fallopian canal, and the digastric ridge as well as the stylomastoid foramen. In order to perform this transmastoid retrolabyrinthine or infralabyrinthine drilling, the neurosurgeon needs a lot of temporal bone dissection exercises and understanding of all neuro-otologic structures. At a minimum, it is recommended for younger neurosurgeons to practice 20 temporal bone dissections to become a skull base expert. Figure 6.22 demonstrates the retrolabyrinthine and infralabyrinthine temporal bone dissection, exposing the posterior temporal tegmen, sinodural angle, and transverse and sigmoid sinus, down to the jugular dome. The most important is the confirmation of the lateral semicircular canal (9 mm length and 15° angle to the basal temporal line), which is easily identified in the mastoid antrum. Anteriorly, the entry corridor to the middle ear named aditus,

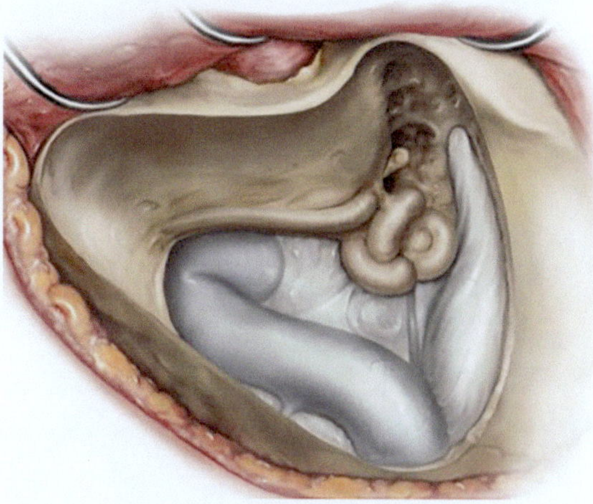

Fig. 6.22 Transmastoid retrolabyrinthine and infralabyrinthine drilling and shaving of the neuro-otologic structures. All eggshell bones must be removed to leave only the soft tissues anteriorly from the aditus, facial recess, incus, and malleus head superiorly, posterior temporal tegmen, the sinodural angle posteriorly, transverse sinus and sigmoid sinus inferior anterior, jugular dome, and digastric ridge. Anterior is just the fallopian canal and the stylomastoid foramen. All skull base neurosurgeons must understand the neuro-otologic structures and need to have the capability of shaving the mastoid toward the facial nerve and labyrinth

short process of incus, malleus head, the facial recess, the genu of the facial nerve, and the descending segment of the fallopian canal as well as the stylomastoid foramen must be identified. In most cases, 12–15 mm of presigmoid dura can be exposed. We can perform presigmoid approach, retrosigmoid approach, or transsigmoid wider exposure. ◘ Figure 6.19a demonstrates the middle fossa dissection of the rhomboid construct, posterior to the trigeminal complex, medial to the greater superficial petrosal nerve (GSPN), and the petrous segment of the carotid artery, anterior to the geniculate ganglion and the posterior semicircular canal. About 5 mm of petrous ridge can be drilled away, and the anterior petrosectomy will expose from the internal auditory canal, postmeatal and premeatal triangle, and all the way to the posterior fossa dura toward the abducens nerve (◘ Fig. 6.19). ◘ Figure 6.19b demonstrates the completion of the extradural dissection, exposure of the middle fossa rhomboid construct, and anterior petrosectomy. ◘ Figure 6.23 illustrates the retrolabyrinthine-combined supra- and infratentorial exposure to identify cranial nerves III, IV, V, VI, VII, VIII, IX, and X and vascular structures.

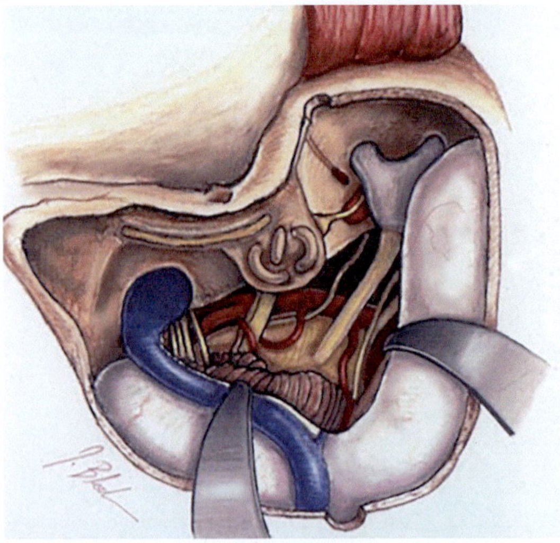

◘ **Fig. 6.23** The typical retrolabyrinthine-combined supratentorial and infratentorial transpetrosal approach exposing the cranial nerves III, IV, V, VI, VII, VIII, and IX-X complex. The incision must be only presigmoid with basal subtemporal incision, and removal of the rhomboid-shaped tentorium will make sufficient operative field toward the basilar trunk and for surgery of petroclival tumors. No incision should be made from the superior petrosal sinus along the transverse sinus because this area is the key point where the posterior temporal vein of Labbe enters

The red line arrow from the superior petrosal sinus along the transverse sinus, this dura must not be incised to protect the vein of Labbe. The combined petrosal dural incision is from the presigmoid to the temporal base dural incision and resection of the superior petrosal sinus and the tentorium. The superior petrosal sinus should be double ligated 10 mm off the transverse sigmoid sinus junction.

Far Lateral Transcondylar Approach (ELITE Technique)

Management of aneurysms located on the vertebral artery, PICA, and vertebrobasilar junction can be operated through the so-called far lateral ELITE approach. This extreme lateral infrajugular transcondylar exposure was developed by Hakuba and Fukushima simultaneously in 1987 in Japan. Fukushima elaborated this ELITE approach to two types of exposure, dorsolateral transcondylar approach and anterolateral transcondylar approach, which is combined with the transjugular and the high cervical exposure.

The transcondylar and transjugular tubercle approach was first described in anatomy research by Prof. Seeger in 1976. Later, his pupil Prof. Bertalanffy performed the first clinical operative series in the mid-1980s. ◘ Figure 6.24a demonstrates the lazy S curvilinear incision 2–3 cm posterior to the body of the mastoid line. Figure 6.24b illustrates the inferior retrosigmoid point; opening of the foramen magnum lateral edge; exposure of the C1 lamina upper edge, C1 condyle J groove, and occipital C1 facet; and identification of the hypoglossal canal and the triangular concept of the condylar triangle as well as the jugular tubercle triangle. In front of the C1 dura, when the occipital condyle is drilled away, for superior medial portion (about 30% of the condylar bone), hypoglossal canal can be exposed slightly cephalad parallel to the facet line and anterior to the C1 dura. From this hypoglossal canal under the jugular bulb, the jugular tubercle extends 25 mm long toward the inferior clivus. Removal of this jugular tubercle is a key step to make flat access to the ventral medulla and to the vertebrobasilar junction. This drilling exercise is extremely difficult not to violate the ninth and tenth lower cranial nerves. Surgeons need microanatomy dissection practice in the laboratory (at least on 10 to 20 specimens). The author performed the ELITE far lateral approach in three cases of basilar trunk giant aneurysm

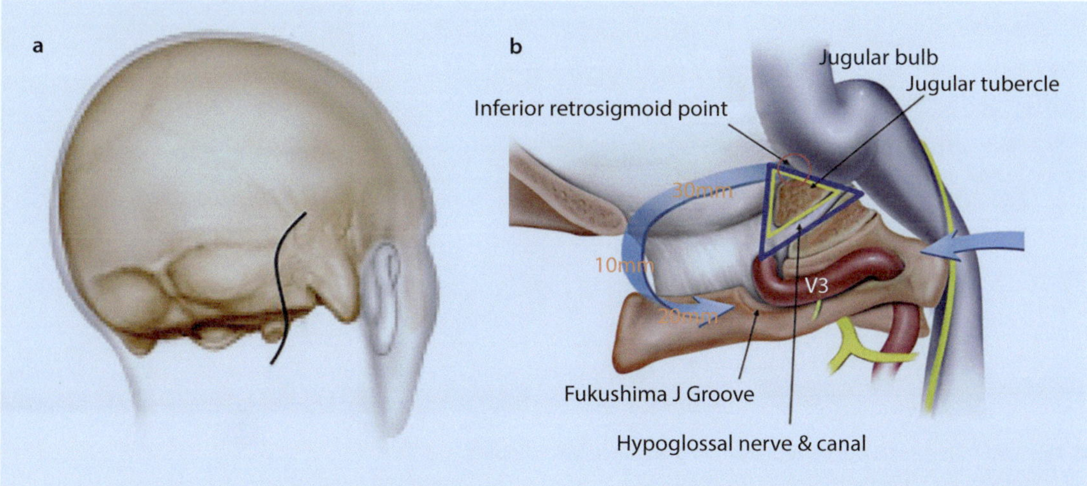

Fig. 6.24 **a** demonstrates the lazy S curvilinear incision 2–3 cm posterior to the body of the mastoid line. **b** The typical scheme of the far lateral transcondylar approach. Important landmarks are infrajugular point, inferior retrosigmoid point, opening of the foramen magnum lateral, and opening of the lateral portion of the foramen magnum. In the majority of patients from the inferior retrosigmoid point, go back 3 cm to the posterior edge of the foramen magnum 10 mm, which indicates the posterior tubercle of the C1 lamina and follows the upper edge of the C1 lamina. There is a definitive J-groove C1 condyle groove where the V3 horizontal segment of the vertebral artery is located. The surgeon needs to identify the anterior border of the C1 dura, vertebral fibrous ring, and the C1 transverse process, vertebral artery foramen, which connects from the V3 to V4 horizontal segment. C2 posterior spinal root and 11th nerve over the internal jugular vein and from the occipital condylar facets, the skull base surgeon must identify the condylar triangle and the jugular tubercle triangle. About 10 mm removal of the occipital condyle medially, superiorly will exposed the hypoglossal canal near the vertebral fibrous ring slightly cephalad, and from this hypoglossal canal, jugular tubercle starts anteriorly toward the clivus about 25 mm length

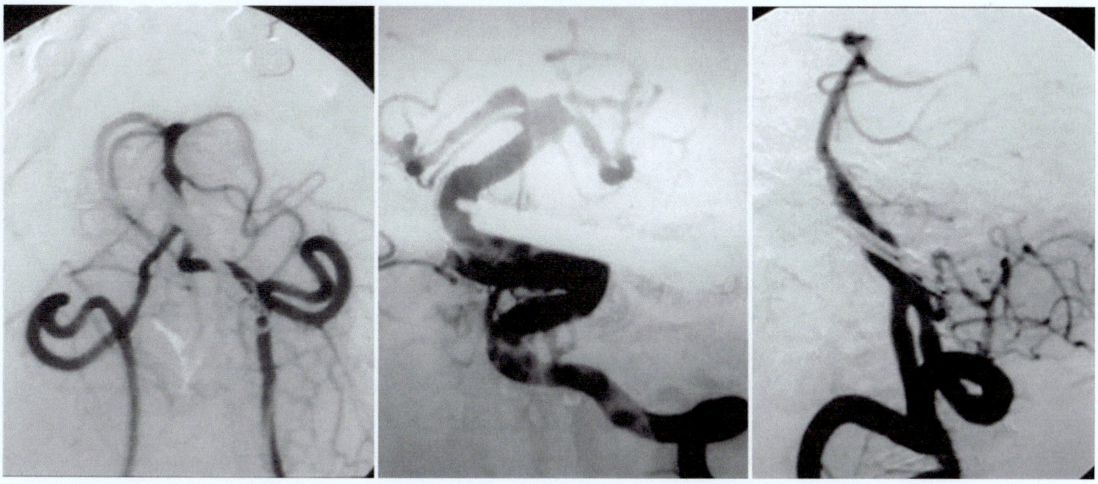

Fig. 6.25 Three cases of basilar trunk giant aneurysm clipping through the far lateral ELITE approach

clipping and 25 cases of vertebral artery giant aneurysm. The majority of vertebral artery giant aneurysms are fusiform, either atherosclerotic origin or dissecans type. Some reports assume of unknown vasculopathies or vascular inflammatory etiology. Figure 6.25 illustrates two cases of clipping of the vertebral artery giant aneurysms. Figure 6.26 demonstrates three cases of vertebral artery giant aneurysm clipping. Figure 6.27 demonstrates three cases of resection of the vertebral giant aneurysm and aneurysmorrhaphy with 7-0 Prolene sutures.

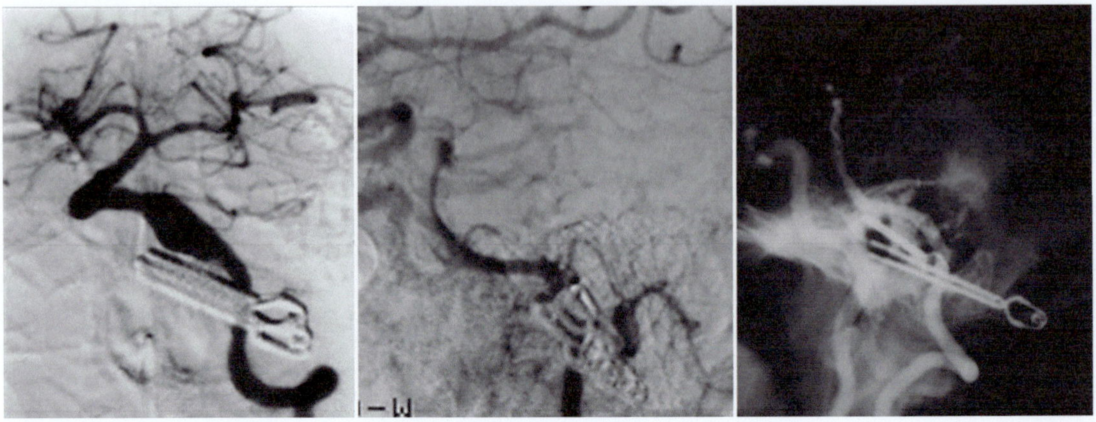

Fig. 6.26 Three cases of vertebral artery giant aneurysm clipping

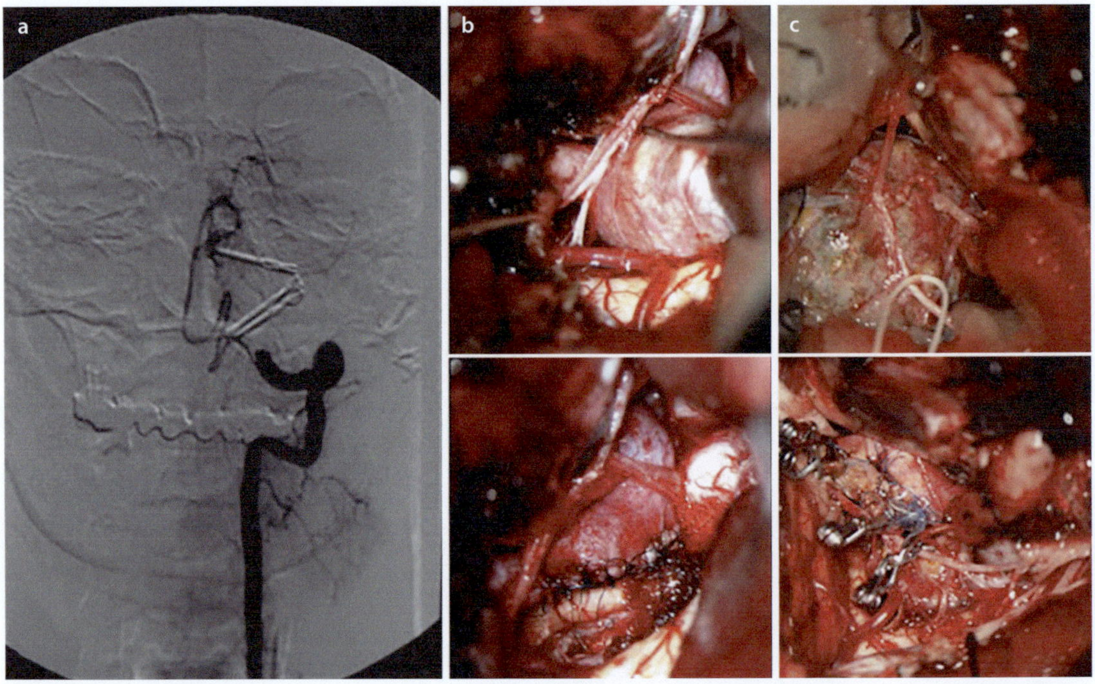

Fig. 6.27 **a** Trapping of the vertebral giant aneurysm with mobilization anastomosis PICA to the distal vertebral artery. **b** The giant aneurysm is excised proximal to the IX-X cranial nerves, and the vertebral artery was sutured, a so-called aneurysmorrhaphy. **c** Complex clipping and aneurysmorrhaphy, mega-giant vertebral artery aneurysm

6.1.5 Evolution of Skull Base Fukushima Bypass (Microsurgical Flow Diversion)

Skull Base Cavernous Bypass (Fukushima Bypass Type 1)

With the report of Dolenc in the early 1980s, it started the development of extradural direct transcavernous surgery [10, 11]. Fukushima established the extradural transcavernous triangular entry corridors in June 1986 (Fig. 6.14). On October 4, 1986, the author operated on a very rare case of bilateral calcified and thrombosed giant aneurysms on a 62-year-old female presented with left eye blindness and oculomotor palsy. Figure 6.28 demonstrates these bilateral calcified and thrombosed giant aneurysms. The left side shows the mega-size giant aneurysm. Because of the left eye

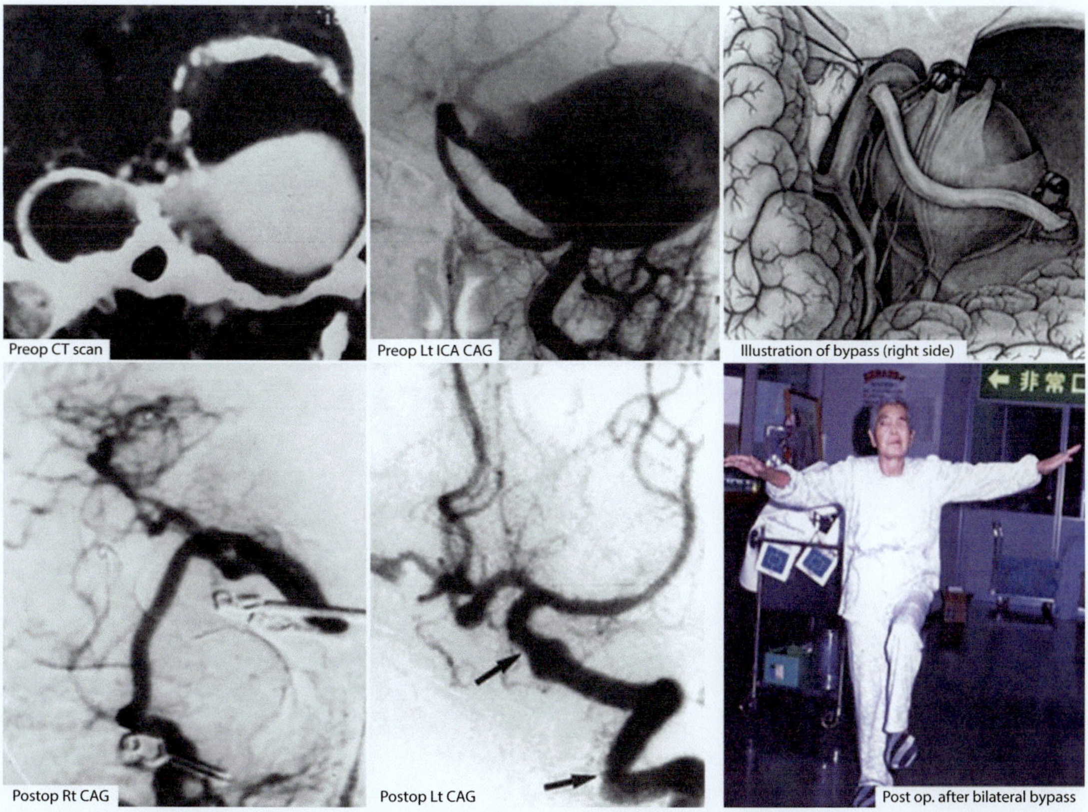

Fig. 6.28 Fukushima's first skull base saphenous vein bypass operated on October 4, 1986. This 62-year-old lady presented with left oculomotor palsy blindness and right hemiparesis due to bilateral calcified and thrombosed paraclinoid aneurysm. At first, the left side of the mega-giant aneurysm was resected with temporary clipping. Unfortunately, I could not reconstruct the cavernous carotid artery. The idea came up in the operation room to use a 6 cm saphenous vein interposition graft from C6 to C2-3 junction bypass anastomosis. After 2 months, I performed the right side operation with a jump bypass without touching the aneurysm. After the bilateral bypass, this patient did very well with recovery of hemiparesis

blindness and oculomotor palsy and right hemiparesis, the author performed resection of this mega-giant aneurysm and planned to perform reconstruction of the cavernous carotid segment. Because of the very severe atherosclerosis and mega-giant aneurysm, following total resection, the author had no way to reconstruct the cavernous carotid artery and quickly elaborated the new idea of placing a saphenous vein interposition graft (7 cm) between C6 petrous carotid to the paraophthalmic segment (C2-3) of the internal carotid artery. The patient tolerated the procedure very well and recovered uneventfully. Two months later, the author performed the right side saphenous vein jump bypass from the C6 petrous carotid artery anastomosed to the paraophthalmic C2-3 junction segment. The patient tolerated the second surgery as well and recovered to with normal neurological condition except for pre-existing left eye blindness and oculomotor palsy. Since this amazing experience, the author performed C6 to C2-3 cavernous carotid bypass in 34 cases of intracavernous giant aneurysms (Fig. 6.2). Analyzing later, the postoperative follow-up of these 34 patients, the author noted three patients (8.8%) had unexpected visual loss, presumably due to the temporary clip on the ophthalmic artery. Also, these types of skull base exposures of the C6 petrous carotid artery, such as anterior clinoidectomy, optic canal decompression, and excision of the distal carotid fibrous ring, were fairly difficult and time-consuming skull base procedures; in three patients the author tried External Carotid to C2-3 paraophthalmic segment long saphenous bypass, which has been designated as Fukushima Bypass Type 3.

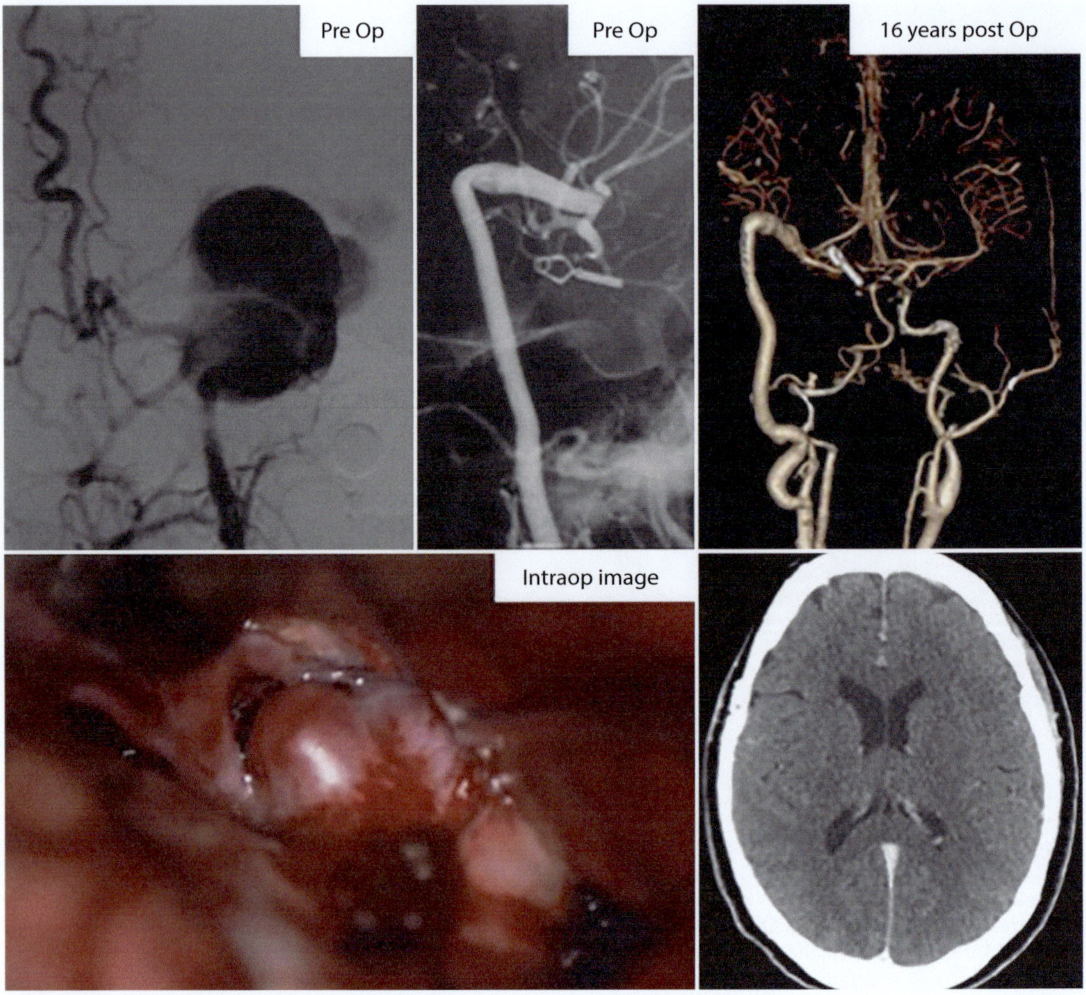

Fig. 6.29 A 21-year-old young female presented with a combination of cavernous sinus giant aneurysm and paraclinoid triple lobule complex aneurysms. This aneurysm is treated with external carotid to M2 bypass and internal carotid ligature in the neck. I could clip proximal to the P-com aneurysm to trap these complex aneurysms. Surgery went very well, and the patient had no deficit. The 16-year postoperative CT and 3-D CT angiogram showed an excellent bypass flow and virtually no damage to the brain. The patient has no neurological deficit

External Carotid M2 Long Saphenous Vein Graft Bypass (Fukushima Bypass Type 4)

Gradually the author switched to the submandibular subzygomatic External Carotid to M2 (posterolateral trunk) long saphenous vein bypass. Figure 6.29 demonstrates a case of young female presented with very complex intracavernous giant aneurysm plus three lobules of paraclinoidal giant aneurysm presented with blurry vision, oculomotor paresis, and abducens nerve paresis. Because of the very complex aneurysm consisting of both intracavernous and paraclinoid giant aneurysms, the author performed External Carotid to M2 bypass with cervical internal carotid ligation and placed a clip just proximal to the P-com branch. The patient did extremely well and recovered all neurological deficits. The 16-year postoperative 3D CT angiogram shows total disappearance of the aneurysm and persistent good flow of the saphenous vein carotid artery replacement.

Type 4 External Carotid to M2 saphenous bypass is performed with opening of the submandibular, carotid triangle exposing the common carotid, external carotid, and internal carotid arteries. Following the exposure of the neck carotid arteries, small frontotemporal and subtemporal craniotomy is performed with extradural exposure of the anterior subtemporal base and the infratemporal fossa between the foramen rotundum and ovale. From this V2-V3 lateral Vidian triangle, a small tunnel is produced while separating the space between the lateral and medial pterygoid muscles. Likewise, submandibular to pterygoid fossa tunnel is made using blunt dissection with a long Kelly hemostat over the digastric muscle. Then, the curved chest trocar tube 25, 26, or 28-gauge is passed from the anterior infratemporal fossa toward the submandibular area above the digastric muscle. Then, through this polyethylene tubing, 0 silk suture is passed toward the infratemporal area. The saphenous vein is passed using this 0 silk through the inside of polyethylene tubing. As soon as the saphenous vein is passed, the polyethylene tube is removed. The saphenous vein is filled with heparinized saline, and two temporary clips are applied to each end of the graft. At first, cervical end of the saphenous vein is anastomosed end-to-side to the external carotid artery using 7-0 or 8-0 nylon sutures. Next, the distal saphenous segment is anastomosed end-to-side to the posterolateral trunk of M2 using 8-0 or 9-0 monofilament nylon sutures. This external carotid to M2 bypass is technically much easier than cavernous sinus interposition graft. There is no need to expose the proximal carotid or cavernous sinus. This bypass was performed in 40 patients (◘ Table 6.2), with extreme

◘ **Table 6.2** Skull base saphenous high-flow Fukushima Bypass (1986 Oct. 4–2016 Dec. 31)

Summary of 136 cases	Lessons learned in three decades	No. of cases
Type I (C6 to C2-3 bypass)	Intracavernous giant aneurysms	*34*
Type II (EC to C6 bypass)	Infratemporal bypass	*16*
	Infratemporal aneurysms	4
	Glomus tumor	7
	Glomus vagal	5
	Carotid body tumor	2
	Infratemporal meningiomas	3
Type III (EC to C2-3 bypass)	Intracavernous giant aneurysms	*3*
Type IV (EC to M2 bypass)		*40*
	MC giants, serpentine	6
	Intracavernous giants	22
	Paraclinoid giants	4
	Fusiform C6	2
	IC-Bifurcation	2
	C3-Siphon	4
Type V (EC to P2 bypass)		*13*
	BA-Tip giants	4
	BA-Trunk	9
	Occlusive disease and tumors	*30*
	C3-4 carotid siphon stenosis	2
	C6-C2-3	1
	EC-M2	1
	Cavernous atypical meningioma	8
	Cavernous sinus malignant tumors (Plasmacytoma, Adenoid Cystic, Sarcoma, SCC)	20

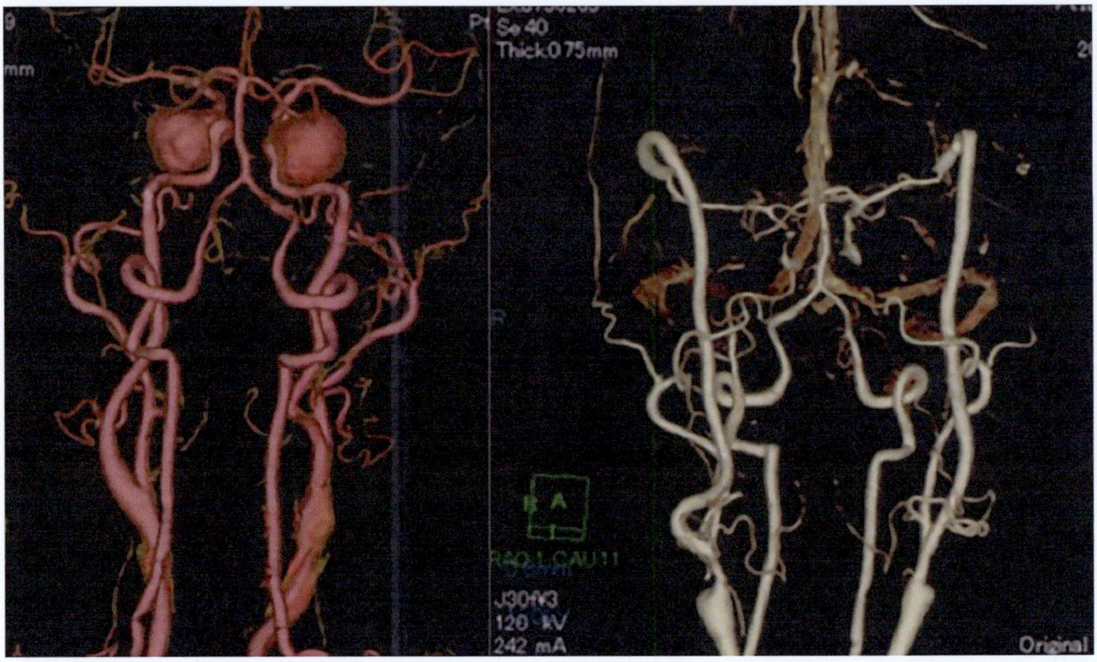

Fig. 6.30 Bilateral cavernous sinus giant aneurysm, right side, presented with VI nerve palsy. The left side illustrates the oculomotor palsy. For safety, the first I performed a right-sided bypass and 3 months later a left-sided bypass. The patient is gradually recovered from abducens nerve and oculomotor palsy

success. Figure 6.30 shows the 72-year-old senior female presented with right abducens palsy and left oculomotor palsy. I performed the bilateral external carotid to M2 trunk saphenous vein microsurgical flow diversion, and the both giant aneurysms were totally eliminated. The patient recovered from all the neurological deficits.

Type 2 bypass is the external carotid to C6 petrous carotid infratemporal bypass. In 1987, the author performed the world's first case of infratemporal bypass in two cases of infratemporal paraganglioma, which engulfed the C7 infratemporal high cervical carotid segment. The author performed total resection of the paraganglioma safely with infratemporal saphenous vein bypass [32]. Since 1987, the author performed 16 cases of infratemporal bypass Type 2 including six infratemporal aneurysms, either atherosclerotic or traumatic origin, and five cases of glomus vagale, two carotid body tumors, and three invasive infratemporal meningiomas. Figure 6.31 demonstrates pre- and postoperative angiograms of two minimally invasive skull base cavernous bypass procedures, passing a 7 cm length saphenous vein under the temporal lobe without opening the dura from C6 petrous carotid to the C2 paraophthalmic segment.

External Carotid to P2 Bypass (Fukushima Bypass Type 5)

Figure 6.32 demonstrates a 60-year-old patient presented with quadriparesis and swallowing disturbance arriving at the hospital in a wheelchair due to a thrombosed giant aneurysm at the basilar trunk as visualized on CT and angiogram. Through the right, combined with the petrosal approach, the author performed right external carotid to right P2 segment of posterior cerebral artery bypass procedure, namely, Fukushima Bypass Type 5 (EC-P2 bypass). A small clip was placed just proximal to the aneurysm origin. This patient did excellent. After rehabilitation of 6 months, the patient recovered in normal neurological condition. Figure 6.33 shows other examples of such basilar trunk giant aneurysm clipped with backup safety bypass of external carotid to P2 bypass.

As shown in Table 6.2, the author performed high-flow skull base Fukushima bypasses in 136 cases in 3 decades between 1986 and 2016. A scheme of the five Fukushima bypass types is demonstrated in Fig. 6.34. Among the type 1 bypasses there are 34 patients, Type 2 infratemporal bypass16 patients, Type 3 three cases, Type 4

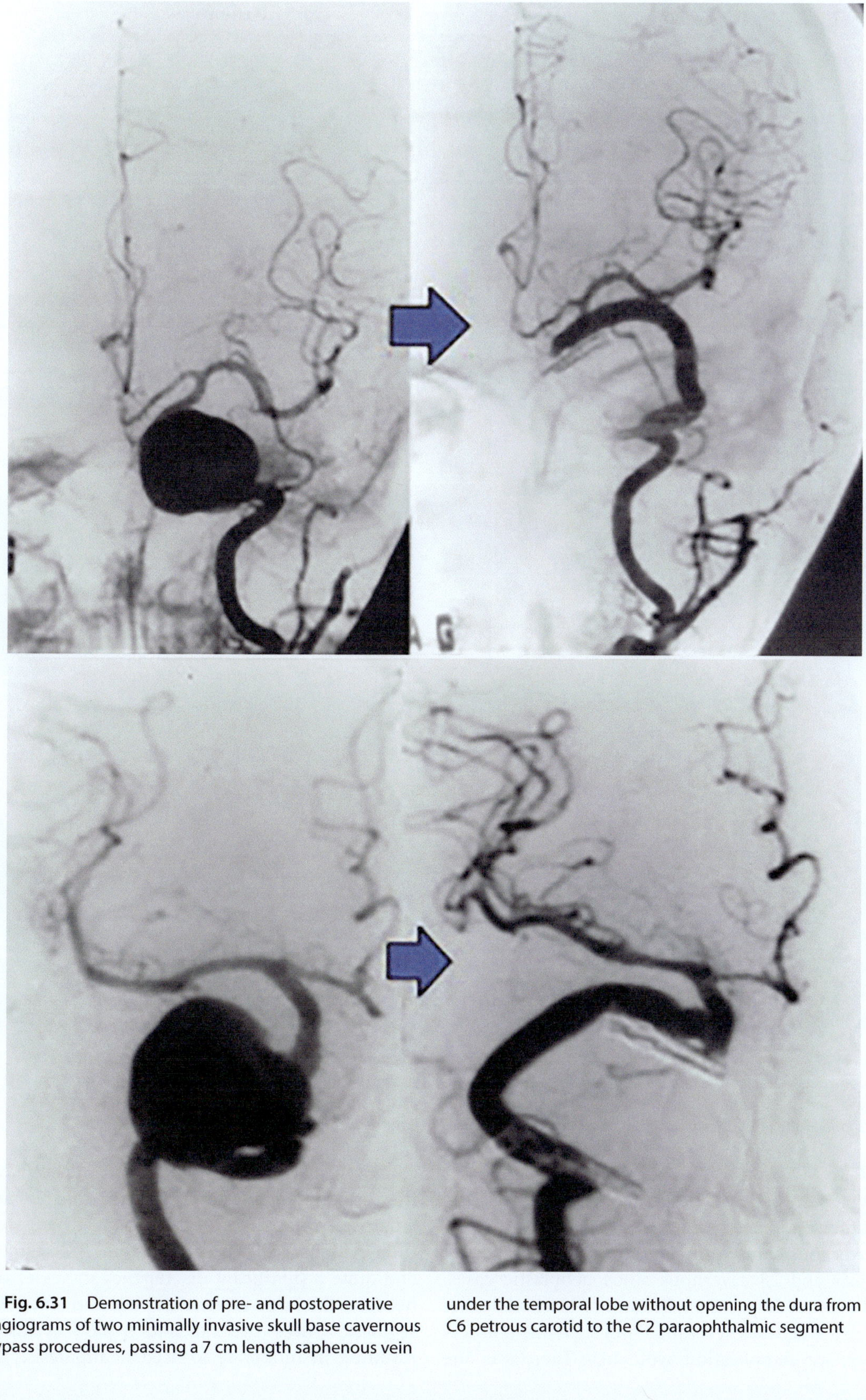

Fig. 6.31 Demonstration of pre- and postoperative angiograms of two minimally invasive skull base cavernous bypass procedures, passing a 7 cm length saphenous vein under the temporal lobe without opening the dura from C6 petrous carotid to the C2 paraophthalmic segment

6

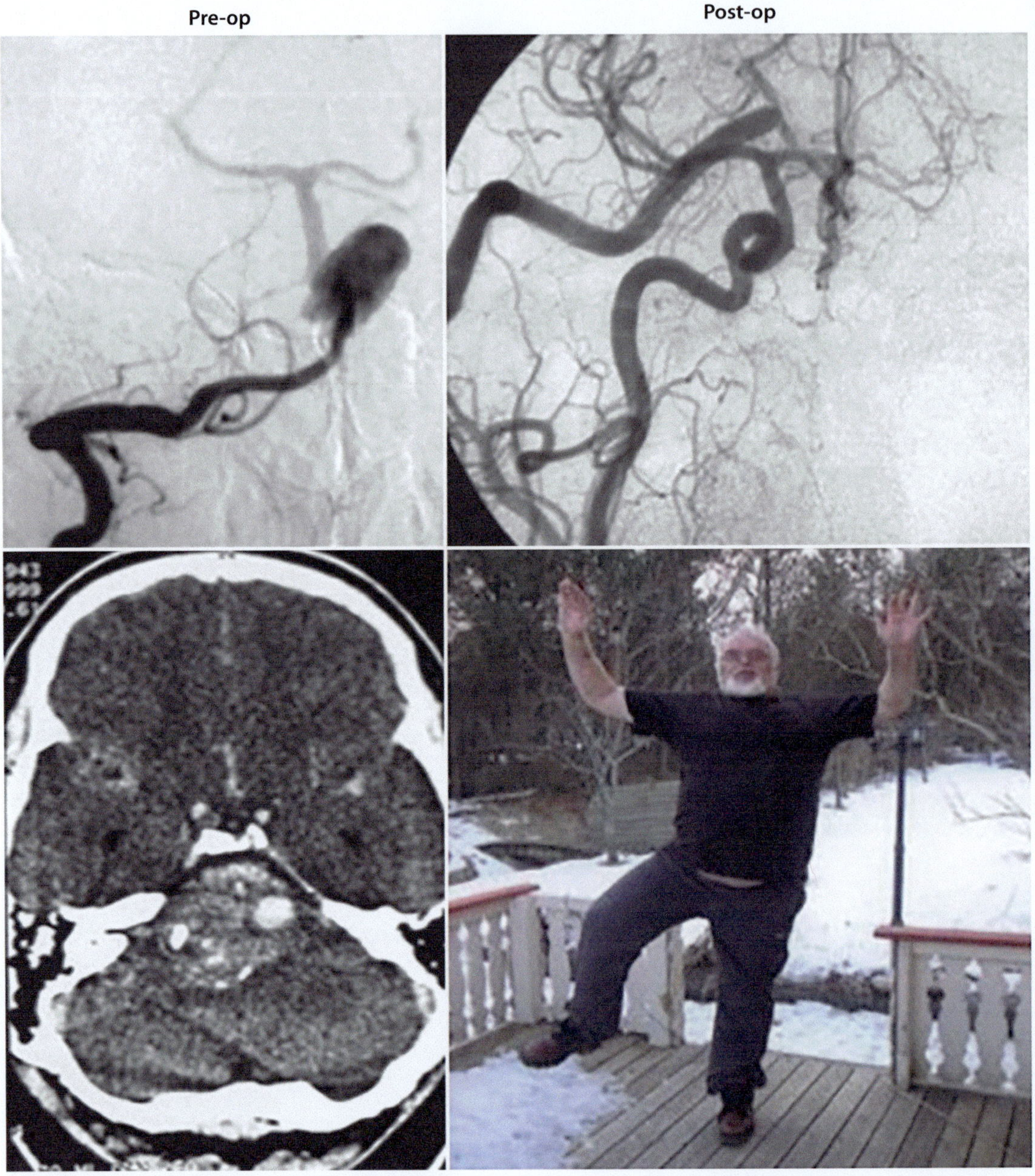

Fig. 6.32 Mega-giant vertebral trunk aneurysm, mostly thrombosed. The patient suffered from swallowing disturbance and quadriparesis. The patient was wheelchair-bound. I performed the right external carotid to P2 bypass. Through the right-sided combined petrosal approach, I placed a proximal small clip onto the basilar artery just proximal to the aneurysm neck. This patient made excellent recovery after 6 months of rehabilitation to a normal condition

EC to M2 bypass 40 patients, and Type 5 EC-P2 bypass 13 patients. Besides aneurysm cases, the author performed saphenous bypass in 2 cases of cavernous sinus segment carotid high-grade stenosis and 28 cavernous sinus neoplastic cases, altogether 30 patients. The author learned during these 3 decades several technical points and lessons for complication avoidance. There was one case of the cavernous bypass occlusion because of the very difficult anastomosis to the calcified and atherosclerotic C2 carotid segment. There were three patients who had a very small M2 segment and quite a significant discrepancy in vessel size between the large saphenous vein and small M2 segment. Three patients had bypass occlusion resulting in moderate to mild hemiparesis. The

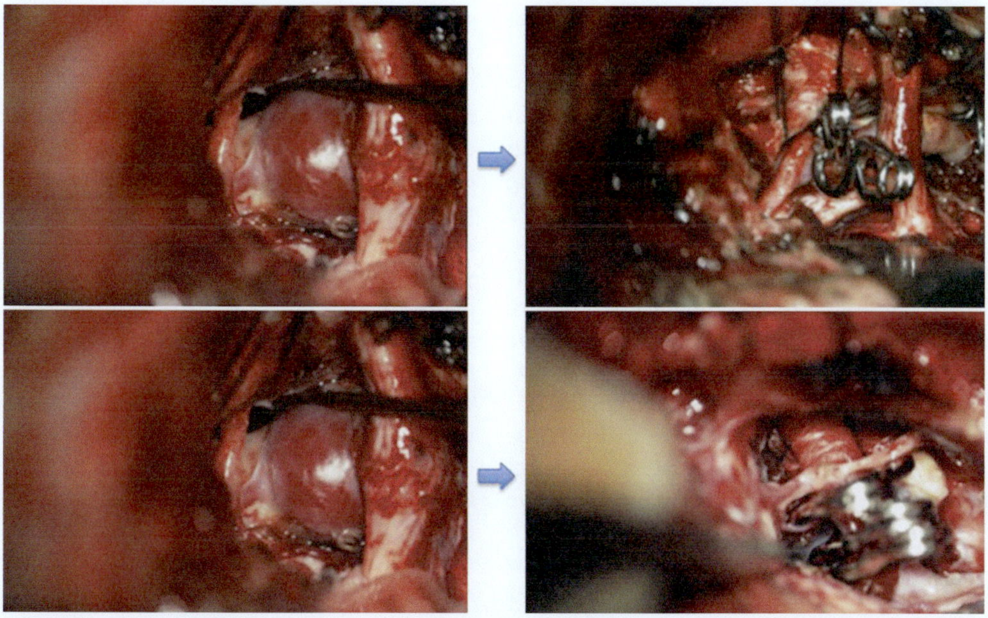

Fig. 6.33 Two cases of clipping of the basilar trunk giant aneurysm with backup external carotid to P2 bypass. Clipping went very well to preserve the basilar artery flow as well as the backup EC-P2 bypass

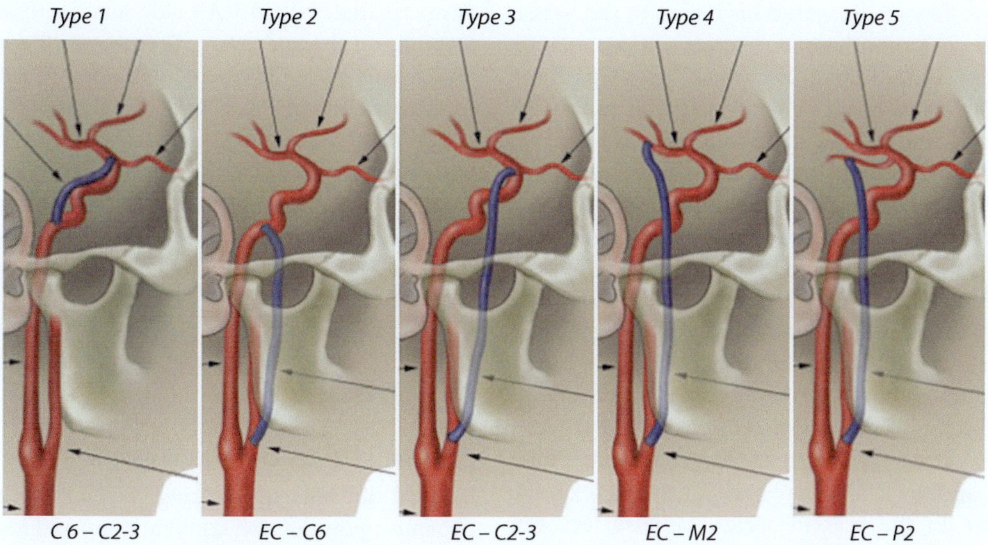

Fig. 6.34 Summary of the five different types of skull base Fukushima Bypass, C6-C3; cavernous carotid jump bypass illustrates external carotid to C6 petrous carotid infratemporal bypass, type III. I have operated only three patients' external carotid to C3 paraophthalmic segment. I have done only three patients of this type of bypass. Type 4, external carotid to M2 bypass is now the major operation for giant aneurysm, intracavernous aneurysms, fusiform aneurysms, and some of the internal carotid bifurcation or siphon aneurysms. In addition, this EC to M2 bypass is now more often performed for radical resection of cavernous sinus tumors. The external carotid to posterior cerebral artery P2 bypass. The majority of this operation is performed through the combined petrosal approach with minimum brain holding. Extradurally, the subtemporal base to expose the free segment of the P2 artery between the P-com junction and P3 peripheral branches. Any perforating branches must be avoided for the anastomosis of the saphenous vein end-to-side. Although the peripheral P3 segment has a lot of collateral circulation, I have two patients with hemiparesis, possibly due to vascularity insufficiency of the posterior choroidal artery, for anastomosis must be done in a very efficient way with two surgeons and four hands microanastomosis, possibly shorter than 15 min while under anesthesia pharmacological brain protection

author had one case of infratemporal clot, and the surgeon must be extremely careful to make subzygomatic pterygoid tunnel and pass the chest trochar polyethylene tubing from the infratemporal fossa to the submandibular areas. Blunt dissection is necessary, and precise hemostasis with long bipolar forceps must be performed. For the P2 segment of posterior cerebral artery, the surgeon must be very careful to select the P2 portion without any perforating arteries (free segment of P2). Saphenous vein graft microanastomosis must be done within 10–15 min for P2 bypass.Otherwise, even under general anesthesia for pharmacological brain protection, some of the P3 and particularly the posterior choroidal artery may get decreased perfusion and may cause postoperative hemiparesis. The author had two patients with hemiparesis, possibly P2 distal perforator low flow and one case of quadriparesis due to basilar perforating artery infarction. In case of EC-P2 bypass, meticulous and careful checking of the basilar trunk with Doppler flow or ICG is essential. When there is some finding of relatively low bypass flow or decreased back flow to the basilar trunk, 2–3 months of moderate anticoagulation therapy is indicated. Nowadays, any lengths of saphenous vein can be harvested with minimally invasive endoscopic technique. The author has been exclusively using the saphenous vein graft over three decades with no complications. Careful selection of the recipient vessel with good caliber is of cardinal importance for the success of skull base Fukushima Bypass. Of these 136 cases, the author had no mortality and no major complications of wheelchair-bound or bedridden conditions. In the literature, some reports advocate the use of a radial artery graft. Harvest of radial artery leaves extremely disfiguring long scar on the forearm, and the artery may have atherosclerosis and spasm. In the present series, radial artery was never used, because the saphenous vein has been available at any length. Saphenous vein graft has been used for coronary artery bypass for nearly half a century and is well established and accepted as donor vessels with adequate efficacy and long-term durability.

Small Vessel Bypass

Many complex and difficult aneurysms cannot be obliterated safely only with the clipping method. Some C/D aneurysms of the anterior cerebral artery and middle cerebral artery can be treated successfully with small vessel backup anastomosis. Long STA to anterior cerebral artery (A3) or A3-A3 side anastomosis is useful for aneurysm resected and aneurysmorrhaphy or for trapping of aneurysms. STA-MCA microanastomosis is an excellent backup bypass for clipping of the complex middle cerebral artery giant aneurysms. ◘ Figure 6.35a shows the case of a 35-year-old young man with calcified and thrombosed M1 giant aneurysm treated with double STA-MCA microanastomosis and trapping of the aneurysm. ◘ Figure 6.35b shows a 60-year-old gentleman with thrombosed M1 giant aneurysm treated with double STA-MCA anastomosis and clipping of the aneurysm. ◘ Figure 6.36 demonstrates an 8 cm mega-giant aneurysm in a 9-year-old boy treated with STA-MCA anastomosis, resection of the mega-giant aneurysm and end-to-end anastomosis reconstruction of the M1-M2 junction. These three cases show excellent results without any neurological sequelae. ◘ Figure 6.37 shows a 27-year-old young man, with callosal bifurcation, calcified, thrombosed, giant aneurysm treated with A3-A3 side anastomosis and trapping of the aneurysm. ◘ Figure 6.38 demonstrates a 60-year-old treated with long STA to A3 microanastomosis, resection of the giant thrombosed aneurysm, and Acom aneurysmorrhaphy with excellent results. These are examples of the small vessel microanastomosis and repair of complex aneurysms. This type of small vessel microsurgical flow diversion was performed in 16 cases (◘ Table 6.1).

6.1.6 Discussion

Classification of Aneurysms

Surgical difficulty of repairing cerebral aneurysms depends upon the size, configuration, and location of the aneurysm. Particularly, size is the key issue. To classify cerebral aneurysms, as mentioned above, there have been several criteria of identifying aneurysm size. The author has been using the basic principle of Fukushima Rule of Three and Triangle concept for all the neurosurgical diseases, conditions, and microanatomy. For the majority of the skull base anatomy and surgical defining operative access and entry, the author determined with triangular corridor concept and, for cerebellopontine angle lesions, upper CP angle through an infratentorial paratrigeminal route, middle CP angle through

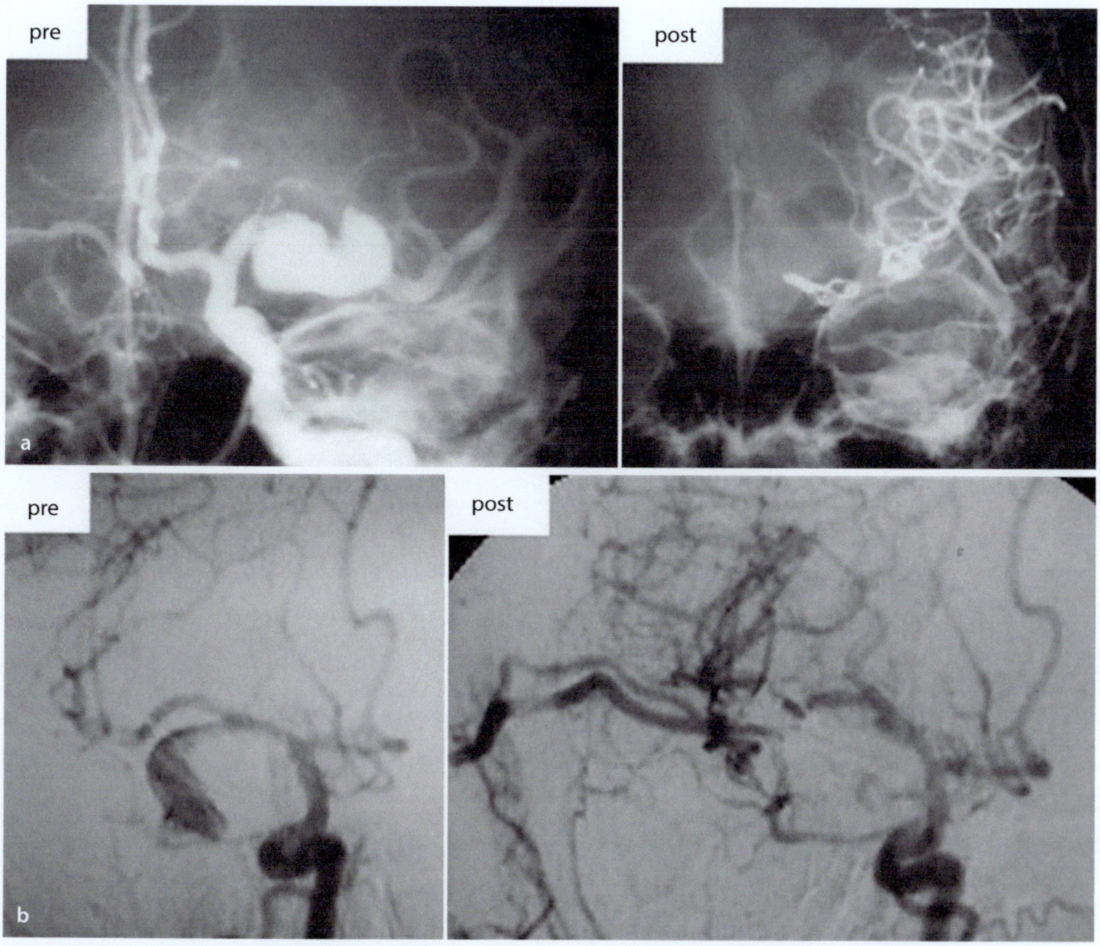

Fig. 6.35 **a** A 35-year-old young man with calcified and thrombosed M1 giant aneurysm treated with double STA-MCA microanastomosis and trapping of the aneurysm. **b** A 60-year-old gentleman with thrombosed M1 giant aneurysm treated with double STA-MCA anastomosis and clipping of the aneurysm

an acoustic route, and lower CP angle through a subcerebellar glossopharyngeal route. For classification of AV malformations, there is a simple Fukushima grading system: Grade 1, simple easy AVMs; Grade 2, difficult AVMs; and Grade 3, inoperable AVMs. For grading of subarachnoid hemorrhage (SAH), conventional Hunt and Hess, Hunt and Kosnik or WHO classification are too complex and hard to apply to clinical patients. Fukushima's grading of subarachnoid hemorrhage is simple based on the Fukushima Rule of Three: SAH Grade 1, good condition patients from awake to slight sleepiness; SAH Grade 2, fair condition patients with definitive drowsiness to stupor; and SAH Grade 3, poor condition patients from semicoma to coma. Likewise, for classification of cerebral aneurysms, the best method is to classify into three categories: category 1, class A aneurysms with average standard small size less than or equal to 10 mm; category 2, class B aneurysm with bulbous, bit bigger aneurysm between 11 and 19 mm; and category 3, class C/D aneurysms, namely, complex and difficult ones, including large fusiform, giant size (≥20 mm) and intracavernous locations. I hope the world of neurosurgery will take this simple classification, and it should become the international neurosurgical standard. According to the nomenclature of cerebral arterial segments, the correct nomenclature for anterior circulation (carotid vascular tree), posterior circulation (vertebrobasilar vascular tree) (Fig. 6.2). The already established Fischer classification should be used over seven decades in the German and Japanese societies: A1, A2, A3, A4; M1, M2, M3, M4; P1, P2, P3, P4; C1, C2, C3, C4, C5, C6, C7; and V1, V2, V3, V4 from the intradural center to the extracranial to periphery (Fig. 6.2).

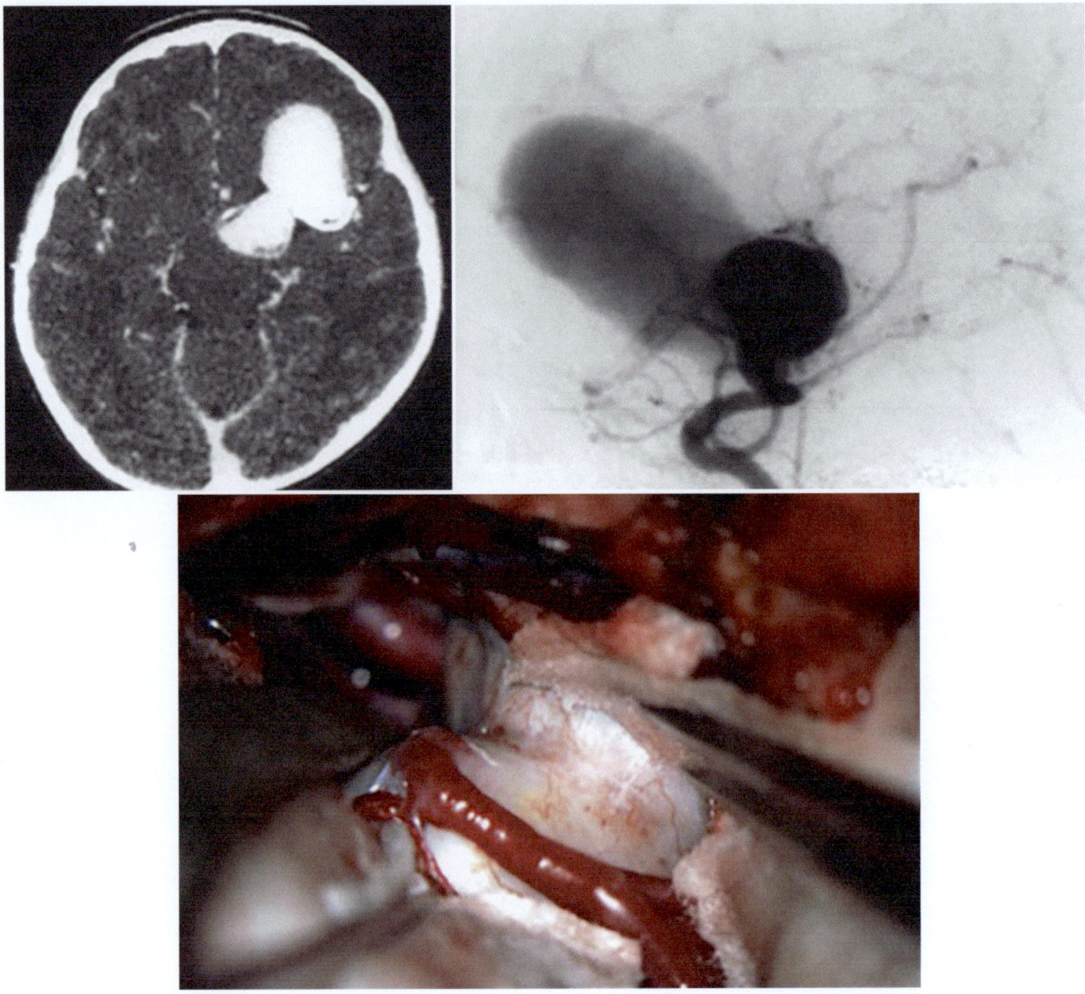

Fig. 6.36 8 cm mega-giant aneurysm in a 9-year-old boy treated with STA-MCA anastomosis, resection of the mega-giant aneurysm and end-to-end anastomosis reconstruction of the M1-M2 junction

The Learning Curve for Microsurgical Aneurysm Repair

Surgical treatment of cerebral aneurysms is a difficult challenge in neurosurgery irrespective of size, configuration, and location. Therefore, surgeons must have ability to perform precise, meticulous and most careful, clean, and sharp dissection. Surgeons need to practice in a laboratory with a number of cadaveric specimens learning microanatomy of the brain, skull base, and cerebral vascular system. In addition, surgeons must have ample clinical operative cases experience. For category A- and B-class aneurysms, micro-operative clip obliteration must demonstrate more than 99% long follow-up total obliteration rate, and surgery should be performed within the 1%–2% range of morbidities. For C/D class aneurysms, the surgeon must have much more superb micro-technical skills and updated refined instrumentation and demonstrate a high volume of personal clinical surgical series of at least more than 500 cases. C/D class neurosurgeons should have the ability of performing complex multiple clipping methods and the capability of all kinds of microvascular anastomosis and skull base high-flow bypass procedures. Younger generation of neurosurgeons must study updated textbooks, first-class atlases, surgical DVDs by experts, and anatomy laboratory practice including cadaveric hands-on courses to obtain cerebrovascular and skull base expertise. Neurosurgeons who wish to become cerebrovascular skull base experts should practice more than 10 times, hopefully 20 times attendance to hands-on courses,

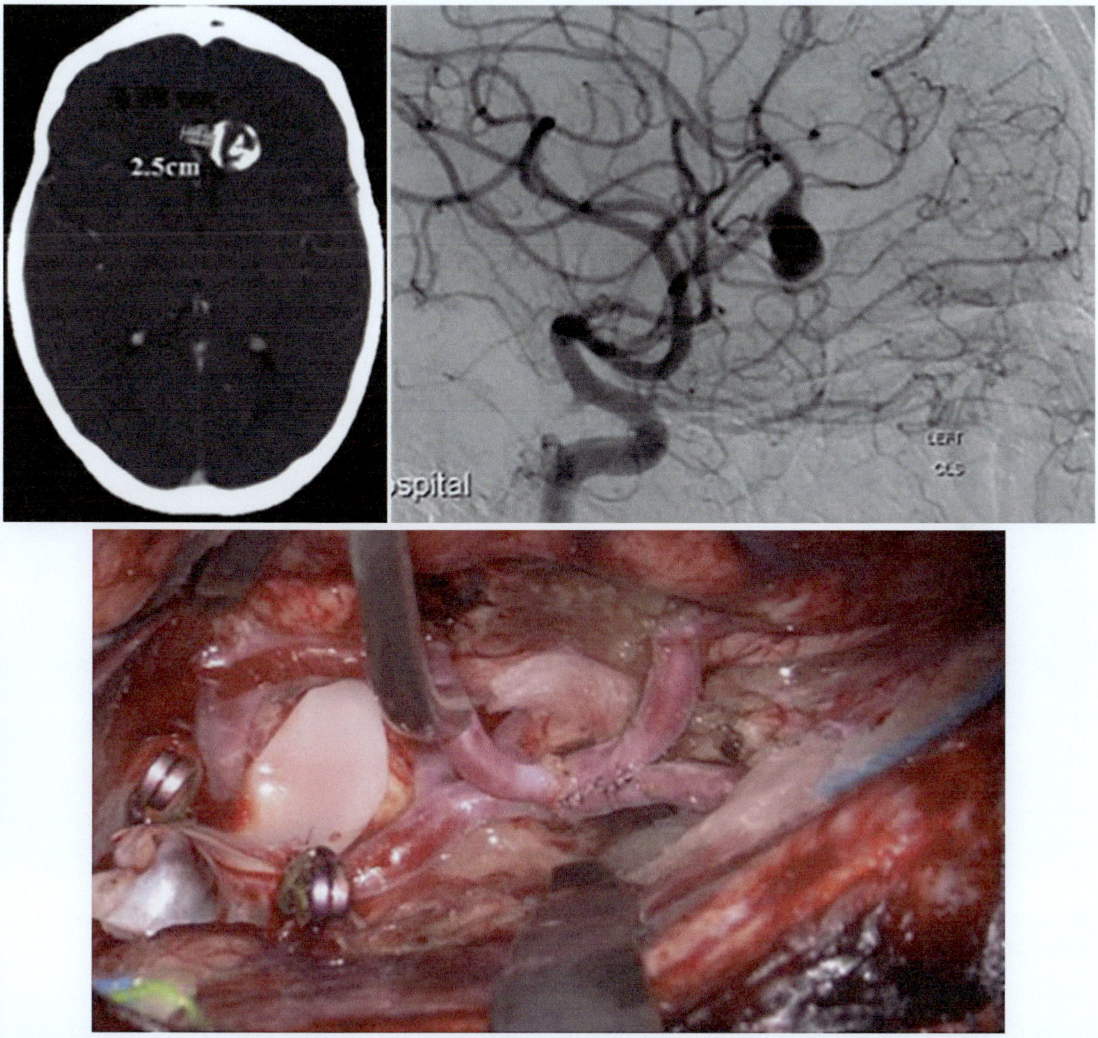

Fig. 6.37 A 27-year-old young man, with callosal bifurcation, calcified, thrombosed, giant aneurysm treated with A3-A3 side anastomosis and trapping of the aneurysm

and visit many hospital ORs in various countries worldwide, to learn on-site from expert surgeons, «how to do it».

Brain Doc Program

Management of subarachnoid hemorrhage due to rupture of cerebral aneurysms is extremely difficult as outlined by Pen Roc Chen's overview article [36]. Morbidity and mortality of ruptured cerebral aneurysms are extremely grave. The best treatment of cerebral aneurysms is to clip for total obliteration to achieve a one-time microsurgical permanent cure. This curative surgery can be done very safely and accurately, while it is small and in non-ruptured condition. In 1990 in Japan, Fukushima advocated general population survey of brain pathology and early detection of intracranial aneurysms using noninvasive MRI and MRA for all people in Japan, from pediatric age to the senior generation. Japan has the most advanced uniform socialized healthcare system, and the cost of medical care is the cheapest of all the countries in the world. The cost of a CT scan is less than $100. The insurance payment of one MRI and MRA examination is $100. Fukushima wrote a public education book as annual brain checkup program named «Brain Doc» in 1990. Since that time, currently, nationwide, a huge number of medical institutions and neurosurgical units have the Brain Doc Program with the drive-through

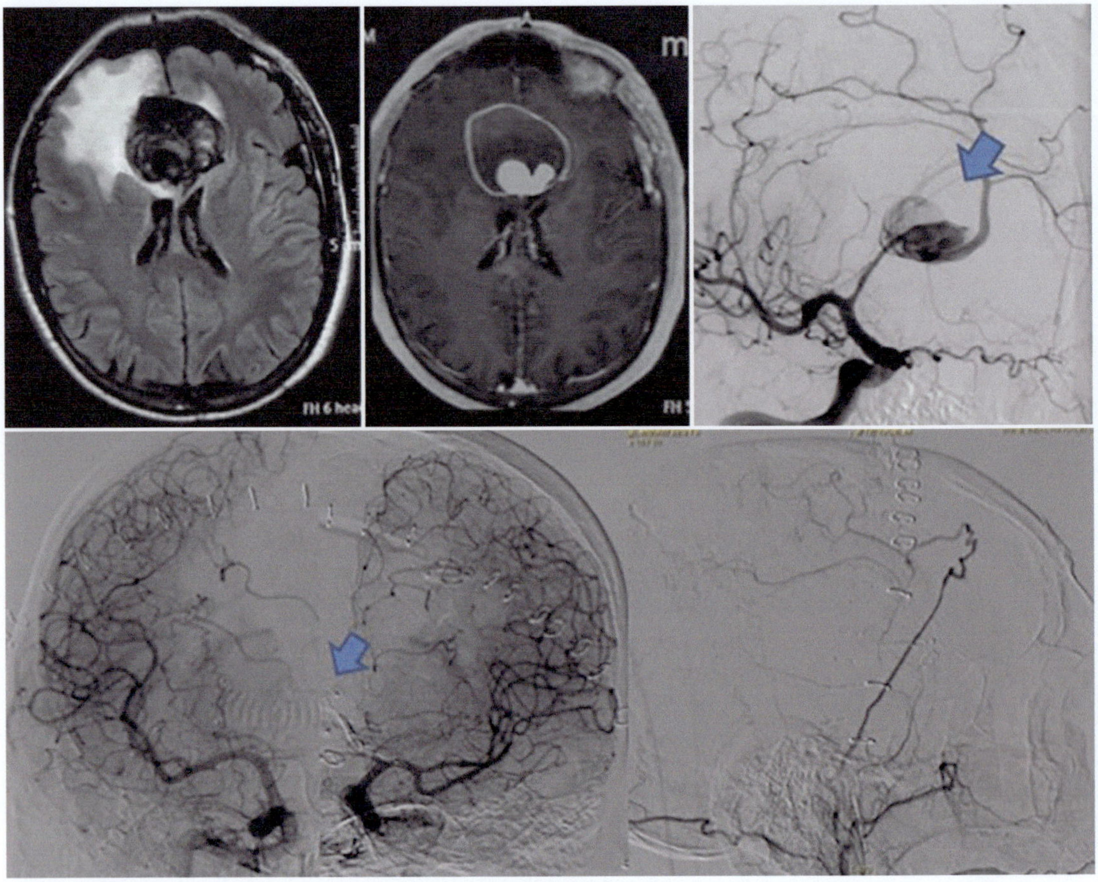

■ **Fig. 6.38** A 60-year-old male treated with long STA to A3 microanastomosis, resection of the giant thrombosed aneurysm, and Acom aneurysmorrhaphy with excellent results

brain checkup using quick MRI and MRA tests at a cost of $200–$300 in Japan. Japan has the largest manpower of neurosurgeons with over 8500 board-certified neurosurgeons. Even in small cities and villages, there is board-certified neurosurgical care available. Currently, the annual number of aneurysm surgeries exceeds 30,000 in Japan. Around 70% of these aneurysm surgeries are for non-ruptured small incidental aneurysms detected by the Brain Doc program. On average, Japan's Brain Doc program detects 3–5% incidence of unruptured aneurysms per 100 people. There are many reports published in Japan, regarding risks of small unruptured aneurysm clipping, which ranges from 1 to 2%, and mortality is extremely rare. I hope this Japan Brain Doc Program will propagate to the entire world to detect cerebral aneurysms while they are small, less than 5 mm. All patients with unruptured small cerebral aneurysms should be treated with a one-time surgical cure using experts' clipping method.

Endovascular Therapy

Over the past 2 decades, since the development of coils and stents as well as recent invention of pipeline stent, endovascular management of cerebral aneurysms has become gradually popular. In European countries, nowadays, endovascular treatment has been done more than microsurgery, because of widespread endovascular Internet announcements and aggressive marketing by the catheter coil medical industry. Many of the endovascular neuroradiologists, neurologists, and even neurosurgeons advocate endovascular treatment, ignoring the presence of super-expert skull base cerebrovascular surgeons who treat complex, difficult, and giant aneurysms far better than endovascular therapy. Recently, Pipeline Flex, Silk, or Fred (so-called flow diverter stents) have been tried, again ignoring the presence of cerebrovascular expert neurosurgeons who are able to operate C/D aneurysms with very low morbidity and with high success rate of one-time surgical cure (microsurgical flow diversion). Some of the aggressive endovascular physicians make very optimistic in adequate dogmatic statements such as «endovascular treatment of very large and giant intracranial aneurysms (≥ 15mm) has largely replaced surgery during the past decades» [42]. The majority of endovascular physicians utilize the discussion of the patient and families to activate their fear of open craniotomy surgery. It is totally opposite. Microsurgical exposure of the aneurysm is performed under direct visual exposure, and aneurysm obliteration is performed accurately under direct visual control. Instead, endovascular therapy is performed indirectly with imaginary radiologic aneurysm shadow. Insertion of coils may rupture an aneurysm. Catheters, guidewires, coils, and stents may cause distal embolism and stenosis. Coils and stents migration and vessel occlusion may occur. Any stents may cause stenosis, occlusion of the perforating branches, or rupture of aneurysm [1, 4, 6–9, 12, 15, 20, 23, 24, 26, 27, 30, 31, 37, 40–43].

Efficacy of coil and stent in the long follow-up study is not known, and durability of the stent has been not yet established. For the management of cerebral aneurysms irrespective of size and location, patient management must be done by teamwork; therefore, neurologists, ER physicians, neurosurgeons, and endovascular radiologists need to establish teamwork and fair discussions. We need to tailor the decision of the best management individually or case by case.

In addition, recurrence due to compaction of the coils or dilatation of the residual necks is significant in more than 20 percent of the coiled aneurysms. Endovascular coil obliteration of the aneurysm is the most successful for the small size with a small neck standard aneurysms (A class), which is very simple to obliterate with microsurgical clipping virtually with 99% long-term total obliteration rate and with negligible morbidities. One noteworthy thing with endovascular therapy is total obliteration rate of aneurysms is poor. For small aneurysms, class A may be 70 or 80% occlusion rate (varying depending upon institutions) and class B aneurysm 60%. Class C and D aneurysms may be less than 30% for total occlusion of the aneurysms, whereas microsurgical clipping in the long follow-up study over 10 years is 99% of total occlusion.

6.2 Dural Arteriovenous Fistulas

A. König, M. Biegler, and U. Spetzger

Dural arteriovenous (AV) fistulas represent a vascular shunt between a meningeal artery and a meningeal vein or a dural venous sinus. Etiology includes previous thrombosis of a dural venous sinus, head injuries, or intracranial surgery, but most fistulas are of idiopathic nature. Dural AV fistulas show a very individual vascular anatomy. Usually they are classified by their venous drainage according to the Borden or Cognard classification. A very common type is the carotid-cavernous fistula. Dural AV fistulas of Borden type II and III can develop aneurysms and lead to an intracerebral hemorrhage; therefore, therapy is indicated in these cases. Endovascular treatment is the best option in most cases. Surgical treatment is indicated if a space-occupying intracerebral hemorrhage occurs.

6.2.1 General Information

Dural arteriovenous (AV) fistulas represent a vascular shunt between a meningeal artery and a meningeal vein or a dural venous sinus. They are often associated with a thrombotic occlusion of the involved dural venous sinus. The arterial blood afflux comes from meningeal branches of the external carotid artery, tentorial branches of the internal carotid artery, meningeal branches of the vertebral artery, and/or pial branches of cerebral arteries [56]. Etiology includes previous thrombosis of a dural venous sinus, head injuries, or intracranial surgery, but most fistulas are of idiopathic nature. The pathophysiology of dural AV fistulas is explained by the widening of naturally occurring microshunts by a raised arterial or venous pressure.

A very common type is the carotid-cavernous fistula (◘ Fig. 6.39). Furthermore, manifestation at the convexity (◘ Figs. 6.40 and 6.41) and at the skull base (◘ Fig. 6.42) are observed.

According to the Borden classification [48], there are three different types of dural AV fistulas characterized by their venous drainage:

- Type I dural AV fistulas drain directly into dural venous sinuses or meningeal veins.
- Type II dural AV fistulas drain into dural sinuses or meningeal veins but also have retrograde drainage into subarachnoid veins.
- Type III dural AV fistulas drain into subarachnoid veins and do not have dural sinus or meningeal venous drainage.

6

Type I fistulas are supplied from meningeal arteries and drain into a dural venous sinus or meningeal veins. The flow within the venous sinus or the draining vein is anterograde. Simple AV fistulas are supplied by a single meningeal artery (type Ia). Complex AV fistulas are supplied by several meningeal arteries (type Ib). Type I fistulas are often asymptomatic; thus, having a low bleeding risk and treatment is not mandatory.

Type II fistulas according to the Borden classification show a high pressure inside that causes a retrograde flow into subarachnoid veins which normally drain into a venous sinus. Since there is an obstruction of drainage within the sinus, the result is the situation described above. The draining veins make up varices and aneurysms with a tendency to hemorrhages; therefore, type II fistula have to be treated.

Type III fistulas drain directly into subarachnoid veins that make up aneurysms and tend to bleed spontaneously. They have to be treated as well to avoid a life-threatening hemorrhage.

As an alternative to the Borden classification, the Cognard classification does not only consider venous drainage but also the clinical course [50]:

- Type I: anterograde drainage into a dural venous sinus, typically after thrombosis
- Type IIa: drainage into a dural venous sinus with reflux into another sinus
- Type IIb: retrograde drainage into cortical veins (10% risk of hemorrhage)
- Type IIc: retrograde drainage into a venous sinus and cortical veins
- Type III: direct drainage into cortical veins without ectasia (40% risk of hemorrhage)
- Type IV: direct drainage into cortical veins with ectasia bigger than 5 mm (65% risk of hemorrhage)
- Type V: drainage into spinal perimedullary veins associated with progressive myelopathy in more than 50%

The carotid-cavernous fistulas (CCF) are classified according to Barrow et al. [47]:

- Type A: direct drainage of the internal carotid artery into the cavernous sinus
- Type B: drainage by meningeal branches from the internal carotid artery into the cavernous sinus
- Type C: drainage by meningeal branches of the external carotid artery into the cavernous sinus
- Type D: drainage by meningeal branches of the external and internal carotid artery into the cavernous sinus

Dural AV fistulas with retrograde drainage into cortical vein show a much higher incidence of intracerebral hemorrhages and venous infarctions [51, 52, 62]. The annual risk of a hemorrhage- or a non-hemorrhage-associated deficit is as high as 8.1% and 6.9%, respectively, which leads to an annual event rate of 15% [51, 62]. In patients with an intracerebral hemorrhage, the risk of rebleeding within the first 2 weeks is 35% [52]. Therefore, dural AV fistulas with cortical venous reflux have to be treated consequently to achieve a complete and definite occlusion of the fistula [51]. Endovascular therapy is the treatment of choice in most cases. Only if this is technically impossible or if the occlusion is incomplete, then microsurgery is indicated. Furthermore, space-occupying intracerebral hemorrhages have to be treated surgically. Usually the fistula is occluded as well during surgery.

6.2.2 Clinical Signs and Symptoms

Clinical symptoms depend on the localization of the fistula. Nonspecific symptoms like headaches and a feeling of pressure inside the head can occur. Dural AV fistulas of the lateral skull base can cause flow-associated ear noise [55].

If intracerebral hemorrhage occurs, focal neurological deficits and even a clouding of consciousness

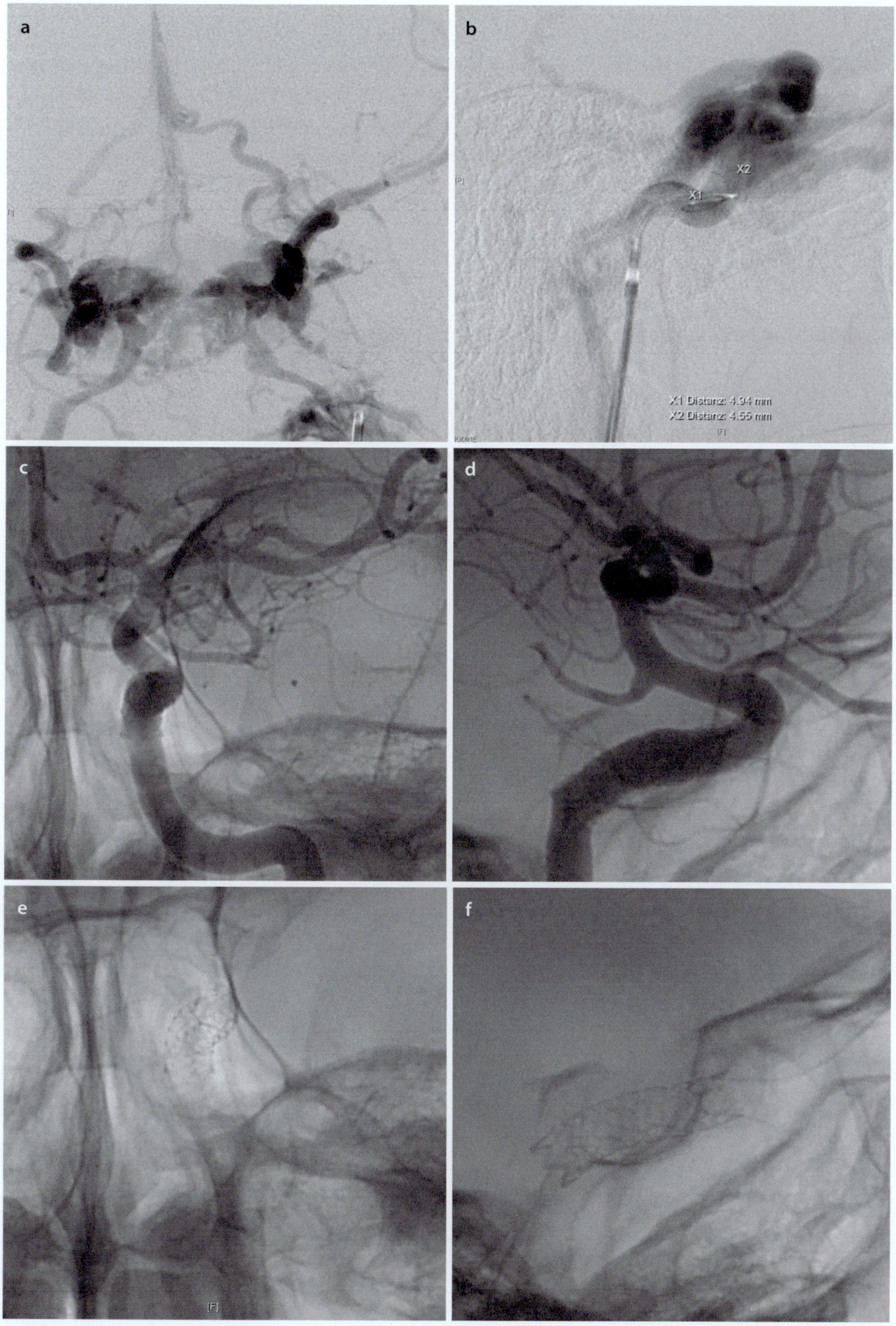

Fig. 6.39 DSA imaging **a**, **b** and intervention **c**–**f** of a CCF Barrow type A. Early filling of the cavernous sinus from direct branches of the left ACI. Venous drainages from the cavernous sinus into supra- and infraophthalmic veins. Occlusion of the fistula by stenting, with **c**, **d** and without contrast agent **e**, **f**. Anterior-posterior **a**, **c**, **e** and lateral **b**, **d**, **f** projections

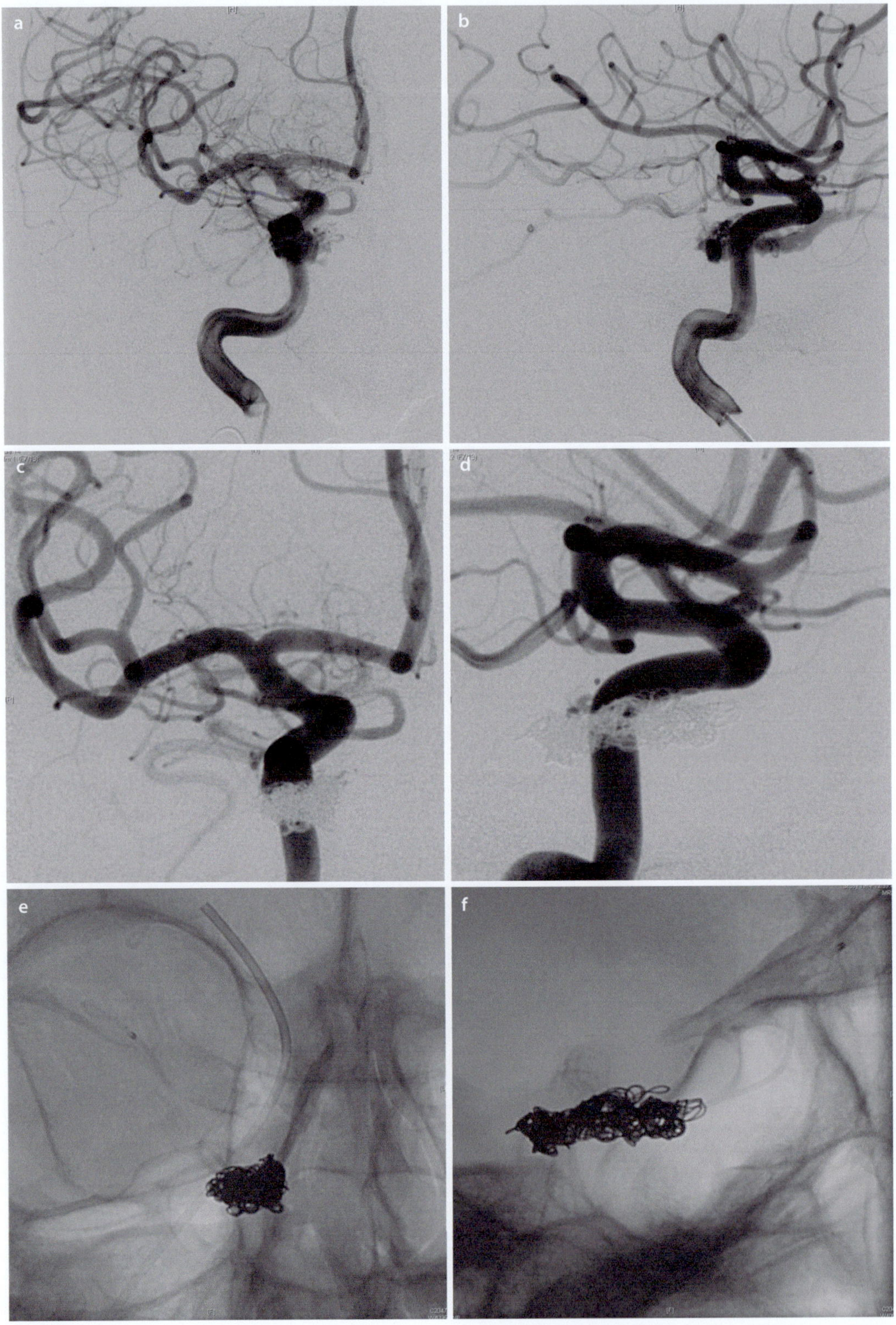

Fig. 6.40 DSA visualization **a**, **b** and intervention **c**–**f** of a Barrow type B fistula from the right ACI. Occlusion of the fistula by coil embolization, images with **c**, **d** and without **e**, **f** contrast agent. Anterior-posterior **a**, **c**, **e** and lateral **b**, **d**, **f** projections

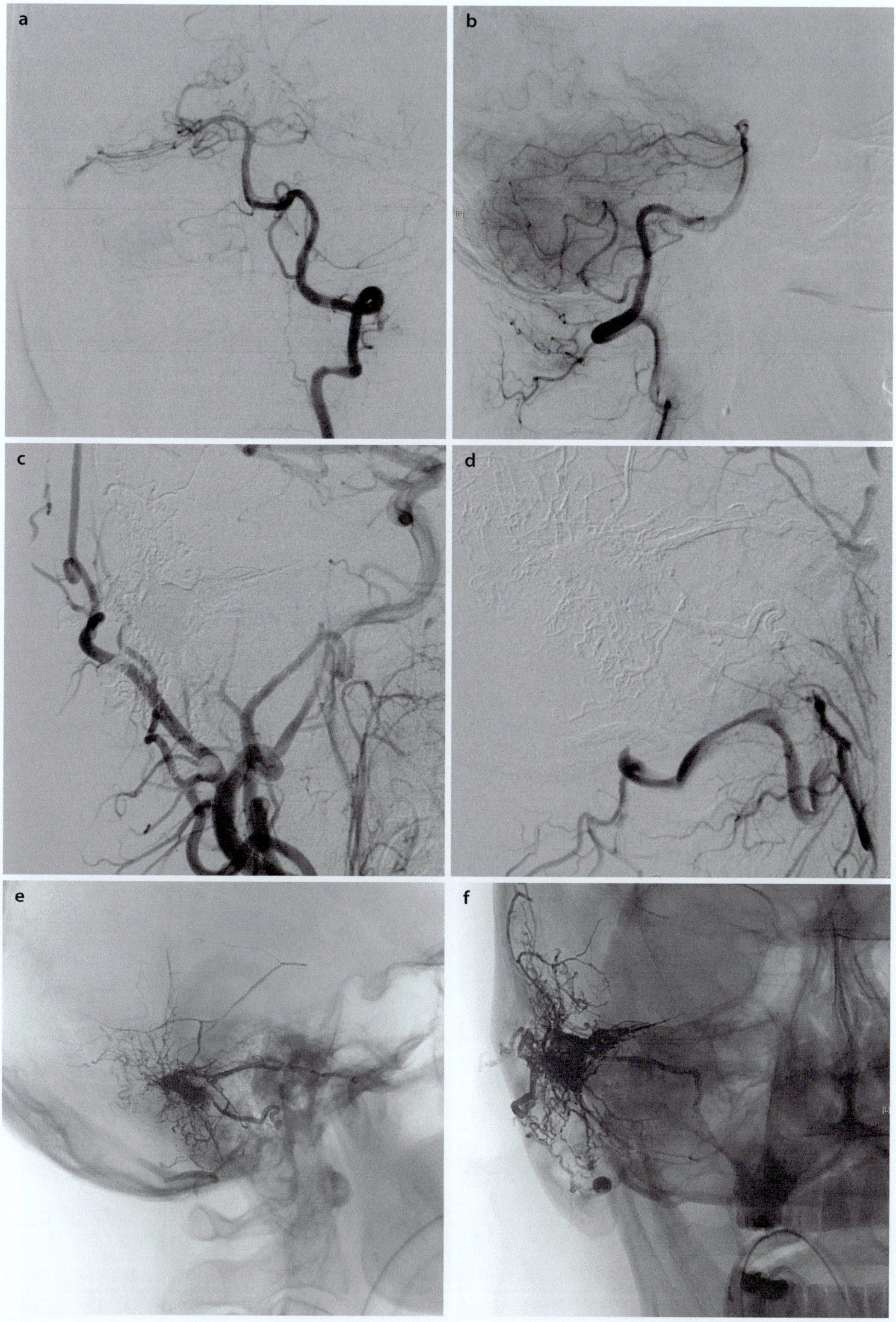

Fig. 6.41 DSA visualization **a**, **b** and intervention **c**–**f** of a dural AV fistula from the right ACI. Occlusion of the fistula by Onyx, images with **c**, **d** and without **e**, **f** contrast agent. Anterior-posterior **a**, **c**, **e** and lateral **b**, **d**, **f** projections

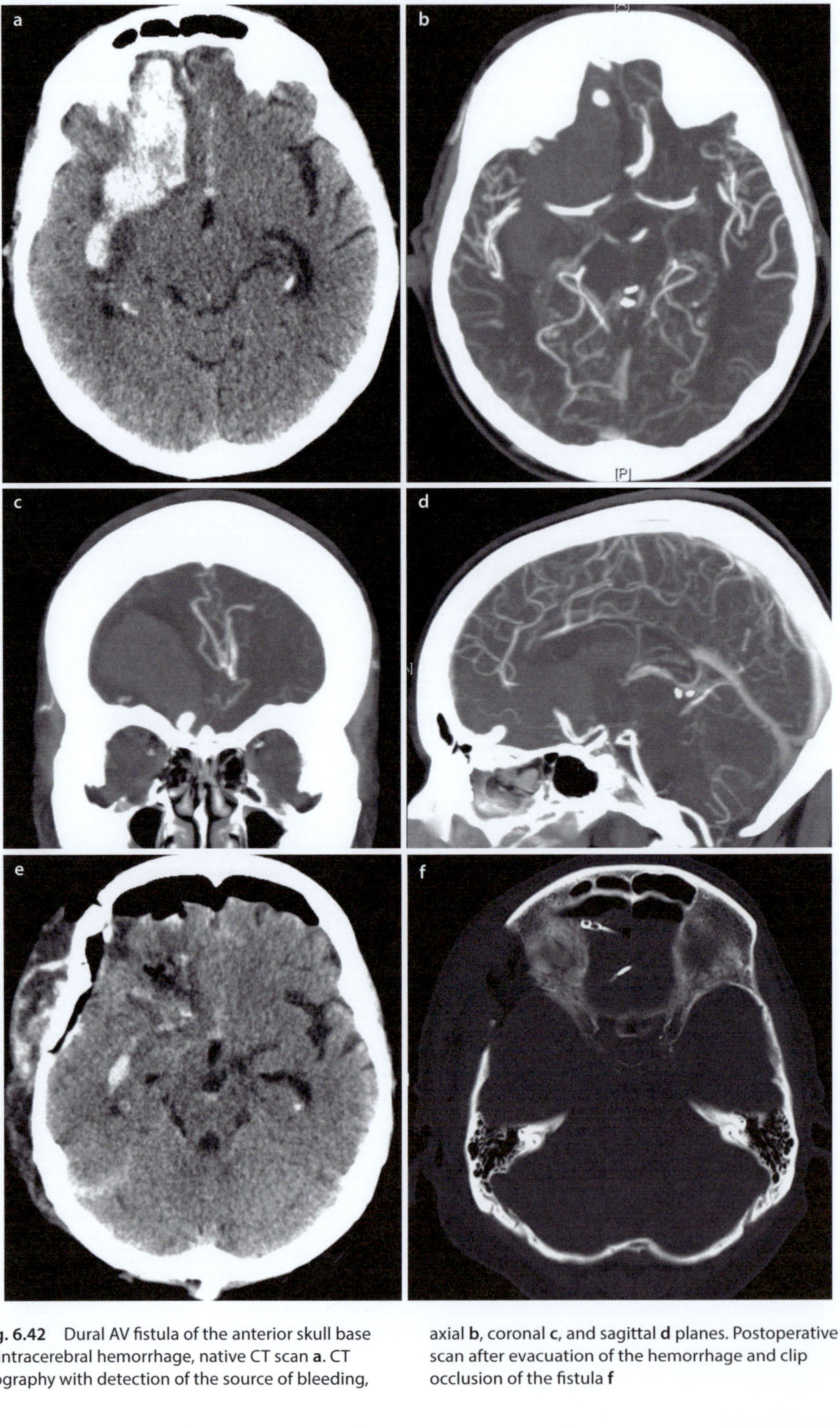

■ **Fig. 6.42** Dural AV fistula of the anterior skull base with intracerebral hemorrhage, native CT scan **a**. CT angiography with detection of the source of bleeding, axial **b**, coronal **c**, and sagittal **d** planes. Postoperative CT scan after evacuation of the hemorrhage and clip occlusion of the fistula **f**

can be observed. In some cases, venous congestion causes encephalopathy with dementia and a Parkinson syndrome [63].

Typical clinical signs for a CCF are:

- Pulsatile exophthalmus
- Chemosis
- Internal and external ophthalmoplegia
- Double vision
- Progressive visual loss
- Papilledema

Investigations

In case of acute clinical symptoms, a CT scan is usually the primary diagnostic. A native CT scan can detect an intracerebral hemorrhage but not the fistula itself. CT angiography can be of help in detecting the dural AV fistula (Fig. 6.42). Especially enlarged veins (enlarged superior ophthalmic veins in CCF cases) and changes in the caliber of veins in the venous phase of CT angiography are direct signs.

In cases of subacute clinical complaints, MRI is the diagnostic of first choice. T1-weighted sequences can show hyperintense thrombus material in a dural venous sinus. T1-weighted images with contrast agent show a diffuse enhancement of the dura in some cases. T2-weighted and FLAIR images visualize confluent hyperintense white matter lesion in cases of a high-grade venous congestion with edema. If there is thrombosis in a dural venous sinus, then TOF MR angiographs show a lack of flow signal within the sinus.

Digital subtraction angiography (DSA) is the method of choice for the direct evidence of a dural AV fistula and the planning of endovascular therapy. The arterial supply and the venous drainage can be visualized to classify the fistula and to estimate the risk of hemorrhage (see above). Afterward the indication for endovascular embolization or surgical occlusion or combined treatment can be made.

6.2.3 Therapeutic Options

Indications for treatment are given in cases of progressive clinical symptoms, significant shunt volumes, and complications (subarachnoid or intracerebral hemorrhage). Usually treatment is indicated for Cognard type IIb or higher grades. Furthermore, a prophylactic intervention to avoid hemorrhage has to be considered, especially for type II and III fistulas according to the Borden classification since they bear an increased risk for hemorrhage due to venous varices and aneurysms.

The mainstay for treatment is endovascular therapy [46, 49, 54, 57, 58]. Depending on size, localization, and configuration of the dural AV fistula embolization, coils or liquid agents such as Onyx (Covidien, Irvine, CA) or stent reconstruction of the ACI in cases of CCF is used (Figs. 6.39, 6.40, and 6.41).

Transvenous coil embolization and transarterial application of n-BCA have become established techniques for the occlusion of dural AV fistulas, whereas Onyx has given proof of being a safe and feasible material with a higher rate of obstruction [53].

Via a transfemoral arterial approach, a diagnostic angiogram of the ACE, ACI, and VA is made. A guiding catheter is used to bring an Onyx-compatible microcatheter close to the fistula, whereas an adequate distance for the reflux of the liquid agent has to be achieved. In cases of very complex supply of the fistula, it might be necessary to perform a multistage intervention to embolize the different arterial feeders [56].

In Borden type II fistulas, the draining sinus and veins have to be embolized. As an alternative, surgical clipping might be indicated if a space-occupying intracerebral hemorrhage has to be evacuated. In Borden type III fistulas, the fistula itself and the draining veins have to be embolized. As an alternative, surgical clipping of draining veins close to the sinus can be performed when the evacuation of an intracerebral hemorrhage is indicated.

Recurrences of dural AV fistulas after embolization with Onyx have been described, but they are asymptomatic in most cases, and the overall neurological outcome after endovascular treatment is very good [46, 54].

Surgery is only indicated in cases of relevant space-occupying hemorrhages or when endovascular treatment achieved only a partial embolization [59–61, 64]. During surgery the fistula usually can be occluded (Fig. 6.42). The craniotomy is planned according to preoperative CT and MRI scans and DSA imaging. A thin-sliced CT scan or MPR-3D MRI scan enables the use of neuronavigation for accurate localization of the hemorrhage and fistula and is useful when planning the size and site of the craniotomy.

Stereotactic radiosurgical treatment can be considered for dural AV fistulas without cortical venous drainage [60, 61] if there is a patient-related contraindication for endovascular or microsurgical treatment.

6.3 Neurovascular Compression Syndromes

N. J. Hopf, R. Reisch, and P. Kurucz

6

Neurovascular compression syndromes (NVCS) of cranial nerves are most commonly affecting the trigeminal nerve causing trigeminal neuralgia. Other recognized NVCS are glossopharyngeal neuralgia, hemifacial spasm, and vestibular paroxysmia. NVCS result from mechanical compression from an artery or less frequent compression from a greater vein at the transition zone of the affected nerve, where it is most vulnerable. Treatment consists of membrane-stabilizing medication as the first choice or local installation of botulinum toxin in hemifacial spasm. In case of inadequate control of symptoms, surgical treatment should be considered. Treatment of the cause of the disease can only be achieved by surgery in form of microvascular decompression. Dependent on the patient's condition and comorbidities, focal lesioning of the affected nerve may be an option. This is performed by thermal, chemical, or mechanical-controlled damage of the Gasserian ganglion via a transfacial route or applying radiosurgery to the cisternal part of the nerve. Currently, endoscopic microvascular decompression has the highest success rates with up to 99% initial pain control and lowest side effects with facial dysesthesia in only 8% and hearing impairment in 1% of the patients.

6.3.1 General Information

Neurovascular compression syndrome (NVCS) is defined as mechanical irritation of nervous tissue by blood vessels. In most instances NVCS consists of a conflict between a cranial nerve and an artery. In rare cases, larger veins can be the offending vessels or distinct parts of the brain itself, the affected nervous tissue [78]. Most commonly, the trigeminal nerve is involved leading to trigeminal neuralgia. Other well-established NVCS are hemifacial spasm caused by affection of the facial nerve or glossopharyngeal neuralgia if the glossopharyngeal nerve is involved in a relevant neurovascular conflict. There is also strong evidence that vestibular paroxysmia is also caused by a neurovascular conflict with consecutive irritation of the vestibulocochlear nerve [74]. Furthermore, vascular compression of the brain stem is thought to be responsible at least in selected cases of idiopathic arterial hypertension (▫ Table 6.3).

▫ Table 6.3 Neurovascular compression syndromes

ANT	Syndrome	Offending vessel
CN V	Trigeminal neuralgia	SCA, AICA, BA, CPV
CN VII	Hemifacial spasm	AICA, PICA, BA, VA
CN VIII	Vestibular paroxysmia	AICA, PICA, BA, VA
CN IX	Glossopharyngeal neuralgia	PICA, VA
Brain stem	Hypertension	PICA, VA

ANT affected nervous tissue, *CN* cranial nerve, *SCA* superior cerebellar artery, *AICA* anterior inferior cerebellar artery, *BA* basilar artery, *SPV* superior petrosal vein, *VA* vertebral artery, *PICA* posterior inferior cerebellar artery

Cranial nerves are most vulnerable for mechanical irritation at their transition zone. This is the area of a cranial nerve, where the axonal insolation changes from central myelin produced by oligodendrocytes to peripheral myelin produced by Schwann cells. The transition zone varies from 1 mm (CN VII & IX) to more than 10 mm (CN VIII) within the cisternal portion of the different cranial nerves (▫ Fig. 6.43) measured from the brain stem [72]. Therefore, it has to be clearly pointed out that the transition zone is not equivalent to the root entry zone [73]. This delicate but important difference needs to be taken into account for adequate interpretation of imaging studies, indication for treatment, and intraoperative judgment.

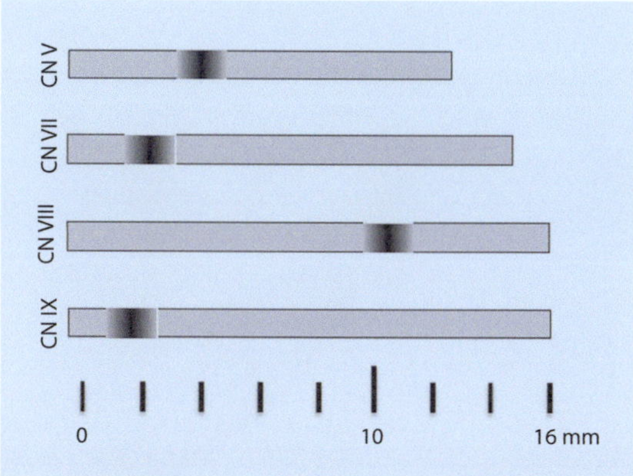

Fig. 6.43 Schematic illustration of the average location of the transition zones in different cranial nerves (From Haller et al. [73])

Primary NVCS are distinguished from symptomatic NVCS (Fig. 6.44). In symptomatic NVCS, symptoms are caused by direct compression of or dislocation of vessels toward the affected nerve. This can be seen in space-occupying lesions or direct affection of nervous tissue by inflammatory or demyelinating diseases. The primary NVCS is typically seen in elderly patients, when arteries become elongated by increasing blood pressure and decreasing elasticity of the vessel wall and is advancing with age. Women are generally more frequently affected, because of the higher life expectancy. Clinical symptoms are according to the involved cranial nerve. Generally, symptoms present as attacks, triggered by specific stimuli or spontaneously.

Pathophysiology and treatment of the most common NVCS, i.e., trigeminal neuralgia, goes back to the pioneering work of Dandy, Gardner, and Miklos [67, 70]. Initially, surgical treatment consisted of partial transection of the sensory root of the trigeminal nerve, sometimes combined with dissection or destruction of the offending vessel. Peter Jannetta introduced in 1967 an entire nondestructive surgical procedure with the goal to treat only the cause of the disease by mere microvascular decompression [76]. Because his method has remained the strategy also of modern surgical treatment of NVCS, this procedure is still referred to as «Jannetta-Operation» throughout the world (Fig. 6.45).

6.3.2 Clinical Signs and Symptoms

Clinical symptoms are according to the involved cranial nerve and consist of neuralgic pain (trigeminal neuralgia, glossopharyngeal neuralgia), involuntary contractions of muscles (hemifacial spasm), or vertigo (vestibular paroxysmia). Generally, symptoms present in recurrent, short episodes of high intensity, which appear spontaneously or triggered by specific stimuli.

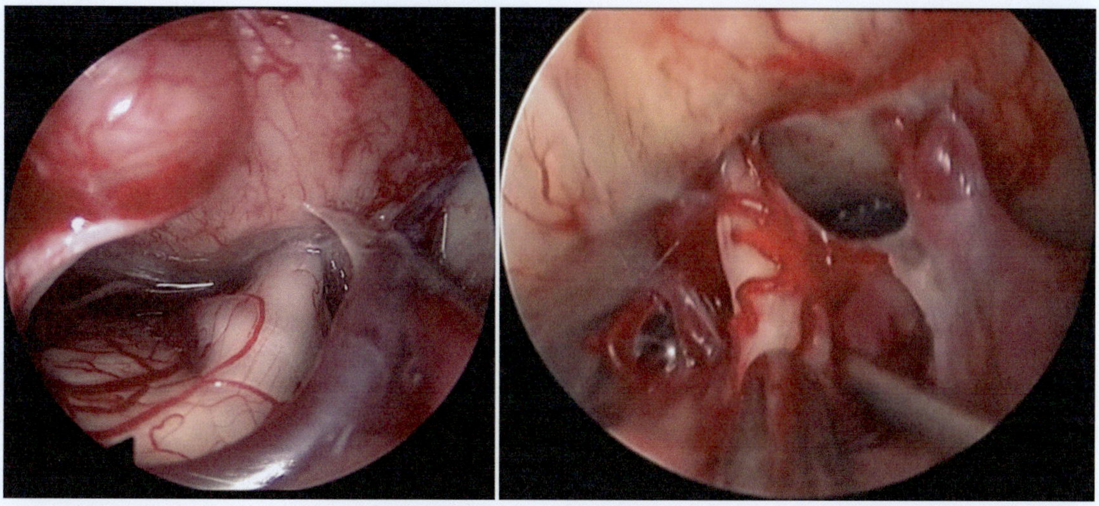

Fig. 6.44 Endoscopic picture of (*left*) a primary neurovascular compression syndrome showing the right trigeminal nerve thinned out by the underlying superior cerebellar artery and (*right*) a symptomatic neurovascular compression syndrome caused by an arteriovenous malformation affecting the right trigeminal nerve

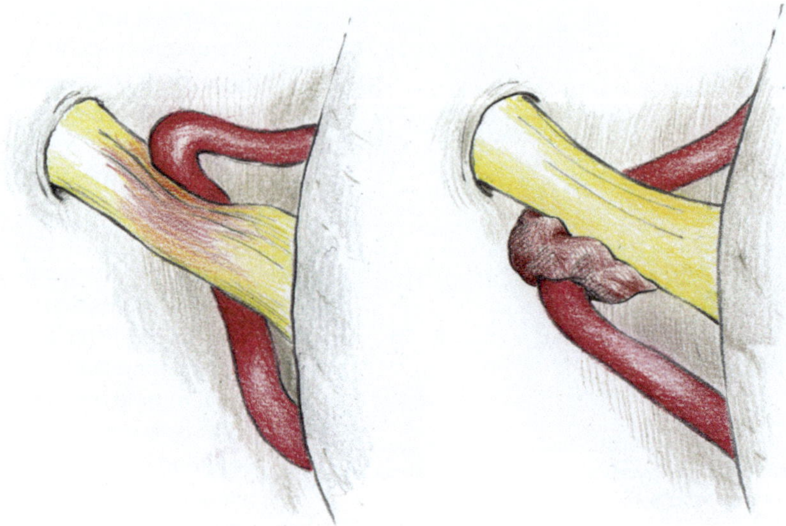

Fig. 6.45 Schematic drawing of a neurovascular conflict (*left*) and causal treatment (*right*) in terms of microvascular decompression with an alloplastic interponate acting as a cushion to prevent transmission of rhythmic arterial pressure

6

Trigeminal Neuralgia

Patients with trigeminal neuralgia experience severe pain attacks in the innervation area of one or multiple branches of the trigeminal nerve. Triggers are typically mechanical stimuli such as chewing, drinking, tooth brushing, talking, or contact with the involved skin (▶ Box 6.1). Frequently, vegetative phenomena such as reddening of the skin in the supply area of the affected trigeminal branch or secretion of the lacrimal or salivary gland follow the pain attacks [68]. Cold temperature seems to increase the stimulus. In the advanced stage of the disease, spontaneous attacks without trigger seem to occur more often, and a dull permanent background pain may be present. The pain is rated generally 10 out of 10 on the visual analogous scale (VAS) with 10 being the strongest pain imaginable. Time from first symptoms to diagnosis does often take many years. Thus, many patients have previously undergone multiple dental procedures. Intensity and inability to anticipate or control the pain do not infrequently lead to suicidal thoughts in affected patients.

Box 6.1 Criteria for Primary (Idiopathic) Trigeminal Neuralgia by the International Headache Society (HIS)

I. Paroxysmic attacks of a frontal or facial pain for seconds up to 2 min
II. The pain shows at least four of the following characteristics:
   - Distribution of one or multiple branches of the trigeminal nerve
   - Sudden, intensive, superficial, radiating of pungent, or burning quality
   - High pain intensity
   - Elicitability in trigger zones or by specific daily activities like eating, talking, washing, tooth brushing
   - Complete pain relief in between the pain attacks
III. No neurological deficit
IV. Stereotype pattern or attacks
V. Exclusion of other causes by medical history, examination, and possibly further investigations

The primary (previously referred to as idiopathic) trigeminal neuralgia is distinguished from the symptomatic trigeminal neuralgia because of relevant differences in timing and selection of the appropriate treatment option.

Primary trigeminal neuralgia typically appears beyond 50 years of age. The second branch is affected most frequently (18%) followed by the third (15%), often mistaken as toothache, or a combination of both (40%). The first branch is affected only rarely as the only branch in primary trigeminal neuralgia; bilateral trigeminal neuralgia is described in 3% of all cases [68].

The incidence for women is 5.9 per 100.000 people per year, for men 3.9. [77]. Symptomatic trigeminal neuralgia accounts for less than 10% of all cases and is caused by space-occupying lesions such as tumors (vestibular schwannomas, epidermoids, meningiomas), vascular lesions (aneurysms, arteriovenous malformations, cavernomas), or demyelinating diseases (multiple sclerosis). In symptomatic trigeminal neuralgia, the first branch is affected more frequently, and patients are often younger at the first onset of symptoms.

Hemifacial Spasm

Hemifacial spasm manifests as involuntary and arrhythmic contractions of the face muscles on one side, regularly beginning in the orbicularis oculi muscle (Fig. 6.46). Contractions occur spontaneously or are triggered by arbitrary innervation of face muscles. Draft, reading, and mental strain increase the symptoms. A facial palsy is usually not present [74]. Patients with hemifacial spasm may be severely disabled by impaired vision due to prolonged closure of the affected eye and do not infrequently draw themselves back from public life. Differential diagnosis includes blepharospasm, facial nerve tics, focal seizures, and oromandibular dystonia [83].

The incidence of hemifacial spasm is 0.8 per 100.000, and the ratio between women and men is 2:1. The time between the beginning of symptoms and diagnosis was found to be more than 8 years in average [83]. Bilateral hemifacial spasm is rare. In 1–5% the hemifacial spasm is secondary to a space-occupying lesion within the cerebellopontine angle or demyelinating diseases such as multiple sclerosis [74].

Vestibular Paroxysmia

Vestibular paroxysmia is characterized by short attacks of rotatory or postural vertigo with instability of posture and gait, frequently lasting for only a few seconds. Attacks are triggered by a particular head position, hyperventilation, or fast movements of eyes or head. The vertigo may be associated with nausea or cochlear nerve symptoms such as unilateral tinnitus or hearing impairment (▶ Box 6.2). Concerning the onset, vestibular paroxysmia shows two peaks in the frequency of occurrence. Onset in an early age is most likely associated with vertebrobasilar vascular anomalies; late onset

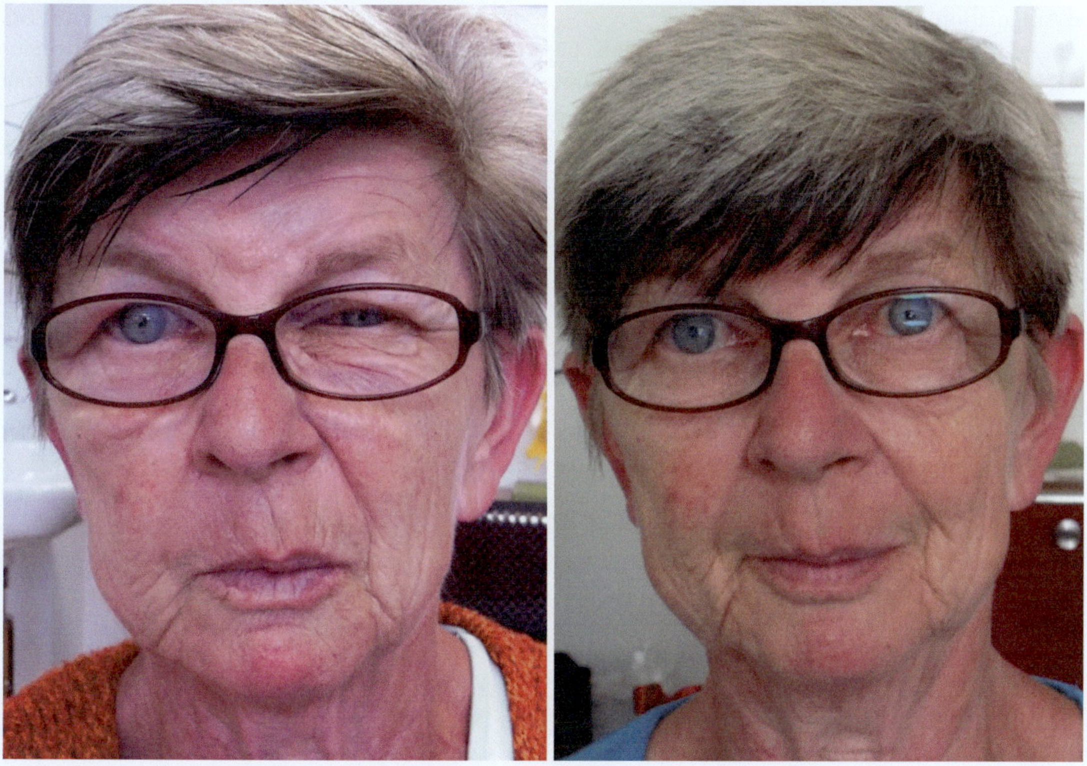

Fig. 6.46 Patient with left-sided hemifacial spasm pre- (*left*) and postoperatively (*right*)

Box 6.2 Criteria for Primary (Idiopathic) Vestibular Paroxysmia

I. Paroxysmic attacks of rotatory or postural vertigo with instability of posture and gait
II. Attacks triggered by particular head positions or hyperventilation
III. Attacks associated with unilateral hypoacusis or tinnitus
IV. Measurable vestibular and/or cochlear deficits increase during attack
V. Symptoms improve by administering carbamazepine
VI. Absence of central vestibular/ocular motor disorders or brain stem signs

between 40 and 70 years of age is thought to be initiated by vascular elongation due to increasing atherosclerosis and stronger pulsations associated with arterial hypertension of old age [66].

Differential diagnosis includes vestibular migraine, benign paroxysmal positional vertigo, superior canal dehiscence syndrome, orthostatic dysregulation, and panic attacks [66].

Assignment of the side of origin can be very difficult in vestibular paroxysmia without associated cochlear nerve symptoms, because electrophysiological work-up shows only in 20–45% of patients abnormalities [66]. Therefore, the diagnosis of vestibular paroxysmia should be based on the combination of clinical examination, neurophysiological, and imaging techniques to define the affected side and differentiate between a deficit syndrome and increased excitability [65].

Glossopharyngeal Neuralgia

Glossopharyngeal neuralgia presents as short, unilateral pain attacks, lasting for seconds up to minutes in the supply area of the glossopharyngeal nerve, most commonly at the ear and in descending frequency of the tonsil, larynx, and tongue. Sometimes, patients report of a longer-lasting dull pain, a feeling of pressure, or burning sensations. In some cases, pain attacks are accompanied by coughing, hoarseness, or hypersalivation, in 10% by bradycardia or cardiac arrest [82]. Pain attacks are triggered by swallowing, chewing, speaking, coughing, contact with the skin of the outer meatus, or even simple movements of the tongue [71].

Glossopharyngeal neuralgia is by far less frequent than trigeminal neuralgia with an incidence of 0.2–0.7 per 100.000 people per year [69, 74]. Female and male are affected equally. Symptomatic glossopharyngeal neuralgia occurs and is caused by either space-occupying lesions within the cerebellopontine angle or focal demyelination.

6.3.3 Investigations

NVCS are generally diagnosed clinically, based on the typical signs and symptoms (see 6.43). However, symptomatic NVCS caused by a space-occupying lesion or demyelination need to be ruled out. Therefore, contrast-enhanced MR imaging is required in any suspected case of NVCS immediately. High-resolution 3D T2-weighted imaging with 3D time-of-flight angiography (◘ Fig. 6.47) and 3D T1-weighted gadolinium-enhanced sequences (◘ Fig. 6.48, left) are considered the standard of reference for the detection of a neurovascular conflict [73].

In addition, high-resolution 3D heavily T2-weighted sequences, including CISS (◘ Fig. 6.48, right) and FIESTA, are helpful from the neurosurgical point of view to visualize the cisternal portion of the affected nerve. Diffusion tensor imaging (DTI) is able to show loss of anisotropy in the trigeminal nerve in several cases of trigeminal neuralgia. However, this does not relevantly contribute to the decision for and type of treatment.

Electrophysiological investigations can be helpful in vestibular paroxysmia to support the diagnosis and screen for a possible lateralization. In trigeminal neuralgia, electrophysiological investigations in form of trigeminal SEP, blink, and masseter reflex should be considered facultative. However, they may pick up subclinical damage of the affected nerve and can be used during postoperative follow-up. In hemifacial spasm, pathognomonic indirect responses to stimulation of individual branches of the facial nerve can be detected [74].

A positive medical treatment trial with carbamazepine or oxcarbazepine is an important puzzle piece for the diagnosis of a NVCS, in particular, in vestibular paroxysmia.

In glossopharyngeal neuralgia, initiation of pain attacks by contact with the tonsil and termination of the pain by application of a local anesthetic, such as 10% lidocaine spray, supports the clinical diagnosis [74].

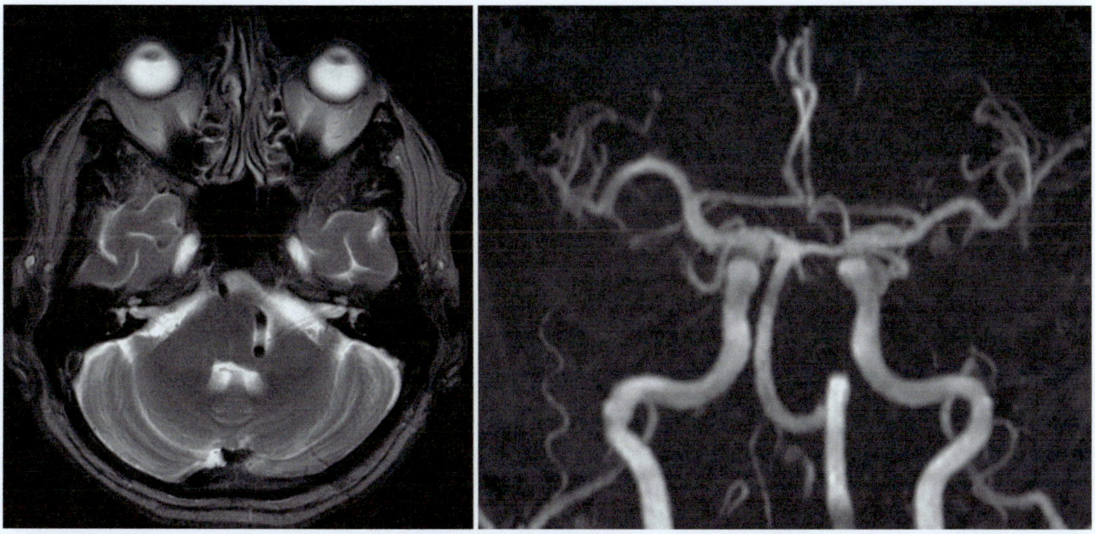

Fig. 6.47 T2-weighted MR image (*left*) and 3D time-of-flight angiography (*right*) of a patient with left-sided hemifacial spasm due to compression of the left facial nerve by the left elongated vertebral artery

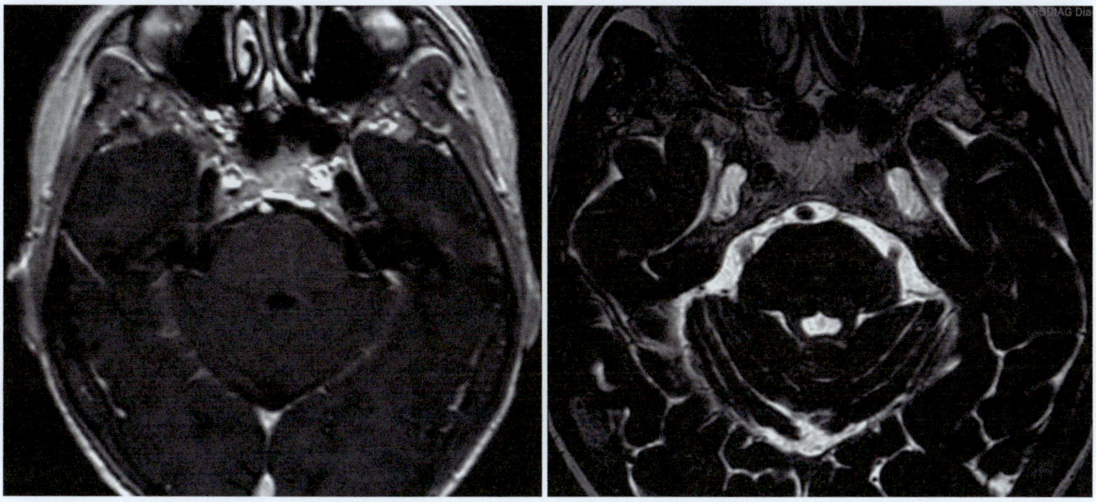

Fig. 6.48 T1-weighted gadolinium-enhanced MRI (*left*) and T2-weighted CISS sequence (*right*) demonstrating a neurovascular conflict between the trigeminal nerve and the superior cerebellar artery on the right side

6.3.4 Therapeutic Options

Generally, NVCS are treated conservatively. Surgery should be considered only in case of failed medical treatment or symptomatic NVCS caused by a space-occupying lesion. Concerning surgical treatment, we distinguish causal, function-preserving methods from symptomatic, destructive-ablative methods. Recently, also Radiosurgery has been proven a successful minimal invasive treatment alternative to surgery in selected cases of NVCS.

Medical treatment consists of antiepileptic drugs. Carbamazepine and oxcarbazepine are the preferred substances for all NVCS. Initially, a daily dosage of 600–1.200 mg is used. The dosage should be gradually increased according to the symptoms and side effects up to a maximal dosage of 2000 mg for carbamazepine and 2400 mg for oxcarbazepine. Drugs of the second choice are phenytoin,

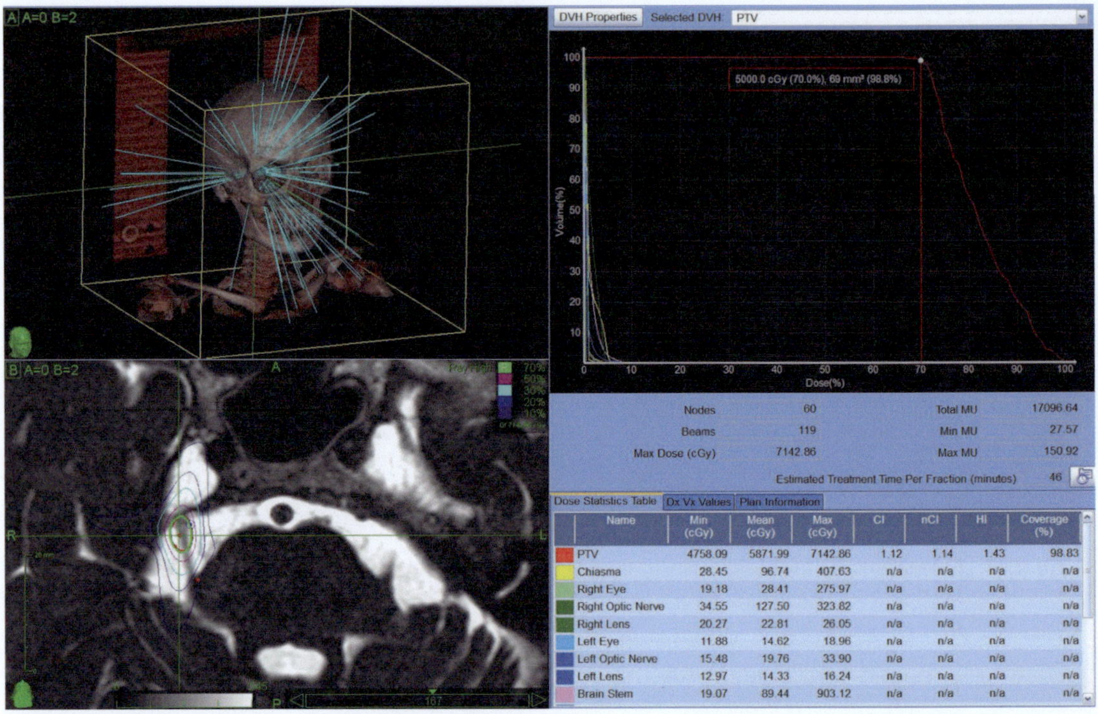

Fig. 6.49 Treatment plan for radiosurgery with the CyberKnife of a patient with recurrent trigeminal neuralgia on the right side showing the planned single beam trajectories (*upper left*), the distribution of isodosis projected on the MRI (*lower left*) and the dosage distribution of the target and critical structures (*lower right*)

lamotrigine, and baclofen [68]. Generally, medical treatment provides satisfactory relief of symptoms in the initial stage of the disease in 90% of the patients. However, in the further course, these results drop to 50% despite maximal daily dosage as described above or even a combined medical treatment. Opiates are less effective and therefore generally not recommended.

Local instillation of botulinum toxin into the orbicularis oculi muscle is the treatment of choice for hemifacial spasm. Good results can be achieved in approximately 80% of patients. The effect lasts for 16–20 weeks. Side effects are transient decrease of the lacrimal gland and incomplete lid closure.

Radiosurgery has been increasingly used for the treatment of trigeminal neuralgia. Even though it is generally known as a noninvasive method, it has to be classified as a destructive-ablative treatment for trigeminal neuralgia. Indication is failed medical treatment in patients that have relative or absolute contraindications for surgery or previously unsuccessful surgical treatment. A high single dosage of up to 90 gray is administered to the trigeminal nerve in an outpatient setting (Fig. 6.49). The success rate is initially high with 70–90% but drops to 50% after 5 years. The effect may appear immediately but normally sets in after days up to weeks. The nerve may appear atrophic during surgery in patients having had radiosurgery (Fig. 6.50) and 10–30% of radiosurgically treated patients experience a sensory deficit due to the destructive-ablative character of this method [80].

6.3.5 Surgical Treatment

Surgical treatment of choice for NVCS is «microvascular decompression» (MVD). MVD is the only causal and function-preserving treatment by separating the offending vessel from the affected cranial nerve or brain tissue. Destructive-ablative surgical treatment options are only used for trigeminal neuralgia and have the goal of controlled damage to the Gasserian ganglion. These procedures should be reserved for patients, who are no good candidates for MVD due to relevant comorbidities or failed previous MVD. Destructive-ablative procedures

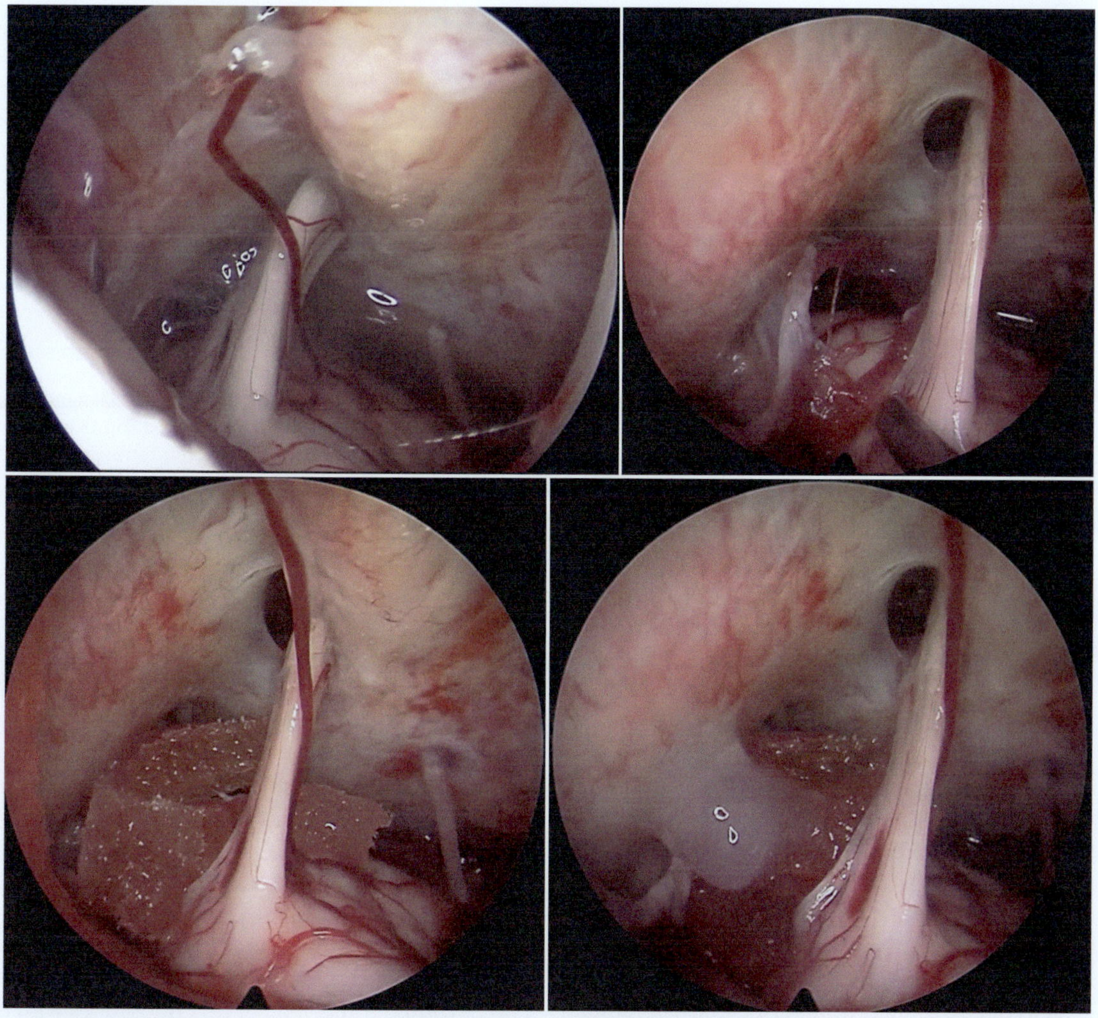

Fig. 6.50 Endoscopic images of a patient with recurrent trigeminal neuralgia after initially successful radiosurgical treatment with the CyberKnife 1 year before showing (*upper left*) the atrophic appearance of the trigeminal nerve, (*upper right*) the offending artery behind the nerve detected only with the 30°-angled endoscope, (*lower left*) Teflon pads interponated between the offending artery and the nerve, in this case because of large subarachnoidal space fixed with tissue glue (*lower right*)

are performed in terms of thermal coagulation, glycerine injection, or balloon compression of the Gasserian ganglion via a transfacial percutaneous route.

Microvascular Decompression

Microvascular decompression (MVD) is generally performed via a retrosigmoid craniotomy or craniectomy in a semi-sitting or park bench position. The offending vessel is separated from the nerve under the operating microscope [78, 84]. This may be difficult because the operating microscope allows only visualization in a straight trajectory, and illumination can be inappropriate due to the deep location of the neurovascular conflict in case of trigeminal neuralgia and hemifacial spasm, in particular, in patients with narrow cisterns. Re-approximation is prevented by interponation of a piece of autologous muscle, alloplastic material, or fixation of the offending vessel at the tentorium or dura of the skull base with tissue adhesive or sutures.

The classic procedure has to be addressed as major surgery with relevant risks for the patient, often being in an advanced age with significant comorbidities. Therefore, MVD was earlier recommended only in a late stage of the disease. Introduction of minimal invasive and endoscopic neurosurgery has changed this significantly. Therefore, endoscopic MVD should be considered as the method of choice in all patients with NVCS, but only performed if sufficient experience and adequate equipment is available.

Endoscopic MVD is by the authors performed with the patient in a supine position, the head of the patient turned approximately 70° to the contralateral side and slightly inclined. The shoulder should not be elevated using a cushion because that will obliterate the best straight view to the neurovascular conflict (◘ Fig. 6.50). In case of impaired neck mobility or stout patients, the OR table may be tilted after securing the patient or a park bench position can be used. In all cases, multimodal electrophysiological neuromonitoring consisting of acoustic evoked potentials (AEP) and free-running electromyogram (EMG) of the facial and trigeminal nerve is strongly recommended for trigeminal neuralgia, hemifacial spasm, and vestibular paroxysmia. In glossopharyngeal neuralgia, additional monitoring of the caudal cranial nerves should be performed [79]. In general, neuronavigation is recommended for optimal placement of the craniotomy but is not a conditio sine qua non.

Using endoscopic technique, a tailored mini-retrosigmoid craniotomy of about 1.5 × 1.5 cm is sufficient via a 3 cm skin incision behind the ipsilateral ear and parallel to the hairline (◘ Fig. 6.51) to approach the region of interest. Shaving is in most instances not necessary. For trigeminal neuralgia a superior retrosigmoidal, for hemifacial spasm and vestibular paroxysmia a central, and for glossopharyngeal neuralgia an inferior retrosigmoidal keyhole craniotomy should be used (◘ Fig. 6.52).

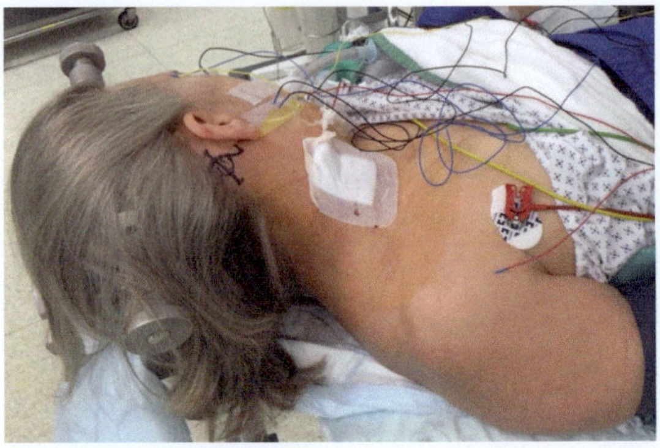

◘ Fig. 6.51 Patient with right-sided trigeminal neuralgia in supine positioning with the head turned approximately 70° to the contralateral side. The superior retrosigmoid keyhole craniotomy and skin incision within the hairline are marked on the patient's skin. Notice, that shaving of the hair was avoided and electrodes for multimodal neuromonitoring (AEP, EMG of facial and trigeminal nerve) were placed

The dura is opened toward the sigmoid sinus and generous CSF egress enabled by opening the cerebellopontine cistern. Using adequate positioning and a well-centered craniotomy, the entire procedure can be performed without any brain retractor. The intradural part of the procedure is performed using an «endoscope-controlled» dissection technique [75] and preferably a 4 mm endoscope with a 0° viewing angle. Even the 0° endoscope provides a panoramic view of the entire area, in particular, toward the brain stem and beyond the affected nerve. Endoscopes with a 30° or 45° viewing angle can be a useful adjunct. This is, in particular, true for hemifacial spasm, where the neurovascular conflict is frequently not in a straight trajectory to the craniotomy

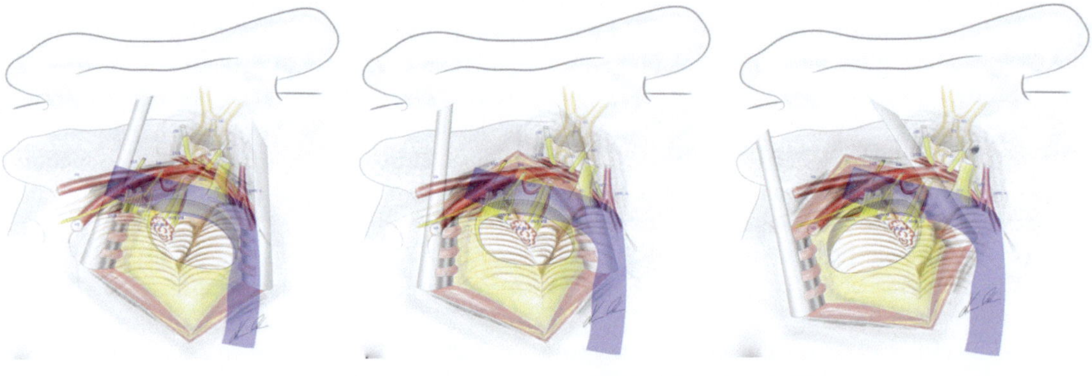

◘ Fig. 6.52 Schematic drawing of a superior (*left*), central (*middle*), and inferior (*right*) retrosigmoid keyhole craniotomy centered over the trigeminal, vestibulocochlear, and caudal cranial nerves, respectively

(◘ Fig. 6.53). Initially, the «one-hand technique» may be used for inspection and simple manipulations (◘ Fig. 6.54 left). However, bimanual endoscopic dissection technique is recommended for sharp or more complex dissection (◘ Fig. 6.54 middle and left, ◘ Fig. 6.55 left). This may be the case if a large vessel, like the vertebral artery or basilar artery (◘ Fig. 6.56), is the offending vessel, if small perforating arteries prevent adequate disposition, or if arachnoidal scaring is present as seen in recurrent cases, in patients having suffered from previous trauma or infection, and sometimes without an obvious reason.

Re-approximation of the offending vessel toward the affected nerve is prevented by interposing autologous or alloplastic material (◘ Fig. 6.53 middle and right, ◘ Fig. 6.54 middle and right) or fixation of the vessel in the disposed position with sutures or tissue adhesive. Soft Teflon pads are ideal because this material does not initiate significant scarring and provides long-term elasticity. The interposed material should be placed in a way that neither the affected nerve nor the offending vessel is compromised. Fixation of the Teflon with glue is an option (◘ Fig. 6.50 lower right) but in most instances not necessary.

Using a supine or park bench position, the subarachnoid space can be filled up with artificial CSF at the end of the procedure to prevent postoperative pneumocephalus. Meticulous sealing of the mastoid and watertight closure of the dura are important to prevent a CSF leak. Refixation of the

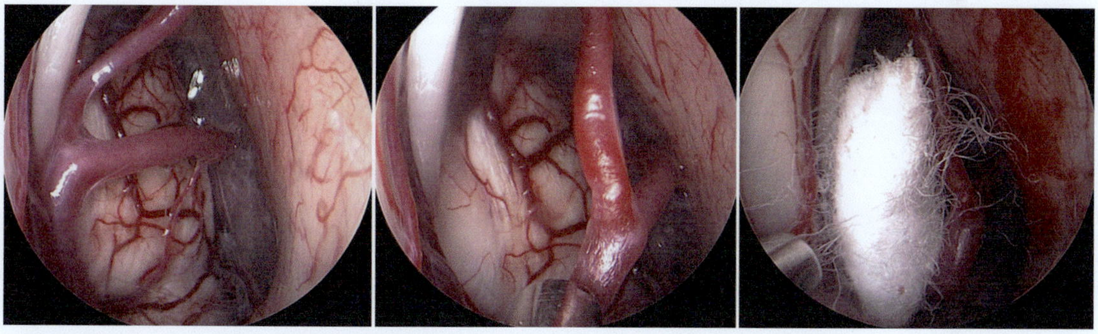

◘ Fig. 6.53 Intraoperative endoscopic images showing (*left*) a neurovascular conflict involving the right facial nerve, (*middle*) the situation after separation of the offending artery from the nerve, and (*left*) after positioning a Teflon pad to prevent readjustment of the vessel via a central retrosigmoid keyhole craniotomy in a patient with right-sided hemifacial spasm

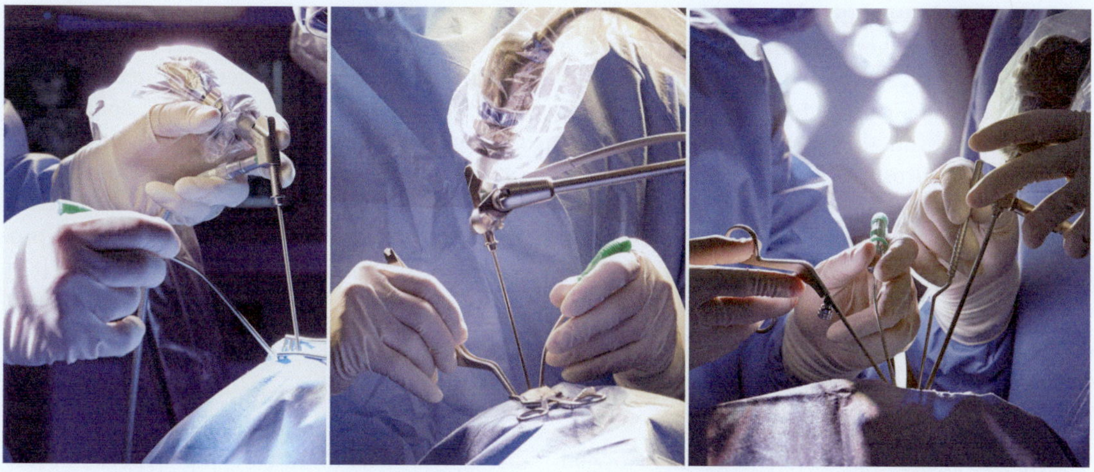

◘ Fig. 6.54 Endoscope-controlled microsurgical dissection techniques showing (*left*) the «one-hand technique» enabling high flexibility concerning inspection of the operation field but only limited to one-handed dissection. Sophisticated bimanual dissection is achieved for a single surgeon by (*middle*) fixation of the endoscope in the operating field or by (*right*) driving the endoscope by a second surgeon

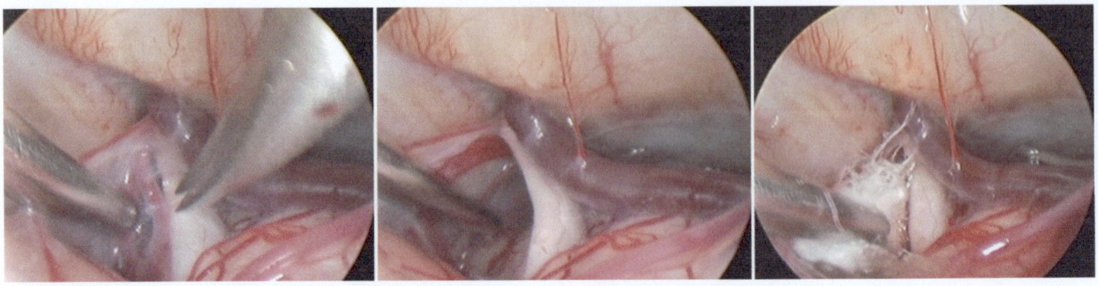

Fig. 6.55 Intraoperative images showing (*left*) endoscopic dissection of the offending superior cerebellar artery along the trigeminal nerve, (*middle*) displacing the vessels toward the tentorium, and (*right*) positioning of a Teflon pad to prevent readjustment of the vessels via a superior retrosigmoid keyhole craniotomy in a patient with right-sided trigeminal neuralgia

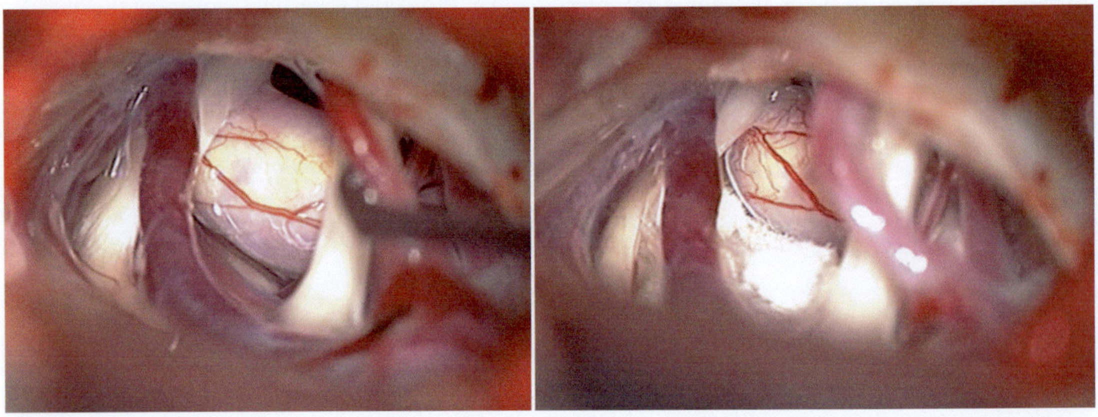

Fig. 6.56 Intraoperative image of a patient with right-sided trigeminal neuralgia caused by an elongated basilar artery (*left*) compressing the trigeminal nerve at its transition zone and (*right*) after separation and interposition of a Teflon pad close to the nerve entering the brain stem

bone flap can be achieved with miniplates or sutures. The skin is best closed with atraumatic sutures or tissue adhesive to enable washing of the hair as soon as 24 h after surgery. Duration of such an endoscopic procedure normally does not exceed 90 min from skin to skin in the hands of an experienced neurosurgeon.

Postoperatively, most patients with trigeminal neuralgia experience an immediate and complete pain relief and generally no new neurological deficits. Thus, prior medical treatment can be terminated at once. In hemifacial spasm, symptoms may fade gradually. Initial management of all patients in an intensive care or intermediate care unit is recommended.

The use of endoscopes, in particular, of angled endoscopes, provides a view far beyond the straight trajectory provided by the operating microscope and therefore leads to a higher detection rate of all offending vessels and consecutively to a better outcome [85].

The success rate of endoscopic MVD for patients with primary trigeminal neuralgia was reported to be as high as 99% of complete or significant pain relief over a follow-up period of 29 months. The overall complication rate was 10.5% (dysesthesia 7.9%, hypacusis 1.7%, wound infection 0.9%) in a series of 113 endoscopic procedures [85]. Others report of similar results [81].

Percutaneous Surgical Procedures at the Gasserian Ganglion

For percutaneous procedures, the Gasserian ganglion is approached by a percutaneous route through the oval foramen using a special needle. This is either done in a freehand technique or guided by fluoroscopy, computed tomography imaging, or stereotactically using frame-based or frame-less technique. Controlled partial destruction is done after prior testing of the correct location of the probe and achieved by thermal, chemical, or mechanical means using a coagulation probe achieving a temperature up to 70 °C, installation of chemicals such as glycerine or pure alcohol, or compressing the ganglion with a balloon catheter.

The procedure is generally performed in local anesthesia or short-lasting total intravenous anesthesia and terminated, when the patient experiences relevant pain relief or numbness of the affected branches. It is of utmost importance in this destructive-ablative procedure to spare the first branch and thus to prevent corneal anesthesia which is associated with a high risk of gradual blindness caused by repetitive injuries of the cornea.

The percutaneous procedures are thought to be less invasive and less risky for the patient compared to MVD. However, if not performed in a freehand technique, which carries higher risks than the guided techniques, it is not so different in terms of operating time and stress for the patients compared to MVD.

The initial success rate of the percutaneous procedures for patients with typical trigeminal neuralgia can be up to 80% with complete or significant pain relief. The complication rate is high with 50% permanent and sometimes very disturbing sensory deficits or paresthesia. Fortunately, anesthesia dolorosa occurs only in 1.5–2% following these procedures [82].

References

Surgery of Complex and Difficult Aneurysms with Skull Base Approaches and Microsurgical Flow Diversion

1. Albayram S, Selcuk H, Kara B, Bozdag E, Uzma O, Kocer N, et al. Thromboembolic events associated with balloon-assisted coil embolization: evaluation with diffusion-weighted MR imaging. AJNR Am J Neuroradiol. 2004;25(10):1768–77.
2. Biondi A, Jean B, Vivas E, Le Jean L, Boch AL, Chiras J, et al. Giant and large peripheral cerebral aneurysms: etiopathologic considerations, endovascular treatment, and long-term follow-up. AJNR Am J Neuroradiol. 2006;27(8):1685–92.
3. Bouthillier A, van Loveren HR, Keller JT. Segments of the internal carotid artery: a new classification. Neurosurgery. 1996;38(3):425–32; discussion 432–423.
4. Cebral JR, Mut F, Raschi M, Scrivano E, Ceratto R, Lylyk P, et al. Aneurysm rupture following treatment with flow-diverting stents: computational hemodynamics analysis of treatment. AJNR Am J Neuroradiol. 2011;32(1):27–33. https://doi.org/10.3174/ajnr.A2398.
5. Choi IS, David C. Giant intracranial aneurysms: development, clinical presentation and treatment. Eur J Radiol. 2003;46(3):178–94.
6. Chow M, McDougall C, O'Kelly C, Ashforth R, Johnson E, Fiorella D. Delayed spontaneous rupture of a posterior inferior cerebellar artery aneurysm following treatment with flow diversion: a clinicopathologic study. AJNR Am J Neuroradiol. 2012;33(4):E46–51. https://doi.org/10.3174/ajnr.A2532.
7. Cruz JP, Chow M, O'Kelly C, Marotta B, Spears J, Montanera W, et al. Delayed ipsilateral parenchymal hemorrhage following flow diversion for the treatment of anterior circulation aneurysms. AJNR Am J Neuroradiol. 2012;33(4):603–8. https://doi.org/10.3174/ajnr.A3065.
8. Darsaut TE, Rayner-Hartley E, Makoyeva A, Salazkin I, Berthelet F, Raymond J. Aneurysm rupture after endovascular flow diversion: the possible role of persistent flows through the transition zone associated with device deformation. Interv Neuroradiol. 2013;19(2):180–5.
9. Derdeyn CP, Cross DT 3rd, Moran CJ, Brown GW, Pilgram TK, Diringer MN, et al. Postprocedure ischemic events after treatment of intracranial aneurysms with Guglielmi detachable coils. J Neurosurg. 2002;96(5):837–43. https://doi.org/10.3171/jns.2002.96.5.0837.
10. Dolenc V. Direct microsurgical repair of intracavernous vascular lesions. J Neurosurg. 1983;58(6):824–31. https://doi.org/10.3171/jns.1983.58.6.0824.
11. Dolenc VV. A combined epi- and subdural direct approach to carotid-ophthalmic artery aneurysms. J Neurosurg. 1985;62(5):667–72. https://doi.org/10.3171/jns.1985.62.5.0667.
12. Fiorella D, Hsu D, Woo HH, Tarr RW, Nelson PK. Very late thrombosis of a pipeline embolization device construct: case report. Neurosurgery. 2010;67(3 Suppl Operative):onsE313–314; discussion onsE314. https://doi.org/10.1227/01.NEU.0000383875.08681.23.
13. Fischer E. Die Lageabweichungen der vorderen himarterie im gefassbild. Zentralbl Neurochir. 1938;(3):300–13.
14. Fukushima T. Direct surgery of the cavernous sinus lesions: summary of 27 cases. The 6th Mt Fuji Workshop on CVD Proceedings vol 6. 1988. p. 169–79.
15. Hampton T, Walsh D, Tolias C, Fiorella D. Mural destabilization after aneurysm treatment with a flow-diverting device: a report of two cases. J Neurointerv Surg. 2011;3(2):167–71. https://doi.org/10.1136/jnis.2010.002873.
16. Hanel RA, Spetzler RF. Surgical treatment of complex intracranial aneurysms. Neurosurgery. 2008;62(6 Suppl 3):1289–1297.; discussion 1297-1289. https://doi.org/10.1227/01.neu.0000333794.13844.d9.
17. Inamasu J, Suga S, Sato S, Onozuka S, Kawase T. Long-term outcome of 17 cases of large-giant posterior fossa aneurysm. Clin Neurol Neurosurg. 2000;102(2):65–71.
18. Juvela S, Porras M, Poussa K. Natural history of unruptured intracranial aneurysms: probability of and risk factors for aneurysm rupture. J Neurosurg. 2000;93(3):379–87. https://doi.org/10.3171/jns.2000.93.3.0379.

19. Juvela S, Poussa K, Porras M. Factors affecting formation and growth of intracranial aneurysms: a long-term follow-up study. Stroke. 2001;32(2):485–91.
20. Kan P, Siddiqui AH, Veznedaroglu E, Liebman KM, Binning MJ, Dumont TM, et al. Early postmarket results after treatment of intracranial aneurysms with the pipeline embolization device: a U.S. multicenter experience. Neurosurgery. 2012;71(6):1080–7; discussion 1087–1088. https://doi.org/10.1227/NEU.0b013e31827060d9.
21. Kassell NF, Torner JC. Size of intracranial aneurysms. Neurosurgery. 1983;12(3):291–7.
22. Khurana VG, Piepgras DG, Whisnant JP. Ruptured giant intracranial aneurysms. Part I. A study of rebleeding. J Neurosurg. 1998;88(3):425–9. https://doi.org/10.3171/jns.1998.88.3.0425.
23. Kim SJ, Choi IS. Midterm outcome of partially thrombosed intracranial aneurysms treated with guglielmi detachable coils. Interv Neuroradiol. 2000;6(1):13–25.
24. Kulcsar Z, Houdart E, Bonafe A, Parker G, Millar J, Goddard AJ, et al. Intra-aneurysmal thrombosis as a possible cause of delayed aneurysm rupture after flow-diversion treatment. AJNR Am J Neuroradiol. 2011;32(1):20–5. https://doi.org/10.3174/ajnr.A2370.
25. Kyoshima K, Shibuya M, Kobayashi S. Surgical Management of Paraclinoid Aneurysm. In: Schmidek HH, Roberts DW, editors. Schmidek & Sweet operative neurosurgical techniques : indications, methods, and results. 5th ed. Philadelphia, PA: Saunders Elsevier; 2006.
26. Lanzino G. Cerebral aneurysm treatment trends. J Neurosurg. 2008a;108(6):1162. https://doi.org/10.3171/JNS/2008/108/6/1162.
27. Lanzino G. Inflammation after embolization of intracranial aneurysms. J Neurosurg. 2008b;108(6):1071–3. https://doi.org/10.3171/JNS/2008/108/6/1071.
28. Lawton MT, Spetzler RF. Surgical management of giant intracranial aneurysms: experience with 171 patients. Clin Neurosurg. 1995;42:245–66.
29. Lemole GJ, Henn JS, Spetzler RF, Rina HA. Surgical management of giant aneurysms. Oper Tech Neurosurg. 2000;3(4):239–54.
30. McAuliffe W, Wycoco V, Rice H, Phatouros C, Singh TJ, Wenderoth J. Immediate and midterm results following treatment of unruptured intracranial aneurysms with the pipeline embolization device. AJNR Am J Neuroradiol. 2012;33(1):164–70. https://doi.org/10.3174/ajnr.A2727.
31. Meyers PM, Lavine SD, Fitzsimmons BF, Commichau C, Parra A, Mayer SA, et al. Chemical meningitis after cerebral aneurysm treatment using two second-generation aneurysm coils: report of two cases. Neurosurgery. 2004;55(5):1222.
32. Miyazaki S, Fukushima T, Fujimaki T. Resection of high-cervical paraganglioma with cervical-to-petrous internal carotid artery saphenous vein bypass. Report of two cases. J Neurosurg. 1990;73(1):141–6. https://doi.org/10.3171/jns.1990.73.1.0141.
33. Morita A, Kirino T, Hashi K, Aoki N, Fukuhara S, et al. The natural course of unruptured cerebral aneurysms in a Japanese cohort. N Engl J Med. 2012;366(26):2474–82. https://doi.org/10.1056/NEJMoa1113260.
34. Morley TP, Barr HW. Giant intracranial aneurysms: diagnosis, course, and management. Clin Neurosurg. 1969;16:73–94.
35. Peerless S. Giant intracranial aneurysms. In: Youmans JR, editor. Neurological surgery : a comprehensive reference guide to the diagnosis and management of neurosurgical problems. 3rd ed. Philadelphia: Saunders; 1990.
36. Roc Chen P. Management of unruptured cerebral aneurysms. In: Schmidek HH, Roberts DW, editors. Schmidek & Sweet operative neurosurgical techniques : indications, methods, and results. 5th ed. Philadelphia, PA: Saunders Elsevier; 2006. p. 1087–98.
37. Soeda A, Sakai N, Murao K, Sakai H, Ihara K, Yamada N, et al. Thromboembolic events associated with Guglielmi detachable coil embolization with use of diffusion-weighted MR imaging. Part II. Detection of the microemboli proximal to cerebral aneurysm. AJNR Am J Neuroradiol. 2003;24(10):2035–8.
38. Solomon RA, Fukushima T. New aneurysm clip appliers for "key-hole" neurosurgery. Neurosurgery. 1991; 28(3):474–6.
39. Spetzler RF, Fukushima T, Martin N, Zabramski JM. Petrous carotid-to-intradural carotid saphenous vein graft for intracavernous giant aneurysm, tumor, and occlusive cerebrovascular disease. J Neurosurg. 1990;73(4):496–501. https://doi.org/10.3171/jns.1990.73.4.0496.
40. Tumialan LM, Zhang YJ, Cawley CM, Dion JE, Tong FC, Barrow DL. Intracranial hemorrhage associated with stent-assisted coil embolization of cerebral aneurysms: a cautionary report. J Neurosurg. 2008;108(6):1122–9. https://doi.org/10.3171/JNS/2008/108/6/1122.
41. Turowski B, Macht S, Kulcsar Z, Hanggi D, Stummer W. Early fatal hemorrhage after endovascular cerebral aneurysm treatment with a flow diverter (SILK-Stent): do we need to rethink our concepts? Neuroradiology. 2011;53(1):37–41. https://doi.org/10.1007/s00234-010-0676-7.
42. van Rooij WJ, Sluzewski M. Endovascular treatment of large and giant aneurysms. AJNR Am J Neuroradiol. 2009;30(1):12–8. https://doi.org/10.3174/ajnr.A1267.
43. Velat GJ, Fargen KM, Lawson MF, Hoh BL, Fiorella D, Mocco J. Delayed intraparenchymal hemorrhage following pipeline embolization device treatment for a giant recanalized ophthalmic aneurysm. J Neurointerv Surg. 2012;4(5):e24. https://doi.org/10.1136/neurintsurg-2011-010129.
44. Wiebers DO, Whisnant JP, Huston J 3rd, Meissner I, Brown RD Jr, Piepgras DG, et al. Unruptured intracranial aneurysms: natural history, clinical outcome, and risks of surgical and endovascular treatment. Lancet. 2003;362(9378):103–10.
45. Zomorodi A, Fukushima T. Two surgeons four-hand microneurosurgery with universal holder system: technical note. Neurosurgical Review. 28 Feb 2017.

Dural Arteriovenous Fistulas

46. Ambekar S, Gaynor BG, Peterson EC, Elhammady MS. Long-term angiographic results of endovascularly "cured" intracranial dural arteriovenous fistulas. J Neurosurg. 2015:1–5.

47. Barrow DL, Spector RH, Braun IF, Landman JA, Tindall SC, Tindall GT. Classification and treatment of spontaneous carotid-cavernous sinus fistulas. J Neurosurg. 1985;62:248–56.
48. Borden JA, Wu JK, Shucart WA. A proposed classification for spinal and cranial dural arteriovenous fistulous malformations and implications for treatment. J Neurosurg. 1995;82(2):166–79.
49. Cannizzaro D, Brinjikji W, Rammos S, Murad MH, Lanzino G. Changing clinical and therapeutic trends in tentorial dural arteriovenous fistulas: a systematic review. AJNR Am J Neuroradiol. 2015;36:1905–11.
50. Cognard C, Gobin YP, Pierot L, Bailly AL, Houdart E, Casasco A, Chiras J, Merland JJ. Cerebral dural arteriovenous fistulas: clinical and angiographic correlation with a revised classification of venous drainage. Radiology. 1995;194:671–80.
51. Cognard C, Januel AC, Silva NA, Tall P. Endovascular treatment of intracranial dural arteriovenous fistulas with cortical venous drainage: new management using onyx. AJNR. 2008;289(2):235–41.
52. Duffau H, Lopes M, Janosevic V, et al. Early rebleeding from intracranial dural arteriovenous fistulas: report of 20 cases and review of the literature. J Neurosurg. 1999;90:78–84.
53. Hu YC, Newman CB, Dashti SR, Albuquerque FC, McDougall CG. Cranial dural arteriovenous fistula: transarterial Onyx embolization experience and technical nuances. J Neurointerv Surg. 2011;3:5–13.
54. Kim B, Jeon P, Kim K, Kim S, Kim H, Byun HS, Jo KI. Predictive factors for response of intracranial dural arteriovenous fistulas to transarterial Onyx embolization: angiographic subgroup analysis of treatment outcomes. World neurosurgery. 2015.
55. Lin TC, Chung HK, Hsu JN. Spontaneous bilateral dural arteriovenous fistulas with pulsatile tinnitus. Ear Nose Throat J. 2015;94:E10–3.
56. Oh JS, Yoon SM, Oh HJ, Shim JJ, Bae HG, Lee KS. Endovascular treatment of dural arteriovenous fistulas: single center experience. J Korean Neurosurg Soc. 2016;59(1):17–25.
57. Pero G, Quilici L, Piano M, Valvassori L, Boccardi E. Onyx embolization of dural arteriovenous fistulas of the cavernous sinus through the superior pharyngeal branch of the ascending pharyngeal artery. J Neurointerv Surg. 2015;7:e16.
58. Robert T, Blanc R, Smajda S, Ciccio G, Redjem H, Bartolini B, Fahed R, Piotin M. Endovascular treatment of cribriform plate dural arteriovenous fistulas: technical difficulties and complications avoidance. J Neurointerv Surg. 2015.
59. Signorelli F, Della Pepa GM, Sabatino G, Marchese E, Maira G, Puca A, Albanese A. Diagnosis and management of dural arteriovenous fistulas: a 10 years single-center experience. Clin Neurol Neurosurg. 2015a;128:123–9.
60. Signorelli F, Gory B, Maduri R, Guyotat J, Pelissou-Guyotat I, Chirchiglia D, Riva R, Turjman F. Intracranial dural arteriovenous fistulas: a review of current management based on emerging knowledge. J Neurosurg Sci. 2015b.
61. Thomas AJ, Ogilvy CS. Treatment of dural arteriovenous fistulas with cortical venous reflux-endovascular therapy and surgery preferred modality of treatment. World Neurosurg. 2015;83:1053–4.
62. van Dijk JM, ter Brugge KG, Willinsky RA, et al. Clinical course of cranial dural arteriovenous fistulas with long-term persistent cortical reflux. Stroke. 2002;33:1233–6.
63. Waragai M, Takeuchi H, Fukushima T, Haisa T, Yonemitsu T. MRI and SPECT studies of dural arteriovenous fistulas presenting as pure progressive dementia with leukoencephalopathy: a cause of treatable dementia. Eur J Neurol. 2006;13:754–9.
64. Zhao J, Xu F, Ren J, Manjila S, Bambakidis NC. Dural arteriovenous fistulas at the craniocervical junction: a systematic review. J Neurointerv Surg. 2015

Neurovascular Compression Syndromes

65. Best C, Gawehn J, Krämer HH, Thömke F, Ibis T, Müller-Forell W, Dieterich M. MRI and neurophysiology in vestibular paroxysmia: contradiction and correlation. J Neurol Neurosurg Psychiatry. 2013;84:1349–56.
66. Brandt T, Strupp M, Dieterich M. Vestibular paroxysmia: a treatable neurovascular cross-compression syndrome. J Neurol. 2016;263:90–6.
67. Dandy WE. Concerning the cause of trigeminal neuralgia. Am J Surg. 1934;24:447–55.
68. DGN. 2005. Leitlinie Trigeminusneuralgie. www.dgn.org/138.0.html.
69. Ferroli P, Fioravanti A, Schiariti M, Tringali G, Franzini A, Calbucci F, Broggi G. Microvascular decompression for glossopharyngeal neuralgia: a long-term retrospective review of the Milan-Bologna experience in 31 consecutive cases. Acta Neurochir. 2009;151(10):1245–50.
70. Gardner WJ, Miklos MV. Response of trigeminal neuralgia to decompression of sensory root: discussion of cause of trigeminal neuralgia. J Am Med Assoc. 1959;170:1773–6.
71. Gaul C, Hastreiter P, Duncker A, Naraghi R. Diagnosis and neurosurgical treatment of glossopharyngeal neuralgia: clinical findings and 3-D visualization of neurovascular compression in 19 consecutive patients. J Headache Pain. 2011;12(5):527–34.
72. Guclu B, Sindou M, Meyronet D, Streichenberger N, Simon E, Mertens P. Cranial nerve vascular compression syndromes of the trigeminal, facial and vago-glossopharyngeal nerves: comparative anatomical study of the central myelin portion and transitional zone—correlations with incidences of corresponding hyperactive dysfunctional syndromes. Acta Neurochir. 2011;153:2365–75.
73. Haller S, Etienne L, Kövari E, Varoquaux AD, Urbach H, Becker M. Imaging of neurovascular compression syndromes: Trigeminal Neuralgia, Hemifacial Spasm, Vestibular Paroxysmia, and Glossopharyngeal Neuralgia. Am J Neuroradiol. 2016.
74. Hopf HC, Kömpf D. Erkrankungen der Hirnnerven. Stuttgart-New York: Georg Thieme Verlag; 2006.
75. Hopf NJ, Perneczky A. Endoscopic neurosurgery and endoscope-assisted microneurosurgery for the treatment of intracranial cysts. Neurosurgery. 1998;43:1330–7.

76. Jannetta PJ. Arterial compression of the trigeminal nerve at the pons in patients with trigeminal neuralgia. J Neurosurg. 1967;26(suppl):159–62.
77. Katusic S, Beard CM, Bergstralh E, Kurland LT. Incidence and clinical features of trigeminal neuralgia, Rochester, Minnesota 1945–1984. Ann Neurol. 1990;27:89–95.
78. Lovely T, Jannetta P. Microvascular decompression for trigeminal neuralgia. Neurosurg Clin N Am. 1997;8:11–29.
79. Musahl C, Weissbach C, Hopf NJ. Neuromonitoring. In: Spetzler, Kalani, Nakaji, editors. Neurovascular surgery. 2nd ed. Stuttgart/New York: Thieme; 2015.
80. Pollock BE, Phuong LK, Gorman DA, Foote RL, Stafford SL. Stereotactic radiosurgery for idiopathic trigeminal neuralgia. J Neurosurg. 2002;97:347–53.
81. Reisch R, Stadie A, Kockro RA, Hopf N. The keyhole concept in neurosurgery. World Neurosurg. 2012;34:34–7.
82. Reisch R, Köchlin N. Trigeminusneuralgie und andere kraniale Neuralgien. In: Agosti, Diener, Limmroth, editors. Migräne & Kopfschmerzen. Basel: Karger; 2015.
83. Rosenstengel C, Matthes M, Baldauf J, Fleck S, Schroeder H. Hemifacial spasm: conservative and surgical treatment options. Dtsch Arztebl Int. 2012;109(41):667–73.
84. Sindou M, Leston J, Howeidy T, Decullier E, Chapuis F. Micro-vascular decompression for primary trigeminal neuralgia (typical or atypical). Long-term effectiveness on pain; prospective study with survival analysis in a consecutive series of 362 patients. Acta Neurochir. 2006;148:1235–45.
85. Teo C, Nakaji P, Mobbs RJ. Endoscope-assisted microvascular decompression for trigeminal neuralgia: technical case report. Neurosurg. 2006;59 (ONS Suppl 4):ONS?

Congenital Disorders of the Skull Base

Alexander König

Electronic Supplementary Material The online version of this chapter (https://doi.org/10.1007/978-3-319-64018-1_7) contains supplementary material, which is available to authorized users.

A. König, U. Spetzger (eds.), *Surgery of the Skull Base*,
https://doi.org/10.1007/978-3-319-64018-1_7

Chiari malformation, basilar impression and Rathke's cleft cysts are congenital disorders at the skull base that can become of therapeutical relevance if clinical symptoms occur. Surgery is the only treatment option in all cases. The indication for treatment is mainly focused on clinical complaints and the consecutive effect on the patient's quality of life. CT and MR imaging findings determine the kind of surgical procedure.

Editor's Comment

The chapter about congenital disorders of the skull base deals with the typical disorders at the craniocervical junction whereupon the classical decompressive surgical methods are described. Since some cases require stabilisation of the craniocervical junction as well, there has been a trend to posterior short-distance fusion in the last few years. Nowadays, these neuro-orthopaedic operations with posterior placement of screws are usually performed with intraoperative electrophysiological monitoring and navigation-guided in selected complex cases. In the future, there will be a further trend of percutaneous placement of screws. Like in the trauma surgery of the cervical spine, there is a trend to transpedicular screw placement instead of the transarticular C1/C2 fusion due to the improvement of instruments and screws and the better biomechanical stability.

7.1 Chiari Malformation

7.1.1 General Information

Chiari malformation represents a developmental disorder of the posterior skull base with a minimised posterior fossa and a consecutive displacement of the cerebellar tonsils through the foramen magnum and into the spinal canal. It was named after the Austrian pathologist Hans Chiari (1851–1916). Depending on the severity of displacement, an internal hydrocephalus can occur. A Chiari malformation can be a secondary phenomenon due to another underlying disease, e.g. Ehlers-Danlos syndrome, craniosynostosis or neurofibromatosis type I.

Chiari [1] defined in his original publication four types of the malformation that were further specified over the years [7]:

- Type I: most frequent appearance with displacement of the cerebellar tonsils into the cervical spinal canal (more than 5 mm below the McRae line) without displacement of the medulla oblongata, often associated with syringomyelia of the cervical or cervicothoracic spinal cord (◘ Fig. 7.1)
- Type II: displacement of the vermis into the cervical spinal canal, displacement of pons and medulla oblongata and elongation of the fourth ventricle, frequently combined with hydrocephalus and syringomyelia
- Type III: inferior displacement of the medulla oblongata and herniation of the cerebellum into a high cervical meningocele
- Type IV: hypoplasia or aplasia of the cerebellum and the tentorium cerebelli.

7.1.2 Clinical Signs and Symptoms

The most frequent type I is usually asymptomatic into adulthood. First, unspecific symptoms like headaches and neck pain occur. The headaches can be amplified by the Valsalva manoeuvre. In the further course of disease, several neurological deficits appear:

- Gait ataxia and coordination disturbances
- Tinnitus
- Nausea
- Nystagmus
- Dysphagia
- Facial pain
- Positive Lhermitte's sign
- Weakness of upper and lower limbs
- A feeling of numbness in the hands and feet
- Dyspnea
- Tachycardia
- Syncopes

7.1.3 Investigations

In the diagnosis of Chiari malformation, the first radiological sign in sagittal MR images is the inferior displacement of cerebellar tonsils through the foramen magnum. They can reach the lamina of the third cervical vertebra. The medulla oblon-

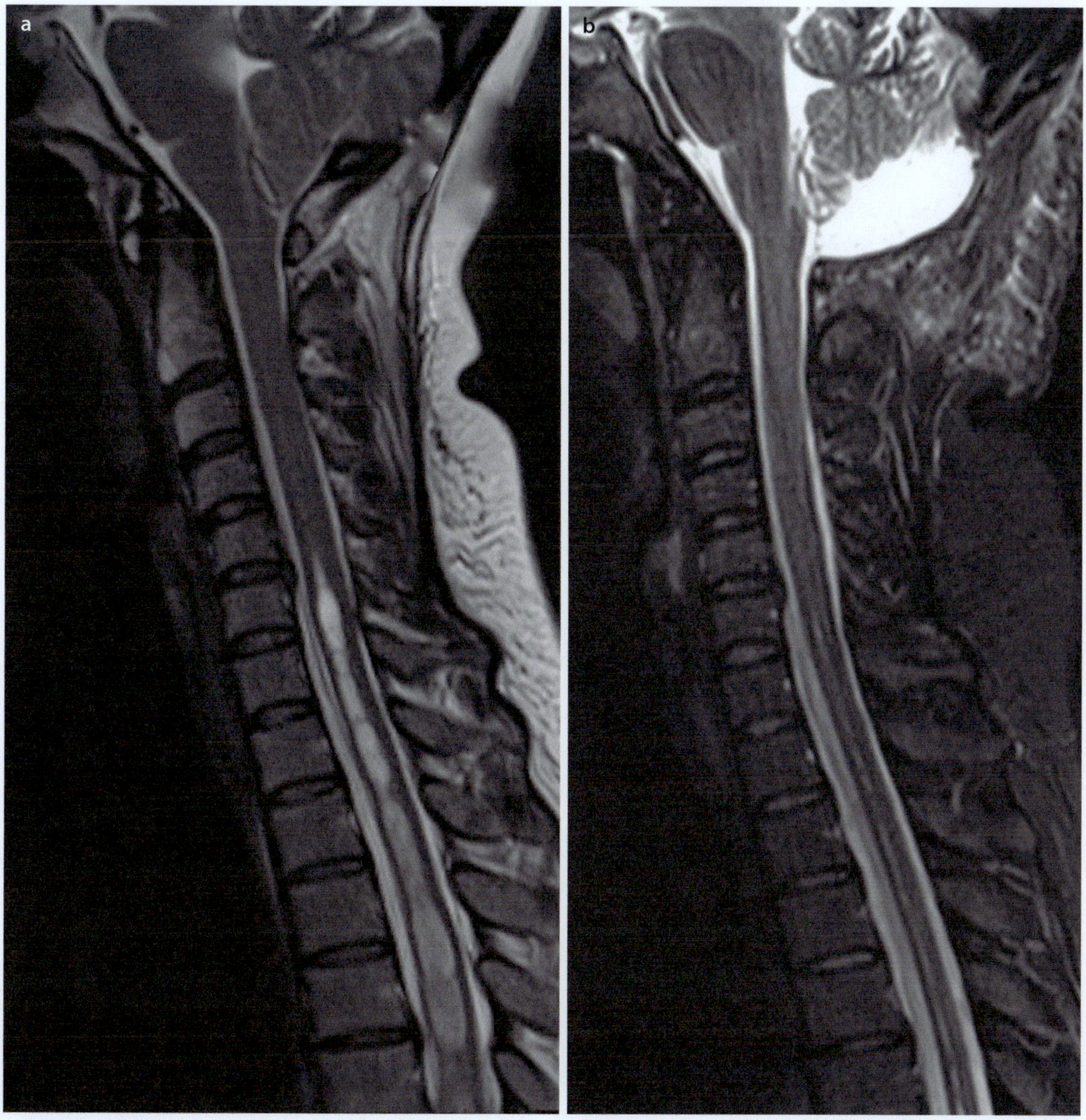

Fig. 7.1 Chiari malformation type I in a T2-weighted sagittal MR image with inferior displacement of the cerebellar tonsil down to the level between the foramen magnum and atlas as well as with a syringomyelia of the cervicothoracic spinal cord **a**. Situation 3 months after suboccipital craniectomy with decompression of the lower cerebellum and medulla oblongata and with remission of the syringomyelia; sagittal T2-weighted MR image **b**

gata, the fourth ventricle and the pons can be elongated and displaced caudally. A typical finding is a syringomyelia of the cervicothoracic spinal cord (Fig. 7.1).

In axial MR images, further dysmorphic features can be detected: a small posterior fossa, a narrowing of the cisterna magna and a displacement of cranial nerves. The cerebellar tonsils are merged with the dorsal and lateral medulla oblongata by meningeal adhesions. Further findings are spina bifida and hydrocephalus [4].

Funduscopy by an ophthalmologist can show papilledema as a sign of raised intracranial pressure in cases of hydrocephalus.

7.1.4 Therapeutical Options

In cases of symptomatic Chiari malformation, especially when neurological deficits occur and radiological signs are typical, surgical treatment should be indicated. Surgery includes suboccipital craniectomy with resection of the C1 lamina for bony decompression and an expansile duraplasty with a dural substitute or autologous tissue. Sometimes the laminae of C2 and C3 as well as the cerebellar tonsils have to be resected. The surgical technique of suboccipital decompression is described in detail in ▶ Sect. 7.1.5.

If symptomatic hydrocephalus occurs, then this has to be treated when persisting after the decompressive surgery. There are two options for the surgical treatment of hydrocephalus: a ventriculoperitoneal shunt or a third ventriculostomy.

7.1.5 Surgical Technique of the Suboccipital Decompressive Craniectomy

The patient is in a prone position, and the inclined head is fixed with a Mayfield clamp. By using a suboccipital midline approach, the suboccipital external table of the skull and the lamina of C1 are exposed (◘ Figs. 7.2, 7.3, 7.4, and 7.5). Only in cases of very deep cerebellar tonsils the laminae of further cervical vertebrae have to be exposed.

Over the posterior fossa, two paramedian and further caudally two lateral burr holes are placed (◘ Fig. 7.6). A curved dissector is used to separate the dural from the internal table of the skull via the burr holes (◘ Fig. 7.7). This has to be done consequently down to the foramen magnum to avoid an early rupture of the dura during craniotomy. The osteoclastic craniotomy (craniectomy) is done with a Kerrison punch or a craniotome starting from the burr holes (◘ Fig. 7.8). When crossing the midline with the craniotome, the surgeon must be aware of a potential occipital dural venous sinus. A rupture of this dural venous sinus has to be closed with sutures.

After elevating the bone flap, a laminectomy of C1 is mandatory (◘ Figs. 7.9 and 7.10). This is a precondition for an adequate dural enlargement and reconstruction. The incision of the dura starts at the C0/C1 level and goes downwards to the upper edge of the C2 lamina. The cranial part of the incision is led over both cerebellar hemispheres resulting in a Y-shaped dural opening

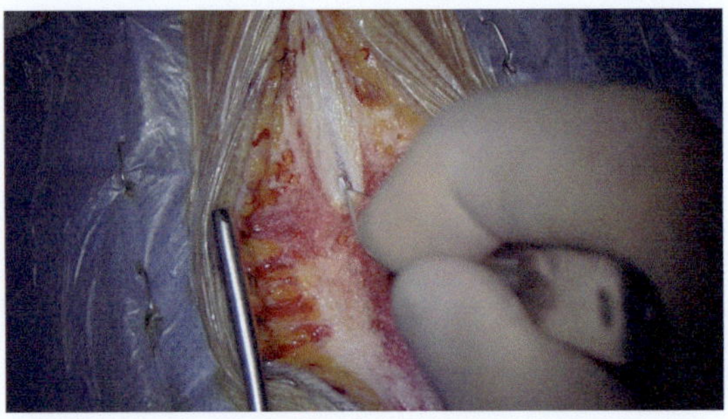

◘ **Fig. 7.2** Incision of the skin and fascia in the midline at the level of the craniocervical junction

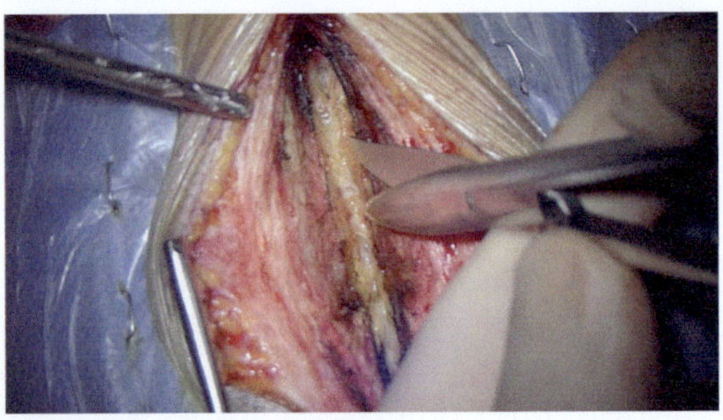

◘ **Fig. 7.3** Dissection of neck muscles in the midline to minimise blood loss and surgical trauma to the muscles

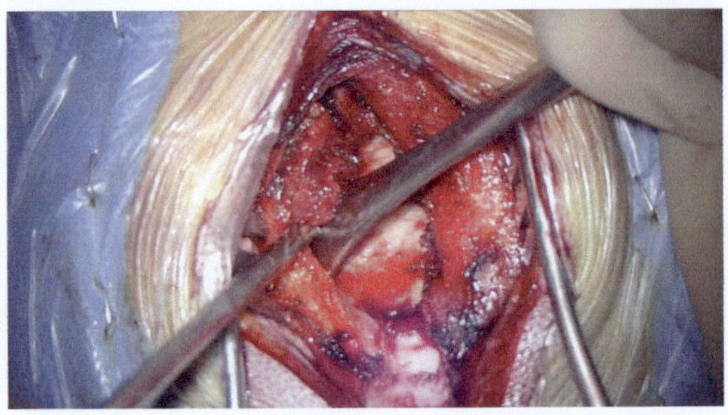

◘ **Fig. 7.4** Dissection of muscles from the suboccipital external table

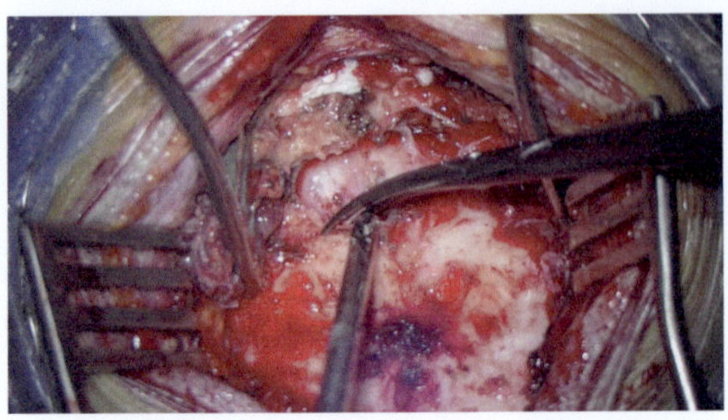

◘ **Fig. 7.5** Exposition and resection of the atlantooccipital membrane between posterior edge of the foramen magnum and lamina of the C1 vertebra

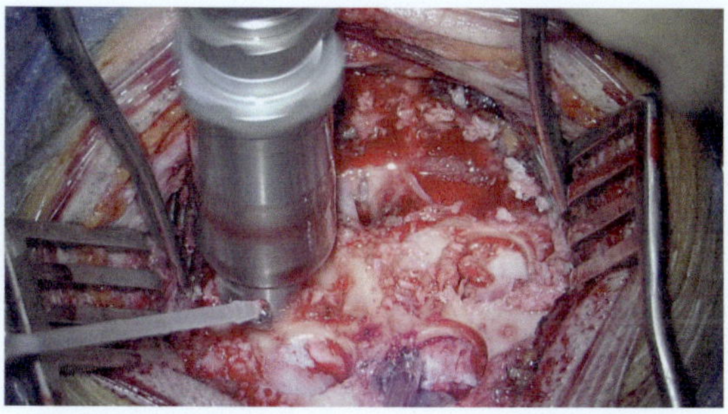

Fig. 7.6 Application of four burr holes over the posterior fossa

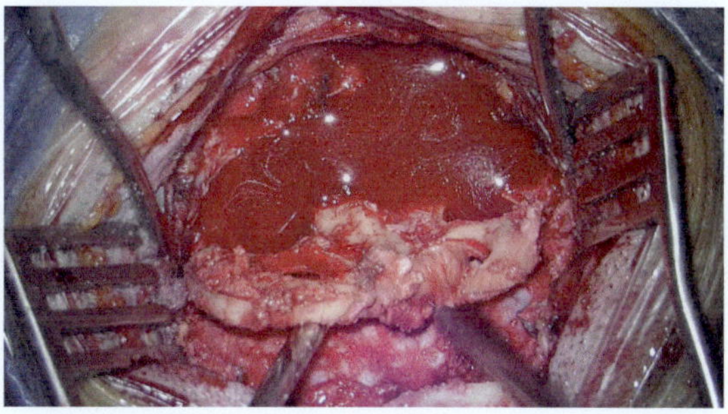

Fig. 7.9 Elevation of the bone flap

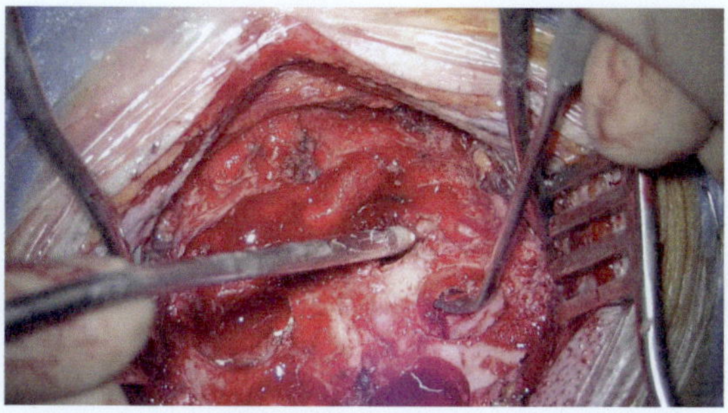

Fig. 7.7 Dissection of the dura away from the internal table of the posterior skull base with a curved dissector

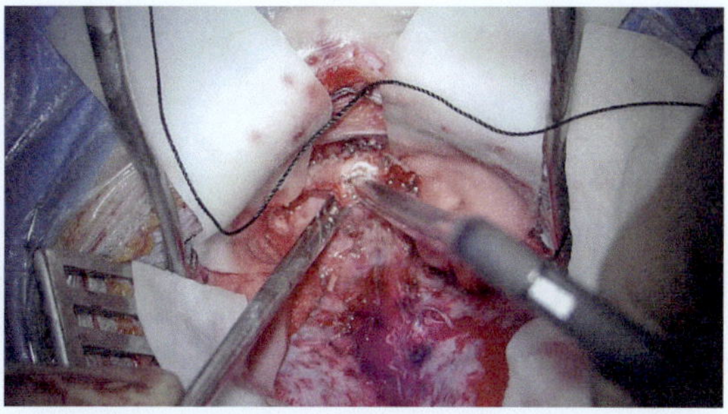

Fig. 7.10 Laminectomy of C1 with a Kerrison punch to achieve an adequate decompression that reaches far enough into the inferior direction

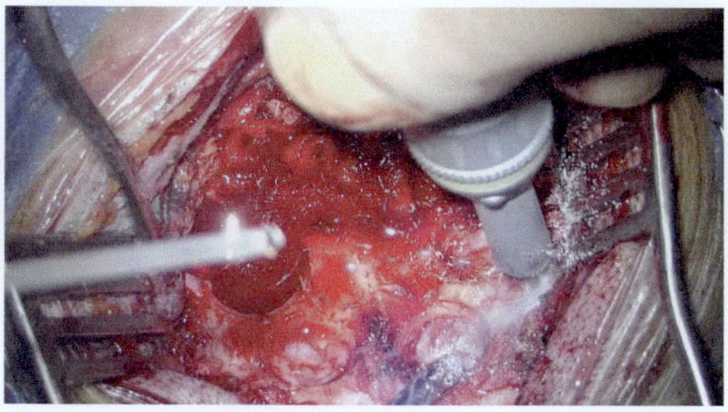

Fig. 7.8 Cutting out a suboccipital bone flap with the craniotome

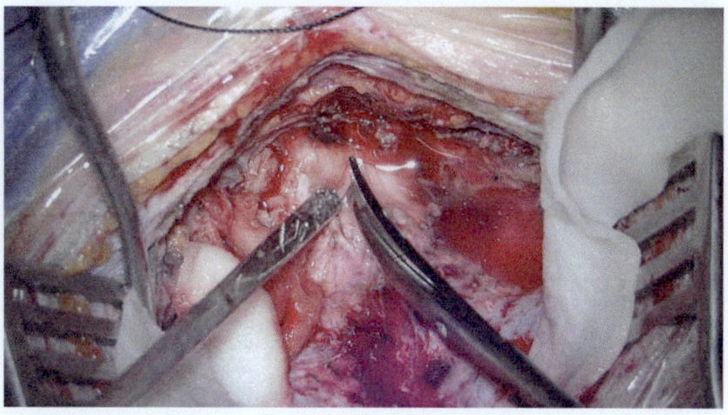

Fig. 7.11 Incision of the dura at the C0/C1 level in the midline

(Figs. 7.11 and 7.12). If this surgical step leads to an opening of a possible occipital venous sinus, the latter has to be closed with Vicryl 4-0 sutures (Johnson & Johnson Medical, Norderstedt, Germany). Further space for the cerebellar tonsils and the medulla oblongata can be gained by separating arachnoid adhesions (Figs. 7.13, 7.14, 7.15, and 7.16).

Afterwards, an expansile duraplasty is recommended. We use the dural substitute Tutopatch (Bess Medizintechnik GmbH, Berlin, Germany). After finishing the sutures, fibrin glue is applied for adequate watertight closure (Figs. 7.17, 7.18, and 7.19). The postoperative result is documented by MRI 3–6 months after surgery (Fig. 7.20).

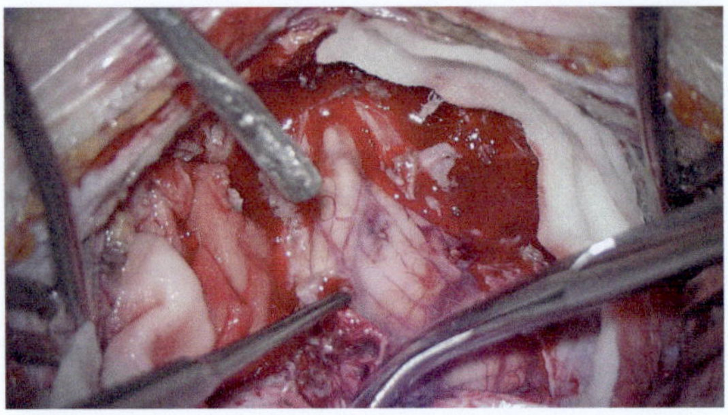

Fig. 7.12 Extension of the dura incision in the superior direction over the cerebellar hemispheres in a Y-shaped fashion

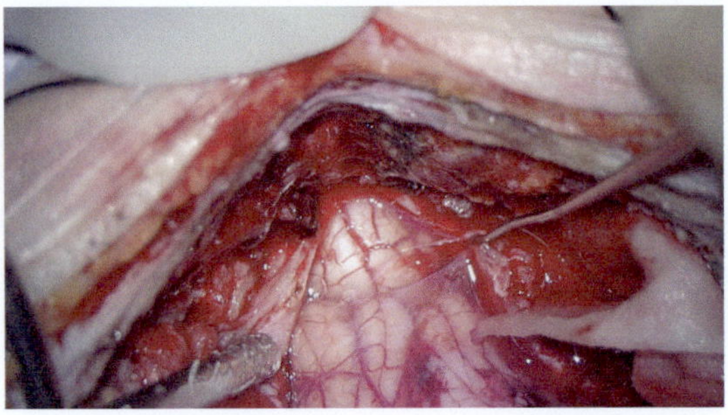

Fig. 7.13 Further gaining of space for the cerebellar tonsils by cutting the arachnoid at the level of the craniocervical junction

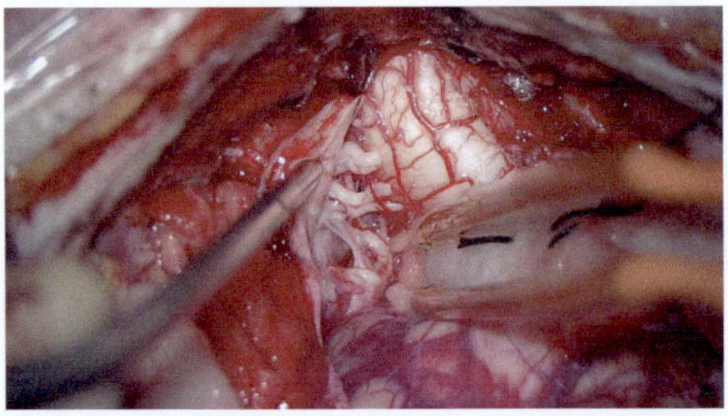

Fig. 7.14 Inspection of the lateral subarachnoid space with exposition of the spinal roof of the accessory nerve

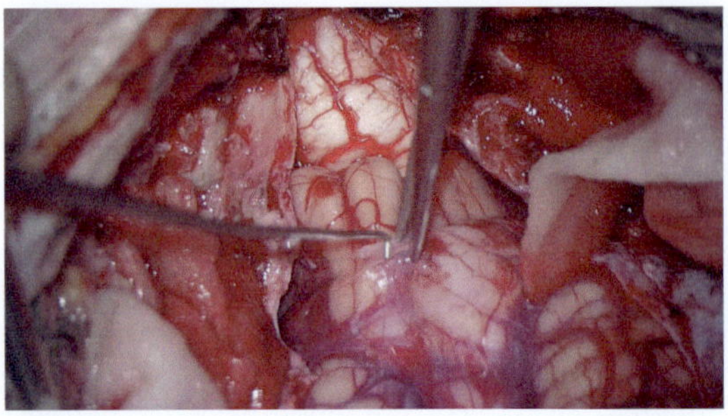

Fig. 7.15 Finishing of the arachnoid incision into the cranial direction

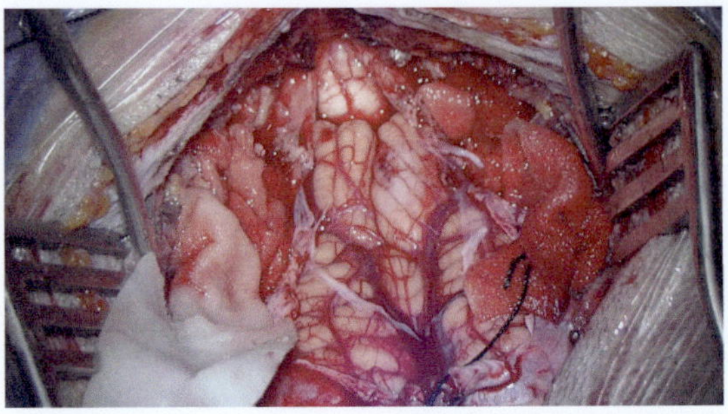

Fig. 7.16 Completed decompression of medulla oblongata, cerebellar tonsils and the lower aspect of the cerebellar hemispheres

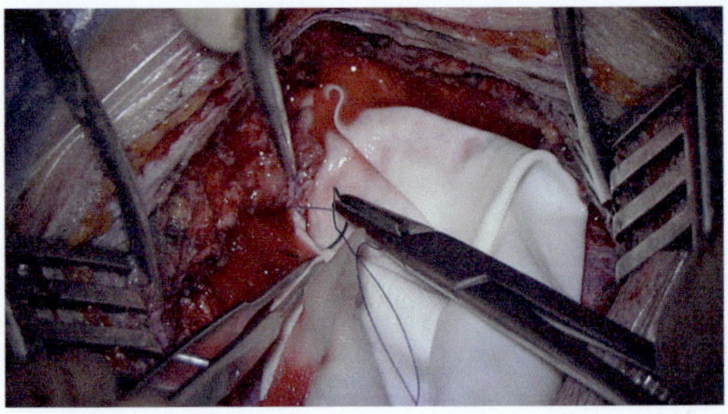

Fig. 7.17 Suturing of the expansile duraplasty with Tutopatch

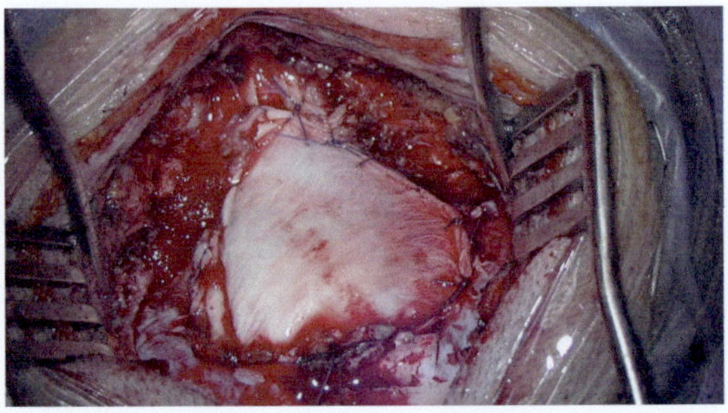

Fig. 7.18 Completed expansile duraplasty

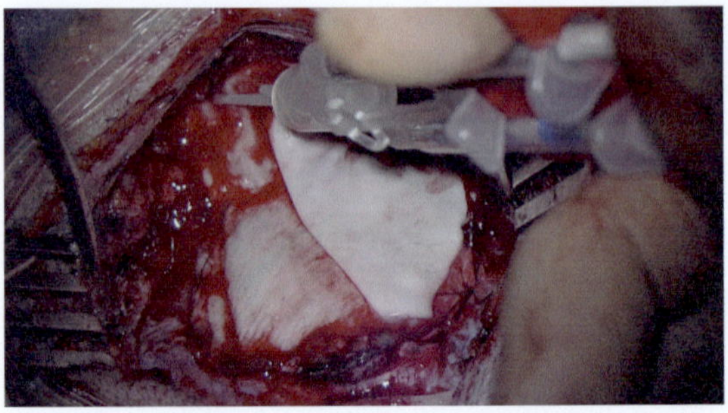

Fig. 7.19 Application of fibrin glue to achieve a watertight closure of the dura

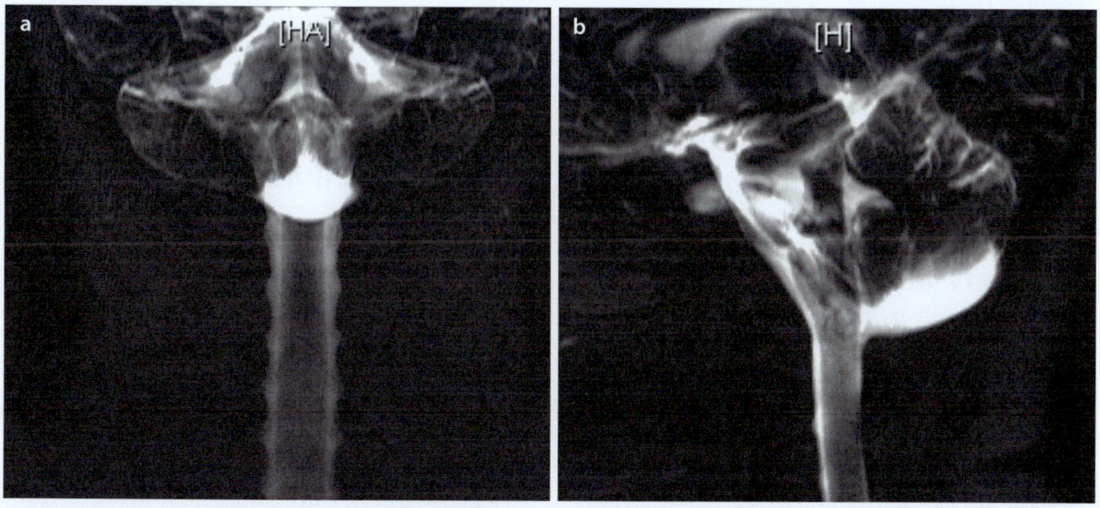

Fig. 7.20 Postoperative MRI after suboccipital decompression, laminectomy of C1 and expansile duraplasty. The achieved expansion of the craniocervical CSF space can be seen in coronal **a** and sagittal **b** RARE myelogram MRI scans

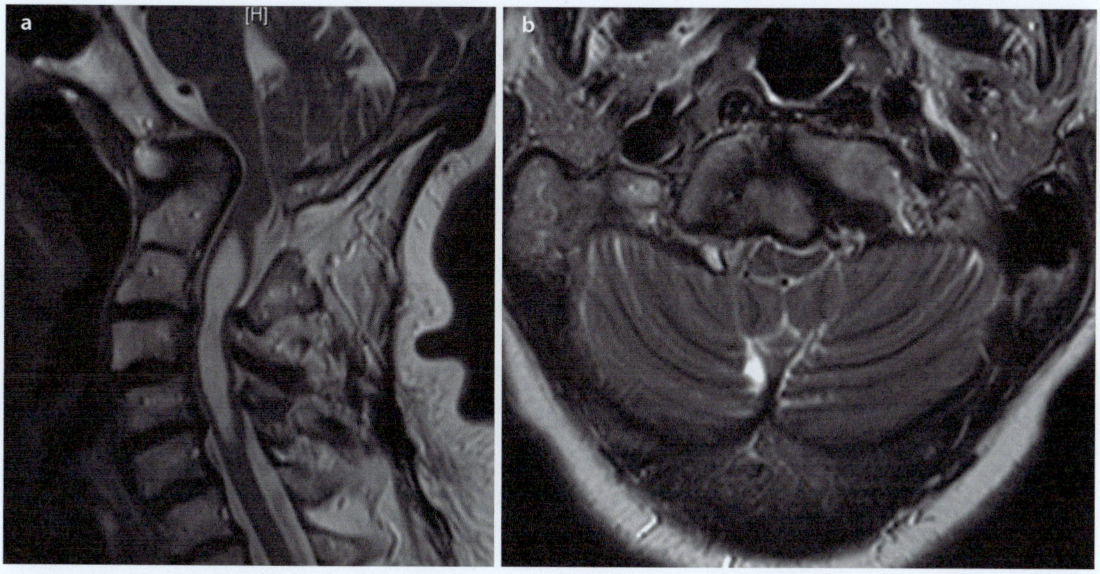

Fig. 7.21 Basilar impression with a cranial displacement of the dens axis, narrowing of the foramen magnum, kinking and compression of the medulla oblongata and an associated syringomyelia of the cervical spinal cord in a T2-weighted sagittal MR image **a**. Axial T2-weighted image just above the foramen magnum showing compression of the medulla oblongata **b**

7.2 Basilar Impression

7.2.1 General Information

Basilar impression or invagination is a condition where the tip of the dens axis extends into the foramen magnum with consecutive narrowing of the foramen and compression of the brainstem (Fig. 7.21). The origin is a flattening of the posterior skull base (platybasia) due to a congenital disorder or an underlying disease.

The Wolf-Hirschhorn syndrome is a genetic disorder often associated with basilar impression. This syndrome is due to a deletion of the short arm of chromosome 4 and causes complex cranial disorders with hypertelorism, microcephaly, coloboma and others. The Down syndrome can also be associated with basilar impression [6].

Hydrocephalus and syringomyelia can be secondary complications of basilar impression due to a chronic congestion of CSF. Especially, a syringomyelia is often observed since almost all patients with Chiari malformation show basilar impression, too. A study by Klekamp [3] investigated several disorders being associated with basilar impression and their frequency of appearance:
- Chiari I malformation, 94%
- Assimilation of the atlas, 46%
- Klippel-Feil syndrome, 30%
- Craniocervical instability, 54%

7.2.2 Clinical Signs and Symptoms

Clinical symptoms result from the compression of the inferior brainstem, the lower cranial nerves, the cerebellum and the upper cervical spinal cord. Most complaints can be aggravated by anterior flexion of the head:
- Headaches and neck pain
- Vertigo
- Dysarthria
- Dysphagia
- Weakness of neck muscles
- Orthostatic syncopes
- Sensory deficits of the limbs
- Tetraparesis
- Positive Lhermitte's sign
- Gait ataxia
- Coordination disorders
- Dissociated disorder of temperature perception of the trunk

7.2.3 Investigations

In the case of clinical signs of brainstem compression, MRI is the diagnostic of first choice. It shows the extension of the dens axis into the foramen magnum and the consecutive compression and kinking of the medulla oblongata (◘ Fig. 7.21).

For the planning of surgical strategy (also compare with ► Sect. 7.2.4), a lateral functional X-ray study of the cervical spine is mandatory to detect or exclude spinal instability at the craniocervical junction. In the case of instability, a lateral X-ray image in neutral position is helpful during stabilisation surgery to estimate the correct position of the head [3].

7.2.4 Therapeutical Options

Basilar impression with neurological deficits has to be treated surgically. Depending on the amount of anterior compression of the medulla oblongata and a potential craniocervical instability, the surgeon has to choose between different surgical procedures [2, 3]:
- In cases without anterior compression of the medulla oblongata and without craniocervical instability, a decompression of the foramen magnum is indicated.
- In cases of moderate anterior compression of the medulla oblongata and proof of craniocervical instability, the decompression of the foramen magnum has to be combined with craniocervical stabilisation.
- In cases of heavy anterior compression of the medulla oblongata with deficits of lower cranial nerves, a transoral resection of the dens has to be combined with posterior decompression of the foramen magnum and craniocervical stabilisation.

The decompression of the foramen magnum is done by a median suboccipital craniectomy and laminectomy of C1 combined with an expansile duraplasty. The surgical technique is described in detail in ► Sect. 7.1.5. Some surgeons reduce the medial cerebellar tonsils in volume by bipolar coagulation or resect the tonsils and inspect Magendie's foramen to exclude an obstruction. These procedures should only be performed in selected cases with massive space-occupying cerebellar tonsils and/or hydrocephalus to avoid unnecessary surgical morbidity.

In cases of craniocervical instability, an occipitocervical fusion is indicated, usually from C0 (occipital bone) to C2 (axis). For the fixation at the occipital bone, a plate is used. Pedicle screws are placed into the C2 vertebra. If dislocation between atlas and axis is observed, then a transarticular C1/C2 screwing should be considered as lower part of the fixation (◘ Fig. 7.22). Before fixing the connective rods to the occipital plate and the C2 pedicle screws, an autologous bone graft is placed between occipital bone and C2

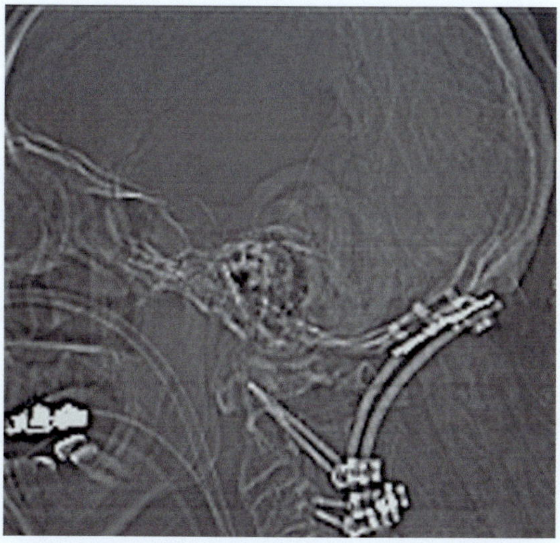

■ **Fig. 7.22** Occipitocervical fusion with transarticular screwing of atlas (C1) and axis (2) and lateral mass screws in the C3 vertebral

lamina to achieve a safe bony fusion in the long term [3].

In case of further subaxial congenital disorders of degenerative disease of the cervical spine, the fusion has to be extended further downwards beyond the C2 vertebra.

As an alternative to posterior fusion for the treatment of basilar impression with atlantoaxial displacement, Xia et al. [8] presented a reduction plate which is placed by using an anterior transoral approach. However, there are only short follow-up data available for this method.

7.3 Rathke's Cleft Cyst

7.3.1 General Information

Rathke's cleft cysts are benign sellar and suprasellar lesions arising from epithelial remnants of Rathke's pouch. The pathogenesis of these lesions is uncertain [5]. They were named after the German anatomist Martin Rathke (1793–1860). The peak incidence is at 30–50 years of age [5]. Most cysts are between 10 and 20 mm in diameter and contain mucoid or gelatinous material encapsulated in a thin cyst wall of simple or pseudostratified cuboidal or columnar epithelium. Incidental lesions are found in 11% of unselected postmortem cases, but symptomatic cases are rare [5]. The craniopharyngioma is a tumour arising from Rathke's pouch, and it is described in detail in ► Sect. 5.5.

7.3.2 Clinical Signs and Symptoms

As described above, most cysts are asymptomatic. Symptomatic patients present with headaches, with visual field disturbances and occasionally with hypopituitarism. All clinical symptoms are a consequence of the compressive effect of the lesion.

7.3.3 Investigations

Disturbances of visual acuity and visual field usually will guide the patient to an ophthalmologist who often diagnoses bitemporal hemianopsia. With these ophthalmological findings, the next step is a cranial MRI which reveals a well-demarcated homogenous lesion with variable intensity that is highly dependent on cyst contents, which can range from clear, CSF-like fluid to thick, mucoid material [5]. Furthermore, the size and configuration of the lesion are of importance for the surgical strategy (■ Fig. 7.23). Another typical finding in the MRI is a displaced optic chiasm.

If a Rathke's cleft cyst has been diagnosed with MRI, it is mandatory to endocrinological checks as well to rule out hypopituitarism.

7.3.4 Therapeutical Options

Symptomatic cysts are treated surgically. Basically, there are two different transnasal procedures: the classical microsurgical or the endoscopical technique. The characteristics as well as advantages and disadvantages of both techniques are discussed in ► Sect. 5.8. In ► Sect. 7.3.5, the transnasal transsphenoidal microsurgical procedure is described.

The goal of surgery is the decompression of the cyst to achieve a relief of pressure by partially resecting the anterior wall of the lesion (■ Fig. 7.24). Through this, an adequate decompression can be achieved, but unnecessary surgical morbidity that could occur during complete resection (CSF leak, injury of the pituitary gland) can be avoided.

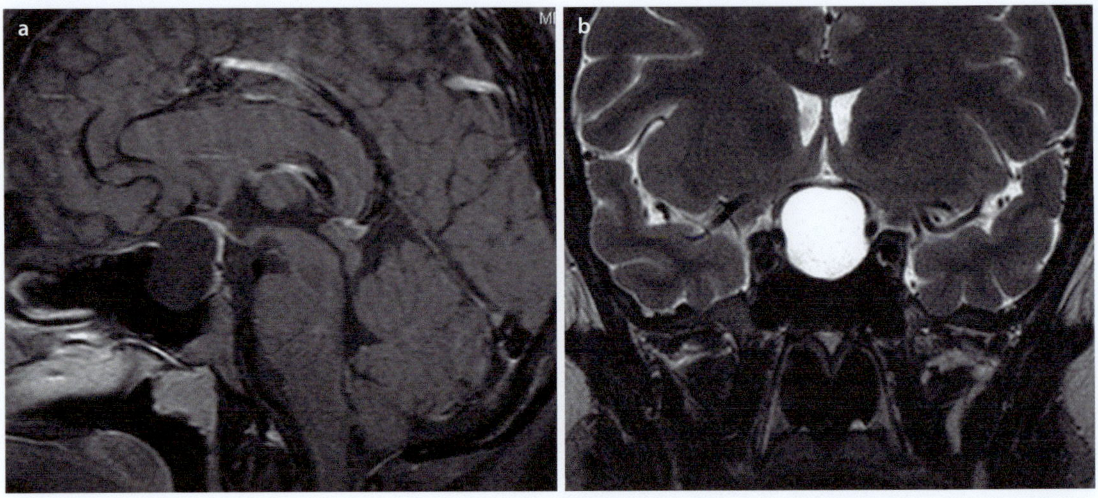

Fig. 7.23 Intra- and suprasellar Rathke's cleft cyst with extension of the pituitary gland **a** and the optic chiasm **b**. T1-weighted sagittal MR image **a** and T2-weighted coronal MR image **b**

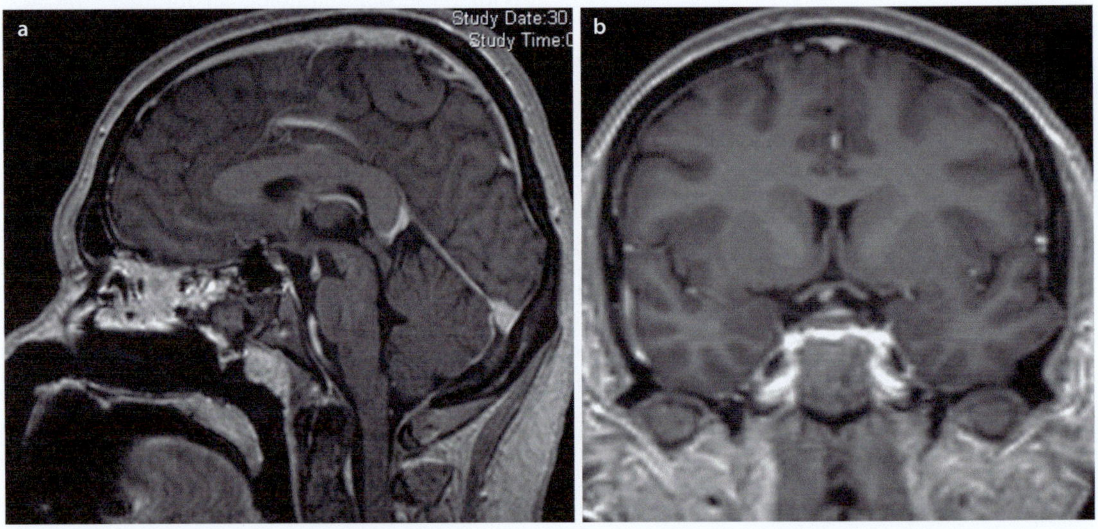

Fig. 7.24 MR imaging after decompression and partial resection of a Rathke's cleft cyst, patient from Fig. 7.21. A sagittal T1-weighted image shows a complete collapsing for the cyst **a**. The optic chiasm is significantly decompressed; T1-weighted coronal image **b**

7.3.5 Surgical Technique for the Decompression of a Rathke's Cleft Cyst

The surgical technique is in accordance with the procedure for the surgical treatment of pituitary adenomas. There is a microsurgical or an endoscopic option for transnasal transsphenoidal surgery. The following section describes the microsurgical procedure. The planning of the approach is usually done with the help of a neuronavigation system.

After an incision at the border between the skin and mucosa over the cartilaginous part of the nasal septum, the mucosa is dissected from the septum until the bony part of it is reached (Figs. 7.25, 7.26, and 7.27).

By using a speculum, the bony septum is pushed to the opposite side to have a better access for the resection of bone until the vomer is

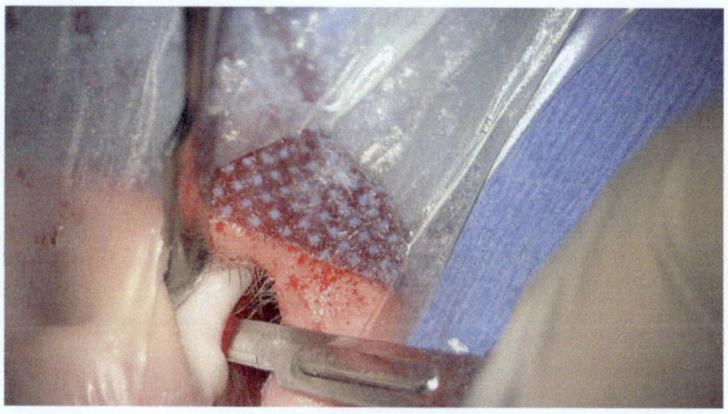

Fig. 7.25 Incision at the border between the skin and mucosa at the medial aspect of the right nasal ostium

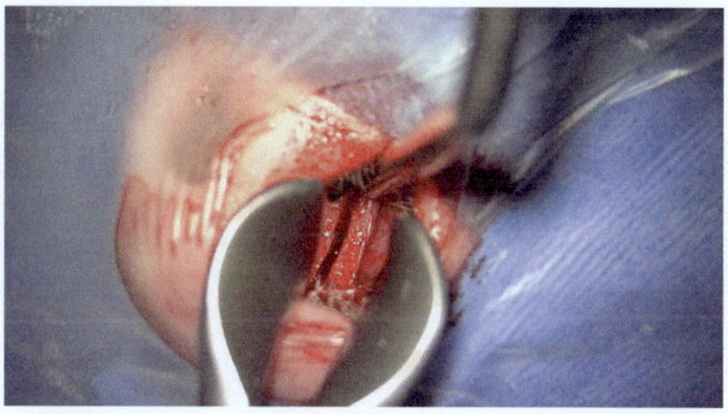

Fig. 7.27 The cartilaginous part of the nasal septum is pushed to the opposite side to be able to expose the bony septum with a speculum

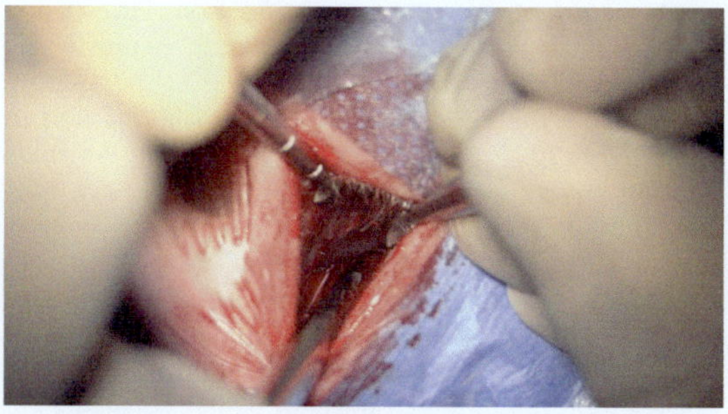

Fig. 7.26 Dissection of the mucosa away from the cartilaginous septum with a dissector

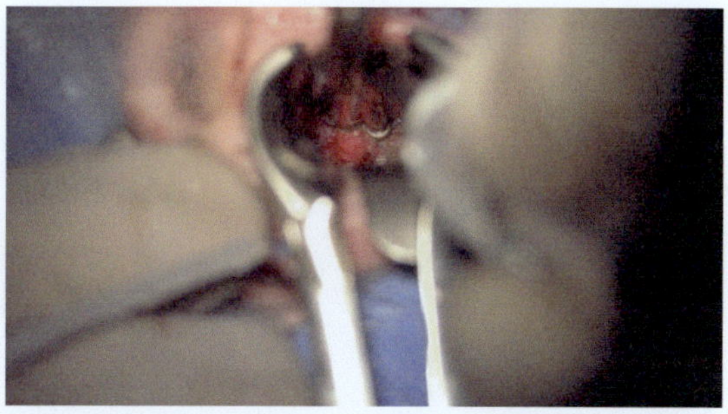

Fig. 7.28 After resection of the bony septum, the anterior wall of the sphenoid sinus is perforated with a diamond drill

reached. A self-retracting speculum is inserted whose position is checked by intraoperative X-ray. Afterwards, the X-ray image is correlated with the navigation to verify the navigation's accuracy. The use of neuronavigation is very useful to estimate the optimum trajectory to the sphenoid sinus and the sella as well as for verifying the midline during surgery.

The anterior wall of the sphenoid sinus is opened with a diamond drill that should have an ankled handpiece for optimum visualisation of the surgical field (Fig. 7.28). The opening of the anterior wall of the sphenoid sinus is enlarged with a Kerrison punch. The septum within the sphenoid sinus is usually in the midline in the anterior part but often deviates to one side or another in the posterior part. Therefore, a subtle analysis of preoperative imaging is necessary to stay in the midline. Furthermore, the right trajectory can be confirmed with neuronavigation.

The bony floor of the sella is also opened with a diamond drill and a small Kerrison punch. Afterwards, the anterior wall of the cyst can be seen (Fig. 7.29), and it is resected with an ankled micro-forceps to open and decompress the cyst. The fluid inside of the cyst is removed with the sucker (Fig. 7.30). After the relief of pressure, the diaphragma sellae bulges out as a sign of adequate decompression (Fig. 7.31).

Now, the multilayer reconstruction of the sellar floor can be started. First, some collagen is applied. Afterwards, some bone chips from previous punching can be placed at the level of the sellar floor and fixed with some fibrin glue. To support the pieces of the bone in their position, another piece of collagen is applied.

In case of an intraoperative CSF leak, a duraplasty with fibrin glue and fascia lata or abdominal fat and possibly with a lumbar drainage is necessary before starting with the skull base reconstruction.

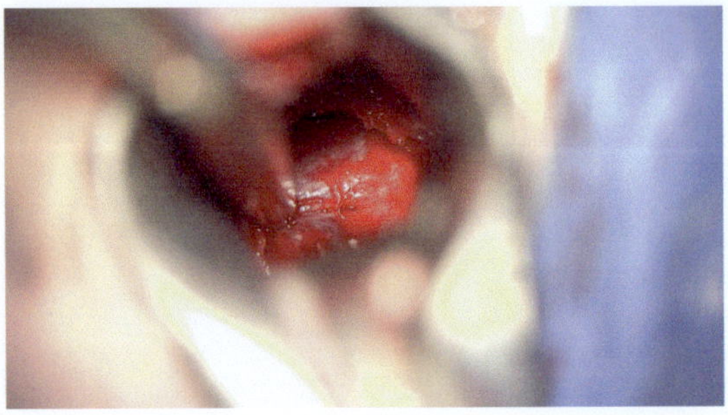

Fig. 7.29 Anterior wall of the sphenoid sinus and sellar floor are resected with a 2-mm Kerrison punch. The intraoperative microscopic view shows the anterior wall of the Rathke's cleft cyst after resection of the sellar floor

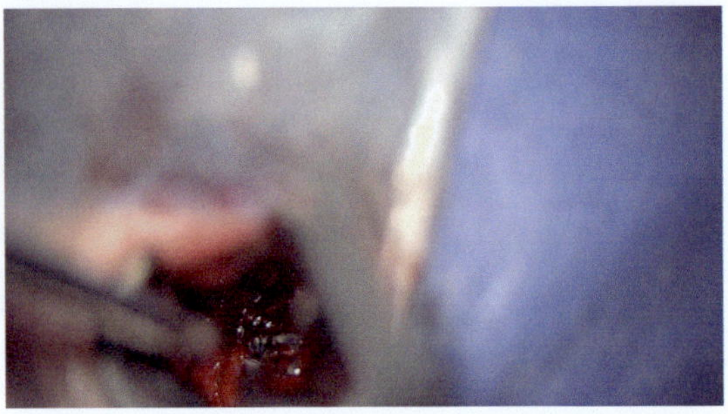

Fig. 7.30 Opening of the Rathke's cleft cyst with ankled microscissors

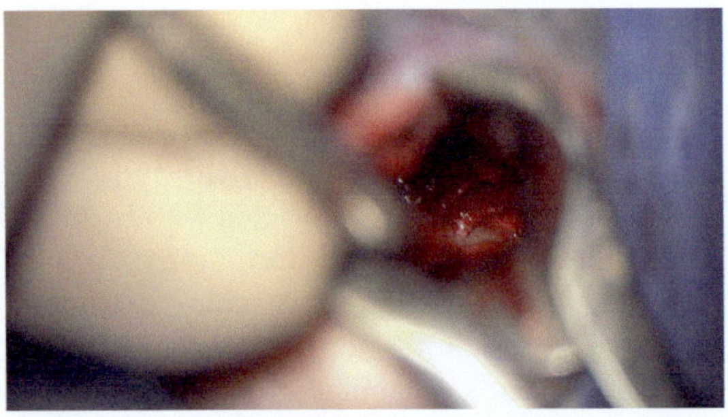

Fig. 7.31 After opening, decompression and partial resection of the Rathke's cleft cyst, the diaphragm immediately reoccupies its normal space. Afterwards, the sellar floor is reconstructed with bone fragments from punching, collagen and fibrin glue

References

1. Chiari H. Über Veränderungen des Kleinhirns infolge von Hydrocephalie des Grosshirns. Dtsch Med Wochenschr. 1891;17:1172–5.
2. Guo SL, Zhou DB, Yu XG, Yin YH, Qiao GY. Posterior C1-C2 screw and rod instrument for reduction and fixation of basilar invagination with atlantoaxial dislocation. Eur Spine J. 2014;23(8):1666–72.
3. Klekamp J. Treatment of basilar invagination. Eur Spine J. 2014;23(8):1656–65.
4. Lang J. Skull base and related structures. Atlas of clinical anatomy. Stuttgart/New York: Schattauer; 2001. p. 22–3.
5. Larkin S, Karavitaki N, Ansorge O. Rathke's cleft cyst. Handb Clin Neurol. 2014;124:255–69.
6. Menezes AH. Craniovertebral junction abnormalities. In: Albright AL, Pollack IF, Adelson PD, editors. Principles and practice of pediatric neurosurgery. New York/Stuttgart: Thieme; 2008.
7. Soleau S, Tubbs RS, Oakes WJ. Chiari malformations. In: Albright AL, Pollack IF, Adelson PD, editors. Principles and practice of pediatric neurosurgery. New York/Stuttgart: Thieme; 2008.
8. Xia H, Yin Q, Ai F, Ma X, Wang J, Wu Z, Zhang K, Liu J, Xu J. Treatment of basilar invagination with atlantoaxial dislocation: atlantoaxial joint distraction and fixation with transoral atlantoaxial reduction plate (TARP) without odontoidectomy. Eur Spine J. 2014;23(8):1648–55.

Future Developments in Skull Base Surgery

Uwe Spetzger

A. König, U. Spetzger (eds.), *Surgery of the Skull Base*,
https://doi.org/10.1007/978-3-319-64018-1_8

Today, modern skull base surgery represents a multidisciplinary, highly specialised collaboration of different medical specialties. The main goal is the treatment of tumorous, traumatic, vascular and congenital pathologies at the skull base while preserving neurological functions. In the last few years, skull base surgery has undergone a continuous development. This mainly regards the modern possibilities of visualisation by the improvement of the operating microscopes and the increasing use of brilliant high-definition endoscopes. But also the refinement of visualising the anatomy by the continuous developing cranial imaging and the navigation technology which is based on imaging has a relevant impact on the development of skull base surgery. The current concept is a function-preserving skull base surgery. Its future development aims a further improvement of treatment results and a continuous reduction of treatment-related morbidity. The future of modern skull base surgery will basically take place and be decided in four sections:

- Technical innovations of equipment
- Planning simulation and visualisation
- Computer assistance and robotics
- Education and training

The technical innovations of the last few years with significant improvement of surgical instruments have an influence on the surgical strategy and also on the further development of microsurgical possibilities. A crucial milestone was the development of tube shaft instruments that fit in much smaller surgical approaches due to their slim design and, thus, allow well-directed surgical manipulations in very narrow spaces without blocking the view onto the surgical field.

The further development of modern endoscopes is also closely associated with the development of surgical instruments. One field is monoportal endoscopy, a surgical concept in which surgical instruments are directed through a single flexible endoscope like in the NOTES procedures in abdominal surgery. It is imaginable that a future generation of such monoportal and flexible endoscopes could be useable in skull base surgery and bring a basic change in the surgical strategy. With such systems, the common straight-line surgical approaches like in current microsurgical and endoscopic procedures would not be necessary anymore, and miniaturised approaches «around the corner» could be possible. With this, for example, an approach to the posterior fossa was possible through the foramen magnum. At the moment, this is definitely impossible due to the lack of technical preconditions. To achieve this, it is necessary to significantly miniaturise the existing systems and to improve the controlling and visualisation as well as to develop so-called snake-robotic systems further that allow grabbing, holding and other manipulations. Furthermore, surgical technique and education as well as practical training would significantly change due to such technology. A whole generation of experienced neurosurgeons had to learn and train new procedures. When comparing this with the slowly ongoing acceptance of neuroendoscopy, it is imaginable that it would take more than one generation of surgeons to establish such a new technology, even in a scenario of perfect technical realisation.

This surgical strategy sounds relatively futuristic but was a completely new concept without the well-known and sometimes formidable approach-related morbidity since minimal burr-hole craniotomies could replace the craniotomies with a bone flap.

Such a strategy is also imaginable for the spinal canal or the ventricular system or the whole cisternal space of the skull base whereupon the existing instruments had to be significantly modified and first of all miniaturised. Some basic strategies like the navigation-guided highly precise approach to the target region and the exact movement within predefined target corridors including an exact return path for the endoscope are already technically realisable.

3D endoscopes are not just realisable in the foreseeable future but are close to clinical use in our daily routine at the skull base. They allow a brilliant high-definition presentation of the target region and, thus, a view into the future era of further miniaturisation of surgical approaches. Furthermore, digital microscopy, especially in combination with neuronavigation and robotic components, will more and more come into clinical practice. This is no future development in the classical sense but has already started getting into neurosurgical reality.

The use of computer-assisted manipulators and robotic systems will get acceptance in skull base surgery, too. Here, active and passive assisting systems will be mainly used. When comparing the use of the robotic da Vinci system in laparoscopic surgeries in abdominal surgery, gynaecology and urology with the market for comparable systems for cranial surgery, then the latter market is much smaller which inhibits the industry-driven development and modification of such systems. Furthermore, the concept that was realised for laparoscopic manipulators is not applicable for cranial operations or skull base surgery, and a complete reorientation and new product development was necessary. Thus, robotic assistance systems for cranial, head and neck surgery will be developed as guided holding systems for endoscopes and for drilling systems.

With the CyberKnife system in stereotactic radiosurgery, there has been an establishment of a robotic system in the treatment concept of skull base tumours. Already in 1999 in the USA, the FDA approved the robotic-guided linear particle accelerator for the treatment of brain and skull tumours. Stereotactic radiosurgery will stay an inherent part of skull base surgery. By now, modern radiosurgery systems allow a highly precise planning and destruction of tumours, even in the craniocervical junction, which was almost impossible a few years ago with the Gamma Knife system. The increasing use of robot-guided radiosurgery systems (CyberKnife) for different skull base lesions is nowadays an established treatment strategy. Thus, in this area, the era of robot-assisted skull base surgery has already begun. The ongoing development of linear particle accelerators and the increasing clinical use as well as the scientific evaluation of proton beam therapy for the treatment of skull base tumours will increase the number of radiosurgical options in the near future.

As a further development of operating microscopes and digital imaging, there will be a near-field microscopy where special staining methods will visualise the tumour margins or the transition zone between pathological and normal tissue. An interlink with near-infrared spectroscopy or even the integration of targeted ablative procedures into the operating microscope was imaginable.

The targeted and exactly controlled energy-driven ablation for the treatment of tumours or vascular lesions at the skull base will be a future development. An already realised project with real clinical applicability is the focused ultrasound (HIFO). Already in the 1950s, this method was presented by William Frey as high-intensity focused ultrasound (HIFO) for application in neurosurgery, and now, many decades later, it seems that it will establish as a therapeutical option for surgery. The advantage of this less invasive method is that after an adequate calculation of the target region, which can be done with modern MR tomography and especially with the further improved thermosensitive sequences, there are no late effects by focused ultrasound like the summation of radiation effects in stereotactic radiosurgery. The risk-free repeatability of this focused therapy will make this technique highly attractive, especially for benign lesions with a tendency for recurrence. The therapy of skull base meningiomas, especially that of recurrent tumours and WHO grade II lesions, will basically change if HIFO will give proof of being an adequate therapeutical method in the future.

Nowadays, computer-assisted skull base surgery is an established part of the whole treatment algorithm and will increase its significance as a central data interface. Here, the navigation data for preoperative simulation including segmentation of structures at risk and the surgical target region as well as trajectories and approach planning are deposited. These digital planning of surgeries can facilitate intraoperative orientation during navigation and, thus, lead to risk minimisation during surgical treatment of a lesion. Computer-assisted surgery and image data are both a platform for the treatment planning and a reference data set for postoperative control. Furthermore, these data are the basis for further treatment modalities, for example, the combination with stereotactic radiosurgery. Intraoperatively positioned markers at the margins of resection can augment the data set with additional landmarks which can be used for the precise target planning and volumetry for stereotactic radiosurgery treatment. Thus, DICOM data for computer-assisted surgery that mainly result from a fusion of CT and MRI data to achieve optimum precision already at present represent a crucial component in the whole multidisciplinary treatment regimen. Due to the ongoing improvement of radiological imaging techniques, these image data will be the precise basis for upcoming robotic surgical operation steps in the future. Especially the resection of bony structures at the skull base with exact guidance of a high-speed drill or a piezo ultrasonic instrument is a foreseeable surgical step in the near future that can be done in a half-automatic way.

The further development and miniaturisation of piezo ultrasonic instruments for the precise resection of bony structures at the skull base will establish itself in the future. With the help of piezo ultrasound, very thin cut lines without significant loss of bone or necroses are applicable which leads to an improvement of cosmetic results. Furthermore, the removal of bone at and around critical neurovascular structures is less risky with piezo ultrasound compared to high-speed drills but also more time-consuming at present.

The fast-paced further development of computer technology presupposed: the possibilities in visualisation and demonstration of complex neuroanatomical structures will improve. Even today, high-resolution 3D atlases are widespread. With the help of dedicated apps, such detailed anatomical images are immediately available on mobile telecommunication devices. Just one example from the continuously increasing number of apps is ▸ upsurgeon.com which delivers a 3D skull atlas with high-resolution images of surgical and anatomical details. By means of such 3D atlases that will be experienceable as holograms or with appropriate equipment as virtual or augmented reality in the future, the learning of anatomy will change. In the future the young skull base surgeon will virtually walk along the anterior skull base, balance over the anterior clinoid process, carefully climb the optic chiasm and bang his head on the anterior communicating artery complex with the help of a specially programmed head-mounted display. Afterwards he or she will slide down the clivus, passing the huge and scary pulsating basilar artery with its covert of perforating arteries, and go down into the spinal canal. Today, such a scenario is not a fiction anymore; I could experience and admire these three-dimensional projections by a specially programmed software for a VR head-mounted display at the Institute of Anthropomatics of the Karlsruhe Institute of Technology (KIT) (◘ Fig. 8.1).

There is a general recognisable change of paradigms in the learning of the young generation that has also reached medical education and especially surgical training. In principle, there is a trend away from active to passive knowledge. In practice this means to know where and how to get information online but not to have the knowledge in detail. The trend is to quickly call the adequate source which delivers the detailed knowledge directly and comprehensively. On one hand, this is reproducible because of the fast-increasing information flood but on the other hand carries the risk that even basic details are not inside the active memory.

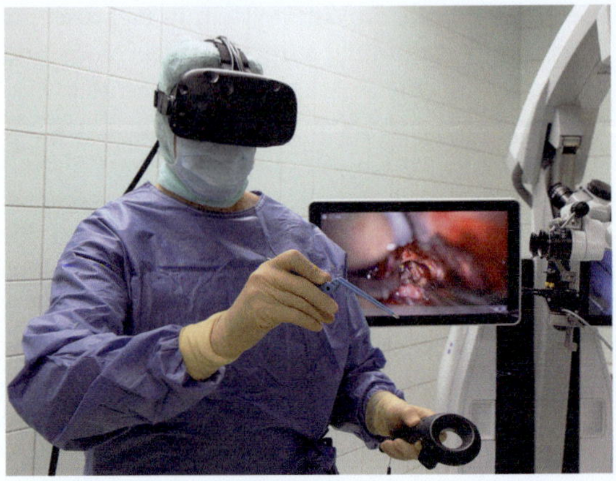

◘ **Fig. 8.1** Head-mounted display for a 3D experience of surgical navigation image data

Following this trend there will be anatomical atlases being integrated into modern navigation systems that can be used for the specific case or patient with the help of special software. The navigation systems themselves will be controlled much more intuitively with the help of voice control and gesture recognition.

Thesaurus functions have been already integrated into many medical devices and this trend will continue. Learning surgical thesaurus systems recording all the information about decision algorithms and the associated surgical steps and their ubiquitary interconnection could deliver standardised recommendations about surgical indications and make the sense of single surgical manoeuvres statistically analysable. Such a continuously growing, knowledge-based digital surgical textbook is the basic requirement for autonomous operations. However, when discussing with leading experts from information technology and humanoid robotics, it seems that we are still far away from autonomously acting surgical robots.

Surgery at the skull base is a difficult procedure that requires complex and intelligent planning and active tactile realisation of this planning in very limited space. Here, situative, fast and experience-based decisions and a continuous adaption to a permanently changing scenario are basic requirements. Despite the huge and permanent advances in the field of artificial intelligence (AI), such complex decision algorithms that lead to an immediate, targeted, situatively logical, highly differentiated manual action are not imaginable to be done by an autonomously acting robot at present. The human brain has a huge performance advance due to its morphology and the given ability of parallel data processing of huge amounts of information compared to programmed machines. The extraordinary skill of the human brain of immediately reacting adequately to a changed situation is a crucial difference to programmed systems. When comparing autonomous driving with skull base surgery, there are massive differences since operating is an active acting in a three-dimensional space. Due to the very small dimensions and the highly precise, haptically controlled and targeted motor skills, it is not comparable with the relatively trivial task of moving a car on a road. Thus, the cybernetic movement control during surgery is much more complex than the control of a vehicle. The recent and the following generation of humanoid robots (the latter being recently under development) are overrated in terms of their performance and will definitely not replace well-trained skull base surgeons in the foreseeable future.

By means of appropriate 3D visualisation using virtual reality (VR), there will be simulations and digital surgical textbooks with realistic 3D animations but the latter with a lack of haptic tactile feedback which is essential for adequate and successful surgical training.

The increasing extension of 3D printing technology opens up further possibilities in teaching and surgical training. Today, by means of thin-sliced CT or MRI data sets, a realistic patient model can be printed in a relatively short period of time. This model which shows a skull base tumour or, for example, a complex aneurysm at the skull base and matches with the actual anatomical situation of the patient enables a realistic surgical training scenario. With such a 3D model depending on the materials being used, a precise simulation of an operation and a realistic surgical training can be conducted. Single surgical steps from positioning to skin incision and craniotomy can be done to finally applicate a clip to an intracranial aneurysm made of thin-walled silicon. From this practical simulation of surgery could be concluded if the chosen craniotomy is big enough and at the right position or if it had to be modified or if the trajectory to the lesion is suitable or if it had to be optimised. Furthermore, it could be checked if the aneurysm clip fits to the aneurysm neck and occludes it properly or if the clip provides complete occlusion without compromising perforating branches. By means of such a model made by 3D printing technology, a training surgery close to reality is absolutely imaginable. This technique would revolutionise neurosurgical education and practical surgical training.

The teaching and further education in the field of skull base surgery is an essential part of maintenance of the subspecialty «skull base surgery». Nowadays, the present generation of young neurosurgeons that are still in training often tends to other specialties. Especially spinal surgery, stereotactic surgery and functional neurosurgery are the subspecialties of most interest by younger colleagues. Furthermore, there is a trend in cerebrovascular neurosurgery to combine endovascular and microsurgical procedures in the training which leads to a separation between the cerebrovascular subspecialisation and tumour surgery of the skull base. Additionally, the stereotactic radiosurgery gains more and more importance in the treatment of skull base tumours, and, thus, in the future perspective, there will be a crossover between stereotactic radiosurgery and oncologic skull base surgery. But it is still a current principle that well-grounded and skilful surgical manipulation on cerebral blood vessels like in aneurysm and angioma surgery is an essential precondition for the dissection and resection of many skull base lesions. Therefore, it is necessary to reconsider if the trend of ongoing differentiation and further subspecialisation in skull base surgery is reasonable.

The number of training courses and practical courses in the field of skull base surgery has increased over the last few years. This leads to an improvement of knowledge among the younger colleagues in this field. In the future, there should be a scaling of the courses with basic courses that teach working on the bone with high-speed drills, the handling of microsurgical instruments and basic microsurgical suture techniques. Furthermore, the basics of craniotomy and simple skull base approaches should be demonstrated and learned. In the advanced courses, complex and combined craniotomies as well as microanastomoses of vessels and nerves for neurovascular reconstruction should be taught. This guided working is optimal under realistic conditions in perfectly equipped training laboratories with operating microscopes, endoscopes, state-of-the-art micro-instruments and cadaveric specimen. However, learning suture and drilling techniques on simple modes can also be of help in improving practical skills. A relatively simple but effective model is the microsurgical drilling of hard-boiled eggs where the eggshell is removed with a fine diamond drill but the egg membrane is dissected and preserved at the same time. Suture techniques can be trained on thin silicon vessels. For microsurgical vascular anastomoses, chicken wings or in vivo exercises on experimental animal models are effective.

In master courses, all the surgical models mentioned above can be further diverse. For example, the drilling of eggshells can be exercised through small tubes with a length of 5 cm and a diameter of 1.5 cm. This experimental setup perfectly simulates the microsurgical opening of the anterior wall of the sphenoid sinus and the sella floor in surgical approaches to pituitary adenomas or clival tumours and can be simply trained with a microscope or endoscope. In the same way, microvascular suturing techniques can be made more difficult by using such small tubes to simulate vascular anastomoses in depth and close to the skull base, respectively. All these practical training models are also applicable in one's own institution. Thus, a well-grounded subspecialisation in skull base surgery can be developed and trained with relatively simple equipment. An important task for established skull base surgeons will be the leading of young and interested colleagues to skull base surgery. For ensuring quality and a highly specialised supply of patients in the future, it will be necessary to do an active acquisition. At present, a decreasing interest in skull base surgery can be recognised whereupon it is likely that there are multifactorial reasons for this. One reason can be found in the social development where many individuals tend to reach a quick success with manageable effort. Furthermore, the strict regulation of working hours and also a certain kind of consumer mentality in the younger generation of physicians and surgeons lead to a decreasing number of colleagues deciding for complex and longsome surgery with setbacks and the mental burden of surgical morbidity. Therefore, we are requested to intensively promote and support the domain of skull base surgery by pointing out the beauty of anatomy, almost unlimited possibilities of computer-assisted surgery and visualisation to enthuse the talented young surgeons for this fascinating surgery.

All these mentioned future developments and technologies will lead from function-preserving to function-improving skull base surgery. Due to the close interdisciplinary collaboration in skull base centres, there has already been a rethinking with questioning the philosophy of radical and maximum surgery, and the establishment of partial resection of complex skull base tumours has been more and more accepted since there are adequate alternative treatment modalities for the subsequent therapy. In general, the concept of function-preserving skull base surgery that came more and more into the foreground has been finally established as an important principle in the treatment of skull base lesions. With the consequent further development and refinement of all modern techniques, the aim of getting from function-preserving to function-improving skull base surgery can be achieved. Special miniaturised endoscopic and also robot-guided techniques, the concept of focused application of energy for highly precise and selective tumour ablation as well as intelligent regenerative methods will make a contribution to this development.

Erratum to: Surgery of the Skull Base

Alexander König and Uwe Spetzger

The updated original online version for this chapter can be found at
https://doi.org/10.1007/978-3-319-64018-1_2
https://doi.org/10.1007/978-3-319-64018-1_5
https://doi.org/10.1007/978-3-319-64018-1_6

A. König, U. Spetzger (eds.), *Surgery of the Skull Base*,
https://doi.org/10.1007/978-3-319-64018-1_9

Errata to:

A. König, U. Spetzger ***Surgery of the Skull Base,*** https://doi.org/10.1007/978-3-319-64018-1

We received the following corrections in chapters 2, 5 and 6 and the same has been updated in the book.

Corrections:

1. In chapter 2, new figure 2.7 was received
2. In chapter 5, new figures 5.46, 5.52 and 5.54 were received
3. In chapter 5, the names of the contributing authors were to be placed under the respective sections in the chapter TOC, chapters and the running heads of the chapter
4. In chapter 6, legend of the box 6.2 was changed to 'Criteria for Primary (Idiopathic) Vestibular Paroxysmia'
5. In chapter 6, the names of the contributing authors were to be placed under the respective sections in the chapter TOC, chapters and the running heads of the chapter

Supplementary Information

A. König, U. Spetzger (eds.), *Surgery of the Skull Base*,
https://doi.org/10.1007/978-3-319-64018-1

Index

MIX
Papier aus verantwortungsvollen Quellen
Paper from responsible sources
FSC® C105338

If you have any concerns about our products,
you can contact us on
ProductSafety@springernature.com

In case Publisher is established outside the EU,
the EU authorized representative is:
Springer Nature Customer Service Center GmbH
Europaplatz 3, 69115 Heidelberg, Germany

Printed by Libri Plureos GmbH
in Hamburg, Germany